Pediatric Nursing

This book is lovingly dedicated:

– to my husband Leon
for supporting and encouraging me throughout this endeavor, as well as many others in our years together.

– to my children Michael, Suzanne, Paul, Thomas, and Barbara
for teaching me a lifetime of parenting and pediatrics surrounded with love.

Pediatric Nursing

PATRICIA A. LESNER

10 9 8 7 6 5 4 3 2 1

LIBRARY OF CONGRESS CATALOG CARD NUMBER: 81-82910
ISBN: 0-8273-1932-0

Printed in the United States of America
Published simultaneously in Canada
by Nelson Canada,
A Division of International Thomson Limited

Preface

The scope of pediatric nursing is expanding in response to increases in knowledge in a variety of disciplines. Indeed, specialization is often a necessity for the nurse practicing in the pediatric field. As a result, the beginning student may be overwhelmed by the breadth and depth of knowledge specific to this age group. Students in a basic educational program must be afforded the tools that allow them to provide safe and effective care to children. Upon completion of such a program, the student who chooses to continue working with children will have a sound base of knowledge from which to work.

The approach used in PEDIATRIC NURSING is based on a developmental continuum that extends from birth through adolescence. A section on the growth and development of each age-group is included, followed by a discussion of the health care needs that are specific to each group. The problems common to that age-group are then presented. The primary focus of the text is on assisting children to attain an optimal state of wellness, taking into consideration their individual strengths and limitations. The nursing approach to any child must, by its very nature, incorporate a knowledge of that child's growth and development as well as the norms for the particular age.

Throughout the text, emphasis is placed on the child and his or her relationship to a family unit. The nurse in the health care setting must establish a positive working relationship with the parents or significant others, as well as with the child.

This multi-dimensional approach allows the student to use the text in a variety of ways. It may be read in its entirety chapter by chapter. Or, by concentrating on the chapters of growth and development and health care needs prior to studying health care problems, it can be used to study the normal child first. These approaches provide a degree of flexibility, accommodating the variety of age-groups encountered in a pediatric unit or in a well-child setting.

PEDIATRIC NURSING is divided into eight sections. The first three sections apply to children of any age. The remaining five sections each identify a developmental age and those diseases that are common, but not exclusive, to that particular age group.

Section I includes the historical aspects of child care, the changing features of the child's life in various cultures, and the agencies and organizations that have effected change.

Section II focuses on prenatal development and those influences that may change the child's state of wellness. This section also includes important information for the care of the neonate, both in the hospital and at home.

Section III addresses the topic of hospitalization. The emphasis is on the nursing process and working with the child and the parents during the child's hospitalization. Information on medications, as well as on preoperative and postoperative care, is provided in this section.

Section IV begins the portion of this text that is based on a developmental continuum. This section addresses the needs of the infant, as well as normal growth and development. A discussion of congenital anomalies and problems that interfere with growth is included.

Section V addresses the health care of the toddler, including such entities as accidents and child abuse. Major respiratory problems are also presented in this section.

Section VI is devoted to the preschooler. Growth and development, as well as the problems of leukemia and nephrosis, are presented. Section VI also contains information on retarded and terminally ill children.

Section VII covers the school-aged child. Communicable diseases, juvenile diabetes, and rheumatoid arthritis are among the subjects addressed. Information on traction and casts is also included in this section.

Section VIII focuses upon the needs of the adolescent. Information on emotional disturbances, along with information on acne, scoliosis, and venereal diseases, is contained in this section.

Accompanying each chapter in this text are objectives, suggested activities, discussion topics, review questions, and a bibliography. A glossary is also included at the end of the text.

The appendix provides a ready reference for such information as growth charts for various age ranges, normal laboratory values, normal vital signs, and the Denver Developmental Screening Test.

About the Author:

Patricia A. Lesner received a baccalaureate degree in nursing from St. John College of Cleveland, Ohio, in 1958. In 1972, she received her master's degree in education from Kent State University, majoring in technical education.

Ms. Lesner has worked in both staff and charge nurse positions in pediatrics. She was appointed to the faculty of Lorain County Community College with the inception of the associate degree nursing program in 1965. She participated in the development of the curriculum as well as of the conceptual framework. During that time, she taught in a variety of content areas with a specialization in pediatrics. This author has presented workshops on child abuse and juvenile diabetes and has conducted review sessions in pediatric nursing. Currently, Ms. Lesner holds the rank of Associate Professor of Associate Degree Nursing, and is a member of the American Nurses' Association and the Ohio State Nurses' Association.

Contents

SECTION VIII THE ADOLESCENT

APPENDICES

Section I

Child Care in History

Chapter 1

Historical Perspectives

OBJECTIVES

Upon completion of this chapter, the student will be able to

- list three influences of earlier civilizations on child care practices.
- identify two changes in child health care practices in the United States that were caused by industrialization.
- describe four concepts of child development that influenced children's care and quality of life.
- discuss the relationship of the various theories of child development to the educational system.

The full scope of pediatrics and the changes that have taken place in that specialty cannot be fully appreciated without considering the events of the past. A broader perspective is thereby gained by the nurse in relation to the changes of the past and the directions of the future.

The original family group consisted of an extended family unit living amidst a given tribe. The roles of the family members were clearly defined and the values and traditions carefully transmitted from one generation to the next. The cycles of birth and death, as well as all related rituals, were carefully observed and preserved by the family members. Then, as now, family problems and priorities reflected local concerns, the availability of local resources, and a preoccupation with local needs. Any changes in these priorities were a result of economic, social, political, or religious influences.

ANCIENT AND MEDIEVAL CIVILIZATIONS

Little direct information is available regarding the care of children in earlier times or the factors which may have influenced that care. However, since the care of children was generally dictated by the culture of a particular society, some information may be gleaned from a study of that culture. Other bits of information may be derived from such sources as the legal codes that were enacted in many areas. Some of these codes even detailed what was to be done for orphans.

Chinese Civilization

The major influence of the Chinese civilization on pediatrics was its concept of filial piety, or a loyal devotion to the family unit. This encompassed both ancestor worship and a profound respect for parental authority. The family was patriarchal, with three to four families living under one roof. This arrangement was typical of an agriculturally based family structure. The group structure was maintained through the mandate of filial piety. Parents were obligated to have many children to perpetuate this ancestor worship. The civil government of the time was viewed as an extension of the family's responsibilities.

Babylonian Civilization

The ancient Hammurabic Code, which contained both civil and criminal law, made references to the adoption of children and included a discussion of the rights and responsibilities of both parties. Within the same culture, there was evidence that the temple priestesses served as wet nurses for infants three years of age and younger. These priestesses also became foster mothers for children whose parents had died. Similarly, the ancient Brehon Laws of Ireland included provisions for the adoption and care of illegitimate children.

The Hebrew culture, guided by strong ethical and moral codes, greatly influenced the lives of children. The many prescriptions within the Mosaic Code governing hygiene and sanitation served to protect the adults within this society, as well as the children.

Greek and Roman Civilizations

Greek civilization before the time of Christ showed concern for both widows and orphans and provided for their care. Hippocrates included information on child care in his writings, as did Celsus. Celsus was the first to recognize that children were not "small adults" and, therefore, required different care.

Prior to the influences of Christianity, the father in Roman families had ultimate control over his family members. His control was so total that he could kill his family or have them killed, sell them into slavery, dictate a marriage contract, or initiate a divorce. A young woman coming into his home as a bride of his son lost all contact with her family of birth and was totally subject to the patriarchal rule of her father-in-law. Young girls six to ten years of age were often selected for service in the temple as vestal virgins.

The rise of Christianity brought with it the concept of charity and a concern for the care of widows, orphans, and the sick. Greater value was placed on human lives. However, hospice care was available only to those injured in battle. The nurses were men, usually from religious orders, and the care was given to men. The care of abandoned children in foundling homes was less than ideal by today's standards.

The rise of feudalism, the Crusades, and the plagues that devastated Europe were among the factors that influenced children's lives. Moreover, an explosion in knowledge, and the process of spreading that knowledge, laid the groundwork for change. The development of a method for printing enabled the production of two early books on pediatrics, one by the English pediatrician, Thomas Phaer, and the other by Felix Wurtz.

HISTORICAL CONCEPTS OF CHILD DEVELOPMENT

In earlier ages, each culture had a particular attitude toward, or concept of, children. These attitudes strongly influenced both the treatment of the child and the child's self-image. Many of these concepts lasted for long periods of time and some are still evident today.

The concept of a child as a miniature adult arose in the sixteenth and seventeenth centuries and was common in colonial America. As soon as children were able to feed and dress themselves, they were expected to take on responsibilities and to work to help maintain the family. The only allowances made were in consideration of the child's physical strength. The practice of allowing children as young as seven and eight years of age to work in the factories, and even younger children to be apprenticed, was consistent with this theory. Sexual abuse, as defined by today's standards, was also practiced prior to 1900.

The concept of children as inherently sinful has its origins in the Bible, and is a reflection of the doctrine of original sin. It was promoted in Europe by Edmund Burke around 1790, and was embraced by the Puritans in colonial America. The moral responsibilities of children were emphasized; harsh and excessive forms of punishment were used to reinforce those responsibilities. The goals of education for children of this era were linked to religious values and the teaching of morality. Many felt that children were unable to internalize morals, and merely acted to avoid punishment. This philosophy is reflected in the descriptions of children in Dickens' writings.

The concept of a child as a "blank slate," advanced by John Locke at the end of the seventeenth century, also led to some difficulties. There was no consideration for innate abilities or individual differences. It was thought that if all children were given the same optimal environment and the same education, all should progress at the same pace, becoming carbon copies of each other. The one advantage of this philosophy was that it emphasized positive experiences, not punishment.

The view of children as inherently good was proposed by Rousseau about 1762. This concept was contrary to the rigid disciplinary measures and harsh punishment that were common at that time. Children were encouraged to develop through activities and enjoyable pastimes until they reached adolescence, when their formal education would begin. Once children were in the school setting, great emphasis was placed on individual reasoning ability.

The concept of a child as chattel, or property, was prevalent in sixteenth-century England, and is still evident in some areas. Exploitation of children was a direct result of this philosophy and its proponents. The value of children was determined by the physical labor they could perform. This was the basis for the apprenticeship of children as young as seven and eight years of age, and for the selling of children as slaves. These practices were officially abolished in England in 1814.

In the United States, the Fair Labor Standards Act of 1938 put a stop to child labor.

The concept of children as developing individuals in their own right was another philosophy that emerged. This philosophy offered a better perspective for children. It acknowledged the gradual physical growth, progression in knowledge, and increase in judgment that occur as a part of the growth process. This theory began with Plato and was described in the writings of Shakespeare. More recently, it has been reaffirmed in the developmental task themes of Erikson and Piaget. This philosophy encourages schooling that is dependent on grade levels as well as abilities. It is the result of scientific research related to child growth and development, and recognizes the individual differences and backgrounds of children.

FAMILY LIFE IN COLONIAL AMERICA

The original United States census taken in 1790 showed a very different family structure than now exists. At that time, a typical family consisted of a father, a mother, and five or more children. This was true for more than one-third of the families included in the census.

Health and Welfare Services

The health care of children in colonial America was given a low priority. The child had no acknowledged legal rights. By 1780, the death rate for children younger than ten years of age was fifty percent. The problems identified at that time included physical and mental illness, lack of parental supervision, inadequate economic support, child abuse or exploitation, care of handicapped children, and care of delinquent children. Many of these problems persist in various forms today.

In colonial America, the economic needs of families unable to provide for themselves were met by a form of "poor relief." Both orphanages and almshouses were available for the care of children. The first private orphanage was established in 1729 in New Orleans by the Ursuline Nuns. Indentured apprenticeships similar to foster home care were also used to provide for these children. If the child was not old enough to qualify for an apprenticeship, the child could be placed in a mixed almshouse. This institution cared for young orphans, aged and indigent adults, and individuals with psychiatric problems.

The child's behavior was considered to be the responsibility of the family. The family was expected to keep the child under control. If children were publicly unruly, they could be removed from their homes by local officials once due warning had been given the family and fines had been levied.

Education

The educational process in colonial America strongly reflected Old World values. Religious, social, economic, and political institutions and organizations in America were based on the traditions and ideals of European cultures. The colonists were not, however, a true cross-section of the society they left behind. They freely selected those traditions and customs they wished to continue and ignored those they wished to abandon.

The philosophies of various groups conflicted in many areas, notably in the education of children. Puritans in New England, among others, believed that the state was responsible for the education of children and set the pattern for colonial New England. Other groups, such as the Anglicans, were convinced that education was the responsibility of the Church. They believed that an education should perpetuate religious tradition through the choice of a curriculum.

Social order also influenced the educational process. The Old World practice of establishing universities was continued in colonial America. The major purpose of these institutions was to prepare a select few for leadership positions. Latin grammar schools prepared individuals for directive positions as lawyers, ministers, and merchants, whereas vernacular schools provided an education for the commoners. The English poor laws of 1601 established the concept of apprenticeships and trade education.

The concept of compulsory education arose in the mid-1600s with the directive that children were to be taught to read and write. They were also to learn the principles of religion and a trade. If the parents or the master were unable to comply with this mandate, the child could be placed with another master who was able to do so. None of these statutes included any provisions for the maintenance of schools or for compulsory attendance. However, by 1671 all of New England had adopted a compulsory education act which detailed local enforcement measures. Many of these laws were repealed near the end of the seventeenth century only to be reinstituted at a later date.

THE FAMILY AND INDUSTRIALIZATION

The use of children in the work force stems from two distinct areas. In the agricultural community, the family farm was a well-established tradition. Children were borne to increase the hands available to help. In an industrial setting, the traditions transplanted from England included the apprenticeship of children as young as seven or eight years of age.

During the 1800s in the United States, children between the ages of four and ten years were working in industrial factories. There was little thought of schooling for these children, as they worked an average of twelve to fourteen hours per shift. Some of the earliest legislation in the 1800s gave the factory owner responsibility for teaching these child-employees the basics of reading and writing. The children were usually employed in textile mills or coal mines.

By the end of the nineteenth century, the first child labor laws were enacted. They restricted the employment of children to those twelve years of age and older. The signed affidavit of a parent was required as proof of the child's age. Children were to have completed a certain grade in school or passed a literacy test. They could work no more than ten hours per shift. At that time, the compulsory school attendance laws had been in effect for some time but were seldom enforced.

Education

During this period parents identified the educational needs of their children. However, the responsibility for educating the children was delegated to other individuals. Some instruction was provided by youth groups as a function of a given church affiliation. Other socializing influences came from organizations such as the Boy Scouts and the Young Men's Christian Association (YMCA).

Attitudes toward the education of children gradually began to change. Education was recognized as being partially the government's responsibility. Private education was surfacing. Philanthropic systems of schooling such as the infant school movement and the subscription societies or the Sunday schools were enthusiastically received.

In the early 1800s, Free School Societies came into being. These schools were designed to provide young people, ages three to ten years, with moral, physical, and intellectual training. However, they existed only in urban areas. In actuality, the economy and industrialization of the time had a greater influence on the child's life than did the schools.

Family Life

Industrialization also had a great impact on the structure of the family. In rural communities, each family provided for their own economic and social needs. Family roles were structured. Family values were reinforced by the extended family group as well as by the isolation imposed by the parceling of large tracts of land.

Urban migration allowed families to take advantage of available work in factories. It was often necessary for every member of the family to work in order for the family to survive. Children contributed their earnings to the parents to help maintain the family. Many outside influences now altered the family value systems. Children could not avoid being affected by the overcrowded living conditions in the areas surrounding the factories. The twelve- and fourteen-hour workdays for parents left little time for family life. The economic demands for survival forced many families to alter or compromise their values.

MODERN INFLUENCES

Subsequent economic changes brought about a dramatic revision of the ineffective child labor laws that had been common earlier. The population shift from rural to urban locations, the increased production generated by technologic advances, and the rising income of families all contributed to the general welfare of children. The increased income of families decreased the family's dependency on the wages of the children. This, in turn, prompted the family to insist on higher education for the children. The depression resulted in even more children leaving the labor market, as adults were vying for the few jobs that were available.

Currently, the child begins mandatory schooling at age six and continues until age sixteen. Many children begin earlier in kindergarten and preschool programs which may or may not be associated with day-care programs. At age sixteen the adolescent remaining in school may enter the job market on a part-time basis after obtaining a work permit through the local Board of Education. A wide variety of programs are available to the young person at both the high school and college level, providing vocational or technical skills as well as purely academic courses.

Literature and Education

A study of children's literature offers some insight into the lives of children, both during this period and in earlier times. Before the Civil War, most children's literature focused on religious instruction and desired social behavior. Biblical teachings and emphasis on the nuclear family were evident in most of the books. Specific roles for family members were also reinforced in the stories. Problems affecting a given family were generally attributed to permissive parents or to the death of a parent or child.

The Puritan work ethic and virtues that would merit salvation in heaven were strongly emphasized in literature. In the early 1900s, however, this system of values underwent a change. Values became relative rather than absolute. The expression of negative feelings became more acceptable in literature. Prior to World War II, books written for amusement rather than instruction became more prevalent than ever before.

Most recently, the changes reflected in children's books have included the recognition of different cultures, values, and social groups, and a decrease in sex stereotyping. The broad scope of behavior presented in current children's books encourages children to consider the consequences of their actions.

Schools also underwent major reforms during this period. They developed their own philosophies as well as corresponding curricula. Initially, trade schools were operated separately. Later, they were integrated into the current system of vocational education.

Health Care of the Child

In the early part of the nineteenth century, there was a rapid increase in the number of existing orphanages. In these institutions, emphasis was placed on strong moral and ethical values. At the same time, placement of children in almshouses continued to decrease steadily, largely because this was considered to be an unacceptable form of care. Children were also being placed in foster homes. An early problem of the foster care approach was the fact that the religious affiliation of the parent was not always taken into consideration.

Many of the agencies that were formed at this time to meet the needs of children focused on identified handicaps, such as blindness, deafness, and mental retardation. The New York Institution for the Deaf and Dumb was an example of one agency operating in the first part of the nineteenth century.

Changes occurred gradually over the latter half of that century. Additional agencies, as well as new legislation, resulted in the legal recognition of adoption. The onset of the White House Conferences, the formation of the Children's Bureau, and later, the funds provided by the Social Security Act all improved various aspects of the child's life.

Many of the problems in child health care persist. Such factors as limited access to needed services, arbitrary decisions by case workers, and the quality of child care in institutions still represent problems. Positive changes include recognition of children's needs as paramount, a search for alternatives to institutional care, and increased involvement of the child recipients in the services.

Family Structure

If the typical family structure of today was to be compared with that of the original census in 1790, only three percent of the families would be found to include a father, mother, and five or more children. Many factors influenced this change, including the shift from a rural to an urban population, a longer life span, decreased fertility rates, an increase in single-parent families, and the rising number of women in the work force. Other factors that contributed to the change included decreased infant mortality rates, a decreased incidence of infectious illnesses because of immunizations and treatments, and improved nutrition.

Currently, there are a number of different family structures in which children may be nurtured. These include the single-career family, the dual-career family, the single-parent household, the remarried nuclear family, the kin family, and the experimental family. Each of these family systems has both strengths and weaknesses. In order to identify the strengths, one must be aware of cultural values, economic potential, availability of support systems, and specific parenting or nurturing roles. Certainly, the commitment of individual family members to the maintenance of the family structure plays a major role in its effectiveness. In caring for children, the nurse should be aware of their family structure and its value system.

SUMMARY

Children evolve within the context of a family group in a given culture. Earlier cultures left little information regarding children's lives, although some information may be extracted from the writings that did survive. The family's perception of the value of children has traditionally played a major part in the treatment of children. Changing social and economic factors, particularly industrialization, have also influenced children's education, health care, and the nature of their family group.

SUGGESTED ACTIVITIES

- Visit a local museum and note the number of paintings that depict family groupings. Share with your group the types of family groupings and the cultural information that is conveyed by the paintings.
- Interview your grandparents or other individuals in the community who are older than seventy years of age. Compare their childhood life-styles with your own. In your study, consider schooling, play activities, responsibilities in the home, and work outside the home. Share this information with your group or class.

DISCUSSION TOPICS

1. Select one civilization and research its attitudes toward children. In your report, identify those aspects of the culture which directly influenced the care of children.
2. Research the history of a local child care institution. What were the identified needs at the time it was established? Has the focus of the agency changed over the years? How do the current goals of the agency differ from those established in the past?

REVIEW

A. Multiple choice. Select the one best answer.

1. The ancient Babylonian legal code that makes reference to the adoption of children is called the
   a. Brehon Laws.
   b. Hammurabic Code.
   c. Mosaic Code.
   d. Hippocratic Code.
2. The Greek philosophers who refer to child care and the individuality of the child in their writings are
   a. Hammurabi and Moses.
   b. Galen and Rousseau.
   c. Hippocrates and Celsus.
   d. Phaer and Galen.
3. The theory of child development that places the greatest emphasis on punishment is the concept of the child as
   a. chattel.
   b. a blank slate.
   c. a developing individual.
   d. inherently sinful.

4. Parental ownership of children is a concept that is closely linked with the view of a child as
   a. chattel.
   b. a blank slate.
   c. a developing individual.
   d. inherently sinful.

5. Which major historic event permitted children to remain at home longer, thereby promoting their education and fostering parental advocacy?
   a. Rise of Christianity
   b. Industrial Revolution
   c. Civil War
   d. Compulsory education laws

B. Short answer. Briefly respond to the following statements.

1. Name two factors that altered the number of children in the work force. Child labor laws compulsory education

2. List three values emphasized by children's literature prior to the Civil War.
   1. religious instruction
   2. desired social behavior
   3. puritan work ethic

BIBLIOGRAPHY

Deloughery, G. L. *History and Trends of Professional Nursing.* St. Louis: C. V. Mosby Company, 1977.

Goldstein, Harold. "Child Labor in America's History." *Children Today*, Vol. 5 (May–June, 1976), pp. 30–35.

Kadushin, Alfred. "Child Welfare Services – Past and Present." *Children Today,* Vol. 5 (May–June, 1976), pp.16–23.

Lystad, Mary. "At Home in America: The Family As Seen in American Books for Children." *Children Today,* Vol. 8 (March–April, 1979), pp. 2–5.

Lystad, Mary. "From Dr. Mather to Dr. Seuss – Over 200 Years of American Children's Books." *Children Today,* Vol. 5 (May–June, 1976), pp. 10–15.

Newman, Barbara M., and Phillip R. Newman. *Infancy and Childhood – Development and Its Contexts.* New York: John Wiley and Sons, 1978.

Norton, Arthur J., and Paul C. Glick. "Changes in American Family Life." *Children Today,* Vol. 5 (May–June, 1976), pp. 2–4.

Sussman, Marvin B. "The Family Today – Is It An Endangered Species?" *Children Today,* Vol. 7 (March–April, 1978), pp. 32–37+.

Waserman, Manfred. "An Overview of Child Health Care in America." *Children Today,* Vol. 5 (May–June, 1976), pp. 24–29+.

Chapter 2

Significant Events and Organizations

OBJECTIVES

Upon completion of this chapter, the student will be able to

- list three rights of the child as identified in the United Nations Declaration of the Rights of the Child.
- describe the White House Conferences.
- identify four issues that were addressed in the Children's Charter of 1930.
- name three official and three voluntary agencies and differentiate between them.

The social, political, and economic changes taking place in the world have a profound influence on the status and well-being of children. The negative influences of several of these changes have aroused such sympathy for the plight of the child that agencies have been founded and monies set aside to improve the health and welfare of children. These issues and agencies, Figure 2-1, are the focus of this chapter.

UNITED NATIONS DECLARATION OF THE RIGHTS OF THE CHILD

Prior to World War I, emphasis was not placed on the rights of the child but on the duties of the child, both to parents and to society in general. Before the onset of the war, an international meeting was held to address children's rights. However, because the war effort soon took precedence over social reform, the meeting had little effect.

Following the long and devastating years of the war, the Save the Children Fund was established in London, England by Eglantyne Jebb. The fund was prompted by Jebb's desire

1790	First public orphanage established
1820	First nursery school for children of working mothers established
1836	First child labor law enacted
1853	The Children's Aid Society of New York established for foster home care
1855	The Children's Hospital of Philadelphia founded
1870	Elementary Education Act instituted, providing free public education
1875	The Society for the Prevention of Cruelty to Animals formed in New York; first case of child abuse reported here
1893	Henry Street Settlement established in New York by Lillian Wald
1899	Children's or juvenile courts established; first one established in Cook County, Illinois
1902	School nurse system begun in New York City
1917	First federal child labor law enacted; was later declared unconstitutional
1919	First law for statewide care of handicapped children enacted in Ohio
1935	Social Security Act passed
1941	Federal law regulating child labor passed
1953	Federal Department of Health, Education, and Welfare established
1962	Vaccination Assistance Program designed to help states develop immunization programs
1963	Social Security Act amended to provide grants for maternal and infant care
1964	Economic Opportunity Act passed to assist unemployed youth
1965	Social Security Act amended to help deprived children needing health care
1966	Child Nutrition and Child Protection Acts passed
1968	Child Abuse Law passed
1969	Office of Child Development established
1971	Comprehensive Child Care Act enacted to provide day care facilities
1972	Women, Infants, and Children (WIC) Program established to provide supplemental food to this population
1974	Child Abuse Prevention and Treatment Act legislated
1975	Social Security Act amended to provide child care and foster care services
1976	Mainstream Act passed, promoting education of all children, regardless of any handicaps
1980	Adoption Assistance and Child Welfare Act promoting a redirection of child welfare programs to a family orientation rather than placement of children.

FIG. 2-1 Chronological list of events and legislation influencing child welfare

to change the misery and catastrophic conditions she had witnessed. Her enthusiasm and motivation led to her meeting with the chairman of the International Committee of the Red Cross in Geneva. The result of the meeting was the creation of the Save the Children International Union on January 6, 1920. Other countries joined the effort, and following World War I, relief actions were begun to relieve the plight of thousands of children.

In an effort to extend the impact of this work, Jebb offered a charter to the International Union. The charter was adopted in September of 1924 by the League of Nations at the Fifth Assembly. The charter was first known as The Declaration of Geneva and later as the Declaration of the Rights of the Child.

The original declaration contained five articles or brief statements of rights owed the child without consideration of race, nationality, or creed. These included physical and spiritual care, care of the destitute and handicapped, priority for relief services, and education for a living, with an emphasis on service to others.

In 1934, the League of Nations approved the principles set forth in the declaration, marking the tenth anniversary of the document's original adoption. The fact that the text of the principles remained unchanged emphasizes the concerns of that time. Of primary concern were the effects of physical neglect, poor nutrition, insufficient education, and economic exploitation on children.

In 1946, the Save the Children International Union merged with the International Association for the Promotion of Child Welfare. Together, these groups formed the International Union for Child Welfare. In 1948, the General Council for this group altered the declaration by adding two new articles and altering two others.

The new principles reflected the social changes and the scientific development of the period. The concepts of the family as an integral unit and the inherent dignity and worth of each individual were added. Aid for the handicapped was incorporated. The need to avoid any type of discrimination, originally mentioned in the preamble of the document, was included as one of the articles in the revised version.

After World War II, the document was presented to the newly formed United Nations for approval. Its presentation coincided with the work of the UN on the Universal Declaration of Human Rights. The Economic and Social Council then drafted a new document in 1950. Finally, in 1957, a compromise document was drafted. This document contained general principles that were considered to be desirable but that were not binding upon ratification by a country.

In 1959, the Third Declaration of the Rights of the Child was unanimously adopted by the General Assembly of the UN. In its final form, the document contained ten principles instead of five articles, but the focus was the same. The original declaration was completely incorporated, and many of the articles were further elaborated for clarification, Figure 2-2.

All three documents are characterized by their simple language, brief statements, and clear presentation of ideas. Each reflects the prevailing socioeconomic conditions of the time. None of the articles in the original document were completely eliminated. Subsequent documents have clarified and expanded the original principles, but not one has been discarded entirely.

DECLARATION OF THE RIGHTS OF THE CHILD

1. All children shall be entitled to these rights without distinction or discrimination.
2. All children shall be entitled to relief and protection in all circumstances.
3. All children shall be entitled to a name and nationality.
4. All children shall be entitled to social security to grow and develop in health.
5. All children shall be entitled to special treatment if handicapped.
6. All children shall be entitled to special protection to develop physically, mentally, and morally.
7. All children shall be entitled to education to develop their abilities and to become useful members of society.
8. All children shall be entitled to be among the first to receive relief in time of disaster.
9. All children shall be entitled to protection against exploitation and employment before minimum age.
10. All children shall be entitled to be brought up in a spirit of friendship among peoples.

FIG. 2-2 The ten principles of the Declaration of the Rights of the Child

UNITED NATIONS INTERNATIONAL YEAR OF THE CHILD

The year 1979 was declared the International Year of the Child by the UN. This special year was the first one ever to be focused on the child. It was a continuation of the efforts of the UN to promote human rights. Previously, the concept of human rights had not been related to the life of the child in many areas. This was an opportunity for all peoples to relate their commitment to human rights and to the life experiences of each child.

The year 1979 was significant because it was the twentieth anniversary of the Declaration of the Rights of the Child. The activities that took place throughout the year encompassed all the professional disciplines involved in child care. In addition, children themselves were often included in the activities, particularly in the study of human rights of children in other lands.

That same year, The American Academy of Pediatrics expanded its activities to include a two-year program called "Speak Up For Children!" This program, which coincided with the Academy's fiftieth anniversary in 1980, was developed to focus on four main areas of child health and welfare: accident prevention, nutrition, immunizations, and health education. The local chapters of the organization concentrated on one or more specific projects, depending on identified local and state needs. All of the projects corresponded to one or more of the four major areas of emphasis.

The logo that was used to designate materials related to the International Year of the Child was significant in itself, Figure 2-3. The child is seen reaching up for help with outstretched arms. The arms of the adult, whether parent, teacher, health care worker, or friend, encircle the child. Both are surrounded by olive branches that symbolize peace.

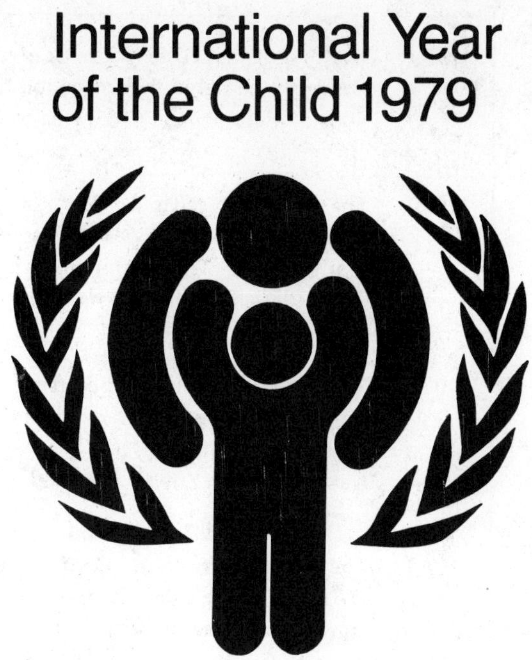

FIG. 2-3 Logo design for the International Year of the Child

WHITE HOUSE CONFERENCES

Problems affecting children were originally considered to be the responsibility of families, religious groups, and local assistance programs. However, in 1909, after recognizing the scope of nationwide problems related to child welfare, President Theodore Roosevelt convened the first White House Conference to address such issues as child labor, infant care, and care of dependent children. Since that time, these conferences have been held every ten years, and have enabled many changes to be made in child health and welfare. These changes include provisions for funding, additional legislation, and a shift in focus from the treatment of specific diseases to preventive well-child care.

The conferences have fostered a dialogue between those individuals specializing in child care and the parents and youth who are recipients of this care. The conferences have also served as a consciousness-raising exercise for the entire nation. Moreover, they have provided the impetus for legislation and funding in many needed programs. The 1930 White House Conference, for example, produced an important document called the Children's Charter. The conference in 1950 resulted in a publication entitled, "A Healthy Personality for Your Child," which is still in use today. The 1970 conference was unique in that young people themselves determined the issues and made recommendations, Figure 2-4. The conference in 1980 was the first on families. A major concern was the negative impact of government policies on families. Other topics addressed at the conference were employment practices for women, needs of the handicapped and unemployed, programs for halting family violence, and family life education programs for children, youth and adults.

1909	The first of the White House Conferences focused on dependent children. This conference was instrumental in the formation of the Children's Bureau several years later. State Divisions of Maternal and Child Health were also developed from this first conference.
1919	The second White House Conference addressed child welfare standards. The socioeconomic basis of the standards was addressed for both mother and child in the regional meetings that followed. This conference triggered the passage of the Sheppard-Towner (Maternal Child) Act and amendments to the Child Labor Law.
1930	The third White House Conference was on child health and protection. The document that evolved from this conference, the Children's Charter, addressed not only the health and protection of children, but also their welfare and education. The Social Security Act and National Health Survey followed this conference.
1940	The fourth White House Conference was devoted to children in a democracy. It addressed the needs of the child under a democratic political system. The Hill-Burton Act on hospital construction was an outgrowth of this conference.
1950	The fifth White House Conference, or the Midcentury Conference, addressed the child's mental health. Its theme was the development of a healthy personality in children. Delinquency and mental retardation were also considered.
1960	The Golden Anniversary, or sixth White House Conference, was devoted simply to children and youth. Its focus was a child's achievement of full potential for a creative life. Problems of minorities, as well as those of the physically handicapped, were discussed.
1970	The seventh White House Conference focused on children and youth amid a changing social scene. This was the first time the conference was divided into two groups. One group consisted of those interested in the care of the child, and the other was composed of young people, ages fourteen to twenty-four years, speaking out for themselves.
1980	The eighth White House Conference directed its attention to families. The issues raised reflected a mandate for change in public policies that affected families. Issues addressed included employment practices which are more flexible, child care facilities, recognition of homemakers, health care in the home for the elderly, repeal of the "marriage tax," and combined efforts of government, schools and the media to combat drug and alcohol abuse.

FIG. 2-4 White House Conference topics

Children's Charter of 1930

Under the guidance of President Herbert Hoover, the White House Conference on Child Health and Protection developed a document known as the Children's Charter. It set forth nineteen goals for the children of America. Considering the time during which it was developed, the document was outstanding in its recognition of the universal needs of children.

The document addressed all aspects of the life of a child. It identified goals such as spiritual and moral training, the security of the child's own home or a foster home, prenatal care, preventive health care and education. The need for a safe home environment was recognized, as was the importance of a safe community and alternative care in nursery schools and kindergartens. The issues of physical and mental handicaps were addressed with the recognition that the costs "should be borne publicly" when they could not be covered by personal income. Family standards of living were considered, as were concerns related to child labor and children who were living in isolated rural areas. The need for a coordinated system of health care involving local, state, and national organizations was also addressed.

HEALTH AGENCIES

Health agencies are divided into two basic types: official or governmental and nonofficial or voluntary. Official agencies function according to a legal mandate and are funded through taxes. Voluntary organizations do not share that tax base.

Official Health Agencies

Health problems over which the government took control were in existence during the founding years of our country. Indeed, many current health programs date from the early beginnings of our country. In 1850, Lemuel Shattuck issued a report to the Sanitary Commission of Massachusetts. The report included suggestions that provided a basis for present programs in sanitation.

Government health responsibilities include those areas over which individuals have little control. Such areas as air and water pollution, impure foods or drugs, and immunization programs to prevent disease are governmental concerns.

Because official agencies are funded by taxes, their budgets are limited. This means that it may take years to incorporate new activities into an existing program. Budget appropriations are based on population data from a given area. Pressure from special-interest groups also plays a part in budget allocations.

World Health Organization. On an international level, the World Health Organization was formed in 1948. Established as a part of the United Nations, it is the official governmental agency in public health. Its primary aims are "to prevent and control disease, promote physical and mental health, expand scientific knowledge, and contribute to the harmony of human relations on a world scale." Its primary objective is disease prevention; its secondary aim is improvement of health. The agency is not directly involved in meeting these goals, however. Rather, it provides assistance to individual nations so that they are able to solve their own problems. Maternal and infant health is considered to be one of the program priorities. Money is spent on food, clothing, medicines, and the eradication of disease in underdeveloped countries.

Federal Agencies. On the national or federal level, health services were, at one time, administered by the Department of Health, Education, and Welfare (HEW). This agency was established in 1935 when the Social Security Act was legislated. Originally, there were many divisions within the department, some with overlapping responsibilities. In 1968, however, the department was reorganized into three main divisions which persist today: Public Health, Human Development, and Social Rehabilitation Services.

In 1980, under President Jimmy Carter, the Department of Health, Education, and Welfare was reorganized. Education was made a separate department at the Cabinet level. The agency responsible for health and welfare concerns was renamed the United States Department of Health and Human Services.

Money for individual programs sponsored by the divisions is made available to the states through federal grants-in-aid. Specific sections of the Social Security Act are referred to as "titles." Child welfare services and services to needy families come under Title IV. Title V provides for maternal and child health services and services to crippled children. Aid to the aged, blind, or disabled is covered under Title XVI. Programs to combat mental retardation may be financed through Title XVII.

All of the divisions touch the lives of children in some way. The oldest, the Public Health Service, was established in 1798 to aid merchant seamen. At this time, its responsibilities include the identification of health hazards in the environment, the delivery of comprehensive health care services, and the support of research. The Division of Social Rehabilitation Services founded in 1968 administers programs that are related to social and rehabilitative programs, as well as those that provide for income maintenance for needy families.

Since the reorganization of HEW in 1980, the Office of Human Development Services includes both the Administration for Children, Youth, and Families and the Children's Bureau. (Under the original reorganization in 1969, the Children's Bureau and the Bureau of Child Development Services, an outgrowth of the national Head Start program, were consolidated.)

At the state level, the departments include Maternal and Child Health, Child Welfare, Education, and Crippled Children's Services. The Department of Maternal and Child Health administers the funds, program planning, education, and research efforts of the Children's Bureau. The only direct service it provides is payment for premature infant care, prenatal clinics, and well-child clinics. The Child Welfare Department also administers Children's Bureau funds, in addition to providing services to families involved in Aid to Dependent Children programs and referral services. Its direct services are related to the needs of poor families, to protective services, and to foster care and adoption. The Education Department administers the National School Lunch Program and the Vocational Rehabilitative Program. The Division of Crippled Children's Services administers funding for crippled children and is involved in the education of professionals and in research. Its direct services include diagnostic clinics and direct payment for hospital and medical costs of crippled children.

The Children's Bureau was established in 1912 as an outgrowth of the first White House Conference in 1909. Lillian Wald, founder of the Henry Street Settlement in New York

City, was instrumental in the development of the Children's Bureau. Julia C. Lathrop served as its first chief. The goals of the bureau are: (1) the setting of standards and the provision of technical assistance to states and agencies for programs for children, (2) the support of research of new programs and the evaluation of existing programs, and (3) education, both of a professional and public nature.

The process of developing standards involves statistical research and data collection on all aspects of children's lives. These data include such factors as the number of births, the number of handicapped children, mortality rates, family incomes, and the number and types of problems affecting children in public and private agencies. This information encompasses all children of all races and from all socioeconomic backgrounds.

The research arm of the Children's Bureau provides federal grants-in-aid to both states and local communities. The monies are used to initiate new programs or services and to train the professional staff. The money may also be used to fund demonstration projects of a research nature that ultimately may improve services in the future. The majority of these grants are provided on a "matching funds" basis in cooperation with the state or local community.

The educational component of the Children's Bureau is best typified by the publication *Children Today* (formerly called *Children*). It is an interdisciplinary journal for professionals and nonprofessionals whose common interest is the care of children. Several other bulletins are also published by the agency. The first publications, *Prenatal Care* and *Infant Care,* were initially published a year after the agency was established. Since then they have undergone many revisions.

Voluntary Health Agencies

The main characteristic of voluntary agencies is the lack of tax-based financial support. Voluntary agencies are supported by outright gifts and a variety of fund-raising activities. With these funds, voluntary agencies provide a variety of services, including research, support of experimental projects, education of both the public and professionals, and support of various types of legislative action. Some voluntary agencies also provide direct payment for services, or provide certain services themselves, such as loans of equipment or supplies, diagnostic testing, and free hospitalization.

Most voluntary agencies arise from an identified need that is not being sufficiently met by official agencies. In many situations, they develop from groups of parents who bond together to address and solve the particular problems of their children. Often, this group support becomes more structured, and fund-raising ensues, first on a small scale and then on a larger scale. Gradually, a viable organization develops. The Easter Seal Society for Crippled Children is just one example of an agency which developed in this fashion. A list of many voluntary agencies can be found in Appendix G.

SUMMARY

Children's lives have been influenced profoundly throughout history by economic and social changes. Increasing national awareness of the special needs of children led to the institution of the White House Conferences.

As an outgrowth of these meetings, the Children's Bureau and the Children's Charter were developed. On an international level, the UN Declaration of the Rights of the Child focused on many of these same issues.

Governmental or official, tax-supported agencies operated on a federal, state, or local level, also contribute significantly to child health and welfare. The gaps in the services provided by these official agencies are often filled by separate voluntary agencies that are privately supported.

SUGGESTED ACTIVITIES

- Visit an official or voluntary local agency. Report on the services provided, the eligibility requirements, and the source of funding for the agency.
- Invite to your class a speaker from the local health department. Ask this person to discuss the services that specifically relate to child health and welfare.
- Attend a pediatric or well-child clinic sponsored by an official agency. Describe to your class the activities you observed and the type of anticipatory guidance given to the parents.

DISCUSSION TOPICS

1. Discuss the various elements of the Children's Charter of 1930. Identify the changes and patterns in society which influenced its content.
2. Discuss the various voluntary agencies in your community. What types of services do they provide for children?
3. Research the life of Lillian Wald or Julia Lathrop. Share your findings with your class.

REVIEW

A. Matching. Match the specific agencies listed in Column I with the type of agency in Column II.

Column I	Column II
1. Children's Bureau	a. Official
2. Child Welfare League	b. Voluntary
3. Office of Child Development Services	
4. American Lung Association	
5. American Celiac Society	
6. Department of Health and Human Services	
7. Division of Crippled Children's Services	

B. Multiple choice. Select the one best answer.

1. The woman who was instrumental in the development and formation of the Children's Bureau was
   a. Clara Barton.
   b. Lillian Wald.
   c. Julia Lathrop.
   d. Eglantyne Jebb.
2. The nationwide meeting that is held every ten years to discuss some aspect of child life is the
   a. White House Conference.
   b. UN Assembly on Children.
   c. Federal Child Advocacy Meeting.
   d. Children's Charter Conference.
3. The document containing nineteen articles that sets forth goals for the health and welfare of American children is the
   a. Declaration of the Rights of the Child.
   b. Child's Bill of Rights.
   c. Children's Charter of 1930.
   d. Children's Bureau Recommendations.
4. The year that was designated the International Year of the Child to focus attention on the care of children everywhere was
   a. 1930.
   b. 1945.
   c. 1953.
   d. 1979.

5. The right to a name and nationality and the right to special care if handicapped are concepts found in the
   a. Children's Bureau Constitution.
   b. Children's Charter.
   c. UN Declaration of the Rights of the Child.
   d. Report of the White House Conference on Children and Youth.

C. Short answer. Briefly respond to the following statements.

1. Describe the relationship between the Save the Children Union and the Declaration of the Rights of the Child. Both the result of the enthusiasm + work of Eglantyne Jebb
2. Describe the three major purposes of the Children's Bureau.

BIBLIOGRAPHY

Axinn, June, and Hermin Levin. *Social Welfare – A History of the American Response to Need.* New York: Dodd, Mead and Company, 1975.

Chanlett, Eliska, and G. M. Morier. "Declaration of the Rights of the Child." *International Child Welfare Review,* Vol. XXII (1968).

Eliot, M. M. "Six Decades of Action for Children." *Children Today,* Vol. 1 (March–April, 1972), p. 2.

Ferro, Frank. "Improving the Child Welfare System." *Children Today,* Vol. 5 (November–December, 1976), p. 1.

Kadushin, Alfred. "Child Welfare Services – Past and Present." *Children Today,* Vol. 5 (May–June, 1976), pp. 16–23.

Marlow, Dorothy R. *Textbook of Pediatric Nursing.* Philadelphia: W. B. Saunders Company, 1977.

Norton, Arthur J., and Paul C. Glick. "Changes in American Family Life." *Children Today,* Vol. 5 (May–June, 1976), pp. 2–4+.

Solnit, Albert J. "Changing Psychological Perspectives About Children and Their Families." *Children Today,* Vol. 5 (May–June, 1976), pp. 5–9+.

Waserman, Manfred. "An Overview of Child Health Care in America." *Children Today,* Vol. 5 (May–June, 1976), pp. 24–29+.

Zigler, Edward F. "The Unmet Needs of America's Children." *Children Today,* Vol. 5 (May–June, 1976), pp. 39–42.

Section II

The Beginning of Life

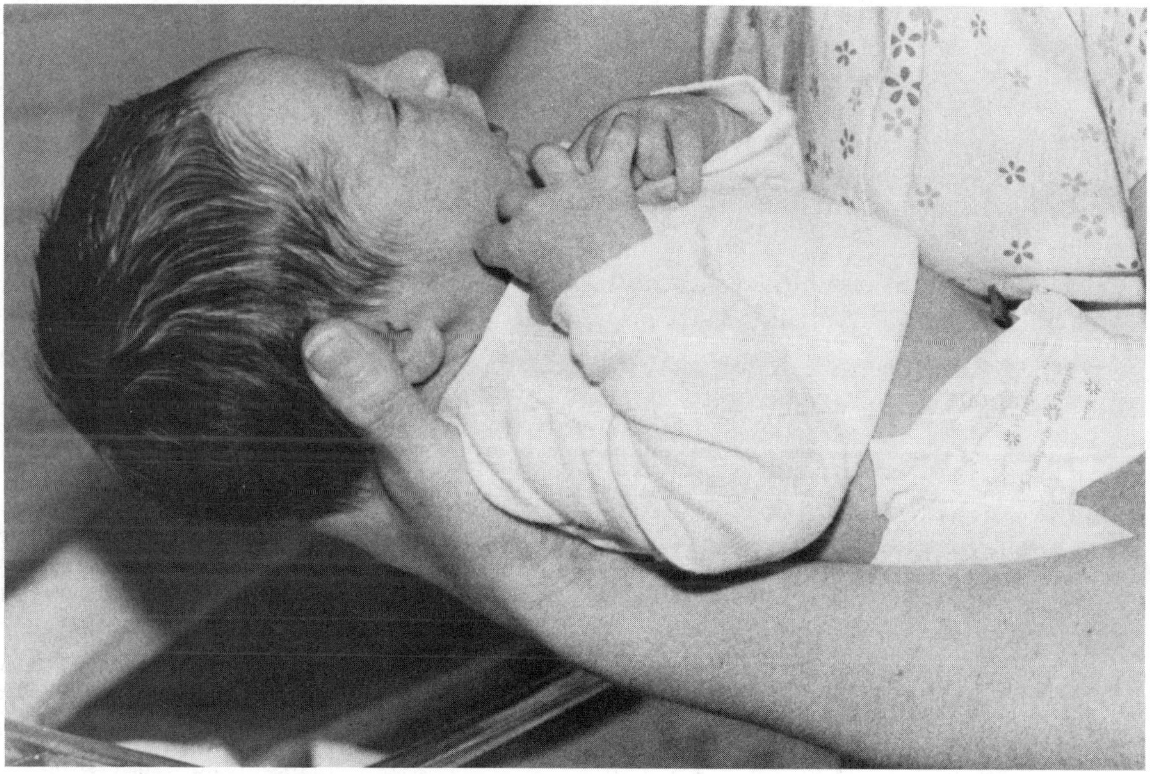

Chapter 3

Prenatal Development

OBJECTIVES

Upon completion of this chapter, the student will be able to

- describe the process by which fertilization and sex differentiation takes place.
- describe the changes that take place during various stages in embryonic and fetal life.
- identify several factors that may negatively affect fetal development.

The prenatal development of any child is dependent on the early health care of the mother as well as a multitude of decisions surrounding that particular pregnancy. Cultural, emotional, developmental, and environmental factors affect not only childbearing as a whole, but each individual pregnancy and each family unit.

EMBRYOGENESIS

The origin of pediatrics is not found in a hospital setting. Rather, it involves the quiet interplay of two mature cells, the ovum and the sperm, as they unite to form a unique individual. In the mature female, the ovum leaves the graafian follicle, propelled by the gentle waves of the fimbriae at the ends of the fallopian tube. This motion directs the ovum toward the distal third of the tube where, if fertilization is to take place, the ovum will meet the sperm.

In the process of coitus, the sperm and seminal fluid are deposited in the vagina near the cervix. Several million sperm are expelled in one ejaculate. This large number of sperm is needed for fertilization because of the many factors that can interfere with their survival. Such conditions as the acid pH of vaginal secretions or heat may lead to their destruction. Once within the vagina, the sperm travel through the uterus and into the distal third of the fallopian tube where the ovum lies.

The protective covering of the ovum, or the zona pellucida, could not be penetrated if hyaluronidase was not secreted by the sperm. This enzyme softens and dissolves the zona pellucida, allowing penetration and fertilization of the ovum by a single sperm cell. The fusion of the male and female pronuclei produces a zygote, Figure 3-1, with a full complement of forty-six chromosomes. Rapid cell division then occurs in a geometric progression, and a cluster of cells, called a morula, is formed. This morula then returns to the uterus, propelled by the cilia and the peristaltic movements of the fallopian tube. As this cell mass increases in size, cells are arranged on the outside of it and a hollow is formed in the center. At this point, the zygote is known as a blastocyst.

The blastocyst then implants itself in the walls of the endometrium with the aid of enzymes. This process is called nidation, and

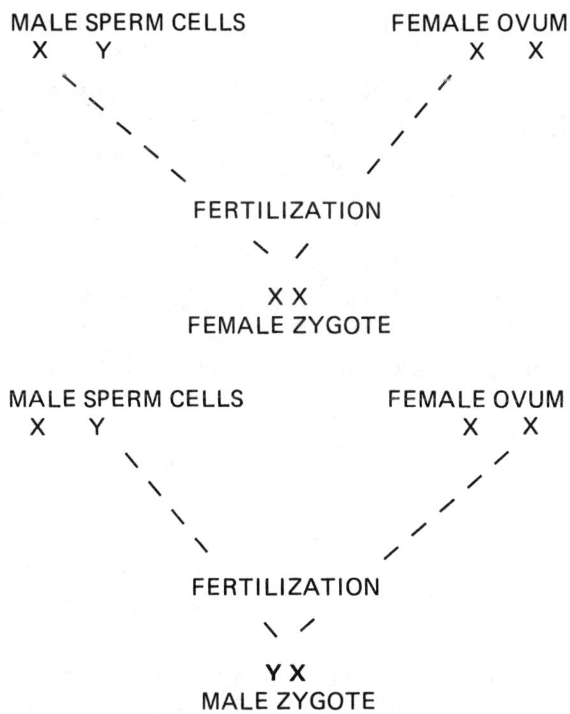

FIG. 3-1 Sex determination

normally occurs in the upper one-third of the uterus on its anterior or posterior wall.

THE PLACENTA

During the weeks following implantation, villi or trophoblasts develop over the surface of the blastocyst. Ultimately, these form the chorionic villi which secrete chorionic gonadotropin. They also synthesize proteins and glucose for nourishment. Those villi that penetrate the endometrium after the first twelve weeks become part of the placenta. They are referred to as the chorion frondosum, and are able to multiply rapidly. The connection formed between the chorion frondosum and the embryo is the umbilical cord.

The amnion is the membrane that lines the chorion and contains the fetus and the amniotic fluid around it. This fluid begins forming during intrauterine life. It is sterile and slightly alkaline in nature, and contains epithelial cells, serum albumin and globulin, white blood cells, and enzymes. It also contains both organic and inorganic salts. During the course of pregnancy, a maximum of 1500 cubic centimeters (cc) of fluid is present at any one time. By the seventh month, however, the amount of fluid begins to decrease gradually until term, when about 700 cubic centimeters are present. Extremes in the amount of amniotic fluid (polyhydramnios and oligohydramnios) may indicate the presence of birth defects. The usual amount of amniotic fluid ranges from 300 to 2000 cubic centimeters.

The placenta begins functioning about the third week of embryonic life. It meets the oxygen, nutritional, and elimination needs of the embryo and fetus. Placental transfer of many substances occurs through a membrane once thought to be selective. Hormone production and antibody transfer are also functions of the placenta.

EMBRYONIC DEVELOPMENT

During the embryonic period, which occurs from the second to the eighth week after fertilization, the germinal tissues differentiate. The three tissue layers are the ectoderm or outermost layer; the mesoderm or middle layer; and the entoderm or innermost layer. The ectoderm evolves into the epidermis and related tissues, including the skin glands, nails and hair, the epithelium of the mouth and anus, as well as the external sense organs and the nervous system. The mesoderm develops into the muscles, connective tissue, blood, cartilage, bone marrow, and lymphatic tissue. It also forms the epithelium of the blood vessels, body cavities, upper genitourinary system, and joint cavities. The entoderm forms the epithelium of the lower respiratory tract (except the nose), the digestive tract, and the lower genitourinary tract.

The development of the embryo proceeds, as with the newborn infant, in a cephalocaudal fashion. It also proceeds from proximal to distal areas (from medial to lateral). This description simply denotes that the development of the upper arm precedes that of the fingers, and that the thigh develops before the foot.

Various areas of the body grow at different rates. The differentiation of body organs and structures is called morphogenesis. The development or formation of distinct tissues is called histogenesis.

The entire pregnancy consists of forty weeks or ten lunar months of twenty-eight days each. The embryonic period is considered to comprise the first eight weeks of pregnancy. By the end of the fourth week

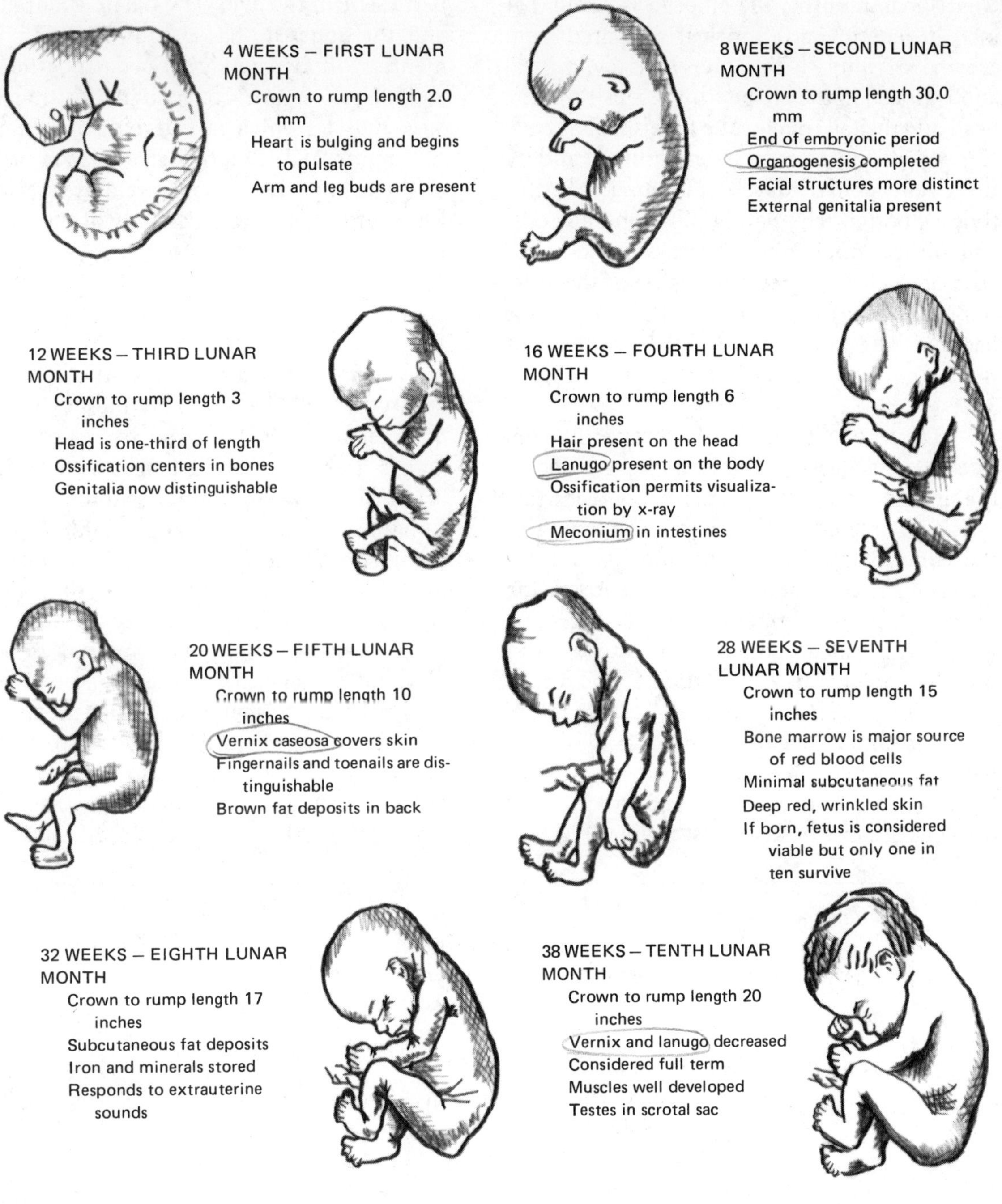

FIG. 3-2 Fetal growth during gestation (*Note:* Relative size has been distorted to better demonstrate correspondence of parts.)

(first lunar month), the embryo is about 1/4 inch in length, or 0.2 inch if measured from crown to rump. The embryo is cylindrical and is flexed in a C shape. In this position, the head and the tail touch. The tube-shaped structure which functions as a heart bulges, and by the twenty-fourth day, is pulsating. At this time, blood is circulating through the fetus and the chorionic villi. The brain and spinal cord are being formed and fusion of the anterior and posterior portions of the neural tube occurs. The limb buds and the precursor of the kidneys are present at this time, Figure 3-2.

The second lunar month brings about considerable changes in the embryo and marks the end of the embryonic period. Organogenesis is completed at this time. The length of the embryo from crown to rump is about 1 inch, or 2.5 centimeters. With the formation of the valves and septa, the heart is completed. At this stage of development, the head is disproportionately large in relation to the rest of the embryo. This is a result of the rapid increase in brain development. In conjunction with this increase in head size, the facial structures become more distinct. The structures of the eye, ear, and nose are discernible. Pigment is present in the eye. The palate is developing and the upper lip has already formed. Rudimentary limbs are developed, and the wrist and elbow are both formed at this time. The large muscles which have developed are capable of contracting. External genitalia are present, but it is impossible to differentiate sex at this time without a histologic study of the developing gonads.

FETAL DEVELOPMENT

After the eighth week the developing embryo is called a fetus. By the twelfth week of pregnancy, the fetus weighs 1/2 to 1 ounce and is approximately 3 inches in length, Figure 3-3. The head continues to be disproportionately large, comprising one-third of the actual linear measurement. The upper and lower eyelids are present at this time, but are still fused. Development of the skeletal system is progressing with the formation of bones and the presence of centers of ossification. Nail beds are formed on the fingers and toes. Enamel-producing cells and dentin combine to form the tooth buds. Also at this time, the external genitalia become distinguishable as male or female. The hematopoietic system

During the first five lunar months:

The length of the fetus in centimeters equals the square of the lunar month. For example, at the end of the third lunar month, the length of the fetus is 9 centimeters.

$$3^2 = 3 \times 3 = 9 \text{ cm}$$

During the second five lunar months:

The length of the fetus in centimeters equals the lunar month times five. For example, at the end of the seventh lunar month, the fetus is 35 centimeters in length.

$$7 \times 5 = 35 \text{ cm}$$

FIG. 3-3 Estimation of fetal growth according to Haase's rule

shows increased development, with the liver providing the majority of red blood cells. The bone marrow also contributes to red blood cell production. The fetus is capable of both spontaneous movements and reflex-type respiratory movements at this point of development.

Throughout the next lunar month (through the sixteenth week), the fetus grows rapidly. Fetal weight is about 4 ounces and the length of the fetus is approximately 6 inches. Lanugo, or fine downy hair, is present on the body of the fetus, and hair is present on the head. The digestive enzymes ptyalin and pepsin begin to be secreted, and carbohydrates and fats are stored. Carbohydrates are used to synthesize the fats. Meconium is present in the intestines. Ossification of the bones is sufficient for radiographic visualization of the fetus. Fetal movements may be detected by the mother during this period of development.

By the twentieth week, or the fifth lunar month, the fetus has doubled its weight to 8 ounces and is about 10 inches long. Lanugo is increasing and the skin is being covered by a cheeselike substance called vernix caseosa. This substance is composed of fatty secretions from the sebaceous glands and dead epidermal cells. Also, increasing amounts of brown fat are being deposited along the infant's back. These deposits are important for heat production during the newborn period. The fingernails and toenails are also distinguishable, and the eyelids and eyebrows are forming. This period of development also marks the beginning of myelinization of the spinal cord.

By the twenty-fourth week, fetal weight is 1 1/2 pounds and the length is 12 inches. The eyelashes and eyebrows are more clearly defined at this time. Surfactant is being produced in the alveolar cells.

By the twenty-eighth week, the fetus weighs 2 1/2 pounds and is 15 inches in length. Outwardly, it resembles a little old man with wrinkled skin, and is deep red in color. At this phase of development, subcutaneous fat is minimal. The bone marrow is now the major source of red blood cells. The brain is still developing, as are the glia cells, and myelinization continues. Glia cell formation continues throughout the first year of life.

Deposits of subcutaneous fat occur by the thirty-second week. The fetus is now about 17 inches in length and weighs 4 pounds. It is able to store iron, calcium, phosphorus, and other minerals. The fetus may also respond noticeably to outside noises or sounds.

During the last two lunar months (the thirty-third to the thirty-eighth week), the fetus undergoes minimal change except for increases in length and weight. By the end of the thirty-eighth week, the fetus is 20 inches long and weighs about 7 pounds. Both the body and limbs have assumed a nicely rounded, unwrinkled appearance because of fat deposits. The vernix caseosa and lanugo both decrease as the fetus approaches term. Well-developed muscles are evident in the flexed limbs. In the male fetus, the testes usually descend about the thirty-sixth week.

DRUGS IN PREGNANCY

Drug use during pregnancy is a cause for increasing alarm. Unfortunately, just as rapidly as the knowledge of the hazards of drug use has increased, so has the number of over-the-counter drugs. The effect of any drug on the fetus is dependent on a number of factors. These factors include the drug itself, its dosage, and the gestational age of the fetus.

In the past, it was thought that the placental barrier prevented harmful substances from entering the fetal circulation. This premise was later found to be incorrect. It is now recognized that enzymes in the placenta, capable of transforming a chemical substance to an active metabolite, allow easy passage of the substance into the fetal tissues. This process, coupled with differences in drug activity within a fetus, can interfere with the normal development of the fetus.

As a drug which may have no toxicity in an adult enters the fetal circulation, the process of its metabolism and excretion is assumed by the immature liver and kidneys. These underdeveloped organs are unequal to the task. As a result, a single dose of a drug, such as thalidomide, administered twenty-eight to forty-eight days after conception can have tragic results.

The fetus is most susceptible to drugs early in the mother's pregnancy. This is the period during which cellular growth and change occur most rapidly; hence, it is the period of greatest vulnerability for the fetus. However, even drugs that are taken prior to the critical period for organ development can cause problems because of their often cumulative effects.

The crucial period of fetal development is considered to be the first eight weeks of pregnancy. If drug ingestion occurs prior to implantation, effects may be minimal or loss of the pregnancy may occur. If drug ingestion occurs within the first eight weeks, severe damage to one or more of the organ systems may prove incompatible with life, and a spontaneous abortion may take place. Although all systems are particularly vulnerable during this eight-week period, it is important to remember that both the central nervous system and the external genitalia of the fetus continue to be vulnerable to drugs throughout the pregnancy. Limited doses of drugs ingested late in the pregnancy may have minimal or transient effects on the fetus. This is the subject of current research. Food additives and other potentially toxic substances may also contribute to fetal abnormalities, as may any interference with maternal nutrition during pregnancy.

OTHER TERATOGENS

A number of infectious organisms have been identified as teratogens. The extent of damage to the fetus or infant may not be known until the time of delivery. The nature and degree of the damage depends on the time during embryonic or fetal development at which the insult, or infection, occurred.

Most teratogenic organisms may be recalled easily by using the abbreviation TORCH. The "T" stands for toxoplasmosis, often transferred from contaminated cat excreta. The "O" refers to other diseases, such as syphilis. The "R" is for rubella, which is a known cause of birth defects. The "C" stands for cytomegalovirus disease, which is responsible for a large percentage of the reported cases of central nervous system damage. The "H" refers to herpes simplex, which often causes central nervous system damage and which is associated with a high infant mortality rate.

Alcohol and radiation are also recognized teratogens. Alcohol has been found to cause developmental delays in infants whose mothers ingest alcohol in large amounts throughout the pregnancy. Part of the problem may stem from the fact that the maternal diet is often poor in this situation, and the alcohol may be the substitute for foods rich in calories and nutrients. Radiation has also been linked to birth defects, and may contribute to the development of cancer or leukemia in later years. As with other teratogens, the risks depend on the amount of radiation as well as the time during which the fetus is exposed. Caffeine, found in coffee and cola beverages, is also considered to be a potential teratogen.

Advanced maternal age and smoking are two other factors which may directly affect the health and survival of the developing embryo or fetus. In mothers over thirty-five years of age there is an increased incidence of chromosomal defects. Newer research suggests that a greater problem in this age-group may be the aging of blood vessels which reduces the uterine blood flow. As a result of the impaired circulation, the fetus receives less nutrients, less oxygen, and ultimately impaired fetal growth. Smoking creates similar problems of reduced blood flow. Placental infarcts or clots which reduce blood flow to areas of the placenta are more common in smokers.

SUMMARY

A knowledge of fetal development is essential for nurses involved in maternal and infant health. The nurse must be able to answer questions about real or potential problems intelligently. Nurses must also take the initiative, through health teaching, to protect the unborn child from inappropriate exposures to teratogens. Drugs, infectious diseases, and alcohol are the leading causes of fatal birth defects. The period of greatest vulnerability to these and other teratogens is the first eight weeks of embryonic life.

SUGGESTED ACTIVITIES

- Interview three pregnant women. Determine what substances they were told to avoid during pregnancy. Find out how they have had to change their life-styles to accommodate this new knowledge. Compile a list of any substances they are taking on a regular or intermittent basis during their pregnancy.
- Visit a health science museum or a coroner's museum. Observe the embryos and fetuses on display. What structures can you identify and what developmental changes are most easily recognized? Using Haase's rule, calculate the approximate length of the fetuses.

DISCUSSION TOPICS

1. Work with your group to prepare an educational program for expectant mothers regarding the use of cigarettes, drugs, and alcohol during pregnancy. Determine when this information could best be used by the mother.
2. Look up three known teratogens and identify their effects on the fetus. Share this information with your class.

REVIEW

A. Matching. Match the developmental milestone in Column I with the fetal age in Column II.

Column I	Column II
1. Surfactant is produced in the alveolar cells.	a. 4th week
2. Lanugo is first present.	b. 8th week
3. Bone marrow is the major source of blood formation.	c. 10th week
4. The embryo is 1/4 inch, or 0.2 inch in length from crown to rump.	d. 16th week
5. The vernix caseosa forms.	e. 20th week
6. Organogenesis is complete.	f. 24th week
7. The fetus responds to external sounds.	g. 28th week
8. Centers of ossification are present.	h. 32nd week

B. Multiple choice. Select the one best answer.

1. The zona pellucida is the
   a. protective covering of the ovum.
   b. protective covering of the sperm.
   c. name given to the fertilized egg.
   d. area where the ovum is implanted.
2. Which of the following combinations would produce a female child?
   a. An ovum with a Y chromosome and a sperm with an X chromosome
   b. An ovum with an X chromosome and a sperm with an X chromosome
   c. An ovum with a Y chromosome and a sperm with a Y chromosome
   d. An ovum with an X chromosome and a sperm with a Y chromosome
3. Another term for nidation is
   a. fertilization.
   b. conception.
   c. implantation.
   d. development.
4. The normal range for the amount of amniotic fluid is
   a. 300 to 2000 cc.
   b. 500 to 1500 cc.
   c. 750 to 1500 cc.
   d. 900 to 2000 cc.
5. The name for the innermost germinal tissue layer is the
   a. mesoderm.
   b. ectoderm.
   c. myoderm.
   d. entoderm.
6. According to Haase's rule, the length of a four-month fetus would be approximately
   a. 9 centimeters.
   b. 12 centimeters.
   c. 16 centimeters.
   d. 20 centimeters.

C. Short answer. Briefly respond to the following statements.

1. Name the two organs or systems that are vulnerable to drug ingestion throughout the entire pregnancy.
2. Identify the period of greatest sensitivity of the fetus to drug ingestion and explain why.

BIBLIOGRAPHY

Blake, Jean P., et al. "Drugs in Pregnancy: Weighing the Risks." *Patient Care,* Vol. 14 (May 30, 1980), pp. 22–37.

Blake, Jean P. "Charting Proved and Suspected Drug Toxicity." *Patient Care,* Vol. 14 (May 30, 1980), pp. 40–67.

Berlin, Cheston M. "Assessing Effects of Maternal Drug Use." *Patient Care,* Vol. 14 (May 30, 1980), pp. 68–111.

Cranley, Mecia S. "Antepartal Fetal Assessment." *American Journal of Nursing,* Vol. 78 (December, 1978), pp. 2098–2102.

Moore, Mary Lou. *Realities in Childbearing.* Philadelphia: W. B. Saunders Company, 1978.

Vaughan, Victor C., et al. *Nelson's Textbook of Pediatrics.* Philadelphia: W. B. Saunders Company, 1979.

Chapter 4

The Neonate

OBJECTIVES

Upon completion of this chapter, the student will be able to

- describe the appearance of both a normal and a premature newborn infant.
- identify the nursing care that is appropriate for a hospitalized neonate.
- differentiate between the assistance given the mother who is breast-feeding and that given one who is bottle-feeding her infant.
- list the various aspects of home care for which the parents must be prepared.

A family's excitement surrounding the arrival of a newborn infant is sometimes dampened by the seemingly overwhelming responsibility of caring for the infant. The nurse in a hospital situation must, therefore, prepare the parents for this responsibility so that they leave the hospital with a positive impression of the childbirth experience and of their role as parents and caregivers.

INITIAL ASSESSMENT AND CARE OF THE NEWBORN INFANT

Assessment of the neonate begins at the point of delivery. On first observation, the nurse should note any obvious anomalies. An assessment by means of an Apgar score is then completed at one minute and at five minutes after birth, Figure 4-1. The scoring should be started fifty-five seconds after delivery so that it is completed at sixty seconds. The timing for the one-minute evaluation begins after the entire infant is delivered. For some infants, it may be performed while the infant is being resuscitated. The score, based on a rating of zero to two for five different parameters, is a

SIGN	SCORE		
	0	1	2
Heart Rate	Absent	Slow (<100)	>100
Respiratory Effort	Absent	Weak cry, hypoventilation	Good, strong cry
Muscle Tone	Limp	Some flexion of extremities	Well-flexed
Reflex Response			
Response to catheter in nostril (tested after oropharynx is clear)	No response	Grimace	Cough or sneeze
Tangential foot slap	No response	Grimace	Cry and withdrawal of foot
Color	Blue, pale	Pink body, blue extremities	Completely pink

FIG. 4-1 The components of an Apgar score for evaluation of the newborn infant. The score is to be determined at 1 minute and at 5 minutes after delivery.

reflection of the baby's adjustment to extrauterine life. A total score of ten is considered to be excellent.

At some time early in the neonatal period, the nurse or the physician performs a complete assessment of the newborn infant. The timing of this evaluation depends on the delivery environment. In the home setting, it may be completed once the mother has been made comfortable. In the hospital setting, it may be done in the delivery room or in the newborn nursery. In a birthing center, the parents may assist with the assessment of the infant. Regardless of the setting, the evaluation must be objective and thorough. If the parents are present, the nurse must be aware of their concerns and should anticipate their questions and comments. The assessment can be an excellent teaching tool if the parents are both present and participating in the evaluative process.

A careful and thorough assessment is performed in order to monitor the status of the infant who has undergone and is undergoing extensive physiologic changes. The initiation of respirations, the change from fetal to neonatal circulatory pathways, the production and conservation of heat, and the increased function of the gastrointestinal and urinary tracts are all major alterations in body processes. An assessment is performed to pinpoint areas of concern in this transitional phase of the infant's life.

General Observations

The assessment begins with a general observation of the infant. Is the baby in a position of flexion as in Figure 4-2, or are arms and legs extended and rather floppy? Is the infant a normal, ruddy color, or is it pale and cyanotic? Is the coloring consistent, or are the

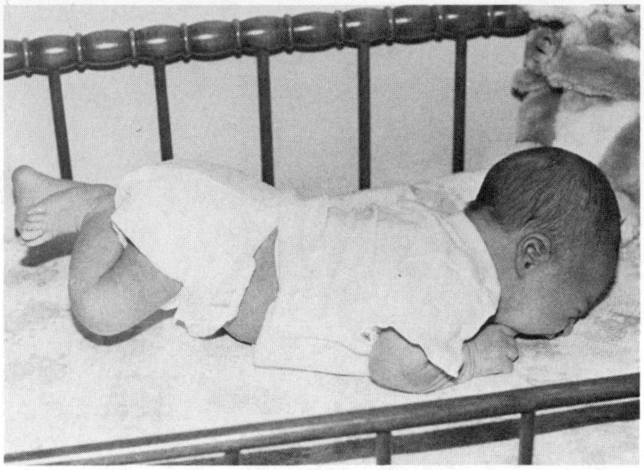

FIG. 4-2 Newborn infant in a normal position of flexion. Crawling movements are typical in this position.

hands and feet cyanotic as in acrocyanosis? Is the baby's cry lusty, or is it weak or shrill? Is the infant making any other noises such as grunting sounds? Are there any signs of respiratory distress such as retractions or nasal flaring?

Vital Signs

The vital signs of the infant should be recorded at this time to establish a baseline for future assessments. The temperature is taken either rectally or by axillary means. This is an important assessment as the infant who is cold and wet and in a cool delivery room loses a great deal of heat. This results in an increased oxygen consumption. The apical pulse rate of the infant, which should be between 120 and 160 beats per minute, is also recorded. For the most accurate reading, it should be taken when the infant is quiet rather than crying. The respiratory rate should also be taken while the infant is quiet. The normal range is from thirty-five to fifty respirations per minute. The respirations will be predominantly abdominal. The presence of cyanosis or dyspnea should be reported immediately.

Head

The infant's head, which comprises one-fourth of the body length, is measured. The head circumference is usually about 13 to 14 1/2 inches, and is generally 2 centimeters larger than the chest. Areas of asymmetry are noted. This may be caused by molding, by scalp edema (known as caput succedaneum), or by a cephalhematoma. The anterior and posterior fontanelles are palpated for size. The infant's face is small and usually round, depending on the birth method. Facial asymmetry may be present as a result of the infant's in utero position or the process of delivery. All areas of the skin on the head should be observed for irritations or actual lacerations. These may be caused by the fetal monitoring devices used.

Eyes, Ears, and Mouth

The appearance of the eyes should be noted. In the neonate, they are usually blue or slate gray in color. Their color will not become apparent until about one year of age. The condition of the eyelids is noted, with particular attention to the presence of edema or purulent drainage. Tears are rarely present until several weeks after birth. The infant is able to see but the vision is less than perfect. The pathways to the brain are not well developed at this time so there is no comprehension of what is being seen.

The ears should be inspected for position, size, and shape. The size and shape of the ears should match. The position may be checked by drawing an imaginary line from the outer canthi of the eyes. The ears should touch the line. Anomalies of the ears are associated with both kidney and chromosomal

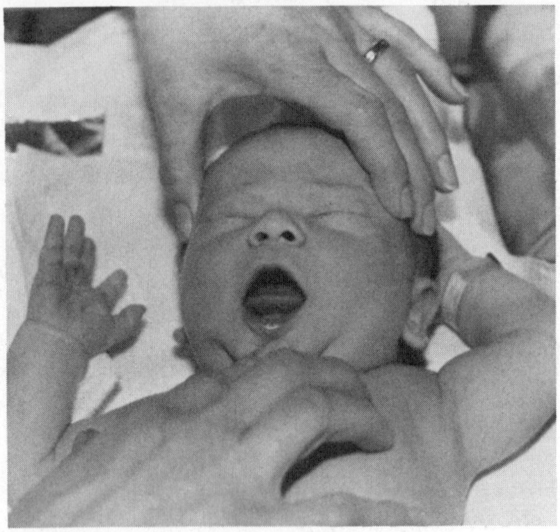

FIG. 4-3 Inspecting the inside of the newborn infant's mouth

abnormalities. The infant's hearing improves within several days as air replaces fluid in the eustachian tubes and the mucus in the middle ear is absorbed.

The mouth is also inspected, with careful evaluation of the lips, gums, and palate, Figure 4-3. Inside the mouth, along the dental ridge, there may be whitish, round areas which the mother may believe are teeth. In reality, these are small white cysts called Epstein's pearls. The cheeks of the infant are thickened with fat pads to aid in sucking.

Chest and Abdomen

The chest and abdomen are inspected next. The chest circumference is measured at a point just above the nipple line. It should be slightly smaller than the head circumference. The breasts may show engorgement from the maternal hormones. The breast fluid that is expressed is sometimes referred to as "witch's

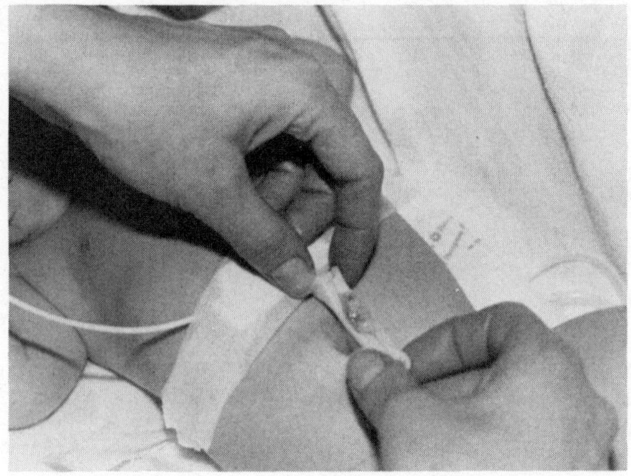

FIG. 4-4 Inspecting the umbilical cord stump. The nurse should also count the number of vessels present.

milk." The engorgement usually resolves spontaneously. The infant's abdomen is rounded and protuberant because of the weakness of the abdominal muscles. The umbilical cord stump should be inspected, Figure 4-4. Moreover, the number of vessels present, normally two arteries and one vein, should be recorded.

Genitalia and Back Region

The infant's genitalia should also be inspected and the presence of normal structures noted. In the female, a vaginal discharge, secondary to the maternal hormones, may be observed. This discharge, as well as any labial swelling, subsides spontaneously. In the male, the position of the urethral opening should be noted. The scrotum usually appears much larger in proportion to the other structures.

The back of the infant is inspected for masses or any other abnormalities. The area of the buttocks and the anal region is of greatest concern. The position of the anal opening is noted and its patency is determined, Figure 4-5. The presence of any dimples in

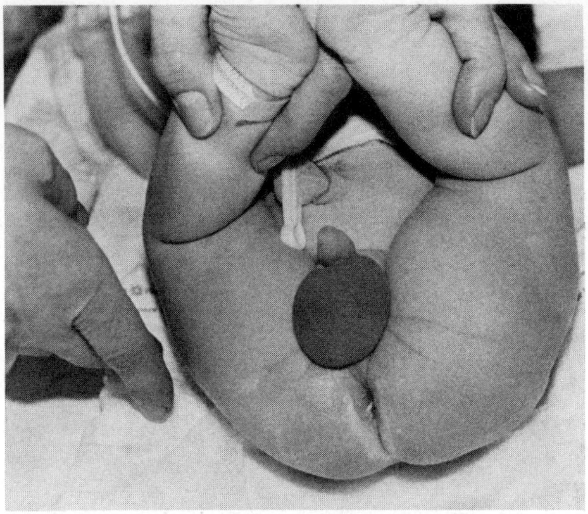

FIG. 4-5 Inspecting the external genitalia and the anus for congenital anomalies

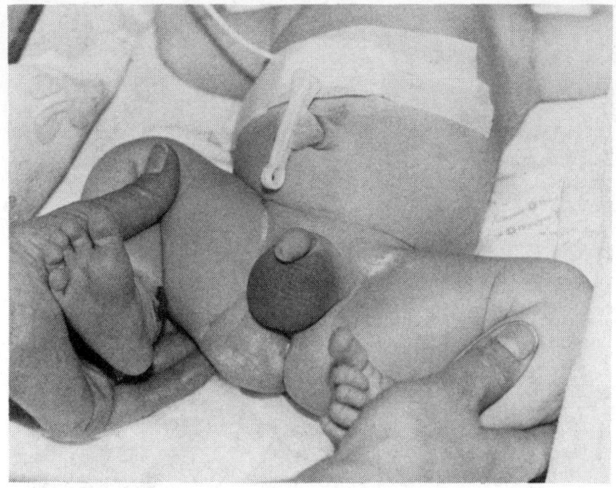

FIG. 4-6 To check for congenital dysplasia of the hip, both hips are abducted 90°. Note the vernix in the creases.

this area is also noted. Dimpling or hair tufts may indicate spina bifida occulta or a dermal sinus tract.

Extremities

The extremities are inspected and compared for size and movement. The hands and fingers, as well as the feet and toes, are inspected for extra digits or webbing. The hips are abducted to assess for possible congenital hip dysplasia, Figure 4-6. The position of the legs and feet are noted. Any bowing that is observed may be due to the infant's position in utero. The criteria for exclusion of an abnormality is whether the foot can be moved into a normal position.

Height and Weight

The infant's length and weight should be determined either at the beginning or at the end of the examination. The average weight range for newborn infants is 5 1/2 to 9 1/2 pounds. Length, which usually ranges from 18 to 22 inches, is also measured. The "textbook average" of height and weight for a normal neonate would be 20 inches and 7 1/2 pounds respectively.

Reflexes

The presence of normal reflexes should also be assessed. The normal infant has the following reflexes: rooting and sucking; tonic neck; grasp, Figure 4-7; Moro or startle, Figure 4-8; and stepping, Figure 4-9. The protective reflexes, such as sneezing, blinking, and yawning, should also be present.

Maintenance of a Normal Temperature

Protection of the infant from heat loss or cold stress is a major concern in the hospital delivery room and the nursery. An

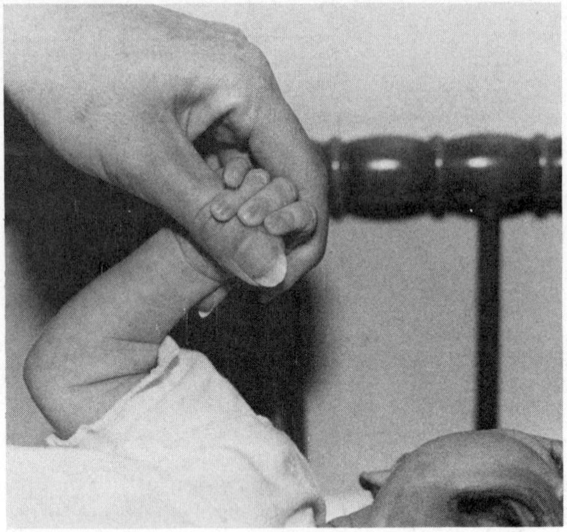

FIG. 4-7 A strong grasp reflex is typical of a full-term infant.

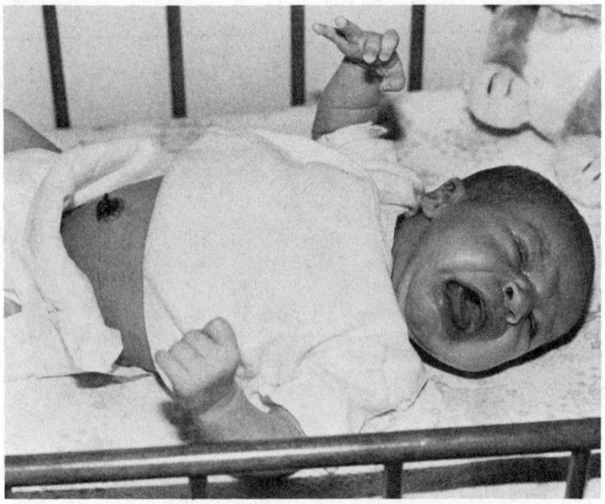

FIG. 4-8 The Moro reflex is exhibited in response to a loud sound. Note the embrace position of the arms and the C position of the right hand.

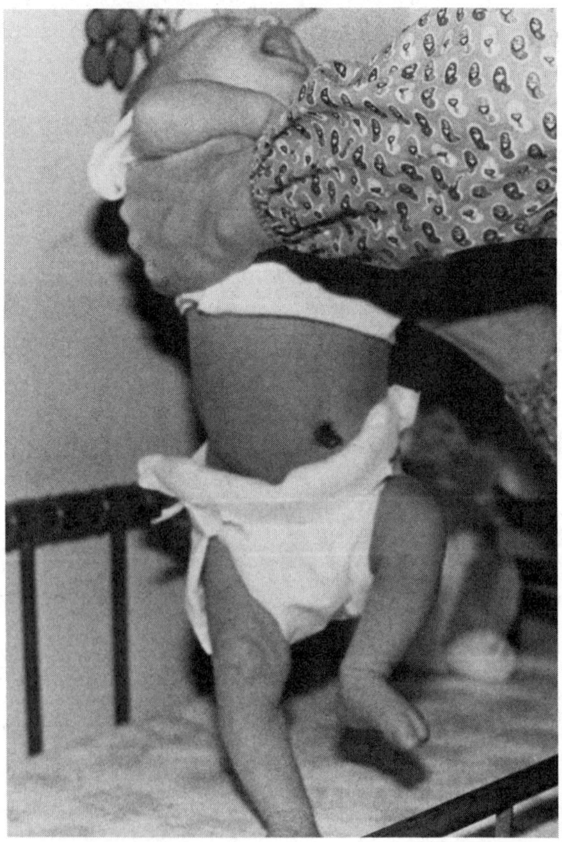

FIG. 4-9 A stepping reflex is elicited by holding the infant in a vertical position so that the feet touch a hard surface.

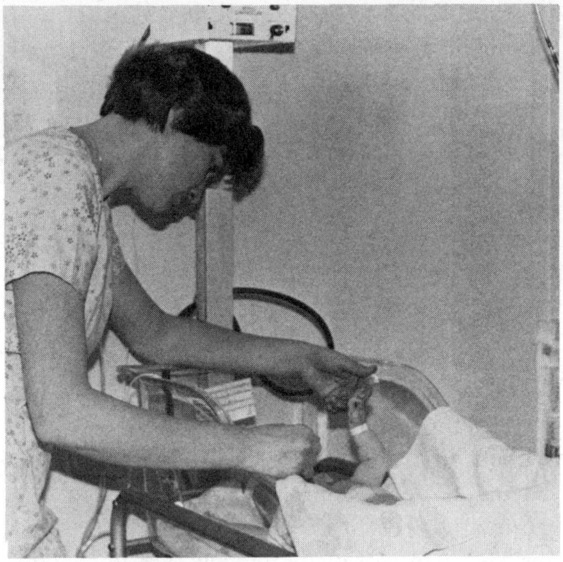

FIG. 4-10 Admission of a newborn infant to the nursery. A warming unit is used to maintain the infant's temperature.

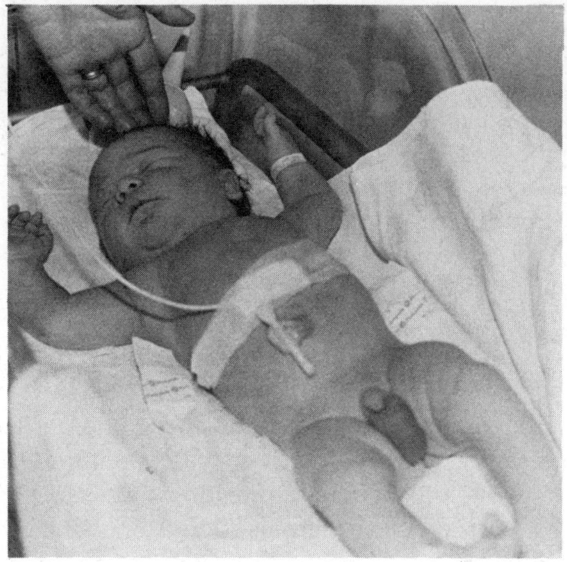

FIG. 4-11 Upon admission to the nursery, a sensor is taped to the neonate's abdomen to regulate the warming hood.

air-conditioned environment may feel comfortable to the adult, but it can cause severe heat loss in the infant through the evaporation of the amniotic fluid on the body surface. In the delivery area, the infant should be dried rapidly, covered with warmed blankets, and placed in a warm incubator or under a warming hood, Figures 4-10 and 4-11.

The problem of heat loss is particularly significant in the infant because of his or her large surface area in relation to body weight. The inability to increase voluntary muscle activity or shiver, as an adult would, is a definite disadvantage. The infant's temperature and vital signs should be stabilized prior to transfer to an open crib in the nursery. For the first twenty-four hours thereafter, the vital signs of the infant should be routinely monitored every two hours for the first eight hours, and then every four hours thereafter.

CARE IN THE NURSERY

Care of the infant in the nursery setting includes a careful initial assessment and an ongoing appraisal of the infant's transition to extrauterine life. Many infants are not taken to the nursery immediately after the delivery. Approximately an hour is spent in a transitional area adjacent to the delivery room. Here the parents and infant can spend a quiet time establishing a bond and getting to know each other. Because the infant is unclothed at this time, it is important to keep it close to the mother's body and wrapped in some way in order to maintain a normal temperature. Many mothers choose to breast-feed the infant at this time.

When the infant arrives in the nursery, protective drops of silver nitrate (two drops of a one-percent solution in each eye) are instilled into the infant's eyes to prevent ophthalmia neonatorum. The baby is then dressed warmly in a shirt and diaper, wrapped in a blanket, and placed in a warm crib. For the first twelve hours, Trendelenburg's position is maintained to allow mucus to drain from the infant's nose and throat.

Parent Teaching

During the period in the nursery or the rooming-in unit, the parents are made to feel comfortable caring for their infant in order to ease the transition to home care. Methods of feeding and bathing are demonstrated to the parents and their participation is encouraged. Whatever the level of preparation, however, having a baby is always a major change in life-style.

Bathing the Infant. When bathing the infant, the parents are instructed to assemble all the necessary items in a warm area that is free of drafts. The infant's face is washed first without using soap. Before the infant's soiled clothing is removed, the head or hair is washed. Each area of the infant's body is washed, rinsed well, and dried before going on to the next area. Careful attention should be given the creases and folds in the neck, the armpits, and the genitalia.

Holding the Infant. In teaching the parents, it is important to reinforce appropriate skills and positive nurturing and parenting behaviors. The baby should be well supported when picked up. The head and neck should be supported with one hand while the buttocks are supported with the other. Cradling the baby in the arms is generally most comfortable. However, when bathing the baby, the use of the football hold is preferred, Figure 4-12. Under no circumstances should the baby be left unattended on a changing table. If the parent has to turn to reach something, one hand should be kept on the baby at all times.

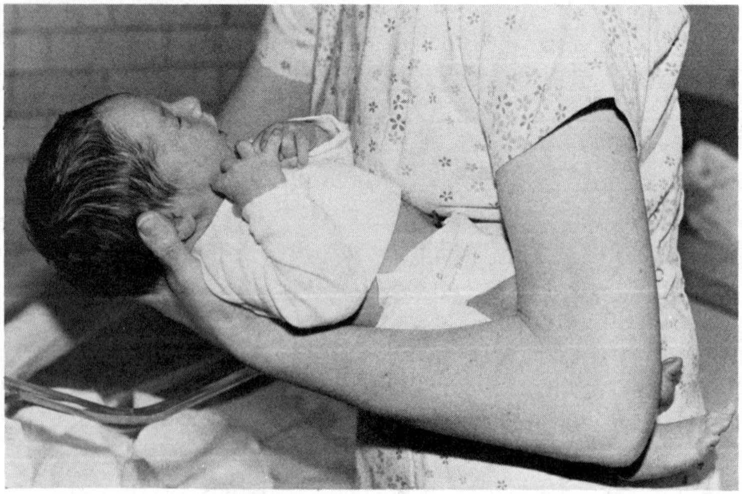

FIG. 4-12 The football hold provides support for the baby and a free hand for the nurse or parent.

If the parent has to leave the area, the baby should be wrapped in a blanket and taken with the parent, or returned to the crib for protection.

Care of the Umbilical Cord. Special care of the umbilical cord stump is provided until the cord falls off and the area is healed. The base of the cord is wiped daily with alcohol. Iodophur preparations or triple dye may be used for cord care. The site is exposed to air in the drying process. Care should be taken to keep diapers and shirts away from the cord until the stump sloughs, Figure 4-13. Umbilical dressings are not used as they allow moisture to remain in contact with the cord. The baby is not given a tub bath until the umbilical area is well healed. The cord clamps applied in the delivery room are usually removed after twenty-four hours, if the cord is sufficiently dry. The cord stump usually falls off between the eighth and the fourteenth day.

Continuing Assessment

Daily evaluation of the infant in the nursery setting should include a weight measurement, an assessment of activity and, an assessment of elimination of urine and meconium. Weight is recorded daily for each infant in the nursery. Infants lose up to fifteen percent of their body weight in the first few days after delivery. This is a result of excess fluid loss and minimal fluid intake during that period. Gradually, the infant begins to gain weight, with increases of 4 to 6 ounces per week for the first six months of life. After that period, the gain is roughly half that amount for the remainder of the first year.

A careful assessment of the elimination process is necessary. Usually, the infant voids shortly after the time of delivery or within the first twelve hours. The first voiding must be charted. If the infant does not void, this is reported, as it may indicate an imperforate meatus or dehydration in a low-birth-weight infant. Infants normally void up to fifteen times daily. The first meconium stool should also be charted. Meconium is a brownish green, tarlike material. The black, tarry stools gradually lighten to yellow as all the meconium is passed. The consistency of the stools is dependent on the method of feeding. Breast-fed babies have a bright yellow, mushy stool which may be eliminated every feeding. Bottle-fed babies have a pale yellow stool that is more solid than that of breast-fed infants.

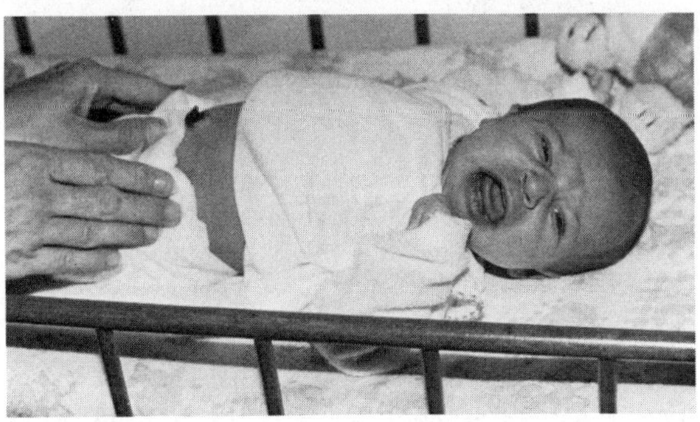

FIG. 4-13 This cord stump is very dry but has not yet sloughed. The diaper is positioned below it in order to prevent wetting of the area.

HOME CARE OF THE NEWBORN INFANT

Meeting the newborn infant's needs at home is often dependent on adequate prenatal preparation for the arrival of the baby. During the latter part of the pregnancy, it is important for the parents to obtain clothing and supplies for the baby and to prepare other siblings for the new arrival, Figure 4-14.

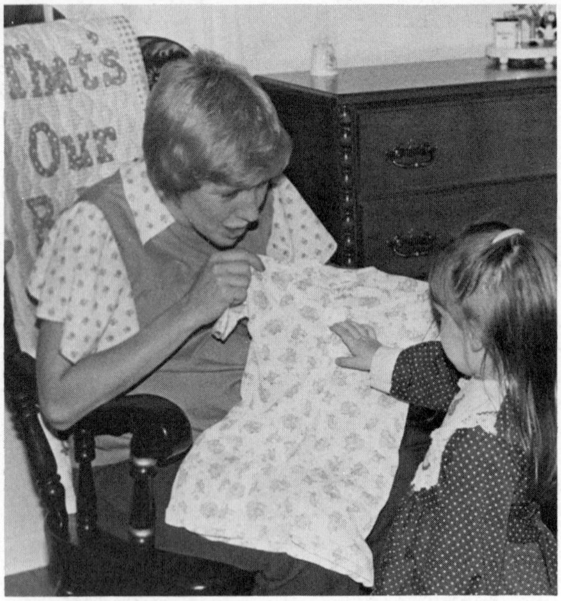

FIG. 4-14 Preparing older children for a new arrival may be facilitated by allowing them to get the baby's things ready.

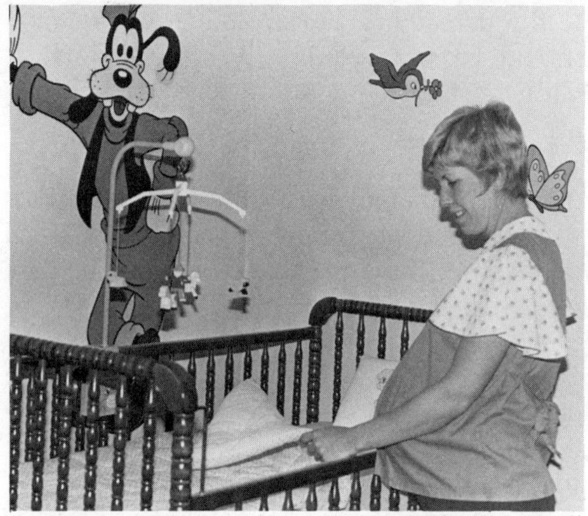

FIG. 4-15 Checking the crib for readiness. Note the close spacing of the spindles of the crib.

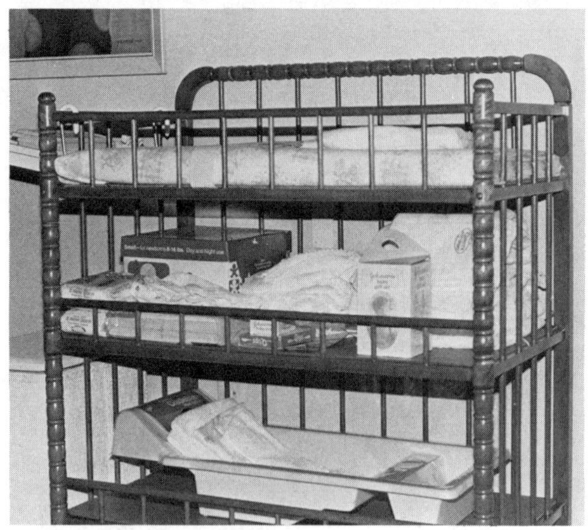

FIG. 4-16 A changing table is optional equipment, but is convenient for holding supplies. Note the accessibility of the hamper.

Equipment

Nursery equipment should be chosen for its durability, safety, and usefulness to the infant. Much of the acquired furniture will continue to be used as the infant grows. In an emergency, a buggy, laundry basket, or drawer may be used as a temporary bed for a newborn infant. However, this arrangement is impractical beyond the first few weeks. If a bassinet is used initially, the covering and liner should be easily washable. When a crib is selected, the bars should be close enough together so that the baby's head cannot be caught in them, Figure 4-15. Recent federal regulations dictate the minimum distance for new crib rails. Individuals borrowing older or used nursery equipment should be certain that it meets these standards. Moreover, the crib should be equipped with a firm mattress and a waterproof covering. Other equipment previously used for siblings and subsequently stored may also present hazards and should be thoroughly checked.

Other useful nursery items include a storage area for the baby's clothes, a diaper pail, and a baby bathtub. A changing table is convenient, but is not a necessity, Figure 4-16.

Selection of clothing for the infant depends on the wishes of the parents as well as on the climate of their locale. Layette items should be easy to launder. Articles of clothing should be easy to put on as well as large enough to accommodate an infant's rapid growth. Parents should be encouraged to purchase a minimal number of items initially and to supplement this supply after the baby is born.

Items that are generally included in the layette are six shirts, six nightgowns or stretch outfits, two or three large towels and washcloths reserved exclusively for the baby's use, four to six receiving blankets, and three to six dozen cloth or disposable diapers. The need for sweater sets, buntings and afghans, or blankets is determined by the climate. Other items which might be obtained include diaper pads, bibs, bath items, and a diaper bag.

Generally, by the time the infant is ready to leave the hospital with the parents, a bond is beginning to form between the parents and the child, Figure 4-17. In certain cases, families may need the privacy of their home to establish this bond. The establishment of this bond begins with the earliest exposure of parents to the infant at the time of the delivery and is an ongoing process. As the father assumes an increasingly important role in the birth process through his participation, he becomes increasingly attached to the infant. As the parents learn how to care for their infant adequately, they will start to recognize and respond to the individualized behavior of their infant.

Mothers demonstrate specific behaviors as the attachment process develops. They usually begin examining the infant on the extremities with their fingertips. Gradually, they move to the trunk, massaging with their entire hand. Affectionate ties are demonstrated by the mother and infant maintaining visual contact in the face-to-face position. Over a period of time a reciprocal interaction forms. Many parents need help in recognizing the patterns of attention and nonattention of the infant as normal behavior.

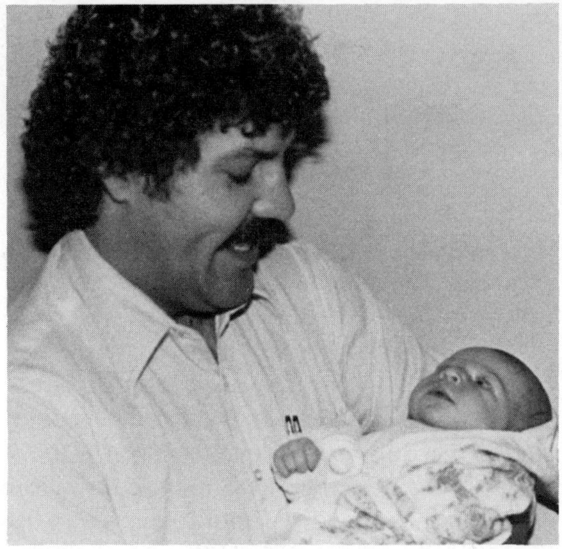

FIG. 4-17 This father's obvious pride and the baby's alert interest in the father's face exemplify the bonding process.

The specific behaviors identified in fathers are often referred to as engrossment. Some characteristics of engrossment include a visual identification of the beauty of the child, a desire to hold the infant, recognition of those features similar to the father's own features, feelings of elation and self-satisfaction, and strong feelings of attraction to the child.

The nurse needs to recognize these as normal behaviors and encourage them both in the delivery or recovery area and on the postpartum unit. Use of the child's name and encouragement of the parent's participation in all aspects of the infant's care enhances the process and aids in the development of parenting skills.

Feeding

Regardless of the feeding method chosen, a comfortable position, an adequate period of time (usually one-half hour), and a private place to allow optimal parent-child interaction are crucial to the success of feeding. During and after the feeding, the infant should be burped periodically. This may be accomplished with the parent in a seated position and the baby placed on the lap or over the shoulder, Figure 4-18. Gentle rubbing of the baby's back usually promotes burping. This is one method of reducing the incidence of regurgitation by the infant.

Bottle-Feeding. The mother who chooses to bottle-feed her infant needs as much direction as the mother who chooses to breast-feed. The choice is an individual one. The nurse should avoid any judgmental comments regarding what "ought to be done." The parents must be taught what to feed the baby, how much to feed, how to prepare the formula, and how to ensure a satisfying experience for themselves and the baby.

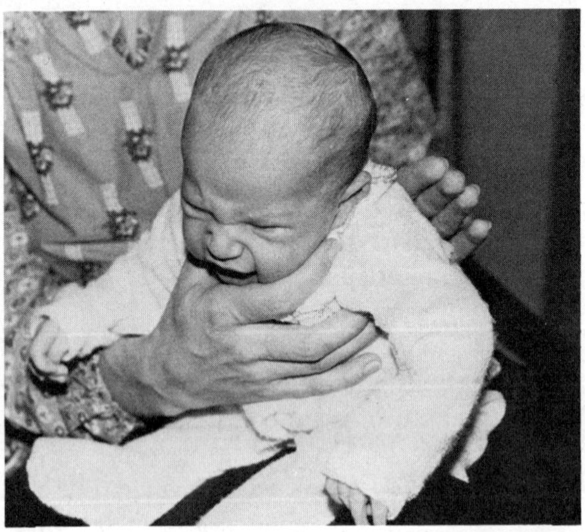

FIG. 4-18 While in a seated position, the baby may be burped effectively by gently rubbing the back.

The type of formula is designated by the pediatrician. The parents choose the preparation method. If a decision has not already been made regarding this matter, the nurse should explore with the parents the options available. Currently, prepackaged formula, cans of ready-to-feed formula, liquid concentrates, and powdered forms are available. The prepackaged and ready-to-feed preparations cost more, with minimal savings in time or ease of preparation.

Formula may be prepared according to the single-bottle method, the aseptic method, or the terminal method. With the single-bottle method, a bottle is washed with hot, soapy water and rinsed well. Sufficient formula powder or concentrated liquid is then mixed in the bottle with cooled, boiled tap water in the correct proportion. The formula is then used to feed the infant. The remainder in the bottle is discarded, and the equipment is rinsed in cold water until the next feeding.

With the aseptic method, all of the equipment, as well as the formula, is sterilized. It is then combined using an aseptic technique. This is the least preferred method of preparation because it is the most involved.

The terminal method involves preparing a twenty-four-hour supply of formula using a clean technique. Closed bottles of formula are placed on a rack in a pan of water to a depth of four inches. (A bottle sterilizer may also be used.) The water is brought to a boil and the formula is processed for twenty-five minutes. It is then cooled and refrigerated.

The methods may be adapted for use with disposable bottle liners. The nipples, rings, and covers are sterilized along with tongs in a dishwasher, or they may be submerged in boiling water for fifteen minutes. The sterile bottle liners should be touched only by the outside tabs. The formula is added and the nipples, rings, and covers are assembled using the tongs.

The amount and frequency of feedings vary with the infant's needs. Most infants are fed every three to four hours as they seem hungry. Initially, 3 ounces is the amount offered per feeding. At some feedings, the infant will consume the entire amount. At other feedings, the infant will lose interest after about 1 1/2 to 2 ounces. Once during a twenty-four-hour period, most infants sleep through a feeding time, allowing about five hours to elapse between feedings. Parents should be informed that these variations are normal. The nurse should help parents to recognize the signs of hunger displayed by the infant.

Breast-Feeding. The decision to breast-feed is also an individual one. Mothers who choose to do so frequently have made up their mind far in advance of the delivery situation. Many have been preparing themselves for breast-feeding by using techniques to toughen the nipples and by expressing some colostrum manually prior to delivery. Interest in breast-feeding has increased recently because of the environmental contaminants and additives, such as sodium, that are present in commercial formulas.

The breast-feeding mother should be supported in her decision by health care workers

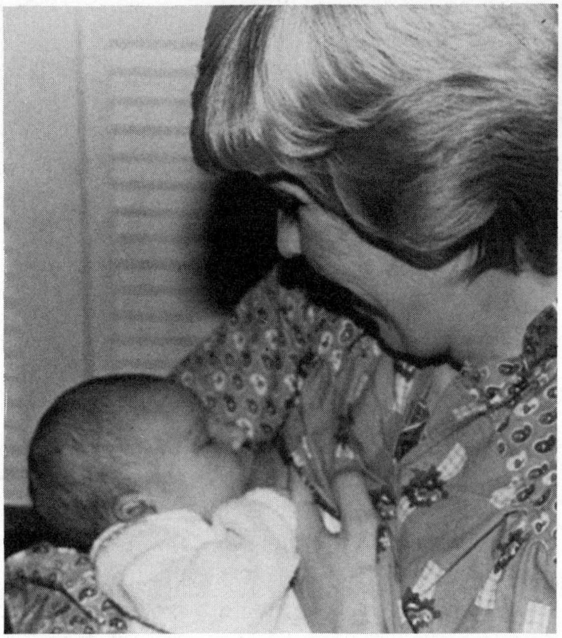

FIG. 4-19 Allowing an infant to eat on demand and assuming a comfortable position facilitate breast-feeding.

as well as by the family. Allowing the baby to eat on demand is very important. The alert, hungry baby is easier to get started on the nipple than one who is sleepy and exhausted from crying, Figure 4-19. The infant must take the entire nipple and the areola into its mouth when nursing. When the mother stops nursing to change breasts, she must break the suction on the nipple by inserting her little finger into the corner of the infant's mouth. Otherwise, the nipples will become cracked, painful, and easily irritated.

The initial sucking of the infant activates the let-down reflex in the mother. This reflex allows milk to flow from the alveoli of the breast into the ducts. After the mother has been breast-feeding for a period of time, she will probably notice that this occurs when she hears the baby cry. Emotional upsets and tension may prevent this reflex release of milk. Changing from a sitting to a reclining position may help in this situation as may reassuring the mother. Support and suggestions are also provided by LaLeche League groups.

Difficult-to-feed Babies. The baby who is difficult to feed presents problems whether the mother is breast-feeding or bottle-feeding. Breast-feeding in this situation may be most difficult, as it is relatively harder for the infant to get the free flow of milk that is desired. Because of this increased work effort, the infant may tire easily and simply stop feeding. If the problem of fatigue is recognized in the bottle-fed baby, a softer nipple or a larger nipple hole can be provided to facilitate the feeding.

Breast shields may be used by mothers with inverted or sore nipples. Other aids for successful feeding include encouraging and supporting the mother. Infants should be wide awake for their feedings. If they appear to be sleepy, changing their position or unwrapping the blankets may wake them. The rooting reflex should be stimulated by touching the infant's cheek with the nipple and encouraging the infant to turn toward it. Sucking may also be encouraged by placement of a small amount of glucose on the nipple. During this persistent effort to improve the baby's intake, the mother should receive the support and encouragement of the nurse.

Waking and Sleeping Behaviors

Initially, neonates awaken only to eat, and may sleep for as many as twenty-two hours per day. As the baby grows, periods of sleep will gradually shorten. During the first weeks at home, infants establish their own schedule of waking and sleeping hours. This may or may not conform to other family activities or schedules. New parents should be helped to distinguish fussy cries from hunger cries, and to provide for their baby's needs appropriately. Increasingly longer waking periods provide an opportunity for parents and child to interact with cuddling, gentle talk, and stroking. If the infant is not being held, he or she should be placed in view and in hearing distance of other family members.

Daily Care

Once the umbilical cord stump has sloughed, the infant may be given tub baths. Parents should be instructed how to give baths and how to protect the infant from a chill. Placing a slippery, wiggling baby in a baby tub may be too stressful for some mothers, and they may elect to use sponge baths for a period of time. Baths given on alternate days with cleansing of the face, hands, and perineum in the interim are also acceptable.

The perineal area under the diaper is continuously exposed to moisture, heat, and urine which breaks down into ammonia. These conditions may cause diaper rash. The rash begins as a slightly reddened area, gradually progressing to macules, papules, and finally, open, moist lesions. The parent should be aware of the condition at the onset and should expose the infant's buttocks to the air. The diapers should be changed as soon as they become wet or soiled. Once the diaper has been removed, the area should be cleansed carefully with water alone or with a bland soap and water, and rinsed carefully. The area is then dried and a clean diaper is applied.

Protective ointments may be used to prevent diaper rash. However, these must be used before the skin breaks down. Soothing ointments are available to help heal diaper rash. Powder should not be used on infants as it causes caking and may act as an irritant if inhaled. If cloth diapers are being used and laundered at home, the technique should be reviewed. A mild laundry soap should be used, and an additional rinse cycle completed. One cup of white vinegar may be added to the final rinse as a fabric softener and as a means of breaking up the ammonia radical that may accumulate in reusable diapers. Exposure to sunshine may also be used for this purpose.

PREMATURITY

A premature infant is defined as a neonate weighing 2500 grams (5 pounds 8 ounces) or less. The gestational age of premature infants may range from twenty-eight to thirty-seven weeks. Occasionally, the term premature is used to describe any infant delivered prior to thirty-seven weeks of gestation. In this case, infants weighing 2500 grams or less are designated as low-birth-weight infants. Regardless of the definition, premature infants have two things in common: high morbidity and high mortality.

Causes of prematurity include multiple births, toxemia, premature rupture of membranes, and antepartum hemorrhage. Moreover, diseases affecting the mother may cause prematurity in the infant. These predisposing conditions include heart disease, diabetes, and endocrine disorders. Socioeconomic and nutritional factors also play a role. For example, a young adolescent who is pregnant may be nutritionally deprived herself, and may therefore deliver a premature infant. Similarly, a woman from a poor socioeconomic background may not seek out adequate prenatal care, thereby increasing her chances of delivering a premature infant.

The goals of prenatal care are not only to identify and treat problems but also to prevent them from occurring. Every pregnant woman must receive good care in order to reduce the number of premature births. Women's health care clinics or maternity clinics are often in a position to provide additional assistance to young women. Nutritional assistance through the Women, Infants and Children (WIC) Program (a federal program providing direct supplements to this population) can often assist these young mothers.

Assessment Techniques

Estimation of Gestational Age. One of the methods used to evaluate gestational age was developed by Dubowitz and colleagues. They assigned scores for age, weight, and physical and neurologic characteristics in order to classify infants. Classifications included small for gestational age (SGA), appropriate for gestational age (AGA), and large for gestational age (LGA).

The assessment of physical findings should be completed within the first few hours after birth. Some of the external signs that are evaluated include the presence of edema; the texture, color, and opacity of the skin; the presence of lanugo; and the plantar creases. Nipple formation and the presence of breast tissue are also noted. The form and firmness of the cartilage of the ear are assessed. The genitalia also have distinctive characteristics.

After the first twenty-four hours of life, a confirmatory neuromuscular assessment is performed on the infants. This includes an evaluation of such factors as muscle tone by observing for the "scarf" sign (position of the elbow when the hand is drawn across the body to the other shoulder), head lag, and body extension. Flexion angles are also noted, particularly in the joints of the popliteal area, the ankle, and the wrist. Reflexes, such as Moro's, tonic neck, sucking, and rooting, are evaluated. This careful assessment permits individualized care to be given the infant with special problems. Infants who are not premature according to the weight classification alone may have had intrauterine growth problems. These infants are high-risk infants with the potential for developing multiple problems. Their special needs must be anticipated.

Infant Behavior. The Neonatal Behavioral Assessment Scale was developed by T. B. Brazelton. It identifies various developmental states as well as the interaction of the neonate with the environment. Considerable time and a trained administrator are required for appropriate testing. The items in the scale are divided into six areas: habituation, orientation, motor maturity, variation, self-quieting activities, and social behavior. The advantage of an assessment of this type is that it recognizes the individualized responses of infants. It can be used to teach parents how to respond most appropriately to their infant, as well as to recognize the infant's responses, Figure 4-20.

This assessment scale has been modified with supplemental scores for use with premature as well as full-term infants. The evaluator should share this information with the parents in order to help them work with the behavior of the infant.

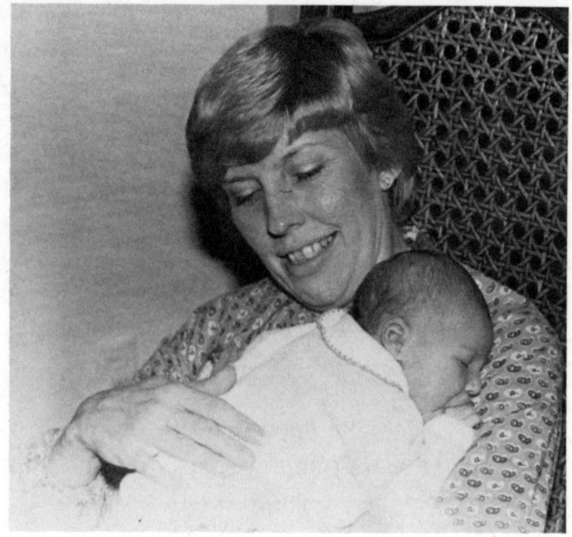

FIG. 4-20 In putting his fist in his mouth, this infant is exhibiting one of the self-satisfying behaviors described by Brazelton.

Physical Characteristics

Premature infants are often described as resembling little old men with wizened expressions, a large head, and thin, wrinkled skin, Figure 4-21. Large amounts of lanugo and minimal vernix are present. The infant's abdomen protrudes and the genitalia are small. The extremities are thin with little muscle mass, and no subcutaneous tissue is evident. The premature infant's cry is feeble and reflexes are depressed or absent.

MAJOR PROBLEMS OF THE PREMATURE INFANT

The major problems of the premature infant relate to temperature control; inadequate development of the respiratory, gastrointestinal, and hematopoietic systems; and susceptibility to infections. Each of these problem

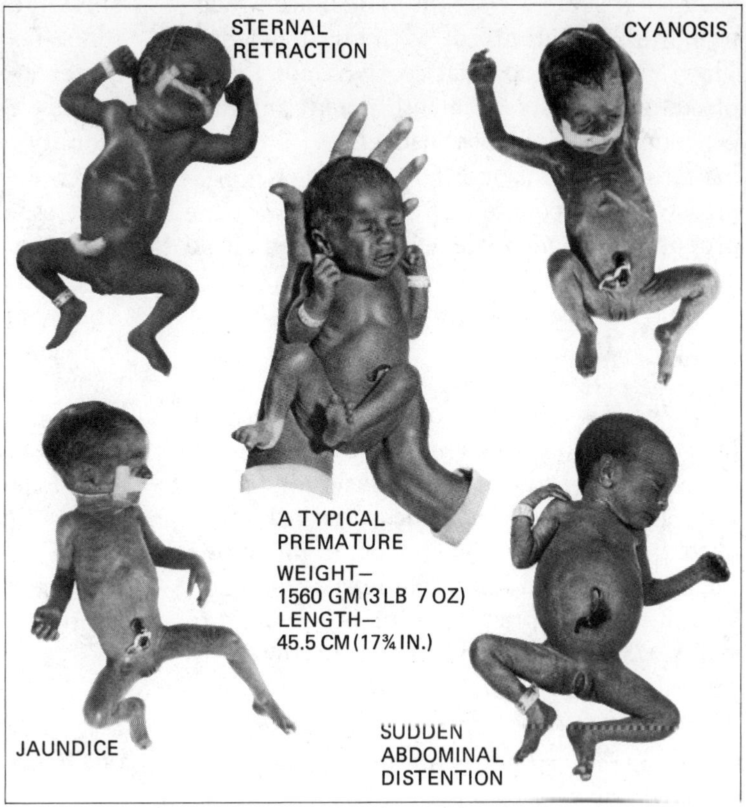

FIG. 4-21 The premature infant (Courtesy of Ross Laboratories)

areas represents a potential threat to the infant's survival.

Temperature Control

Poor temperature control is common in neonates, but represents a major hazard in premature infants. It stems from several sources. The premature infant lacks the subcutaneous fat that usually helps maintain a normal temperature. Moreover, the heat-regulating center in the brain stem is not functioning optimally because of the immaturity of the brain itself. The amount of body surface area in relation to weight is even greater in premature infants. Their lack of muscular activity, as well as their low metabolic rate, prevents these Infants from protecting themselves.

Immature Body Systems

The immaturity of the respiratory, gastrointestinal, and hematopoietic systems of premature infants causes major interrelated problems. The immaturity of the lungs and the weak muscle development of the thorax, as well as of the accessory muscles of respiration, increase the difficulty with which an adequate gas exchange may be achieved. Disorders of the gastrointestinal system include poor sucking and swallowing reflexes, resulting in feeding difficulties. Premature infants are unable to absorb fat-soluble vitamins and so are predisposed to symptoms of vitamin deficiency. They may develop a lack of vitamin D and bleeding disorders from insufficient amounts of vitamin K. Moreover, inadequate iron stores may lead to anemia, as slight blood losses coupled with inadequate iron supplies thwart the production of adequate numbers of red blood cells.

Immune Deficiency

The susceptibility of the premature infant to infection is a direct result of poor globulin synthesis and inadequate antibody formation. The immune substances that are transmitted from the mother to the infant during the last weeks of a full-term pregnancy are not available to the premature infant. Immature skin surfaces also provide a poor barrier to infection.

NURSING CARE OF THE PREMATURE INFANT

The majority of premature infants in the United States are cared for in regional premature centers. This practice has been found to improve their survival.

Maintenance of respirations and prevention of anoxia are the initial concerns upon the delivery of a premature infant. Gentle suctioning to remove mucus from the airway is necessary. Mechanical ventilation may have to be instituted if the infant is hypoxic. Transcutaneous monitoring of arterial pressure (PO_2) is an effective means of identifying hypoxia without subjecting the sick infant to repeated blood sampling with its attendant difficulties. Positioning is also important in premature infants. A supine position with the head slightly elevated provides the best gas exchange with the least amount of impedance from the abdominal contents. Oxygen should be monitored with an analyzer every four hours and should be maintained at 30 percent, Figure 4-22A. Apnea monitors are used routinely in these infants. Narcotic antagonists may be given to reduce the respiratory depression caused by drugs given the mother during labor or delivery.

Maintaining the infant's fluid and nutritional status is accomplished by tube feeding, as in Figure 4-22B, or by hyperalimentation. Initially, the infant receives nothing by mouth until he or she is stabilized. Then, an oral feeding tube may be inserted as the least stressful means of providing nutrients for the infant. Often, feeding tubes are positioned directly in the jejunum. However, problems of gastric reflux, intestinal perforation, and necrotizing enterocolitis may occur with this method. Some advocate the insertion of the feeding tube only as far as the duodenum. Good results and decreased risk have been achieved with this method. Once the infant's reflexes are well established, oral feedings of as little as two to three milliliters every two hours may be initiated. At this time, a formula containing thirteen calories per ounce and an iron supplement may be given.

Prevention of infection is a major concern of the nursing staff in any high-risk or premature nursery. These infants are incapable of protecting themselves from the organisms in the environment. Facilities for each infant should be kept separate. Careful handwashing by personnel is essential. Usually, the same staff member is assigned to a particular infant over a period of time in order to establish a routine, to provide interaction, and to reduce exposure to multiple organisms.

Gentle handling is also important in the care of premature infants. Nursing measures should be organized around feeding times to provide maximal periods of rest for the infant.

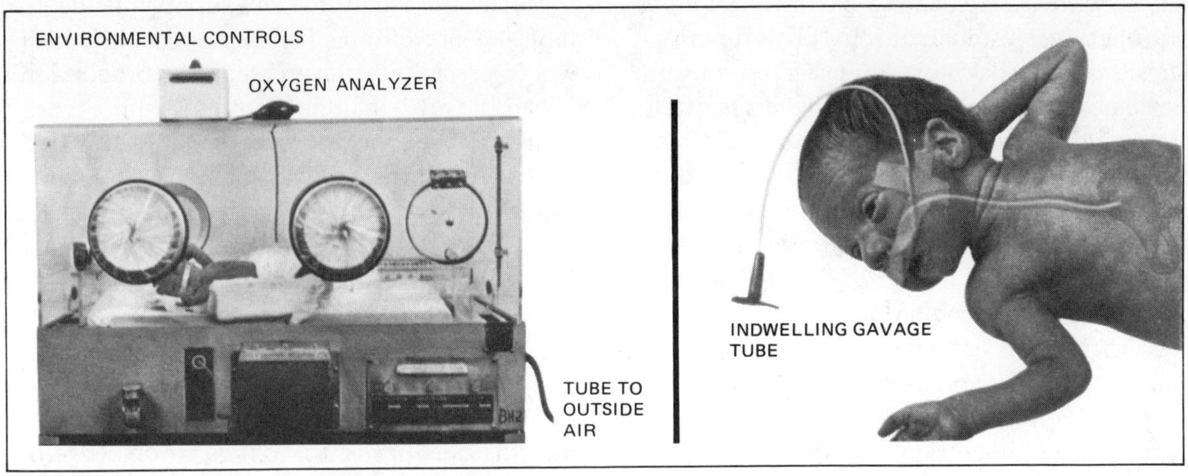

FIG. 4-22 Oxygen analyzer (A) and feeding tube (B) for the premature infant (Courtesy of Ross Laboratories)

Gentle handling also prevents skin breakdown and reduces the risk of infections.

Parental Involvement

It is important to involve parents in the care and nurturing of a premature infant as soon as possible so as not to disrupt the bonding process. This is quite easy to arrange when the mother and infant are hospitalized in the same area. It is far more difficult to accomplish when the infant is transported to a regional neonatal care center some distance away.

Parents should be encouraged to come in and see the infant and to participate in the infant's care in whatever ways possible. The nursing staff can facilitate the bonding process by pointing out the positive achievements of the infant as well as the individualized behavior noted. If the parents are unable to be present, they should be encouraged to send in a few items of clothing that can be placed on the infant or to tape their voices so that the tape can be played for the infant. Parents may need a lot of support and assistance to overcome the fear of getting attached to an infant that may not survive. They may also go through a grieving process for their less-than-perfect baby. A nurse's nonjudgmental attitude and positive support can be instrumental in helping the parents to accept this fact.

COMPLICATIONS OF PREMATURITY

Respiratory Distress Syndrome (RDS)

Respiratory distress syndrome, or hyaline membrane disease as it is also called, is a disease of pulmonary immaturity. The incomplete maturation of the lungs includes inadequate amounts of pulmonary surfactant, the lipid substance lining the alveoli.

Fluid fills the fetal alveoli until the first breath. The first breath causes a high, negative intrathoracic pressure causing the lungs to open and allow entrance of air. Expiration is only partial with the remaining portion becoming the functional residual capacity. This functional residual capacity allows for easier respirations in the normal infant which require less negative pressure than the first breath. The infant with respiratory distress does not retain that residual air because the high surface tension of the alveoli causes the aveoli to collapse with each expiration. Each breath is then taken with the same pressures as were required for the first one.

Tachypnea or increased respiratory rate of more than 60 respirations per minute is a major sign. Increasing difficulty is evidenced by nasal flaring, thoracic retractions, expiratory grunting, and cyanosis. Apneic episodes may occur, lasting for twenty seconds or more and associated with cyanosis and bradycardia. Increasing exhaustion identifies the infant's inability to compensate for the respiratory difficulty.

Any physiologic problem in the infant that decreases the amount of surfactant may cause respiratory distress. The most common problem is prematurity but respiratory distress can also occur with hypothermia, acidosis, hypovolemia, and high concentrations of oxygen. The process begins with the unstable alveoli from a lack of surfactant. This instability leads to alveolar collapse and the formation of areas of atelectasis. The atelectasis causes hypoxia. Arterial-venous shunting then occurs which causes acidosis. The acidosis compounds the problem by causing an increase in vasoconstriction and a decrease in the production of surfactant. This process increases the areas of atelectasis. Both the hypoxia and the high pressures within the chest promote the movement of fluid containing fibrin and damaged cells into the alveoli. The alveolar ducts are then lined with a membrane, hence the original name of the disease, hyaline membrane disease.

The treatment involves support of the infant and preventon of those conditions which would precipitate a decrease in the production of surfactant. Included in this infant's treatment is oxygen therapy with or without assisted ventilation; intravenous therapy to meet nutriitional needs and correct metabolic deficits; and prevention of complications such as infection and necrotizing enterocolitis.

Nursing Care

The primary care of this infant involves meeting the needs for oxygenation. Careful removal of mucus from the mouth is necessary. This can be done with a small rubber bulb syringe periodically and is less traumatic to the infant. The infant is placed in the supine position with head and chest slightly higher than the abdomen to allow for good chest expansion. Turning can be done from side to side but the prone position is avoided.

An infant with severe respiratory distress will require either assisted or controlled ventilation. Constant-positive-airway pressure (CPAP) and positive-end-expiratory pressure (PEEP) are two means of increasing the functional residual capacity in the infant's lungs, improving the oxygenation, and decreasing the arterial-venous shunting of blood. Either of the methods can be delivered through the use of nasal prongs, a nasotracheal or endotracheal tube, and a face mask. PEEP most nearly simulates the grunting mechanism by which infants initially maintain their own oxygenation. The disadvantage of this method is the decrease in cardiac output that can occur.

The infant needing a high concentration without assisted ventilation is usually placed in an oxygen hood. The Isolette provides oxygen concentrations up to 40 percent, however, the hood can administer up to 97 percent oxygen, if necessary. The determination of the oxygen concentration needed should be based on continuous accurate monitoring of arterial blood gases. Assessment for color or cyanosis is not an accurate indicator of true oxygen levels. The thickness of the skin, the hemoglobin and bilirubin levels, and the number of capillaries influence the degree of cyanosis evident. Monitoring of blood gases can be done through an umbilical arterial line or through the use of a transcutaneous monitor which is noninvasive and can give a truer reflection of subtle change as it is done continuously. The oxygen concentrations in both the head hood and the Isolette should be monitored and recorded on an hourly basis with the use of an oxygen analyzer. Prolonged high oxygen concentrations may lead to retrolental fibroplasia in the infant.

During this time the nurse is responsible for continuous assessment of the infant's status. Observations are made regarding the color of the skin and buccal mucosa, the apical rate, spontaneous activity, reflex responses, temperature, and urinary output. Respiratory observations include the presence or absence of nasal flaring, retractions, and grunting. Documentation is made regarding the synchronization of the respiratory effort as well as the presence of periodic breathing or any apneic episodes.

Acidosis in this infant can be precipitated by cold stress. The combination of the infant's large surface area, minimal subcutaneous fat, and poor temperature regulation increases the risk of cold stress. The temperature can be maintained in an Isolette, however the nurse needs to be aware of increases or losses occurring as a result of frequent entrances into the portholes, the position near the room's heating or cooling vents, and other factors which prevent this from being a constant temperature. Computerized thermal regulation is used in some units. The infant in an oxygen hood is usually placed under the radiant warmer with the probe placed on the abdomen covered by a heat reflective material, such as foil, to enhance accuracy of the temperature control. The nurse must monitor the temperature every thirty minutes initially and then every hour and assess the infant for excess drying of the skin and overheating. Avoid use of oils because of potential burns to the skin.

Daily care routines are also monitored to prevent undue loss of heat. After cleansing, the infant's skin should always be dried thoroughly. A soft diaper or blanket is always placed between the infant and the scale or the x-ray plate. Isolettes and radiant warmers are always prewarmed before use. Stockinette caps may be used to prevent heat loss.

Intravenous infusions of a 10 percent dextrose solution are used to combat hypoglycemia in this infant. These may be administered by way of an umbilical intra-arterial line. An infusion pump is always used with this method. Because of the risk of hypertension from the catheter placement, this infant should have routine assessment of blood pressure using an ultrasound device. A solution of sodium bicarbonate may be administered through this line to correct acidosis.

Hyperalimentation can be used to feed an infant who has severe difficulty or prolonged problems. Other infants may be fed with a gavage tube to conserve energy and provide adequate nutrition. The nurse must be familiar with both of these methods as a part of the care of this infant.

Respiratory distress syndrome occurs within the first or second day of the infant's life. Because of the critical nature of the care, the parents may have inadequate time for bonding. It is important that the nurse assists the parents in knowing about the infant and encourages their involvement in care, even if it is limited to touching and talking rather than holding the infant.

Necrotizing Enterocolitis

This condition is a life-threatening problem in the premature infant, caused by necrosis of the intestinal mucosa. These infants usually weigh less than two kilograms and have suffered a degree of hypoxia in the perinatal period. Even a brief period of hypoxia causes shunting of blood from the intestines to the vital organs. This results in ischemia, invasion of gram-negative bacteria such as Escherichia coli, Salmonella or Klebsiella, proliferation of bacteria, and damage to the intestinal wall including perforation.

Predisposing prenatal factors include toxemia, maternal sepsis and fever, placental problems such as abruptio or premature separation, and prolonged rupture of membranes. Postnatal factors include prematurity or low birth weight, an Apgar score below 6, exchange transfusions and umbilical catheterization, congenital anomalies such as patent ductus arteriosus, congenital heart disease, hyaline membrane disease, hypoglycemia, and hypothermia. The high-solute feedings and overfeeding in the premature infant provide an ideal media for the bacterial growth.

Necrotizing enterocolitis can occur at any time within the first two weeks of life. It often occurs between the fourth and seventh days at a time when the infant appears to be tolerating the feedings. The first signs are related to a delay in gastric emptying. The residual which is checked prior to each tube feeding begins to increase. On closer inspection the infant usually shows a slight degree of abdominal distention. Occult blood is usually present in the stools. Other signs include vomiting, bile-stained emesis, poor feeding, and diarrhea. Urinary output decreases and specific gravity increases. Jaundice, apnea, and temperature instability may also be present.

The diagnosis of NEC is based on the x-ray findings of the disease. The bowel appears distended and thickened. Bubbles appear in the bowel wall (intramural gas or pneumatosis intestinalis), and free air will be present in the abdomen, if a perforation has occurred. Other diagnostic work includes blood work such as electrolytes, glucose, and bilirubin levels. Blood and stool cultures are also done to determine the specific bacteria present.

Treatment involves gastric decompression with a nasogastric tube, hyperalimentation to meet nutritional needs, and antibiotic therapy to treat the infection. If this treatment is not effective, a resection of the necrotic portion of the bowel is done. The amount of bowel resected may have lifelong implications in the form of malabsorption syndrome, bowel strictures, and Vitamin B_{12} deficiency.

Nursing care includes use of an incubator to provide warmth and oxygen, maintaining nutrition with hyperalimentation or intralipids, and continuing gastric decompression. Careful monitoring of vital signs and of the gastrointestinal changes is necessary.

Measurement of the abdomen for increasing girth is a routine part of this child's care. At this time, the abdomen is also gently palpated for hardness and auscultated with a stethoscope for bowel sounds. The surface is inspected for erythema or shininess which would indicate peritonitis. Any form of pressure on the abdomen is avoided. This would include diapers as well as positioning the infant on the abdomen. Rectal temperatures are avoided because of the danger of perforation.

Some nurseries may isolate this infant. Others may simply separate the infant and avoid any type of cross contamination of equipment used. Because iodophor preparations are effective against gram-negative organisms, they are usually preferred for the careful handwashing when caring for this child.

CONGENITAL ANOMALIES

The congenital anomalies that appear in the newborn period include those that are incompatible with life unless emergency treatment is rendered. These include such conditions as esophageal atresia, intestinal atresia, imperforate anus, and choanal atresia. In these situations, the nursery staff should identify the problem and notify the physician. Once the diagnostic work is completed, these infants are usually scheduled for surgical correction of the problem.

The parents' joy in the birth of their infant is suddenly tempered with the fear that this infant may not survive. Indeed, the anomaly may not even be apparent to them. Parental responses to this situation are often in stages from denial to anger and, eventually, to acceptance of the information provided by the physician. Parents usually need some time to talk openly about their fears for their infant. An objective "outsider" with some knowledge of the problem can listen to their thoughts and feelings and can clarify information. Nurses and parent groups are extremely effective in providing this emotional support.

Prior to the corrective surgery, the parents should be allowed to spend a few minutes with the infant, if possible. At that time, the nurse can tell the parents what they should expect to see when the infant returns to the intensive care nursery. This gradual sharing of information facilitates the adjustment of the parents to the situation.

Upon completion of the corrective surgery, the parents should have the opportunity to meet with the surgeon and to ask questions regarding the infant. Designating one person in the nursery to serve as a contact for the parents to answer their questions ensures continuity and clarity of the information that is shared.

SPECIFIC ANOMALIES

The specific anomalies discussed here are those which are identified in the delivery room or nursery setting. Most require early intervention for the health of the newborn. Anomalies such as cleft lip and palate, congenital heart disease and orthopedic anomalies are not incompatible with life and so are discussed in later chapters.

Esophageal Atresias and Tracheoesophageal Fistulas

Esophageal atresia occurs in embryonic life when the primitive trachea must separate from the esophagus. This defect in differentiation of tissues occurs in one infant out of 3000 to 4500 live births. Approximately 75 percent of these children have an associated tracheoesophageal fistula which usually occurs at the level of the bifurcation of the trachea.

There are five identified types of this anomaly, Table 4-1. This anomaly occurs more often in premature infants and in those mothers having a history of polyhydramnios. Signs of the problem include an inability to pass a resuscitating catheter in the delivery room, excessive drooling of mucus secretions from the mouth and pharynx, inability to

TABLE 4-1 Classification of Esophageal Atresia

Type	Description	Incidence
I	Proximal and distal segments of esophagus end in blind pouches. No connecting fistula.	8%
II	Proximal segment of esophagus connected to trachea by fistula. Distal segment of esophagus is a blind pouch.	1% or less
III	Proximal segment of esophagus ends in a blind pouch. Distal segment of esophagus connected to trachea by way of fistula.	87%
IV	Proximal and distal segments of esophagus each connect to trachea with a separate fistula.	1% or less
V	No esophageal atresia. Fistula connects esophagus and trachea. H-type anomaly. Usually diagnosed later in infancy or even toddler period.	4%

feed without coughing, choking, and cyanotic episodes. Aspiration pneumonitis can occur in these infants in several ways. Formula in the proximal esophagus or mucous secretions may spill over into the airway and be aspirated. A greater risk is the aspiration of gastric contents through a distal fistula. Abdominal distention of varying degrees can occur as air moves from the respiratory tract through the fistula and into the distal esophagus.

When the nurse suspects this diagnosis, oral feedings should be stopped and the physician notified immediately. The diagnosis is confirmed by the inability to pass a catheter into the stomach. Radiographs demonstrate the catheter coiled in the proximal esophageal pouch. Air in the abdomen can also be visualized and indicates the presence of a fistula connecting to the distal portion. Any contrast media used should be water soluble and withdrawn after the pictures are taken.

Preoperatively, the infant is kept in a prone position to minimize aspiration of gastric contents. Continuous low suction is used on the upper esophagus. Vital signs and the respiratory tract are carefully monitored. The corrective surgery may be done in stages. The initial surgery includes ligation of the fistula and the insertion of a gastrostomy feeding tube. The anastamosis of the two parts may be done much later. Long-term problems include stricture formation requiring dilatation, gastric reflux with aspiration, and esophagitis.

Nursing care preoperatively involves identification of the infant's problem, with particular attention to the infant's response to the first oral feedings and identification of the excessive drooling and mucous secretions. Positioning of the infant with the head elevated thirty degrees is a necessity. Maintaining and monitoring intravenous fluids as ordered and carrying out preoperative routines are also nursing responsibilities.

Postoperatively, the infant with a gastrostomy feeding tube in place may receive small amounts of clear fluids every two hours.

These feedings will continue until the esophagus is well-healed. Formula will be substituted for clear liquids as the infant's tolerance improves.

The nurse must be aware of the type of surgery performed on the infant to administer adequate care. Infants having a thoracic approach to the surgical site will return to the unit with a closed chest drainage system in operation. It is the responsibility of the nurse to monitor the system and to accurately record the amount and type of drainage.

Maintenance of temperature control and provision for oxygenation is usually through the use of an Isolette for a baby who is this small. It provides for constancy of the environment, ease of care, and observation.

Abdominal Wall Defects

Visible defects in the abdominal wall include an omphalocele and gastroschisis. The omphalocele involves the layers of the peritoneum, muscle, and ectoderm. There is a transparent membrane that covers the bowel and the solid viscera. It may be very small in size or so large that all viscera in the abdomen are involved. Gastroschisis involves a defect at the base of the umbilical stalk with a normal abdominal wall. The viscera may protrude through this defect and float freely in the amniotic fluid prior to delivery.

Immediately after delivery continuous, moist, sterile saline compresses should be initiated and maintained on this child until surgery is done. The viscera may be only partially replaced or the skin may be sewn over the abdominal contents. Immediate return of a large amount of viscera to the abdomen may cause problems of respiratory distress in the infant.

Intestinal Atresia

The intestinal tract itself may be the site of various anomalies. An atresia or a failure of a lumen to develop can occur at any point in the intestinal tract. There are three variations of atresias that are seen in infants. In some, the intestinal lumen is blocked by a thin membrane; in others, the intestinal tract ends in blind pouches with no connection to the distal portion; and some are connected by stenotic or cordlike bands.

The characteristic symptoms in the infant include absence of meconium stools, vomiting including the presence of bile, and abdominal distention. The higher in the gastrointestinal tract the lesion occurs, the earlier the symptoms will be recognized. The nurse must be responsible for recognizing the symptoms and reporting them promptly.

After the X rays confirm the diagnosis, surgery is indicated. The extent of the surgery and possible subsequent surgeries are dependent on the degree of the anomaly present.

Imperforate Anus

Normally, the gastrointestinal tract is a continuous tube from mouth to anus. During the latter part of embryonic life the membrane separating the rectum from the anus is absorbed to provide this continuity. In some infants the membrane may remain intact and the infant is born with a defect that is incompatible with life. The specific signs identifying the problem include the absence of an anal opening on visual inspection, the inability to insert a rectal thermometer, the absence of meconium stools, and abdominal distention. In some infants flecks of meconium may appear in the urine or be noted near the urethra or vaginal orifice. This is the result of a fistula extending from the gastrointestinal tract to any of the adjacent structures in the pelvis.

The diagnosis is based on the identified signs and radiographic documentation of the problem. The infant is supported in a knee-chest position to allow air to extend as far as possible in the intestinal tract. An opaque object is held at the site of the anal dimple allowing the distance between the two sites to be measured accurately.

If only a thin membrane exists, the physician may perforate it and correct the problem. If a large distance is found, however, a colostomy is performed. An abdominal-perineal procedure may be done at a later time.

Nursing responsibilities include careful assessment and recognition of the group of symptoms which indicate a need for immediate notification of the physician. Postoperative care is dependent on the procedure of choice. After the perforation of the membrane the perineal area is kept uncovered and is cleansed gently after each stool. Nothing is inserted into the rectum (including thermometers) to avoid perforation and potential infection. Colostomy care requires special attention to skin care. Ointments containing zinc oxide paste or karaya powder can be used around the stoma. Infant- and pediatric-size appliances are available but must be fitted correctly to the ostomy. Parents must be well prepared to care for the child and the colostomy prior to the child's discharge from the hospital. At a later date the infant is usually returned for correction of the anomaly and closure of the colostomy.

Urethral Misalignments

Both hypospadius and epispadius involve deviations from the normal position of the urethra in the male. Hypospadius is a condition in which the urethral opening is located behind the glans penis or anywhere along the shaft. It may also be located on the perineum. Chordee, or ventral bowing, may also occur caused by a fibrous band of tissue causing constriction of the penis.

Epispadius involves the urethral opening on the dorsal surface of the penis. Its most severe form is associated with exstrophy of the bladder.

The surgical correction is not an emergency. The goals of treatment are to allow the child to void in the normal standing position, to achieve as normal an appearance as possible, and to ultimately achieve normal sexual functioning.

Surgical correction is usually done at about age two. It may be done in several stages as well. This child should not be circumcised while in infancy as some of this tissue may be needed when the urethroplasty is done.

Nursing responsibilities involve recognition and reporting of the anomaly, assisting parents with questions and care of the infant, and recognition of potential problems with the delay of the corrective surgery until the late toddler or early preschool period. Fears of separation and mutilation make this a difficult time for the child to cope with surgery on the genitalia.

Exstrophy of the Bladder

This condition results from a failure of the abdominal wall and the ventral wall of the bladder to fuse during embryonic life. The entire lower urinary tract is exposed and the anomaly is easily identified upon visual inspection. It is three times as common in males as in females and is usually associated with epispadius, undescended testes, and inguinal hernia. Separation of the pubic bones which later causes a waddling gait is also associated with this defect. In the female, the clitoris, labia, and vagina may have anomalies.

The two major problems related to care in the infant are the skin breakdown from the continuous seepage of urine and the potential for ascending urinary tract infection. The degree of the anomaly as well as involvement of other structures will dictate the correction. In some children there is sufficient abdominal wall to close both the bladder and the abdomen with few problems. In others, the procedure of choice is ileal diversion.

One nursing responsibility is to aid the parents in the acceptance of this very visible defect. Collection of urine specimens usually includes holding the infant over a sterile container and allowing the urine to drip into the basin. The skin adjacent to the defect is protected with ointments containing zinc oxide paste. The area may be covered with gauze impregnated with petroleum jelly and then covered with plastic. A diaper is then covered over the whole area.

Stabilization of the pelvis may be done at the time of the corrective surgery on the bladder. More than one surgery may be necessary for the correction.

SUMMARY

The care of the neonate is a challenge to the nurse from the time of the infant's delivery to his or her discharge from the hospital. Accurate and ongoing assessment of the infant, parent teaching and support, resuscitation techniques, and an awareness of such potential problems as heat loss and congenital anomalies are essential for optimal nursing care of the neonate.

Premature neonates have special problems that require skilled nursing care in the intensive care nursery or high-risk nursery. It is especially important for the parents of these infants to gradually assume responsibility for the infant's care and well-being prior to the baby's discharge from the hospital. Nurses play an instrumental role in this process.

SUGGESTED ACTIVITIES

- Develop a teaching program on methods of feeding or infant care using audiovisual materials. Present your program to new parents and evaluate their responses.
- After obtaining permission, visit your nearest neonatal regional care center. Share your experiences and observations with your class.
- Arrange to visit the home of a new mother upon discharge of her infant from the hospital. Observe her home care practices. Reinforce proper methods of care and be prepared to lend support and encouragement. Share your experiences with the class.
- Identify legislation that governs the safety and quality of newborn equipment, such as cribs, clothing, and auto restraint devices. Write a letter to your legislator to express either your approval and support of the legislation or your dissatisfaction with any deficiencies that you find in it.

DISCUSSION TOPICS

1. Research the life of Dr. Virginia Apgar and write a report on her method of neonatal appraisal.
2. Research the bonding process that occurs between parents and infants. Discuss with your class the various nursing practices that can facilitate this process.

3. Trace the development of the LaLeche League and discuss their goals and principles.
4. Research the signs, treatment, and complications of three congenital anomalies. Present your findings to the class.

REVIEW

A. Matching. Match the characteristic in Column I with the term in Column II.

Column I	Column II
1. Weight of 7 1/2 pounds	a. Premature infant
2. Reddened, wrinkled appearance	b. Full-term infant
3. Length of 21 inches	
4. Weight of less than 2500 grams	
5. Pink color with lusty cry	
6. Position of flexion	
7. Limp with little motor activity	

B. Multiple choice. Select the best answer.

1. Judy Grey weighs 7 pounds, 6 ounces at birth. At her four-week check-up, Judy weighs 8 pounds, 14 ounces. Since she should gain about 4 to 6 ounces per week for the first six months, you determine that Judy is
   a. not gaining enough weight.
   b. gaining weight normally.
   c. gaining more weight than expected.
2. Mrs. Grey tells you that her baby sometimes takes half a bottle of milk and then stops. She asks whether it is all right to save that bottle for the next feeding. Your *best* reply is
   a. "It is usually best to discard any leftover milk."
   b. "Be sure to put it in the refrigerator."
   c. "Milk will keep for four hours before it needs to be discarded."
   d. "Be sure to reheat it before you give it to the baby the second time."
3. You know that the Brazelton Neonatal Assessment Scale was used to evaluate Judy. This test is done to
   a. check the infant's gestational age.
   b. determine whether the infant is premature.
   c. assess the infant's behavior and interaction with the environment.
   d. assess the infant's neuromuscular function.
4. The problem that occurs most commonly in premature infants is
   a. slow weight gain.
   b. an allergic response to formula.
   c. a resistance to infection.
   d. an immaturity of organ systems.

C. Short answer. Briefly respond to the following statements.

1. List three reflexes that are present in the normal newborn infant.
2. List three methods of formula preparation.

BIBLIOGRAPHY

Bake, Melissa K. "When the Down's Syndrome Baby is Yours." *RN*, Vol. 40 (July, 1977), pp. 67–69.

Brazelton, T. Berry. "Reaching Out to New Parents." *Children Today,* Vol. 7 (July–August, 1978), p. 27.

Capobianco, Julia A. "How to Safeguard the Infant Against Life-Threatening Heat Loss." *Nursing 80,* Vol. 10 (May, 1980), pp. 64–67.

Dingle, Rebecca E., et al. "Continuous Transcutaneous Monitoring in the Neonate." *American Journal of Nursing,* Vol. 80 (May, 1980), pp. 890–893.

Dunn, Janice, et al. "Preemie Care: Stretch the Rules in the Family's Favor." *Nursing 77,* Vol. 7 (December, 1977), pp. 50–53.

Fuller, Randi, and Martha Petering. "A Letter from Tommy." *Nursing 79,* Vol. 9 (November, 1979), pp. 54–56.

Garvey, Judith. "Infant Respiratory Distress Syndrome." *American Journal of Nursing,* Vol. 75 (April, 1975), pp. 614–617.

Gennaro, Susan. "Necrotizing Enterocolitis: Detecting It and Treating It." *Nursing 80,* Vol. 10 (January, 1980), pp. 52–55.

Gunn, Suzanne. "The Bottle-feeding Mother Needs Your Help Too." *RN,* Vol. 42 (February, 1979), p. 53.

Harris, Chandie. "Helping the Breast-Feeding Mother Whose Baby Refuses to Suckle." *Nursing 79,* Vol. 9 (May, 1979), pp. 96–97.

Hersh, Stephen P., and Karen Levin. "How Love Begins Between Parent and Child." *Children Today,* Vol. 7 (March–April, 1978), pp. 2–6+.

Kasper, Mary Ann, and Barbara Jane Clancy. "Breast-Feeding and Drugs: Nursing Implications." *Issues in Comprehensive Pediatric Nursing,* Vol. 3 (November, 1978), pp. 25–35.

Lum, Sister Barbara, et al. "Reappraising Newborn Eye Care." *American Journal of Nursing,* Vol. 80 (September, 1980), pp. 1602–1603.

Moore, Mary Lou. *Realities in Childbearing.* Philadelphia: W. B. Saunders Company, 1978.

Nalepka, Claire D. "The Oxygen Hood for Newborns in Respiratory Distress." *American Journal of Nursing,* Vol. 75 (December, 1975), pp. 2185–2187.

Porth, Carol M., and Leone E. Kaylor. "Temperature Regulation in the Newborn." *American Journal of Nursing,* Vol. 78 (October, 1978), pp. 1691–1693.

Reeder, Sharon J., et al. *Maternity Nursing.* Philadelphia: J. B. Lippincott Company, 1980.

Rothfeder, Barbara, and Mary Tiedeman. "Feeding the Low-Birth-Weight Neonate." *Nursing 77,* Vol. 7 (October, 1977), pp. 58–59.

Vaughan, Victor C., et al. *Nelson's Textbook of Pediatrics.* Philadelphia: W. B. Saunders Company, 1979.

Section III

The Hospitalized Child

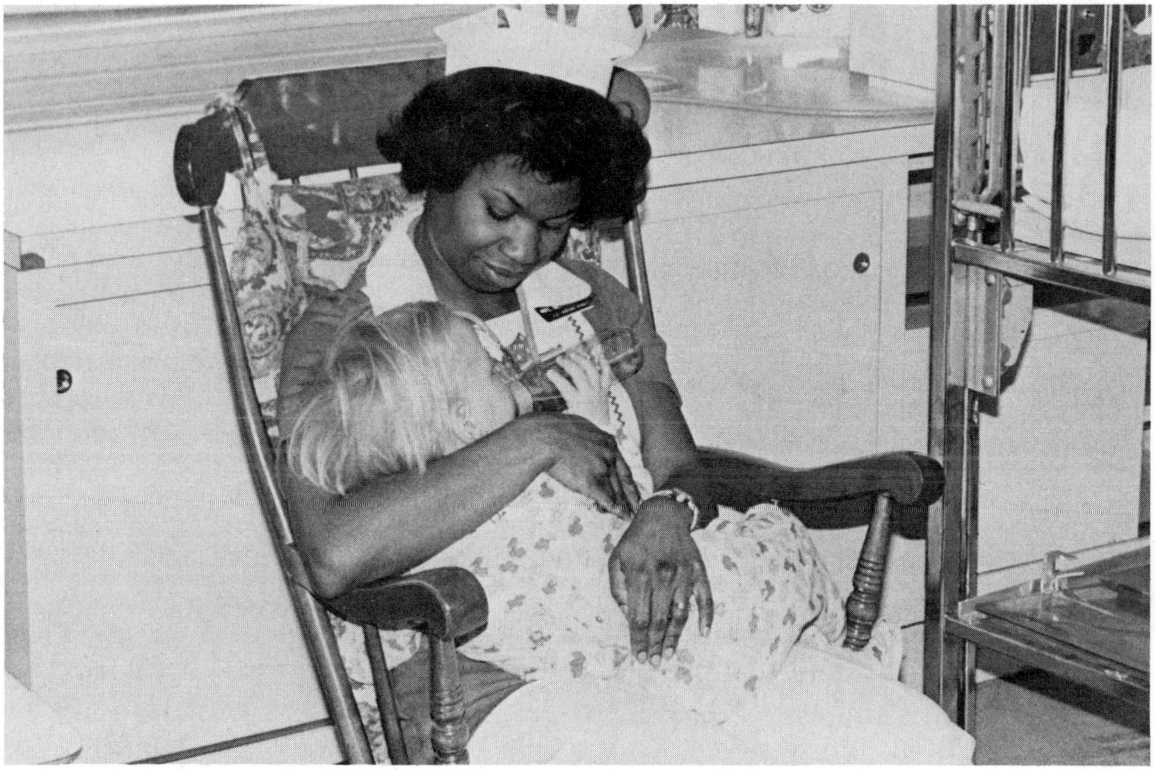

Chapter 5

The Hospital Experience

OBJECTIVES

Upon completion of this chapter, the student will be able to

- describe the adaptations that must be made in the pediatric hospital environment, as well as the admission procedure for a child.
- identify and distinguish between the pre-admission procedures and the in-hospital routines that can be implemented to make hospitalization a positive experience for both parents and child.
- identify several types of play activities that are appropriate for each age-group, including group and solitary play.
- describe the fears and anxieties that are specific to hospitalized children of various ages.

PREPARATION FOR HOSPITALIZATION

Admission to the hospital is anxiety-producing for both children and adults. For most children, it is a very traumatic experience that can only be made less traumatic by adequate preparation and knowledge about what is going to happen during the course of hospitalization. Infants and very young children do not understand all that is happening, but sense their parents' fears and concerns. For children in this age-group, separation from the parent is a greater source of fear than is any strange environment.

Scheduled Admissions

Children who are scheduled in advance for surgery have time to be prepared for the experience by both their parents and the hospital staff. After an explanation of the surgical procedure has been given by the physician, the parents can then share or reinforce this information by re-explaining it to the child in simple, age-appropriate terms. The time interval between the planning of the admission and the actual admission procedure provides an

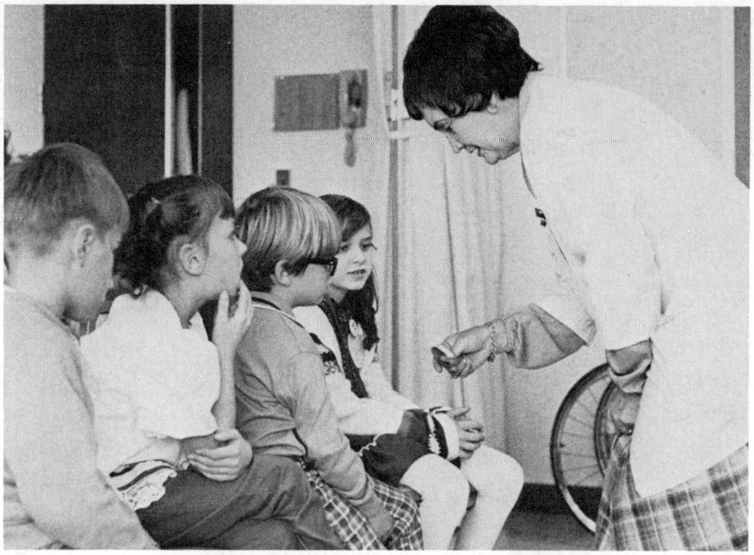

FIG. 5-1 The hospital identification band is inspected by this group at the preadmission party.

opportunity for parents and children to talk about what is going to happen and their feelings in response to the anticipated events.

Planned Preadmission Programs. Any planned orientation program must be based on knowledge and understanding of the child's developmental level. This must include an awareness of the child's perception of reality, as well as his or her fantasies. The program usually includes tours, visual aids, and an explanation of the actual items to be used in the care of the child, Figure 5-1. All of the materials used in the preadmission program should emphasize what is familiar to the child and should avoid or minimize those aspects of the hospitalization that may be frightening or unfamiliar, Figure 5-2.

A preadmission program familiarizes children with the hospital surroundings and also provides information that will help guide the children's behavior later. The program allows children to perceive nurses and the other members of the hospital staff as helpful, caring

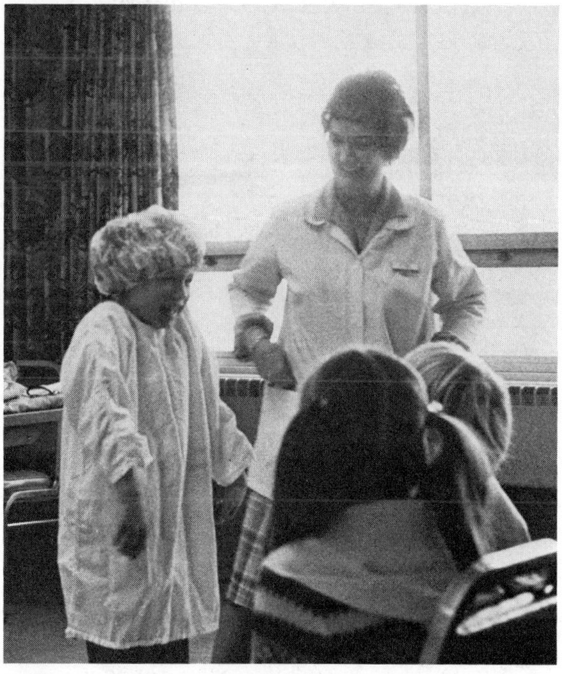

FIG. 5-2 An opportunity to wear a surgical gown and cap elicits peals of laughter from one young girl.

individuals who are much like their own family members in their concern. Children can be helped to identify the routines that are similar to those at home as well as those that differ. The program assists children in recognizing that they will have some choices in the hospital environment just as they do at home. For example, they may be allowed to choose when they take a bath or to select their food from a hot cart.

During the program, children should have ample opportunities to manipulate equipment at their own pace and in their own manner, Figure 5-3. At this time, they may also be encouraged to talk about what they are doing and what they have seen. This exchange helps the nurse to identify areas that require further clarification and to develop a trusting relationship.

At the completion of the preadmission program, a storybook or coloring book that focuses on the experience may be provided. This helps to reinforce the information and to promote further communication between parent and child about the forthcoming hospital experience. The book may also assist the parent in answering the child's questions.

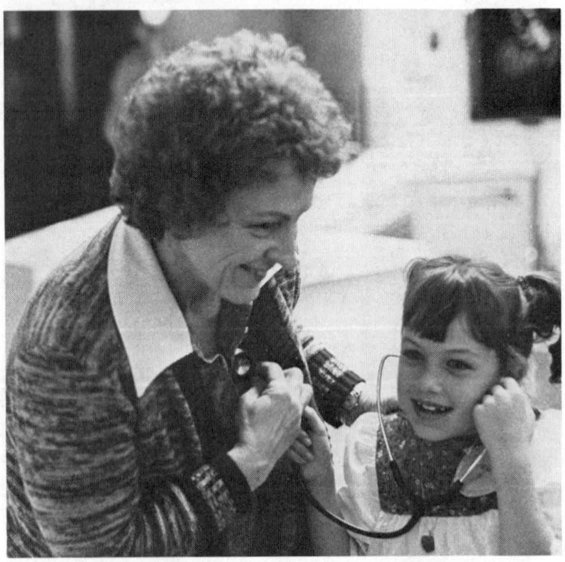

FIG. 5-3 Taking the nurse's apical pulse

The timing of the program is important. It should be scheduled far enough in advance to allow the child to absorb the information, but not so far in advance that he or she becomes bored with it or forgets it. Preschool and school-aged children usually attend the preadmission program one to two weeks prior to hospitalization. Younger children require less time than do older children for assimilation of the information.

Parents also benefit from the planned preadmission program. It provides them with accurate information about what will happen to their child in the hospital and helps them to clarify their role and responsibility during their child's hospitalization. They may also have the opportunity to see members of the hospital staff interact in a caring manner with children, which may relieve some of their fears regarding the quality of care their child will receive.

Emergency Admissions

Emergency or unplanned admissions are especially traumatic for a child. Situations that prompt an emergency admission develop very suddenly, as in the case of an accident, and involve pain and fear on the part of both parents and child. Children who are acutely ill have little energy with which to cope with unfamiliar or frightening experiences. Their coping abilities are often further diminished by the loss of parental support as a result of the emergency situation. For instance, an infant will respond to the separation from the mother by feeling helpless without her. Although the coping mechanisms of adolescents are more highly developed than those of an infant, the adolescent's response may be inappropriate because of a high anxiety level. Frequently, the adolescent will suppress or minimize symptoms to avoid showing weakness.

The early separation from the parent as well as the number of painful procedures and approaches by a large number of strangers are the issues which need to be addressed by the nursing staff. Information about what will happen is a necessity for both parent and child. As the information is provided, the nurse should assess the parents ability to be supportive in the situation. Parents usually respond well to specific directions regarding how they can help the child.

Separation will occur during many procedures because of the nature of the procedures. The parent needs to know that the nurse will be the child's support temporarily. Parent and child should be reunited as quickly as possible. Use of the child's favorite toy (if brought to the hospital), or a hand puppet aids the young child in mastering anxiety over what is happening.

THE HOSPITAL ENVIRONMENT

The equipment and surroundings of the pediatric unit should reflect its main concern – the care of children. A cheerful, homelike atmosphere reduces the anxiety of both the child and parents. The use of bright colors, pictures or cartoon characters on the walls, and homelike furnishings contribute to this atmosphere.

In individual rooms, an easy chair or rocking chair should be provided for the parents, placed near the child's bed. For infants or toddlers, the room may be equipped with highchairs, playpens, potty chairs, and cribs or bassinets. Sufficient space should be provided to allow the child to play in the room once he or she is ambulatory. This avoids disruptive play in the halls or in busy traffic areas, and promotes the child's safety.

Providing familiar equipment for the transport of children within the hospital helps to create a positive environment. For example, a little red wagon, buggy, or stroller may be used to transport the child to and from the radiology or physiotherapy department or to and from other areas of the hospital. Children are much less frightened of these familiar pieces of equipment than they are of carts or wheelchairs. In some situations, it may be necessary to transport a child in his or her own crib for safety reasons. In these cases, familiar toys and blankets can accompany the child. **Caution:** To ensure their protection, all children should be restrained adequately for transport.

Members of the Staff

The appearance of the staff on the pediatric unit should also reflect a homelike atmosphere. In many hospitals, nurses wear brightly colored uniforms or cheery smocks over their uniforms. In some pediatric hospitals, street clothes are worn to normalize the hospital environment even further.

Nurses are the individuals who have the most contact with hospitalized children. They are responsible for implementing the medical and nursing orders, and for treating, feeding, bathing, and observing the children on the unit. Although nurses are very much involved in comforting and caring for the child, they are not intended to be parent-substitutes. Rather, they provide support to both the parents and the child. In order to provide this support, nurses should show warmth, concern, knowledge, and skill in the care of the children on the unit.

The total care of the hospitalized child must be considered within the context of the family unit. The nurse administering primary care to a pediatric patient cannot interview the child exclusively for the assessment. The data provided by the caregiver within the family, along with information regarding the nurturing, as well as the environment contribute significantly to the plan of care.

Both the physical and psychologic facets of the child must be recognized by the nurse. Long-range planning and the preventive aspects of health maintenance are a necessity in pediatric care and are a shared responsibility of the nurse and the physician.

The nurse in pediatrics must have a strong commitment to patient and parent teaching as an integral part of the care. The child will be dependent on the caregiver in the home setting. The caregiver must be well prepared to deal with immediate health problems and the normal changes which are occurring as a part of the child's growth and development. The nurse helps parents recognize their own need for assistance in many situations. This educational process is a major focus in pediatric units.

THE ADMISSION PROCEDURE

The relationship between hospital staff, parents, and children is aided by a positive, concerned manner right from the point of admission. The admission procedure for planned hospitalization consists of two parts: the admission interview and the actual admission to the unit.

Admission Interview

The admission interview is conducted in the admitting office of the hospital. This interview provides an opportunity for legal and financial matters to be discussed and settled privately. At this time, the parents are asked to sign a form permitting treatment or surgery, or both. It is during this time that an identification band is attached to the child's wrist or ankle, and the designated unit will be notified that the child will arrive shortly. In the admitting office, the parents also receive printed information regarding hospital rules and regulations.

Admission to the Unit

In this part of the admission procedure, the child is taken to the pediatric unit and introduced to the nurse responsible for the admission. The selection of a unit is based on the child's age and the diagnosis. The child and parents are greeted by name and are welcomed to the unit in a calm, unhurried manner, Figure 5-4.

Room Assignment. The parents and child are escorted to the admission treatment room or to the assigned room. Children younger than five years of age are usually placed in a crib. Children five years of age or older may be placed in a large bed with side rails. The child may be assigned to a room with other children who are undergoing the same type of surgery or who have the same diagnosis.

Clothing. Once admitted to the unit, the child is assisted by the parent or nurse in undressing

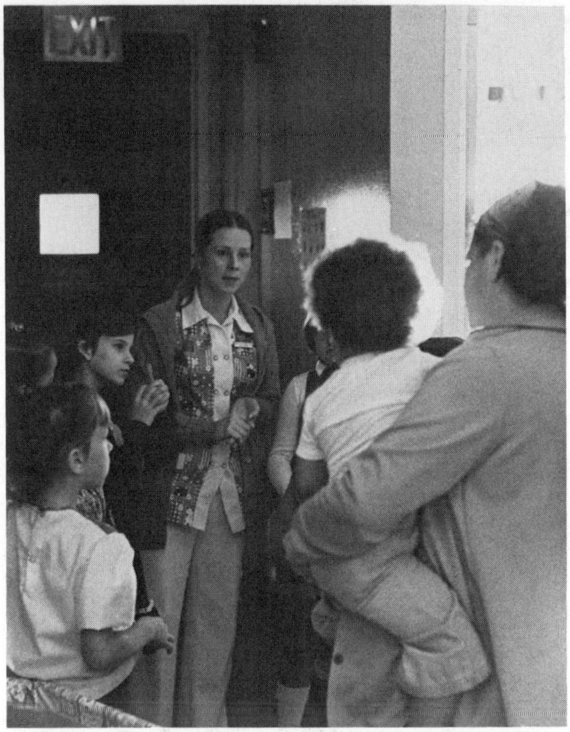

FIG. 5-4 A welcoming committee joins the head nurse to greet the new patient and his mother.

and putting on his or her own pajamas or hospital clothing. The privacy of older children should be respected during this procedure. The child's clothing can be sent home with the parents. If this is not possible at this time, clothing should be labeled and placed in a safe location until the parent can take it home later. The strangeness of the hospital environment may be reduced somewhat if the child is permitted to wear his or her own pajamas, slippers, and robe. *Note:* If the child is to be isolated for a communicable or contagious disease, this practice should not be permitted.

Assessment

Information about the admitted child is obtained during assessment. Prior to admission, the parents may have completed a questionnaire about the child's routines at home, likes and dislikes, and special needs, Figure 5-5. This is helpful to the health care team in planning the child's care and in meeting the child's needs. In the case of toddlers and preschoolers it is important for the nurse to learn any nicknames or special words used by the children in order to facilitate their care. The nurse should also seek some knowledge about the family so that the child can more easily be regarded as a unique person.

The child's past health history and information regarding previous hospitalizations are also significant. Is this the first admission? Has the child frequently been ill? Have many hospital admissions been necessary in the past? Is the child fearful because of past experiences? All of this information helps the nurse form some ideas about the child's needs and how they can best be met by the nursing staff.

Assessing Physical Status. Evaluation of the child's physical status should include a measurement of height and weight. A single measurement is meaningless unless it is plotted on a growth chart, Figure 5-6, and compared with normal patterns. If the child was admitted previously, the current measurements may be compared with the former ones to evaluate the child's pattern of growth. A healthy child follows a consistent pattern, whereas one who is frequently sick may show marked deviations from a normal pattern because of the type or frequency of the illnesses.

Upon admission of the child, the nurse should also note the general mannerisms and

Patient's Name: ROBERT SMITH

Admission Diagnosis: BRONCHO PNEUMONIA

Date: 1-10-81 Time: 2:30 PM

Admitted from: ADM. OFFICE Mode:

Accompanied by: FATHER & MOTHER

Age: 3 Religion: CATHOLIC Baptized: YES — Previous hospitalizations: NONE

Nickname: BOBBI Schoolgrade: -

No. of Siblings: (4) 21 - 17 - 14 - 11

T. 102° AP 110 R 30 B/P 90/50 ARM: Rt — Surgery: NONE

Ht. Wt. Hd.

Born at: ST. JOSEPH Birth Wt.: 9# 1/2 OZ — Fears of hospitalization: NONE APPARENT

Complications: JAUNDICE

Congenital Anomaly: NONE — Childs' Behavior: QUIET

Allergies: NONE

Drugs: NONE — Relationship to mother: GOOD INTERACTION

Foods: NONE other: —

Medication taken today: TYLENOL (children's) — Mother: ANN Age: 44 Father: JACK Age: 47

routinely: MULTIVITAMIN — Family hx of Ca, CVA, diabetes, ht. disease etc. DIABETES - MATERNAL GRANDFATHER

Baby Shots: (Yes) No How Many COMPLETE Next one due: 4 YRS.

Contagious disease hx:				Growth and	Independent	With	Dependent
Has pt. had	Vaccine	Disease	Exposure	Development		Assistance	
Chicken pox	—			Ambulate	✓		
German measles	YES			Sit	✓		
Measles				Turn	✓		
Mumps				Feed	✓		
Polio				Bathe		✓	
Small Pox				Dress		✓	
Tuberculosis				Talk	✓		
Other:				Play	✓		

Food habits: Diet: REGULAR TABLE Formula: NO

Bottle: NO Cup: YES Appetite: GOOD

Likes/~~dislikes~~: PEANUT BUTTER oral hygiene: BRUSHES AM & PM

Elimination: Bm pattern: 1X DAY Wears diapers: NO training pants: NO

toilet trained for bm: YES Urine: YES Uses potty chair: NO toilet: YES

taken to toilet during day YES night NO specify: —

takes what laxative: NO Menstruation: — L.M.P. —

Miscellaneous needs: No. hrs. of sleep: 10-12 Bedtime hour: 7 30 P.M.

Naps taken: YES Time: 12 30 - 2 Language spoken: ENGLISH

Favorite toy: SNOOPY here: YES

FIG. 5-5 Prior to admission, a nursing history form should be completed in order to familiarize the staff with the child's normal home routine.

PHYSICAL NEEDS	yes	no	PHYSICAL NEEDS	yes	no
glasses – contacts		✓	brace		✓
hearing – aide		✓	corrective shoes		✓
speech defect ARTICULATION	✓		hip splint		✓
orthodontal device		✓	crutches		✓
other:			other:		

oriented to unit YES routine YES urine obtained YES

explained to parents: visiting hours YES mealtimes YES

safety precautions YES isolation technique NA

Demonstrated room equipment YES given info booklets YES

Nursing Assessment

Patient/Parent complaints: MOTHER STATES THAT CHILD HAS A COLD WHICH HAS GOTTEN WORSE. MEDICATIONS (AMPICILLIN) AND VAPORIZER AT HOME DID NOT HELP SO CHILD WAS ADMITTED.

LOC ALERT & ORIENTED

NIV

Diarrhea 2 LOOSE STOOLS AT HOME

Resp/Circ Status: FREQUENT, HARSH COUGH - FACE FLUSHED RESPIRATIONS RAPID BUT NO RETRACTIONS OR NASAL FLARING NOTED.

Condition of skin: DRY - WARM TO TOUCH CLEAN - GOOD CONDITION - NO LESIONS

Color: PALE

other:

Ellen Guffett RN

Nurses' Signature

FIG. 5-5 Continued

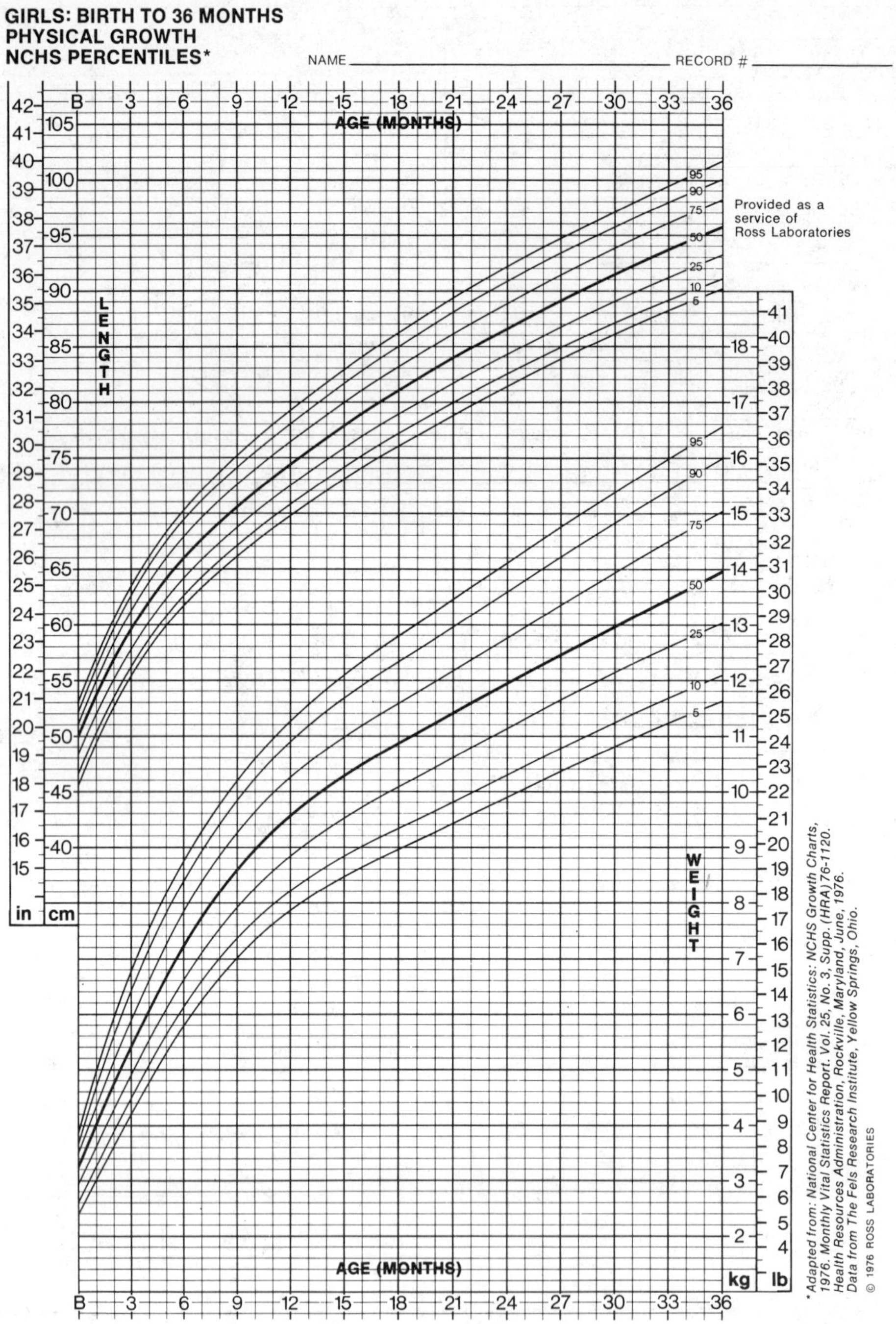

FIG. 5-6 A growth chart from the National Center for Health Statistics (Courtesy of Ross Laboratories)

appearance of the child. Does the child use both arms and legs? Do the extremities appear to be equal in size and length? Does the abdomen appear to be unusually large? Does the child have difficulty moving the head or extremities? Does the child appear to be able to see and hear normally? Can the child follow simple directions? Does the skin appear to be unusually flushed or pale? Does the skin have a bluish tinge, such as in cyanosis? Are cuts, bruises, or burns evident?

Vital Signs. The vital signs of temperature, pulse, and blood pressure are included in the assessment. They are necessary to identify the child's current status, as well as to provide a baseline for future measurements.

Rectal temperatures are taken on all children younger than seven years of age unless contraindicated by a health problem. After proper lubrication and insertion, the thermometer is held in place until the procedure is completed. The child should never be left unattended when the thermometer is in place.

The pulse is taken for a full minute. Any irregularities in volume, rate, or rhythm are noted. An apical pulse is taken routinely in all children, using a stethoscope on the chest at the apex of the heart. An infant who is crying or fussing can be held by the nurse while the position of the stethoscope on the chest is maintained with one hand.

Respirations are also counted for a full minute and assessed for rate, depth, and quality. In infants, the movements of the abdomen, as well as those of the chest, are observed when measuring respirations. Blood pressure readings in infants and toddlers are taken according to hospital policy or when specifically ordered. It is important to use a cuff of correct size in order to obtain an accurate reading. A cuff that is too narrow produces a very high reading, whereas one that is too wide will produce a low reading. A cuff that is 1 to 1 1/2 inches in width is used for infants one year of age or younger. A 3-inch cuff is used for toddlers. The cuff should cover 2/3 the length of the upper arm.

Laboratory Specimens. The hospital laboratory is usually responsible for obtaining blood specimens from children. Nurses may assist in this process by helping to comfort a child or by providing restraint, if necessary. The collection of urine and stool specimens is the responsibility of the nurses on the pediatric unit. To obtain a urine specimen from an infant or young child who is not toilet-trained, it is necessary to use some type of collection device. The most commonly used type is the plastic disposable urine collector, Figure 5-7. Prior

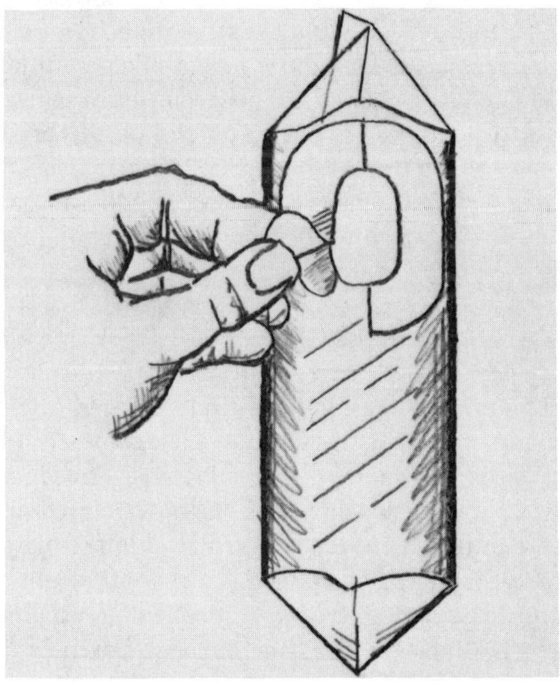

FIG. 5-7 Pediatric urine collector

to the application of the specimen collector, the infant's perineum is cleansed and dried carefully. The gummed backing is then removed from both sides of the device's opening and the adhesive portion is placed firmly against the infant's perineum. The collector remains in place beneath the diaper until a sufficient amount of urine has been obtained. It should not be applied to any infant whose skin is raw or damaged from diaper rash as the adhesive will cause further irritation.

The method used for stool specimen collection depends on the reason for collection. When stools are collected for the determination of the presence of fat, blood and milk antibodies, a small amount of the stool is removed from the diaper with a tongue blade and placed in a specimen cup. The lid is secured and after proper labeling, it is sent to the laboratory. Stool cultures are often obtained by swabbing the anal orifice with a cotton applicator and returning it to a culture media in a test tube or similar container. Stool specimens obtained for a pediatric patient to determine the presence of ova or parasites are collected in a specimen cup but must be kept warm and are usually transported to the laboratory immediately to be placed in the incubator.

Orientation to the Unit

Equipment. Hospitalized children and their parents need to know about the equipment in their nursing unit. If the bed is large, how does it operate? How are the side rails operated on the crib? Can the child be placed in the highchair to be fed or to play? How are the lights, curtains, and television controlled? Most importantly, how does the child or parent call for the nurse? Each of these questions should be answered and the equipment demonstrated for parents and children to make sure they understand its operation. In addition, children (who are old enough) and parents need to know what activities are to be restricted, what children are permitted to do, and what the usual daily routine is on the unit.

Visiting Privileges. Visiting privileges also should be explained to the parents. Most hospitals offer unlimited (free) visiting hours for parents. Many encourage rooming-in for the parents of infants, toddlers, and preschoolers. Some hospitals have home-care facilities in their pediatric units. These facilities allow the parent to take responsibility for the general care and comfort of the child. The nursing staff provides necessary support and assistance, monitors the child's progress, and administers medications and other treatments. If the parents are unable to remain with the child or to visit frequently, some family members such as a grandparent, an aunt, or even a teenage brother or sister should be encouraged to do so. In some agencies, senior citizens volunteer to provide this needed support for individual young children.

Meals. Mealtime is an important part of a child's day. During the orientation period, the time for meals, the type of diet, and the way in which the meal is served should be discussed with the child and parents. Many pediatric units serve meals or snacks in a group setting for those children who are ambulatory, Figure 5-8. In other units, all the children in a single room may eat at small tables provided in that room. Hot food carts that are taken from room to room allow children to make choices regarding the type of food they might like for a meal. This is an excellent means of allowing children some choice when they are on a regular or soft diet.

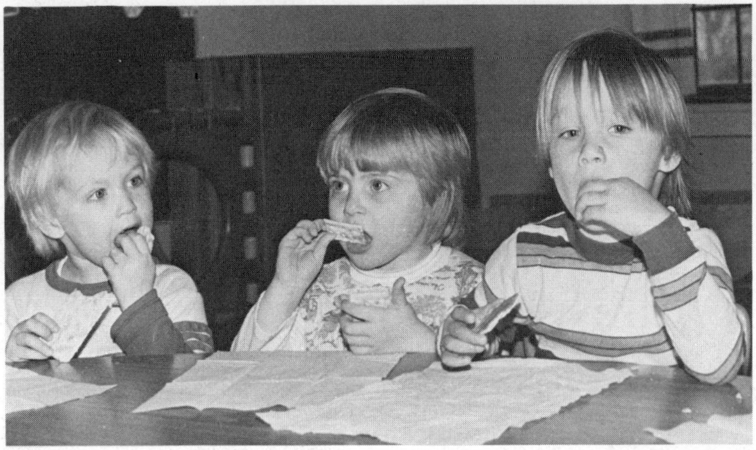

FIG. 5-8 Snacks are enjoyed with friends in the playroom.

Play Activities. The activity program and use of the playroom are also of interest to both parent and child. Play is often called "the work of children." Play allows the child to develop new skills and interests; it provides a distraction from pain and discomfort; it aids in mastering fears; and it helps pass the time. A planned activity or play program is conducted by an occupational therapist, a play therapist, or a child-life worker. In addition to providing a diversion, the toys and games in the playroom should stimulate the imagination. There should be a sufficient number and variety of toys and games to meet the needs of all age-groups. Infants enjoy bright mobiles, musical toys, rattles, and stuffed animals. Toddlers are attracted to pull-toys, toy telephones, musical jack-in-the-boxes, and blocks. Preschoolers find crayons, clay, simple puzzles, books, trucks, and cars to their liking. The school-aged child enjoys puzzles, simple hobbies, games, toy models, and craft kits. Parents may also want to bring one or two of the child's favorite toys from home if this is possible.

Safety. The safety needs of the child must be explored during orientation to the unit. A child's behavior may be unpredictable, especially in the strange environment of a hospital. The child's growth and development level is the clue for concerns regarding safety. It is important to instruct the parent in methods of raising and lowering the side rail correctly, calling for assistance when needed, and keeping all hazardous objects away from the child. The parent should also be taught to inspect the infant's toys for sharp edges and breakable or removable parts, and to determine whether or not they are washable. An explanation should be offered the parents regarding the rationale for careful supervision and the operation of safety belts when a child is in a wheelchair or a highchair, Figure 5-9.

WORKING WITH THE CHILD

In working with children, the nurse must consider two additional areas of concern: effective communication and fears related to hospitalization. These concerns are uniquely challenging in pediatrics because they are based on the developmental level of the individual child.

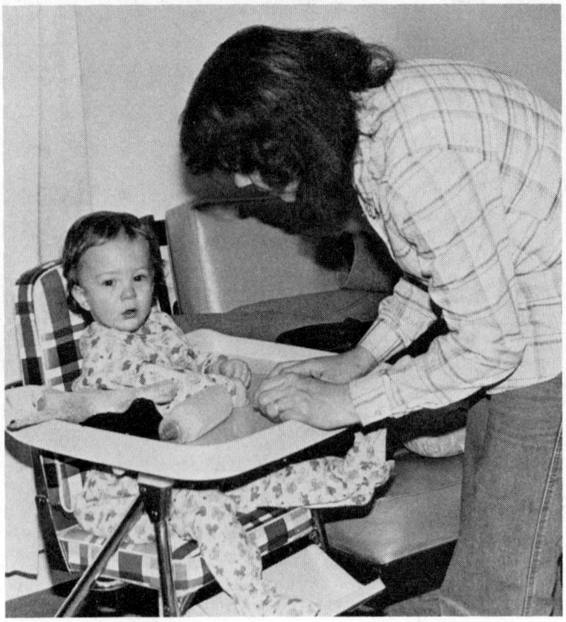

FIG. 5-9 Children should be carefully supervised when sitting in a highchair.

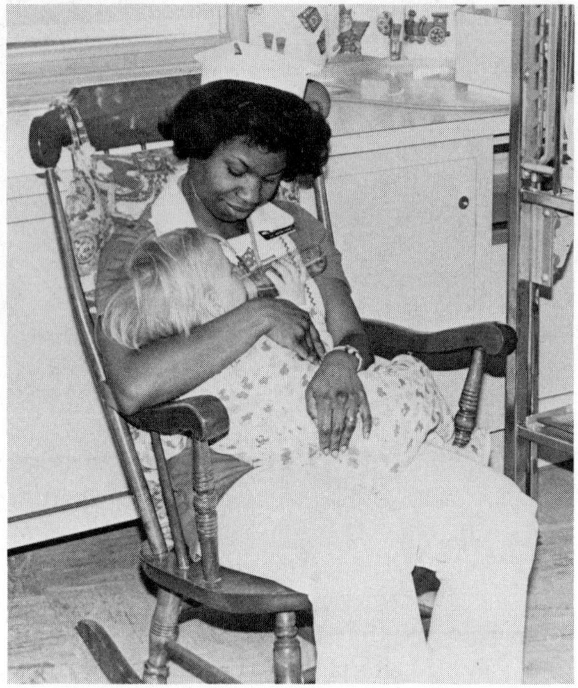

FIG. 5-10 Cuddling and rocking are important aspects of the nursing care of a hospitalized child.

Communicating with Children

Infants voice their complaints of hunger, pain, and separation by crying loudly until the parent or parent-substitute comforts them. Gentle talking, cuddling, and rocking are all important aspects of care, Figure 5-10. When approaching an infant, the nurse should avoid moving rapidly or making loud noises. Nonthreatening communication is made easier by talking to the infant or approaching gently when the infant is secure in the parent's arms. Rapport with an infant is established mainly on a nonverbal level. Therefore, spending time with and handling the infant at times other than during routine care enhances the infant's sense of trust.

Toddlers and preschoolers need the same warm concern conveyed to them even though they are able to communicate verbally. A casual approach that demonstrates knowledge of and interest in the child and his or her concerns enhances the nurse's relationship with the child. At first, the child may exhibit anger or aggressive behavior. This should be acknowledged and dealt with through play therapy. If it becomes a safety problem, then firm limits should be set as kindly as possible.

School-aged children communicate more easily than do preschoolers because of their command of speech. Ill children need the constancy of repeated contacts with the same nurse. These children respond to the nurse's genuine concern for their well-being. As they develop a sense of confidence in the nurse, they will feel more comfortable sharing their

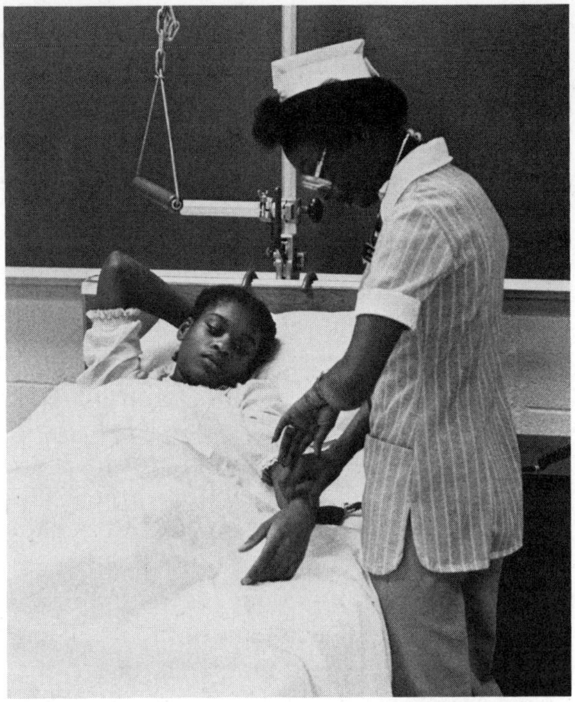

FIG. 5-11 This adolescent shows an interest in her vital signs.

thoughts and feelings. This sharing may include those concerns that they cannot comfortably discuss with their parents. Nurses indirectly affect the personality and character formation of the children through showing concern.

Adolescents communicate a great deal of information through their posture, appearance, and dress, as well as by their verbal responses. They, too, need the understanding and warmth of the nursing staff. The nurse's initial approach to the adolescent is crucial as it may influence the adolescent's entire response to the hospitalization. Adolescents need to feel involved in their care, Figure 5-11. They should be encouraged to question, to express their feelings, and to participate in decisions regarding their care. When communicating with adolescent patients, nurses should be accepting and supportive of the adolescents' efforts to increase control over their environment.

Fears Related to Hospitalization

For infants and toddlers, the greatest fear related to hospitalization is separation from parents. This is commonly referred to as separation anxiety. An infant's response to separation may range from crying episodes to stark terror. If the separation continues for a long period of time, the infant may panic or else become apathetic and depressed.

The three stages identified in studies of the hospitalized child include protest, despair, and denial. In the stage of protest the child cries frequently and may often shake the crib. The child has an urgent desire to find the mother-figure and expects that she will answer his cries. During this time the child often rejects the attention of the nursing staff. In the stage of despair the child may cry monotonously or even intermittently but is hopeless about finding the mother-figure. By the stage of denial the child has repressed all feelings about the mother, seldom crying even when she leaves. The child may appear more attached to the nursing staff during this time but actually appears to find little satisfaction in any relationships with other people.

Hospitalized preschoolers are also concerned with abandonment. They view separation from parents as a punishment for bad thoughts or anger directed at the parent. In addition, they may be concerned with the soundness of their bodies. They often reason that if clothing can fall apart and the stuffing can come out of a doll, the same could happen to them. They may also have heard adults express fears related to hospitalization and may assume these concerns as well. Their limited experiences often result in a misunderstanding of what will happen during their hospitalization. For example, the child may think that the surgeon will have to cut off his or her head in order to remove diseased tonsils. This represents a fear of mutilation. Many children develop fantasies related to the illness or the treatment.

School-aged children have somewhat different fears. They do not fear abandonment but they fear being replaced. The fear that a sibling will assume their place of importance in the family or that a classmate will take their place in the classroom is all too real to them. They may also fear disability and death. During the hospitalization, these fears may be present even though the child is not seriously ill. Phobias are very common in this age-group.

Parents of hospitalized children are beset by other fears. They may dread the financial burden of a potentially prolonged hospitalization. Frequently, they are fearful about procedures that are painful to their child, perhaps recalling their own childhood hospitalization. Parents may also fear that the hospital staff will not care for their child properly, or may simply be concerned about the child's comfort and well-being. The nurse can relieve the latter fear by continually demonstrating genuine concern for the child and by delivering knowledgeable care.

Maintaining Home Contact. A child's fears may be compounded by separation from the parents at some point during the hospitalization. This separation may be the result of other parental responsibilities, transportation difficulties, or perhaps illness of other family members. The child's response depends on several factors, including the developmental age of the child and the child's previous experiences with separation.

During the period of hospitalization, the nurse should encourage parents to be honest about when they will visit and when they must leave. Trust will be lost if the parents tell a child that they are leaving to go to lunch, only to disappear until the following day. Parents may have used this method in the past, believing it to be less upsetting to the child. The nurse must encourage the parents to maintain the child's trust. Staying with a young child and reassuring the child of the parents' love and concern are prime responsibilities of the nurse. The parents' responsibility in this situation is to return at the stated time.

Several methods may be used to help young children maintain attachment to the family group. Personal items belonging to parents, such as a purse, scarf, pair of gloves, or photograph can strengthen this bond. Another item that may be used effectively is a tape recording. For young children, a tape offers an opportunity to hear their parents' voices when the parents cannot physically be present. For older children, particularly those anticipating a lengthy hospitalization or those who are admitted to a hospital that is a great distance from home, tapes may supplement letters from home. Parents and other members of the family can tape messages about daily events and send them to the child. The child, in turn, may be able to tape messages to return to the family. For adolescents, peer contacts are essential. Peer contacts can be maintained through letters, telephone calls, and visits as well as tapes, Figure 5-12.

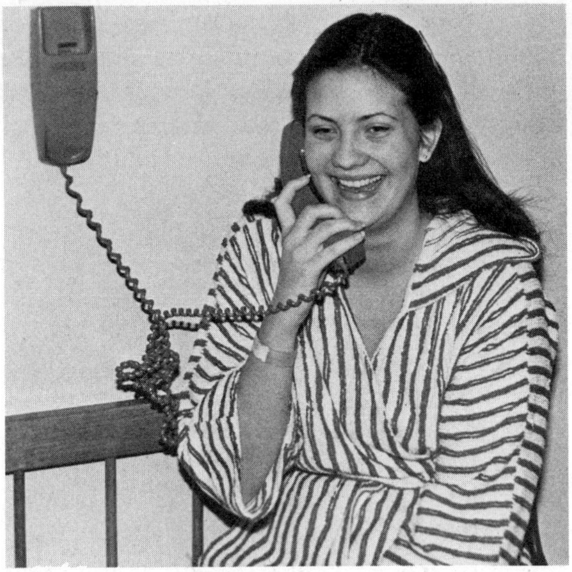

FIG. 5-12 A hospitalized teenager maintains contact with peers by using the telephone.

Throughout this stressful period of hospitalization, the nurse should encourage all children to talk about their home, friends, pets, and schooling. It is important to remind children that their parents and friends miss them. In this way, the child's coping mechanisms are strengthened rather than weakened by the hospital experience. Moreover, the nurse should encourage and facilitate adolescents' contacts with their peers, and should remind them of their eventual return to the peer support group.

WORKING COOPERATIVELY WITH PARENTS

The nurse should realize that all families do not function in the same way. Some parents may not share information with their child as they have been encouraged to do by the health care team. The dynamics within a family situation influence the behavior of a hospitalized child. With some families, conflicts in care and in the presentation of information may arise if the nurse shares information with persons other than the dominant controlling member. Other families may have strong religious views that conflict with certain medical or surgical treatments. Their vehemence in protecting their own beliefs may cause staff resentment or avoidance.

Other families may deliberately use chaos and deception to control the child's behavior. With chaotic families, hospital visitors are often numerous and may be overly emotional in response to what may be a minor illness in the child. Deceptive families are likely to emphasize the availability of ice cream in the hospital and to ignore the tonsillectomy.

During the period of hospitalization, it is imperative that nurses anticipate parents' questions and answer them knowledgeably. This helps to allay some of the parents' anxieties. Hospital routines are foreign to the parent. A warm, trusting relationship with members of the nursing staff may take a little time to form. The nurse should continue to provide basic orientation information and to explain the rationale for treatments, restrictions, and the like until the parents appear to be comfortable with their knowledge of the situation and the routines.

Initially, many of the parents' questions are related to the routines of the unit and to scheduled diagnostic tests. Later, the questions focus on the knowledge of the diagnosis or clarification of information shared by the physician. Gradually, parents' concern shifts toward home-going or discharge activities and the limitations or restrictions that might be imposed on the child. Any parent who will be delivering some type of nursing care in the home should participate in these care activities during the child's hospitalization. Preparation for this responsibility begins shortly after admission of the child.

Parents should be given ample opportunity to talk about their concerns about the child and his or her hospitalization. This is particularly true with emergency admissions related to accidents or sudden illness. Talking about the situation helps the parents to minimize the stress that they feel as a result of the situation. It allows them to clarify and define their anxieties as well as to consider possible solutions to problems. If they express a great deal of anger regarding the present situation, the nurse should avoid making defensive statements. The anger or hostility that may be expressed should be recognized by the nurse as the parents' means of minimizing emotional tension or stress. Once parents have worked through these feelings, they can cooperate productively with the staff to support the child.

During the child's hospitalization, the nurse should be able to recognize the positive parenting and nurturing behavior used by the parents. At times, parents may experience guilt feelings about minor problems with their child. As parents gain confidence in the level of care and concern demonstrated by members of the hospital staff, they may become more willing to share other areas of concern. Therapeutic communication techniques should be used by the nurse to allow parents to express concerns and to make their own decisions. The nursing or medical staff can make recommendations or suggestions for care, but the ultimate decision lies with the parents. This may be particularly difficult to accept when a conflict exists between the life-style or culture of the nursing staff and that of the parents.

It is extremely important for the nurse to keep the lines of communication open with the families. At all times, the nurse must be nonjudgmental toward the parents, and must provide support for both parents and child.

SUMMARY

The pediatric nurse has a unique role in the hospital experience of a child. Children are admitted to the hospital with varying degrees of preparation for the experience. It is the nurse's responsibility to identify these children's informational needs, to help familiarize them with care routines, and to provide support and comfort. The nurse should demonstrate genuine concern for hospitalized children, both to the child and to the parents.

SUGGESTED ACTIVITIES

- Attend a preadmission party for preschoolers. Report on the types of questions that were asked by parents at the program, what equipment was shown to the children, and the comments and questions of the children who attended.
- Interview the parents of four children admitted to the hospital within the last week. Determine the parents' and children's preparation for the hospitalization. Find out what and who helped parents and children the most in their adjustment to the hospital situation.
- Observe a child being admitted through the emergency room to the pediatric unit. Identify ways in which nurses can be supportive to the parents and child. Describe what procedures or situations increased the parents' anxiety level.
- Talk with three preschool and school-aged children who recently have undergone surgery. Ask them to describe, in their own terms, what happened to them. Ask them to draw one picture about their hospital experience.

DISCUSSION TOPICS

1. Discuss various means by which the nurse can promote patient participation in health care decisions.
2. Research the developmental tasks identified by Erik Erikson for each age-group. Discuss the fears and anxieties of hospitalized children in relation to these tasks.

REVIEW

A. Matching. Match the activity of the hospitalized child in Column I with the time it should occur in Column II.

Column I	Column II
1. Touring the pediatric unit with other children	a. Preadmission program
2. Having vital signs taken by the nurse	b. Hospital admission
3. Playing with the stethoscope, tongue blades, and blood pressure cuff	
4. Having blood drawn by a laboratory technician	

B. Multiple choice. Select the one best answer.

Situation: There are children of various ages on your pediatric unit. They include:

Jimmy — a nine-month-old infant
Bobby — a twenty-two months of age toddler
Danny — a four-year-old preschooler
Susan — an eight-year-old school-aged child
Mike — a thirteen years of age adolescent

1. An appropriate toy for Jimmy would be
   a. blocks.
   b. toy telephone.
   c. bright mobile.
   d. simple puzzle.
2. Craft kits or puzzles would provide diversion for
   a. Jimmy.
   b. Bobby.
   c. Danny.
   d. Susan.
3. Fear of separation from the mother is greatest in
   a. Susan.
   b. Mike.
   c. Danny.
   d. Jimmy.
4. A preschool child such as Danny may fear he
   a. is being isolated.
   b. is being punished for bad thoughts.
   c. will be disabled or die.
   d. will be replaced by siblings.
5. The nurse can help strengthen home contacts for hospitalized children by
   1. calling the parents frequently about the child's condition.
   2. encouraging the parents to be honest about when they plan to leave.
   3. suggesting the parents leave some personal item with the child.
   4. strictly enforcing the visiting regulations with parents.

   a. 1 only
   b. 2 and 3
   c. 1, 2, 3, and 4
   d. 1 and 4 only
6. During morning care for Susan, the nurse notices she is very tearful. When asked if she is homesick, Susan begins to sob loudly. The nurse should comfort her and should also
   1. avoid talking about home.
   2. remind Susan that her parents miss her.
   3. change the subject to something more pleasant.
   4. ask her if she would like to call home.

   a. 1 and 3
   b. 3 only
   c. 2 and 4
   d. 1, 2, 3 and 4

C. Short answer. Briefly respond to the following statements.

1. List three things parents should know about safety in the hospital.
2. List three common fears parents have regarding their child's hospitalization.
3. Describe those items which should be included in the admission of a fifteen-month-old child for repair of an umbilical hernia.

BIBLIOGRAPHY

Abbott, Nancy, et al. "Dress Rehearsal for the Hospital." *American Journal of Nursing,* Vol. 70 (November, 1970), pp. 2360–2362.

Broadribb, Violet. *Foundations of Pediatric Nursing.* Philadelphia: J. B. Lippincott Company, 1973.

Chadwick, Barbara J., et al. "Maintaining the Hospitalized Child's Home Ties." *American Journal of Nursing,* Vol. 78 (August, 1978), pp. 1360–1362.

Galligan, Ann. "Books for the Hospitalized Child." *American Journal of Nursing,* Vol. 75 (December, 1975), pp. 2164–2166.

Isler, Charlotte. "The Fine Art of Handling a Hospitalized Child." *RN,* Vol. 41 (March, 1978), pp. 41–45.

Johnston, Marcene, and Mary Salzer. "Pre-admission Program for Rehospitalized Children." *American Journal of Nursing,* Vol. 79 (August, 1979), pp. 1420–1422.

Leifer, Gloria. *Principles and Techniques in Pediatric Nursing,* Philadelphia: W. B. Saunders Company, 1977.

Petrillo, Madeline, and Sirgay Sanger. *Emotional Care of Hospitalized Children.* Philadelphia: J. B. Lippincott Company, 1980.

Smitherman, Colleen H. "Parents of Hospitalized Children Have Needs Too." *American Journal of Nursing,* Vol. 79 (August, 1979), pp. 1423–1424.

Waechter, Eugenia, and Florence Blake. *Nursing Care of Children.* Philadelphia: J. B. Lippincott Company, 1976.

5/31/84

Chapter 6

The Nursing Process and Its Pediatric Applications

OBJECTIVES

Upon completion of this chapter, the student will be able to

- name and compare the components in the nursing process.
- describe the process of physical assessment that might be carried out in a pediatric unit.
- explain the type of information that should be included in a patient's chart.
- identify some cultural elements that might influence a child's care.

COMPONENTS OF THE NURSING PROCESS

The nursing process is the application of a problem-solving method to the care of a patient. It involves four major components: assessment, planning, implementation, and evaluation, Figure 6-1. Each of these elements has an integral part in the process and each is interrelated. Initially, the process proceeds in the sequence just outlined. However, new information or feedback may indicate the need for further assessment or a different mode of implementation.

Assessment

Assessment of a hospitalized child involves an orderly and systematic identification of the child's problem. It is a process of data collection. The sources of the data are many and varied. Data may be gathered from the patient or the family, from observations by health team members, from textbook information regarding the diagnosis or disease process, or from the admission interview itself. All of these sources are used to gain a perspective on the child's problem.

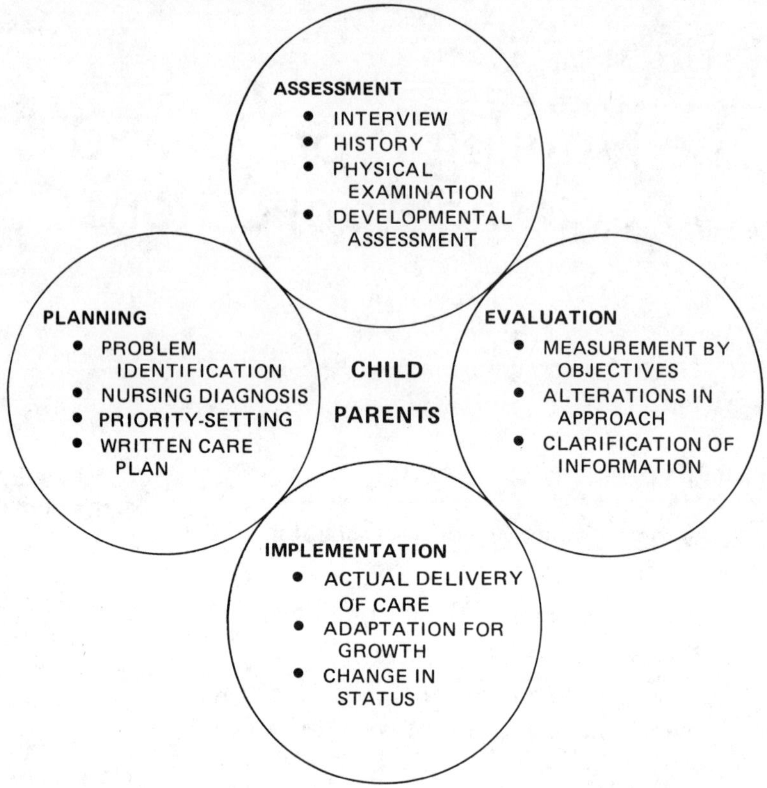

FIG. 6-1 The nursing process in pediatrics

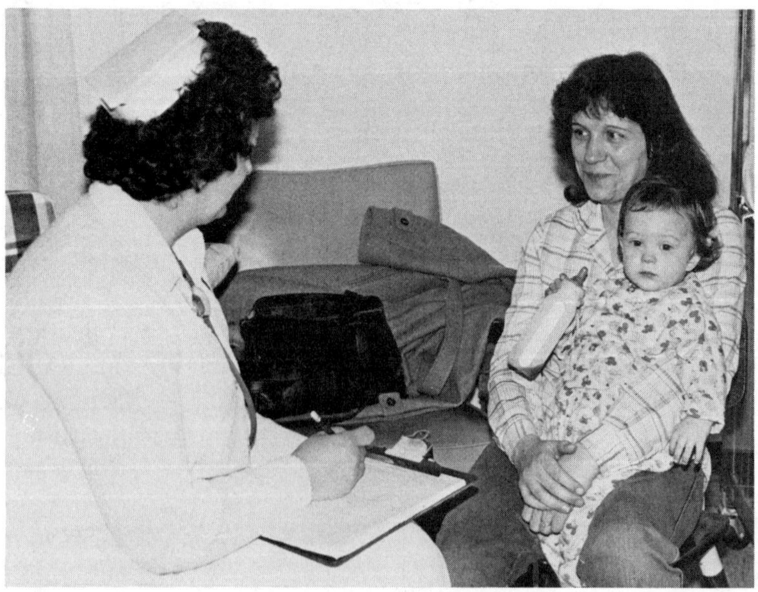

FIG. 6-2 The nurse begins the interview in a comfortable and relaxed environment.

The admission interview is a crucial part of this assessment process. It is often referred to as the original encounter with the child and family, and as such, is extremely important. During this time, the nurse must demonstrate a high degree of empathy and sensitivity to the needs of the child and the parents.

Initially, some provisions should be made for the comfort of the child and parents, such as offering them a comfortable seat, Figure 6-2. The nurse should also be seated to make eye contact easier. Moreover, the setting must provide some measure of privacy in order to promote effective interviewing.

During the interview, the nurse should remember that the perceptions of both the parents and the child depend on past experiences, both good and bad. The parents heightened level of anxiety during the interview may result in some informational inaccuracies or an inability to recall specific facts. The nurse may express this possibility to the parents or child, offering a subsequent opportunity for the parents to share additional information, Figure 6-3.

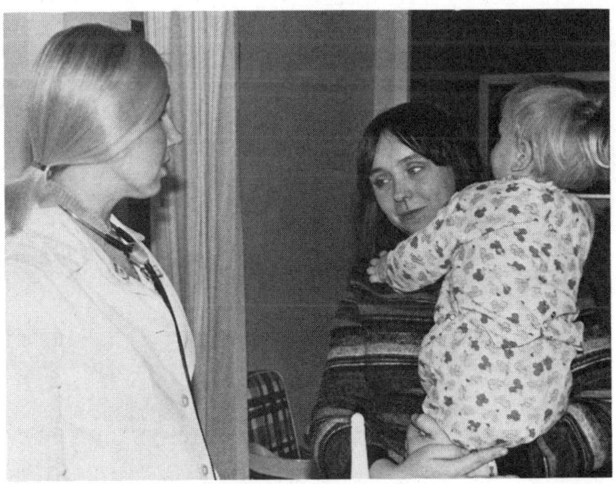

FIG. 6-3 The nurse's approach to assessment begins with questions for the parents.

During this period of high anxiety for the parents, children may also exhibit behavior that is indicative of their own anxiety level. This behavior may simply reflect the parents' tenseness rather than the child's normal temperament.

Planning

The planning part of the nursing process involves sifting and sorting the data gathered and validating the identified needs of the child. The nurse should realize that all needs may not be met for every patient. The nurse must focus on those needs that are most urgent or those that are most relevant to the child's well-being. It may be helpful to classify the identified problems as actual, probable, or potential in order to set priorities for planning. According to Maslow's hierarchy of needs, physiologic needs are the first priority, followed by safety needs. The patient's physiologic needs may be so demanding, as with a respiratory obstruction, that even a slight disruption of care or attention will jeopardize the child's health. In ascending order, Maslow's hierarchy of needs are:

1. Physiological: for air, food, drink, and rest to achieve balance within the body.
2. Safety: for security; stability; and freedom from fear, anxiety, and chaos.
3. Belongingness and love: for affection and intimacy, to be provided by family, friends, and significant others.
4. Esteem: for self-respect and the respect of others.
5. Self-actualization: the sense that one is doing what one is individually suited for and capable of, "true to one's own nature."

The identified problems or concerns reflect the child's or parents' feelings at a given point in time. They may be concerned with a physiologic problem, such as hematuria or edema. Or, the problem may be emotional or social, such as in the case of an obese teenager with a poor self-concept. The nursing diagnosis may focus on adaptation to feeding, as in the adjustment of a child and family to a child's cleft lip and palate.

A part of the planning process is the creation of a written nursing care plan. The plan should include a statement of the problem, the approach to be used in resolving it, and the means by which the health team will know the need is met. A care plan should be written for all hospitalized children and their families. In this way, continuity of care can be ensured regardless of the time of day or the individual who is taking care of a particular patient. Both short-term and long-term goals are identified in the plan. Short-term goals may be achieved in a matter of days; in fact, several may be accomplished before a long-term goal is reached. Short-term problems occur early in the hospitalization period.

Statements of goals and the means of achieving them should be brief, containing only what is to be done, when it is to be done, how it is to be done, and by whom. The words used should be clearly understood by the members of the staff. For the pediatric patient, additional considerations include the child's level of growth and development, his or her position in the family structure, and individual socioeconomic or cultural influences, as well as the pathophysiologic problem. The written care plan is used by all health team members in charting. Charting documents the plan of care and helps to identify new goals or priorities.

Implementation

The process of implementation involves giving direct care to the child and providing for activities that meet both the child's and the parents' needs. During this period of implementation, the parent and child are observed carefully. Some needs may be met with one or two contacts with the child. Other needs may not yet be recognized. During this period of implementation, the nurse should be aware of the cultural and adaptive behaviors of both the child and the parents. Feedback regarding the effectiveness of implementation aids in completing the last aspect of the nursing process.

Evaluation

The evaluative process determines the degree to which the predetermined goals have been attained. It also helps to identify new goals, expanded or altered information, and changes in perception regarding the original problem. For instance, the condition of the patient may have changed considerably since the initial assessment, even if only a few hours have elapsed. This feedback mechanism may then show the need for further information regarding the disease process, the culture, or the knowledge base of the child or parents. It may also identify goals that were not clearly stated or those that were unrealistic for the patient.

Advantages

One advantage of using the nursing process is a sense of satisfaction for the members of the health team. The setting of realistic goals, the achievement of these goals, and a knowledge of having worked together for better health creates a sense of accomplishment for the health team, the child, and the family.

When the patient is ready to be discharged or transferred to another agency, the care plan eases the transfer. The care plan provides a detailed account of what was done during the hospitalization, how it was done, and the outcome. It may also indicate what has been left unfinished and what must still be completed. The family is thus spared the trouble of explaining to another agency exactly what occurred in the hospital setting.

PHYSICAL ASSESSMENT

The process of physical assessment must be adapted to the particular child being evaluated. In examining young children, any procedures that cause discomfort should be postponed until last. In very young infants, this practice also applies to examination of the head. The mother's lap is an ideal setting for examining the infant. The mother provides for the safety and sense of security of the child, and the examiner has a more cooperative patient, Figure 6-4. Forceful restraint of the child should be avoided whenever possible as it represents a significant threat to the child and increases the child's anxiety level.

Provisions should be made for the environment in which the assessment takes place. The examining room should be reasonably warm, as the child wearing a limited amount of clothing becomes chilled easily. Older children should be afforded some measure of privacy for the examination. They should be permitted to dress and undress without undue exposure, and the time lapse between disrobing and the actual examination should be minimized.

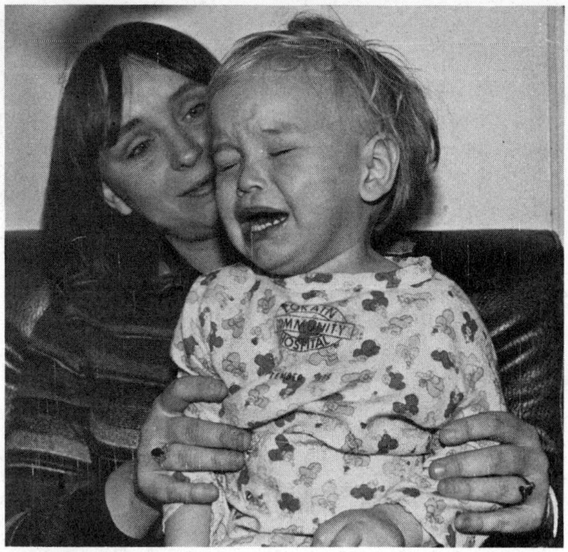

FIG. 6-4 Virtually every toddler responds to the beginning of an examination with some form of protest.

Linear Measurements

The initial portion of the physical assessment is devoted to body measurements or linear measurements of the child. These measurements include height, weight, and head and chest circumferences. The head circumference is most significant in infants younger than one year of age and in those with hydrocephalus, Figure 6-5. In infancy, the circumferences of the head and chest are about equal. The presence or absence of the fontanelles – both anterior and posterior – should also be noted when the head circumference is measured.

Linear measurements should be plotted on a growth chart for accuracy. However, a rough estimate of normal height in inches may be obtained by multiplying the child's age in years by two and adding thirty-two. The

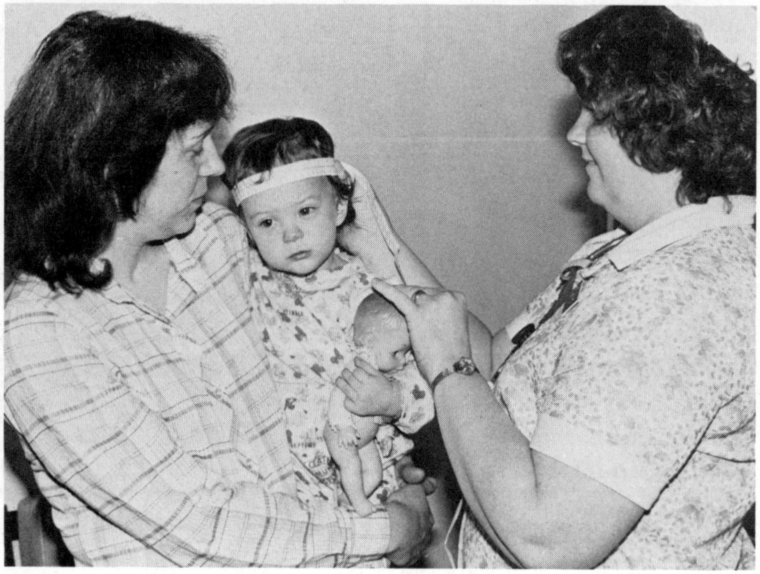

FIG. 6-5 Measuring the child's head is easier when the mother holds the child and the child is given a favorite toy to distract him.

average weight can also be estimated for different age-groups. For infants younger than one year of age, the normal weight in pounds may be approximated by adding eleven to the child's age in months. For any child older than one year of age, the sum of the child's age in years plus eighteen equals the average normal weight in pounds for that age-group.

Vital Signs

The vital signs are recorded for all children. These signs include temperature, pulse, respiratory rate, and blood pressure. Temperature may be determined by the oral, rectal, or axillary method, depending on the age and condition of the child. In general, the temperature of children younger than seven years of age is taken rectally unless a condition such as a rectal prolapse contraindicates this method. In children, the apical pulse is most accurate. However, this should not preclude an assessment of the pulses bilaterally. Respirations should be counted for a full minute. Additionally, the quality, as well as the chest excursion, should be noted. The blood pressure should be measured in every child, regardless of size. In choosing a blood pressure cuff, the child's size should be considered. If taking the blood pressure in the upper extremities proves to be difficult, the lower extremities may be used. Systolic measurements in children one year of age or younger are normally equal in both upper and lower extremities. In children older than one year of age, systolic readings in the lower extremities are generally 40 mm Hg higher than the upper extremity reading. Diastolic measurements are usually the same in both upper and lower extremities throughout childhood. Children with patent ductus arteriosus, coarctation of the aorta, or hypertension may have significantly widened pulse pressures.

General Assessment

Skin. The overall appearance of the child's skin should be noted. Observations should include the condition of the skin, its texture, and hydration status. The color of the skin, including variations of color as with pallor or cyanosis or increased intensity of color as in flushing, should be noted. Textural abnormalities, including the presence of dryness, scaling, or any isolated lesions, should be documented. The presence of old or healing scars should also be noted. The stage of healing of any identified bruises is also noteworthy. Observations of tissue turgor and elasticity which indicate the adequacy of hydration should be recorded.

Hair and Nails. Along with inspection of the skin, the condition of the child's hair and nails should be noted. Is the hair very fine and dry? Does it break easily? Does it appear very oily? Does it lack luster? Are the nails normal in thickness and appearance? Do they appear to be discolored? Are there obvious signs of infection around the nailbeds?

Face. On inspecting the child's face, the nurse should note whether the facial expression of the child indicates an interest and responsiveness to others. Is the responsiveness appropriate for the child's age? The relationship between the outer canthus of the eye and the position of the ears should be noted. Are the responses to light touch equal on both sides of the face? When the child is smiling, crying, or frowning, are the muscles used symmetrically? If not, are there obvious signs of paralysis on one side? Are any areas of edema present, particularly in the periorbital area of the infant and young child?

Eyes. Examination of a child's eyes should include an assessment for any obvious signs of drainage. Is the sclera a normal color? Do the eyes appear to be equal in size and shape? Is excessive tearing or light sensitivity present? Does the child observe an object adequately when one eye is covered? Does the child notice objects in the peripheral field of vision? Is the child able to move the eyes vertically and horizontally in all visual fields? When a penlight is positioned at a distance of two feet from the child, does the light reflect back from the center of the pupil in both eyes? If the child is a preschooler, is he or she able to distinguish between various colors? Is the conjunctiva moist? Are the eyelids a normal dark pink? Does the child blink excessively?

Nose. The nares should be inspected visually. Is any discharge present? If so, the color and amount should be recorded. Patency of the nares is determined by obstructing each side in turn and assessing the airflow through the other nostril. If the child is of preschool age or older, the child may be asked to close his or her eyes and to identify specific substances by odor. This is an indication of nerve function.

Mouth and Throat. The mouth and throat are next in the sequence of the assessment. The inside of the mouth should be inspected using a flashlight and a tongue blade, Figure 6-6. The condition of the teeth should be evaluated. Does the child have a normal complement of teeth for his or her age? Are they in good condition, or are caries present? Is the tongue a normal pink color and uncoated? Are the gums a dark pink color and firm without any visible lesions? Are the buccal membranes normal in color? Are any signs of buccal irritation present?

The pharynx should also be examined and any evidence of drainage in the back of the throat noted. The size of the tonsils should be evaluated and any sign of inflammation noted. The tonsils may be large normally,

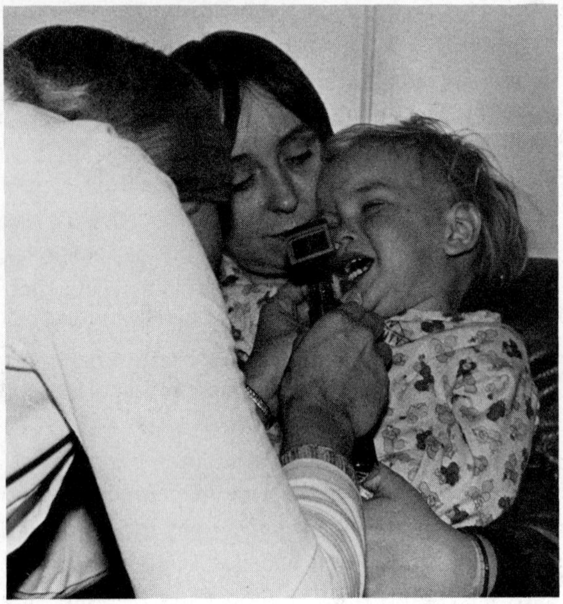

FIG. 6-6 Inspection of the mouth is a routine part of the physical assessment.

depending on the age of the child, but they should not be inflamed. The presence of any odors and the amount of salivation should also be noted. The presence of the gag reflex and the ability to swallow and to move the tongue freely in all directions should also be documented.

Ears. The ears should be inspected using an otoscope, Figure 6-7. The placement of the ears should be noted. Is the top of the ear in a direct line from the outer canthus of the eye, as is normal? Is the color of the outer ear a normal fleshtone or is it unusually waxy in appearance? When looking in the ear, is it free of foreign bodies and discharge in the canal? (Wax is normally present in moderate amounts.) Does the tympanic membrane have a gray, opaque appearance without any signs of redness or irritation? Does the infant or toddler respond to sounds occurring outside

FIG. 6-7 Using an otoscope to inspect the ears

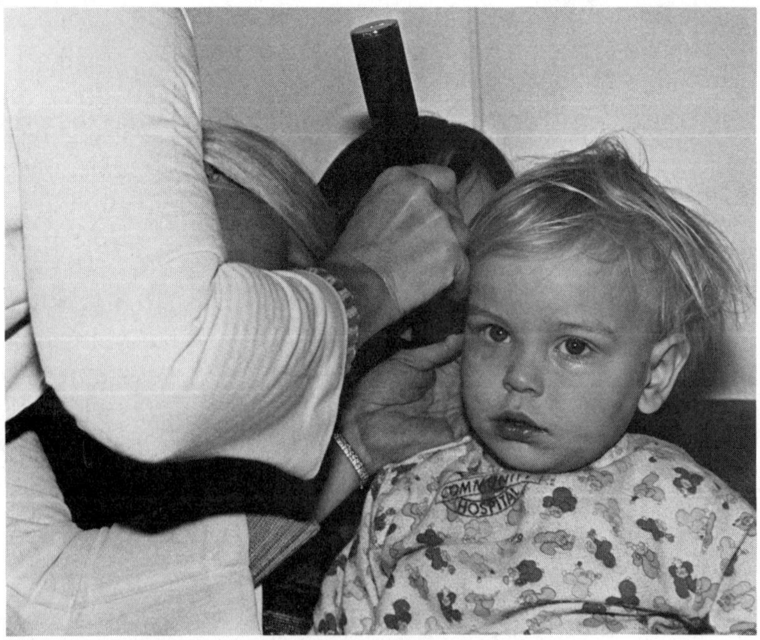

the field of vision? If examining an older child, is there a history of poor school performance? Does the child respond to the sound of fingers being rubbed together in front of each ear? Does the child hear the ticking of a watch? Audiometric testing may be done if there is any question about the child's hearing ability.

Neck. The appearance and condition of the neck is the next part of the assessment. The position of the neck in relation to the head should be noted. Is the child able to move the neck in a full range of motion? Are the neck muscles of equal strength? Is the child able to turn his or her head against the resistance of a hand? Is the child able to raise the shoulders against resistance? Can the trachea, larynx, and thyroid be palpated in the midline? Are the pulsations in the carotid arteries equally strong? Are palpable cervical nodes present?

Chest. The condition of the chest should also be evaluated. Do the nipples and breast tissue appear to be normal for the child's age? It should be remembered that both male and female infants may have some discharge and swelling of the breast tissue. Moreover, during puberty, breast tissue may be somewhat enlarged in the male as well as in the female. Are the axillary lymph nodes palpable? If a chest measurement is taken, it should be measured at the nipple level. The chest measurement is usually smaller than is the head circumference in infants younger than five months of age.

Heart. A stethoscope is used to listen to the heart, Figure 6-8. The position in which the apical beat is the loudest should be noted. This is usually at the mid-clavicular line and at the lower rib margin. The rate, rhythm, and intensity of the heartbeat should be evaluated. Any unusual sounds or murmurs should be noted. Heart sounds are easiest to hear in cooperative children who are able to exhale and hold their breath for several seconds on request.

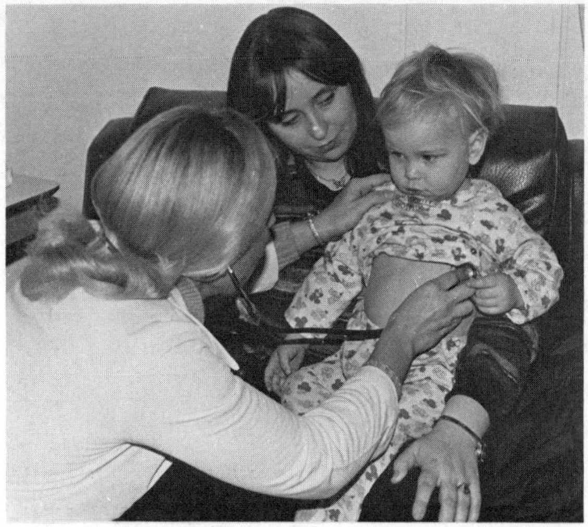

FIG. 6-8 A stethoscope is used for heart and lung assessment.

Respirations. The respiratory movements of the chest are also evaluated. Do both sides of the chest appear to be equal during expansion? Do the lower costal margins flare slightly? This is normal until the onset of puberty. The breath sounds are evaluated using a stethoscope. The duration of the inspiratory and expiratory phases of respiration should be noted. The expiratory phase should be approximately twice as long as the inspiratory phase. The nurse should listen to three breaths in each area and should compare both sides of the chest. Differences in sounds that occur during deep breathing and coughing, as well as inspiration and expiration, should be noted.

Abdomen. The size and contour of the abdomen should be assessed. Respiratory movements are visible in the abdominal area of infants and toddlers, particularly when they are sleeping. Is the abdomen symmetric, without any unusual protrusions? Toddlers normally have protuberant abdomens. Is the umbilicus normal according to the child's age? Are the femoral pulses equal on both sides? Using a stethoscope, can the gentle rumbling of bowel sounds be heard?

Genitalia. The genitalia should be inspected for any abnormalities. Are the normal structures of the external genitalia present? Are the structures appropriate in size and configuration for the child's age? Is there any evidence of lesions, areas of irritation, or infection? The configuration of the anus and the condition of the perineum should also be noted.

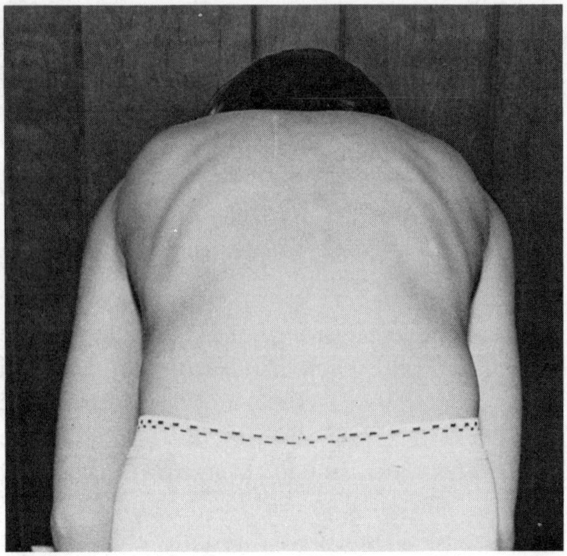

FIG. 6-9 Checking the level and symmetry of the shoulders is an important aspect of the assessment of an older child. The slight prominence of the left rib cage is evident in this child.

Back and Extremities. The condition of the back and the extremities should be noted as well. The symmetry and use of the back should be observed while the child is sitting, standing, and walking. The child should be asked to touch the toes, and the shoulders should be observed for symmetry as he or she slowly becomes erect, Figure 6-9. The extremities should be examined for any evidence of edema, color or temperature changes, or lesions. If the presence of the pulses in the extremities has not yet been documented, it should be checked at this time. The appearance and color of the nail beds are observed, as is the speed of color return after pressure has been applied and released. The muscles should be inspected for equality in size, strength, and tone. Normal range of motion without discomfort should be present in all joints. In a young infant, particular attention is paid to the spine. The presence of spina bifida or a pilonidal sinus is often indicated by an abnormal tuft of hair.

Nurse's Role

The pediatric nurse is in an excellent position to observe normal characteristics and any deviations from normal, both of which should be charted. The child should then be referred to the physician for additional evaluation. As the physical assessment is part of the initial contact with the child, he or she may not be entirely cooperative. Many of the observations may be repeated and documented as the child is given daily care. This approach provides a more relaxed situation and the accuracy of observations may be improved.

CHARTING

All of the observations made during the physical assessment should be included in the patient's chart. In some agencies, the information gained from the physical assessment is included on the admission sheet. In other agencies, this information becomes a part of the initial charting note. These charted observations influence the nursing process by documenting or excluding potential or actual problems. The objectives for a patient are altered on the basis of the observations made by the nurse.

Information obtained should be recorded in the chart as soon as possible. In this way, the information is not altered by omissions or inaccurate interpretations on the part of the nurse.

All observations recorded in the patient's chart should be clear, concise, factual, and specific. An inexperienced nurse may write a great deal on the chart, only to find that the information is of little value. A guideline for recording information is simply to write what can be seen, heard, smelled, or felt. Such objective observations are important in documenting the child's condition. Frequent observations of the child aid in accurate documentation. The parent-child interaction is also included in the observation and documentation.

What Can Be Seen. The nurse should check for bleeding in a postoperative patient. The amount of blood, its color, and the rate of flow are important observations to document. If the child returned from surgery with a clean and intact dressing, saturation of the dressing with bright blood or other discharge within one hour is a significant finding. The rate of saturation is also important.

The general appearance of the patient should be described. Is the child unusually pale or ashen? Is the child generally alert, or does he or she seem unusually sleepy or lethargic?

What Can Be Heard. The nurse should document what is heard as well as what is seen. This is very important in pediatrics because the child may not be able to or may not be inclined to share concerns with the health team. Rather, the child may share concerns exclusively with the parents. The parents, in turn, should be encouraged to share the child's feelings and concerns with members of the health team.

The cry of a young child is as significant as a verbalized complaint. Is the cry high-pitched? Is it continuous or intermittent? Does the child cry only when placed in certain positions? Does the crying occur only when the abdomen is touched? Do the child's respirations sound labored?

The absence of sound may be equally significant. Is the child unusually quiet? Is a verbal response to pain absent? Are breath sounds absent over a lower lobe of the lung where wheezing had been obvious before?

What Can Be Smelled. The nurse should also document what can be smelled. For instance, the odor of acetone on a child's breath should be documented. If the urine of an infant is particularly foul-smelling, that, too, should be reported. Charting of such information frequently reinforces subsequent laboratory reports. For example, foul-smelling urine may be the first sign of a urinary tract infection. A subsequent urine culture and sensitivity report may indicate a high bacterial count, thereby confirming the nurse's suspicions. Moreover, although drainage from a wound is usually described, its smell should also be noted.

What Can Be Felt. What the nurse can feel is just as important as other observations. A distended abdomen may be detected by touch. Palpable differences in skin temperature between one extremity and another should also be identified and charted. Increased skin temperature around an injury generally precedes swelling or redness.

Ambiguity. The use of vague general terms makes it difficult to document a child's condition. The statement that an infant had a "poor night" is an example of ambiguous charting. Does this mean that the infant did not sleep at all, or that the infant cried all night? Does it mean that the infant was obviously hungry and fussing most of the night as a result of a restricted fluid intake?

The terms *appear* and *apparently* also tend to confuse the chart reader. When the nurse observes a maculopapular eruption over the anterior trunk, does the chart read that the patient "appears to have" this skin condition? If the nurse observed it, then the skin eruption was indeed present. The terms used should state what was observed, without qualification.

Systems of Charting

The system within which the charting is done will vary from agency to agency. One of the more commonly used methods for organization of the child's chart is the Problem-oriented Record. The initial data base is collected and a problems list is established. Each of the problems is given an identifying number. Referral to any problem thereafter is according to number. A numbered list of both active and inactive problems is usually located at the front of the chart for a common reference. The charting then addresses the specific problems and documents progress, resolution, and recurrence of problems.

The progress notes in this system have an S-O-A-P format. The entry note begins with the identified problem and then progresses through (S) subjective data; (O) objective data; (A) assessment of the previous data; and (P) plan of care. The plan should include not only the diagnostic and treatment plan but also the patient or parent teaching that must be done.

INFLUENCES ON THE CARE OF HOSPITALIZED CHILDREN

Multiple factors influence the care of the hospitalized child. Some of these factors have a direct influence, whereas others have a more subtle effect. The two major factors that have a direct bearing on a child's hospitalization are the family structure and the cultural beliefs of the family. It is important for the nurse to recognize the part each of these factors plays in a particular child's life, and to include these considerations in the application of the nursing process.

Family Structure

The term *family* is generally used to refer to the nuclear family which is composed of the father, the mother, and their biologic children. Since the late 1950s, the rate at which marriages have dissolved has drastically increased the number of children living in single-parent homes. At the present time, fifteen percent of the pediatric population fit this category. The majority of these children are living with their mothers. However, this pattern is also changing as the number of men seeking and obtaining custody of their children is rapidly increasing.

Single-parent families may or may not have additional potential for influencing the care of a hospitalized child. Certainly this possibility should not be assumed as a natural outgrowth of the single-parent situation. Rather, the nurse should be aware of the potential for problems and should remain alert to clues that would indicate the need for additional help in some areas and referral in others.

One of the most common sources of problems in single-parent families is income. Single parents who are employed may be functioning at the poverty level. The combination of a low salary and the prohibitive cost of babysitting or day-care services may present severe economic problems, especially for the family of a hospitalized child.

Within the single-parent family, a reshifting of roles and a reshifting of family relationships usually occurs. Financial arrangements usually undergo a similar transition.

At times, the single parent may feel overwhelmed by the total responsibility of the family. The hospitalization of a child may increase these feelings of helplessness. In this situation, both parent and child must shoulder additional responsibilities.

The children generally serve as the link between divorced or separated parents. They may, in fact, be the link between two opposing forces. They may find themselves the recipients of gifts and treats from the absent parent. This may contribute to their perception of their respective parents' homes as the "haves" and the "have-nots." Thus, the children, as the link, may foster either a positive or a negative relationship, which in turn may influence their response to hospitalization.

Cultural Background

The cultural background of the family directly influences the child in a hospital setting. The priorities of a given culture may differ significantly from those of the nurse. Nurses must, therefore, be able to recognize the concerns and priorities of other cultures. They must also recognize those aspects of the family's culture that are similar to their own so that the bonds between the two cultures are identified and strengthened. Work with the family then can proceed in a nonjudgmental, accepting fashion.

Black American Families. Children are valued in this culture, and often assume adult roles very early in life. The child's relationship with the parents is generally quite close. This closeness may extend to the more distant family of aunts, uncles, and other relatives. Increasing mobility of a geographic and socioeconomic nature interferes with this extended family concept and adds to stress.

Multiple health concerns exist for Black American families. There is a high infant and maternal mortality among this population. Hypertension is much more common in Black Americans, particularly in the younger age-groups, than in other segments of the population. Sickle cell anemia causes major health problems for Black American children. The death rate from respiratory problems associated with substandard living conditions is high. Lead poisoning continues to afflict children in ghetto areas. Individual families may not seek health care until the problem is serious. In certain segments of the population, home remedies and folk medicine are strong influences on health care.

Nursing Implications. Multiple implications for nursing care may be derived from a knowledge of the Black American family. When assessing the skin of a Black American, it is important to use daylight, if possible. Cyanosis is not always visible by observing the skin, but may be detected in the oral mucosa. Jaundice is difficult to detect in this population unless the sclera of the eyes is examined carefully. Inflammatory areas of the skin may not be visible, but may be recognized on the basis of pain, warmth, or tenderness. Mongolian spots or discolored patches over the lumbar or sacral areas of the back are frequently present in Black American infants and children, and are of no significance.

Hair care in this population is another concern for the nursing staff. Immediately after washing and towel-drying the hair, an oil or lubricant should be applied to the hair and scalp prior to combing. The hair is then combed and allowed to dry.

The type of food served in the hospital may present additional problems for the Black child. The child may be used to eating particular types of food at home, such as pork or food that is highly seasoned. The food offered in the hospital setting may not appeal to the child because of its unfamiliarity and blandness. If the child refuses to eat, the parents may be encouraged to bring in some foods from home that are compatible with the child's diet.

Mexican American Families. The Mexican American family is typically patriarchal in its structure, with decisions generally being made by the husband or father. The father is disciplinarian while the mother nutures. There is a strong sense of family identification. The parents are usually indulgent with younger children. Traditionally, the family's welfare is the first priority, followed by consideration of the needs of the individual family member. Values are clearly defined in this population, and close adherence to behavioral patterns is the norm. Mexican American families are also generally oriented to the present.

Cultural values in this population have a strong influence on health care. Mexican American families may be isolated by choice within their own cultural communities and may seek outside assistance infrequently. The health practices of certain segments of the population are rooted in folk medicine and faith healing. For many Mexican Americans, religious beliefs also affect their health care directly. Some believe that God is responsible for all suffering and illness. Others may seek treatment from the folk healer prior to seeking formalized medical assistance.

Nursing Implications. Nurses may encounter some unusual health beliefs and practices in working with Mexican Americans. Parents may be particularly concerned with "fallen" fontanelles, drafts, or the "evil eye." The condition referred to as fallen fontanelles *(mollera caida)* is accompanied by symptoms of gastroenteritis with dehydration. It is viewed as the result of pulling the nipple out of the child's mouth too rapidly. Holding the child by the feet and pushing on the palate is believed to cure this condition. Another cure for this condition is thought to be an egg white and soap poultice which is placed on the child's fontanelle in order to "draw it out." The child may be admitted to the hospital with the poultice still on the head.

Drafts *(sereno)* are thought by some to be caused by evil spirits present in the night air. These drafts are believed to cause fever and respiratory infections. To prevent these complications, the child is covered before being taken outside, regardless of the temperature.

Health care workers may also encounter Mexican Americans who believe in the effects of the evil eye *(mal de ojo)*. According to this belief, a woman who admires a child must also touch it in some way. Otherwise, she may be suspected of giving the child the evil eye. The child will then become ill with vomiting, fever, and irritability unless a cure is effected immediately. The cure consists of rubbing the child all over with a whole raw egg. The egg is then broken and placed in a dish under the child's bed overnight. Inspection of the egg in the morning confirms the cure.

Puerto Rican Families. Puerto Rican families are generally Spanish-speaking and are of Spanish and Black descent. Religion is generally a major influence within this group. This population shares some of the beliefs of the Mexican Americans, but the values, attitudes, and life-style of Puerto Ricans are generally distinct to their culture and should not be confused with those of the Mexican American family. The extended family structure that is common in this population exerts a major influence and may tend to isolate families from contacts outside the group. Adherence to traditional cultural beliefs decreases in those families with increased socioeconomical status and with a greater length of time in this country.

Nursing Implications. High infant mortality and a high incidence of respiratory diseases, such as tuberculosis, are common among Puerto Ricans because of poor nutrition and the suboptimal living conditions in many areas. Parasitic diseases, such as hookworm, are also common in this group, particularly new arrivals in the United States. Faith healers can play a significant role in the community and should not be disregarded when teaching the family about health care.

Asian Families. This cultural group comprises several different groups. Asian families often form a very close unit which includes the extended family. They may be quite patriarchal in nature and some of the more traditional families do not speak English. It is not uncommon for several families to reside in a single-family dwelling within a community.

Nursing Implications. This cultural group utilizes acupuncture, but the concept of energy flow and balance as crucial to health is a more important influence. Major health problems of this group include tuberculosis, malnutrition, communicable diseases, and mental illness. Some families will not seek medical assistance, preferring to trust folk medicine. Others may believe that blood cannot be replaced once it is removed and are, therefore, fearful of blood tests. As the hospital diet may be unacceptable to the child, the family may be encouraged to bring in food that the child will eat. Some Asian communities have built their own hospitals in order to preserve the traditions yet provide good health care. These hospitals provide excellent resources for nurses working with Asian families.

SUMMARY

The nursing process provides an organized basis for collecting data and giving care according to established priorities. The quality of care and its continuity for both the child and the parents are dependent on its use.

A complete physical assessment adds to the data base. All information should be recorded accurately and concisely as soon as it is obtained. A complete assessment evaluates both the physical growth of the child and his or her developmental level.

The information provided by the parents and child, which is then incorporated into the nursing process, is influenced significantly by the cultural values and attitudes of the family. The nurse must be accepting of these cultural values and must work within their context in delivering care to the child.

SUGGESTED ACTIVITIES

- Complete a physical assessment of a child assigned to your unit. Determine whether the child is within the normal range of growth and development for the appropriate age group. Note the areas you questioned. Was the information recorded accurately?
- Develop a nursing care plan for one child on your unit. Take into account the health problem of the child, the child's growth and developmental level, and his or her cultural background.

DISCUSSION TOPICS

1. Spend several hours with a parent and child from a culture different from your own. Get to know the other family's customs, interests, likes, and dislikes, particularly with regard to health care practices. Share your findings with your class.
2. Separate your class into small groups. Have each group review the nursing notes of an individual patient's chart. Discuss the objectivity and usefulness of the observations recorded. Explain how you could improve the clarity or conciseness of the information.

REVIEW

A. Matching. Match the activity in Column I with the proper phase of the nursing process in Column II.

Column I	Column II
1. Sorting and validating the identified needs of the patient to set priorities	a. Assessment
2. Determining that the identified goals have been attained	b. Planning
3. Providing direct care to the child	c. Implementation
4. Identifying the child's problems through data collection	d. Evaluation

B. Multiple choice. Select the one best answer.

Situation: You are assigned to care for Anna, a three-year-old patient who is scheduled for an operation. Upon meeting her, you begin forming a plan for care. The components of your nursing care plan include:

A. revising the nursing care plan
B. prescribing nursing actions
C. identifying the patient's needs and concerns
D. evaluating the nursing care plan
E. implementing the nursing care plan
F. writing the objectives for nursing care

1. The usual sequence for performance of these actions would be
   a. F, C, B, D, A, E.
   b. C, F, B, E, D, A.
   c. B, F, C, E, A, D.
   d. E, A, F, D, B, C.
2. Your physical assessment of Anna should include
   1. linear measurements.
   2. laboratory tests.
   3. systematic observation.
   4. vital signs.
   a. 1 only
   b. 1 and 2
   c. 2, 3, and 4
   d. 1, 3, and 4

C. Short answer. Briefly respond to the following statements.

1. List three health problems that are more prevalent in Black American families than in the general population.
2. Describe an assessment for cyanosis in a Black American child.
3. Identify three characteristics of good charting.

BIBLIOGRAPHY

Bello, Teresa A. "The Third Dimension: Cultural Sensitivity in Nursing Practice." *Imprint,* Vol. 23 (1976), pp. 36–38.

Billingsley, A. *Black Families in White America.* Englewood Cliffs, NJ: Prentice-Hall, Inc., 1968.

Chinn, Peggy L., and Cynthia J. Leitch. *Child Health Maintenance: A Guide to Clinical Assessment.* St. Louis: C. V. Mosby Company, 1974.

Ferholt, J., and Deborah Lott. *Clinical Assessment of Children.* Philadelphia: J. B. Lippincott Company, 1980.

Hymovich, Debra P., and Martha U. Barnard. *Family Health Care: General Perspectives,* 2nd ed. New York: Mc-Graw Hill Book Company, 1979.

Little, Dolores E., and Doris L. Carnevali. *Nursing Care Planning,* 2nd ed. Philadelphia: J. B. Lippincott Company, 1976.

Scipien, Gladys M., et al. *Comprehensive Pediatric Nursing.* New York: McGraw-Hill Book Company, 1975.

U.S. Bureau of Census. "Marital Status and Living Arrangements." *Current Population Reports.* Series P-20, No. 306. Washington, D.C., 1977.

Watson, Annita, and Marlene Mayers. *Nursing Care Planning: Chronic Problem—Stat Solution.* Stockton, CA: K/P Company, Medical Systems, 1976.

Chapter 7

Oral and Parenteral Medications

OBJECTIVES

Upon completion of this chapter, the student will be able to

- calculate pediatric doses of medications according to Clark's, Fried's, and Cowling's rules.
- identify the intramuscular injection sites used for infants and children and explain the rationale for their use.
- describe the nursing responsibilities related to medication administration and intravenous therapy in pediatric patients.
- estimate fluid requirements for a given child using the formula that is based on the relationship between metabolic function and weight in kilograms.

ADMINISTRATION OF MEDICATIONS

Guidelines for the administration of medications to pediatric patients are somewhat similar to those established for the administration of medications to adult patients. However, there are additional factors that must be considered when treating children. Adjustments must be made for the child's size as well as for his or her level of comprehension.

In all situations, the nurse must make certain that the order that appears on the medicine ticket or the medication record sheet is identical to that which is written on the physician's order sheet. According to individual hospital policy, patients must be positively identified prior to administering any medication. The container label or the unit dose package should be compared with the ticket or medication record often enough to ensure the accuracy of both the medication and the dosage strength, Figure 7-1. Medications prepared by a nurse may only be administered by that same nurse.

Oral Medications

When administering oral medications to a child, the nurse must enlist the child's cooper-

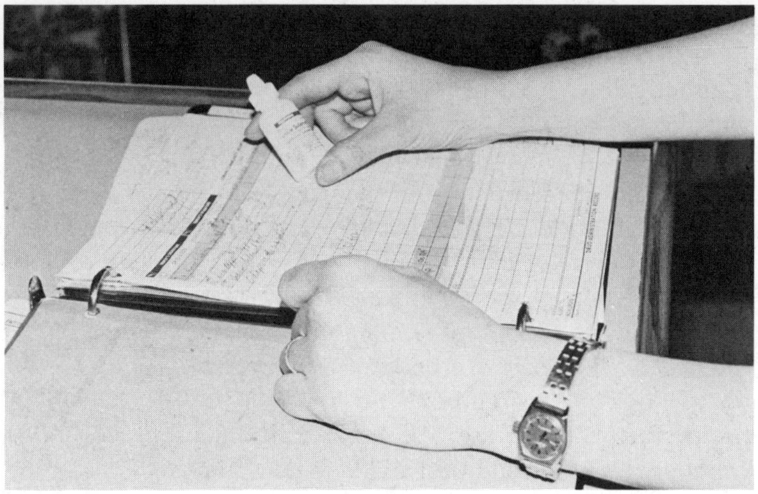

FIG. 7-1 Checking the prescribed medication against the written order

ation with the administration procedure. The nurse's approach should reflect an awareness of the child's level of development. The child should be approached in a firm but friendly manner, and should be informed that it is time to take the medication. This is not a situation in which the child has any choice. Therefore, the nurse should avoid statements such as, "Would you like to take your medicine now?" Frequently, the child does not want to take the medication, and if a choice is implied, it will only strengthen the negative response. If possible, medications should not be administered immediately upon arousing the child from sleep. Rather, the child should be given a few minutes in which to become fully awake so that he or she can focus on the request to take the medication.

Technique of Administration. When administering oral medications to a small child or infant, a plastic dropper or syringe may be used. The liquid should be directed toward the inner aspect of the child's cheek and released slowly. If it is directed across the tongue or at the back of the throat, the infant may aspirate the medication, or the cough reflex may be stimulated, thereby preventing the child from receiving any medication. Oral medications should never be forced on a child because of the danger of aspiration and subsequent pneumonia.

For administration of oral medications, the position of a young child is the same as that used in feeding an infant. The child is held securely on the nurse's lap. One of the nurse's arms is used to support the child's head and neck and to secure the child's free arm. An infant's head or child's head should always be elevated when liquid medications are being given. Older children may sit up to receive the medication or raise their head if the sitting position is impossible or contraindicated.

If the medication is only available in tablet form it must be crushed unless it is an enteric-coated tablet. The crushed tablet is then mixed with a syrup or liquid that will mask the taste. If the child can tolerate semisolid foods, applesauce may be used. The nurse should be sure to use a relatively small amount as the child may refuse even the applesauce after one or two spoonfuls. Whatever the food or liquid used to deliver the medication, it should be compatible with the child's diet and should not interfere with the absorption of the drug. For example, many antibiotics are not absorbed properly in the presence of milk or milk products and should not be given with these products.

After taking medication, children should be praised for their cooperation and complimented on the positive aspects of their behavior. This serves to reinforce the positive behavior further. The use of a bribe or reward for cooperation should be avoided as it implies that the medication is either bad or a punishment and that the child should receive some compensation for the activity. If the positive reinforcement approach is used consistently, children are usually well-behaved about taking medications, even when the taste is not to their liking.

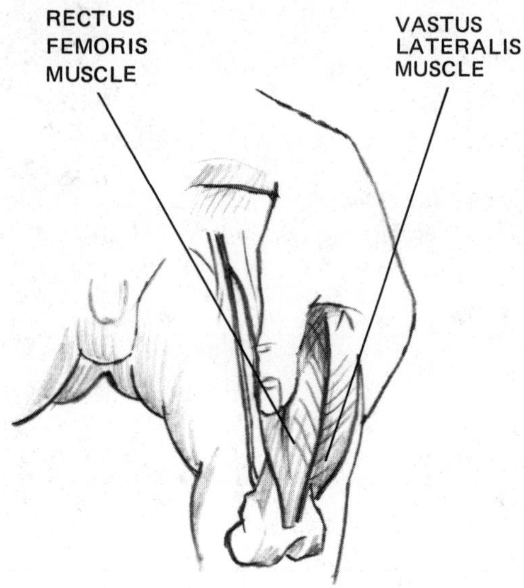

FIG. 7-2 Vastus lateralis muscle in the infant (Adapted from *Intramuscular Injections,* Wyeth Laboratories)

Injectable Medications

Intramuscular injections in infants and children require a sound knowledge of anatomic differences. Nurses must select injection sites carefully so that damage to major nerves and blood vessels is avoided. The administration of injections is most difficult in infants and young toddlers. This difficulty is not because of their inability to cooperate, but rather because of their small muscle mass and the limited number of injection sites available.

Injection in the Thigh. In the infant, the largest muscle group is the quadriceps femoris, which is located in the anterolateral thigh. The chief and largest muscle of this group is the vastus lateralis, which is situated on the anterior surface of the midlateral thigh, Figure 7-2. If this site is used for injection, none of the major nerves and blood vessels will be damaged.

The infant should be in a supine position. The muscle tissue at the upper aspect of the thigh is then compressed with the palm of the nurse's hand, with the fingers directed toward the child's feet, Figure 7-3. The needle is then inserted at a 90-degree angle, directed front to back. The needle should not be inserted to its hub. This is to prevent its complete disappearance should the needle break. The maximal length of a needle for an infant should be one inch. Needle length should be determined according to the weight of the child and the properties of the medication.

An alternative site for injection in the child is the anterolateral surface of the upper

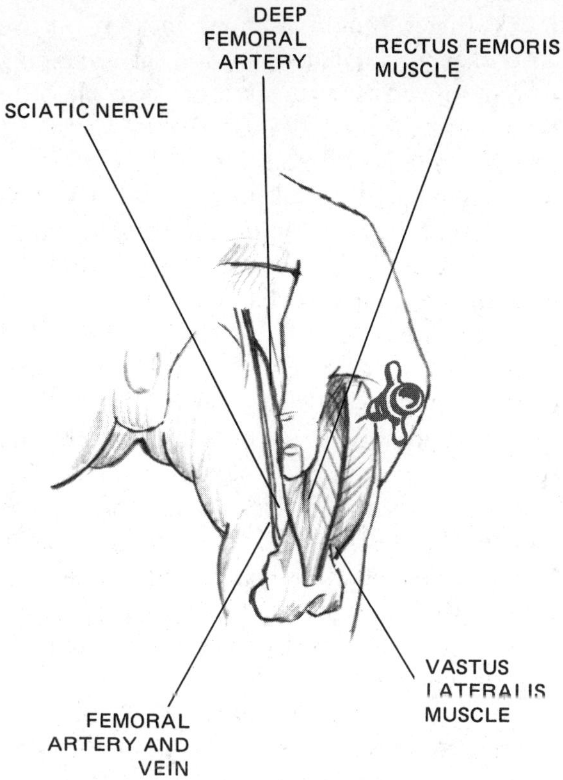

FIG. 7-3 Vastus lateralis site for injections in infants (Adapted from *Intramuscular Injections*, Wyeth Laboratories)

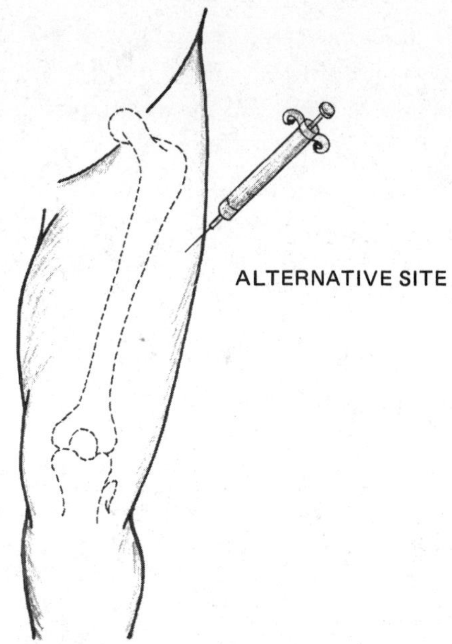

FIG. 7-4 Alternative injection site. Note the 45° angle of the needle. (Adapted from *Intramuscular Injections,* Wyeth Laboratories)

thigh, Figure 7-4. When this site is used, the needle must be inserted at a 45-degree angle with the needle directed toward the knee. As with all others, this site should be inspected prior to injection to rule out tenderness or undue firmness on palpation.

Injection in the Deltoid Muscle. The deltoid muscle may also be used selectively in infants and children. It is usually a last choice and is not used if another site is available. Because of its limited size, use of the deltoid muscle is restricted to certain volumes and types of medications. Generally, the medications are aqueous preparations and the volume does not exceed 1/2 cubic centimeter. The advantage of the deltoid muscle site is that it is accessible regardless of the position of the patient. The exact site of injection should coincide with the largest portion of the muscle. The landmarks to be identified include the acromion process and the axilla in the posterolateral aspect. The muscle mass is compressed between the fingers, and the needle is directed slightly upward toward the shoulder, Figure 7-5.

Injection in the Gluteal Region. The gluteal site for injections includes the ventrogluteal and posterolateral regions in older children. The selection criteria for this site is how long

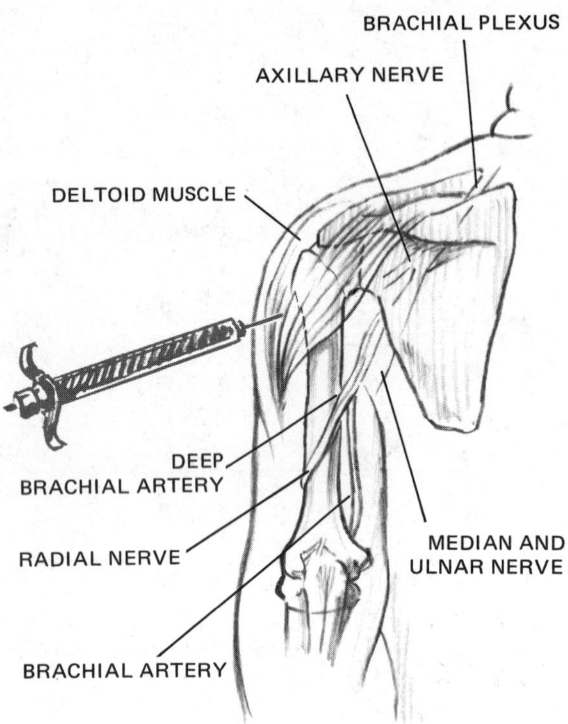

FIG. 7-5 Deltoid site for injections in children (Adapted from *Intramuscular Injections,* Wyeth Laboratories)

the child has been walking rather than age. Any child who has been walking for at least one year has developed sufficient muscle in the gluteal area to allow its use as an injection site. These injection sites do not include the buttocks, which should never be used for injections.

When using the ventrogluteal site, specific landmarks may be identified. These include the greater trochanter, the anterior superior iliac line, and the iliac crest. The nurse should place the palm of the hand over the greater trochanter with the thumb directed toward the anterior surface of the patient's body. The index finger should then be located on the anterior superior iliac spine and the remaining fingers moved as far posterior as possible. The fingers thus form a triangle within which the injection site is centered, Figure 7-6.

The posterolateral portion of the gluteal region that is used for injections is bounded by the posterior superior iliac spine and the head of the greater trochanter, Figure 7-7. The injection site is superior to the imaginary line between these landmarks. The injection is given with the patient in the prone position. The syringe should be perpendicular to the surface upon which the patient is lying. The medication is then injected into the gluteus medius. Suggesting that the child point in the toes will also help to relax the gluteal musculature. This injection site is not usually used in infants or young children because of the location of the sciatic nerve.

Nursing Approach. The nurse can help minimize injection trauma in a number of ways. It is important to be matter-of-fact about the child's cooperation. The nurse should assume that the child will cooperate, but at the same time, should recognize that he or she may not be able to hold still for the procedure. The person administering the medication must, therefore, have assistance to help keep the child still. A minimal amount of time should elapse between the time the child is told of the injectable medication and the time it is administered. The medication should be brought to the child's room already prepared, and it should be placed outside the child's visual field. If the child is old enough to cooperate, a wrapped ice cube may be held over the injection site several minutes prior to the injection in order to minimize discomfort. During the actual injection, dis-

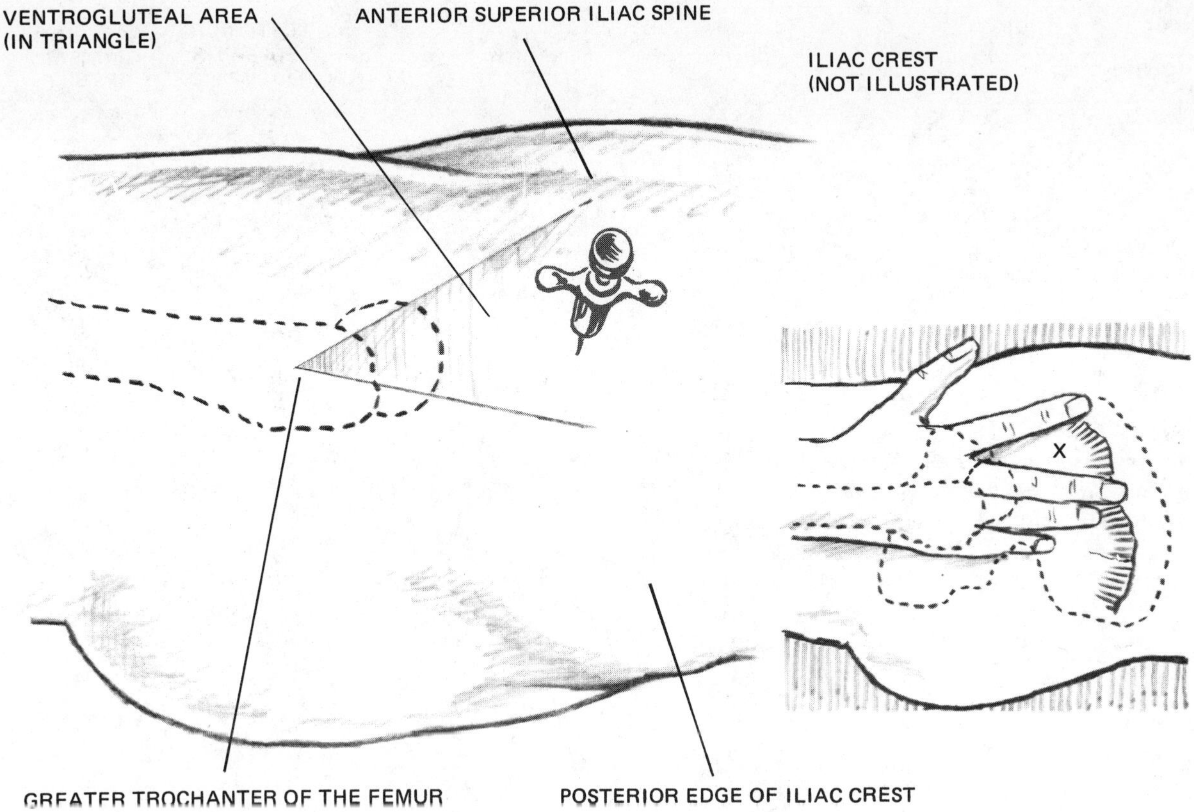

FIG. 7-6 Ventrogluteal site for injection in children. The inset shows the correct placement of the nurse's hand. (Adapted from *Intramuscular Injections*, Wyeth Laboratories)

tractions may prove effective with children. Allowing the child to open a Band-Aid as the injection is being given, or encouraging the child to count, recite the alphabet, sing a nursery rhyme, or shout loudly while holding very still may enhance cooperation.

Following the injection, children should be reassured that they were helpful and that their cooperation was appreciated. Young children may require additional comforting from the nurse. When reassuring the child, the terms "good" and "bad" should be avoided. The child may be sincerely complimented for positive behavior, such as bravery, cooperation, and helpfulness, but no mention should be made of any negative behavior.

Calculation of Dosages

Pediatric dosages of medication are calculated in a variety of ways. Such calculations are primarily the responsibility of the physician ordering the medication. However, the nurse who is administering the medication should verify that the dose that is being given is accurate. The rules for calculating dosage are

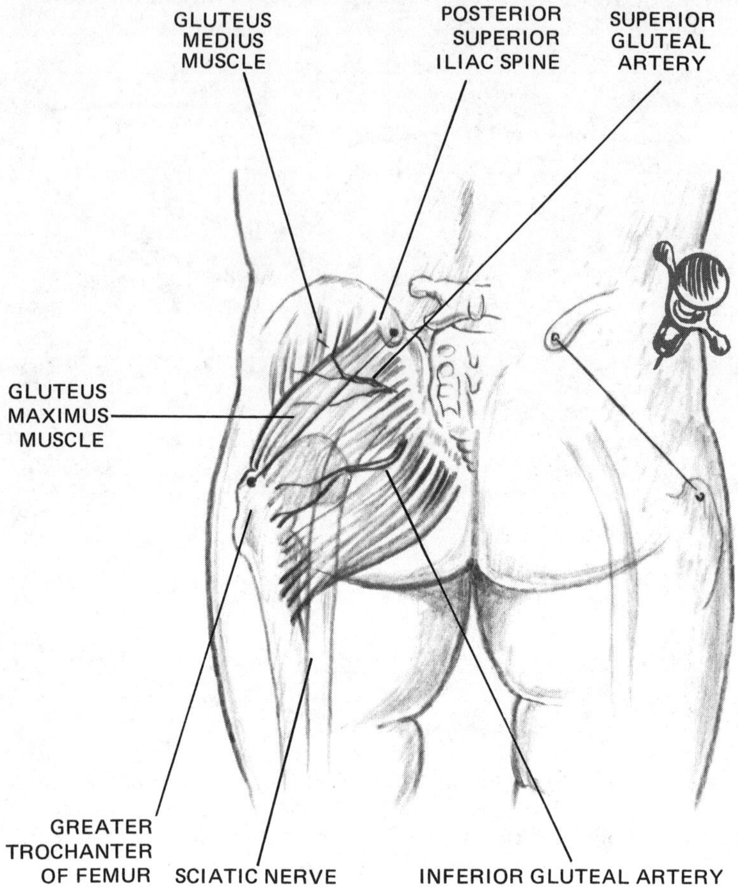

FIG. 7-7 Posterolateral gluteal site for injections in children (Adapted from ***Intramuscular Injections,*** **Wyeth Laboratories)**

based on the age, weight, and body surface area of the child. These rules serve as guidelines and do not take into account the variables of certain pathologic conditions or the physiology of individual infants, toddlers, or adolescents.

The three rules used to calculate dosages according to age are outlined in Table 7-1. The wide variations in height and weight of infants and children of all ages make this method the least reliable. Dosage rules based on body weight are more reliable indicators of the appropriate dosage level, Table 7-2.

The most reliable method of determining dosage is based on the body mass of the child which takes into consideration both height and weight, Table 7-3. Body surface area may be determined with the aid of a nomogram.

INTRAVENOUS THERAPY IN CHILDREN

Intravenous therapy for pediatric patients is a challenge for the nursing staff. Helping the child to accept the treatment, assisting the parents to cope with its restrictions, and main-

Know

TABLE 7-1 Calculation of Dosage According to Age

RULE	EQUATION
Cowling's rule	$\text{Dosage} = \dfrac{\text{age at next birthday} \times \text{adult dose}}{24}$
Fried's rule (for children younger than one year of age only)	$\text{Dosage} = \dfrac{\text{age in months} \times \text{adult dose}}{150}$
Young's rule	$\text{Dosage} = \dfrac{\text{age in years} \times \text{adult dose}}{\text{age in years plus 12}}$

TABLE 7-2 Calculation of Dosage According to Body Weight

RULE	EQUATION
Clark's rule	$\text{Dosage} = \dfrac{\text{weight in pounds} \times \text{adult dose}}{150}$
Dosage in kilograms (kg)	Dosage = dose per kilogram X weight of child in kilograms

TABLE 7-3 Calculation of Dosage According to Body Surface Area

RULE	EQUATION
Based on Clark's rule	$\text{Dosage} = \dfrac{\text{body surface area in square meters} \times \text{adult dose}}{1.73}$
Dosage in square meters	Dosage = dose per square meter X body surface area in square meters

taining the prescribed flow rate with or without additional medications are all parts of that challenge. Intravenous fluid therapy is used for pediatric patients to replace fluid when there is a deficit, such as that caused by vomiting, diarrhea, and other conditions that lead to dehydration. It is frequently used to maintain the patient's current status and to prevent dehydration or electrolyte imbalances. These fluid disorders may occur in patients undergoing surgery who will not be able to consume sufficient amounts of fluids postoperatively.

Intravenous therapy is also used as a supplement or as the primary therapy in treating specific conditions. For example, an oncology patient may require treatment with a chemotherapeutic agent that is only effective when given intravenously.

Of major concern in the use of intravenous therapy in the pediatric population are the differences that exist between adults and children. The metabolic rate of children is vastly different from that of adults. In children, a large proportion of fluids are used in the metabolically active tissues, such as those found in the brain. This explains why the metabolic rate in young children, as well as their fluid needs, is three times that of an adult. As infants and young children grow, the balance shifts gradually. The bone and muscle tissues, which are metabolically less active, start growing rapidly and the growth of the brain and liver tissues tapers somewhat. The high fluid needs of the infant gradually diminish with age until adolescence, when the fluid requirements approximate those of an adult. Both temperature elevations and changes in kidney function alter the metabolic rate and fluid requirement.

General Considerations

The acceptance of intravenous therapy by a child depends not only on physiologic considerations, but more importantly on developmental considerations. Some nursing measures and actions apply equally to all children, regardless of their developmental level. An explanation of the rationale for intravenous therapy, the restriction of mobility, and the need for parental support applies to all children. Pediatric patients receiving intravenous therapy are automatically placed on a regimen of daily weight measurements and strict intake and output recording. Prior to starting the intravenous line, the nurse should assess the hydration status of the patient. This is done by evaluating the child's vital signs, weight, and skin turgor, as well as the condition of the mucous membranes, eyes, and fontanelles, when applicable. The specific gravity of the urine is also determined. Parents may be helpful in supplying information regarding the child's normal pattern of intake and output and hand dominance. If an extremity is chosen as the site for intravenous therapy, the least dominant one is preferred.

Developmental Considerations

Infants. Small infants are totally dependent on others for their needs. The parents of infants should be given an explanation for the use of intravenous therapy, a description of the appearance of the child, and encouragement to comfort and cuddle the child. Parents should be told whether or not they may hold the child, and how to do it safely without dislodging the intravenous line. An explanation of the function of any restraints used for anchoring, as well as the reason for their use, is also warranted. Parents should be alert to the child's swinging of arms or legs, which may cause tension on the intravenous tubing and subsequent needle dislodgement.

In this age-group, scalp vein insertions are well tolerated and are usually the least difficult intravenous sites to maintain. Sandbags are used to maintain the position of the head or to restrain an extremity. When the infant's arm or leg is used, the extremity may be anchored to a sandbag rather than to an armboard. The nurse should make sure that the sandbag is heavy enough to restrain the limb.

Prior to starting intravenous therapy, the infant should receive nothing by mouth for at least one-half hour. This prevents possible vomiting and aspiration during the procedure and reduces the risk to the infant. Some infants may be satisfied with a pacifier during and after the procedure, particularly if oral food and fluids will be withheld for a long period of time.

Toddlers. In toddlers, it is essential that the intravenous line be anchored securely and the needle and insertion site protected. A commercial cover or a medicine cup that has been split vertically and taped, as in Figure 7-8, may be used for this purpose. Minimal restraint should be used with this age-group. Parents have an important role in comforting the child after the intravenous line has been inserted and as the therapy is continued. The child should be reassured frequently by a supportive staff person rather than a parent throughout the insertion procedure.

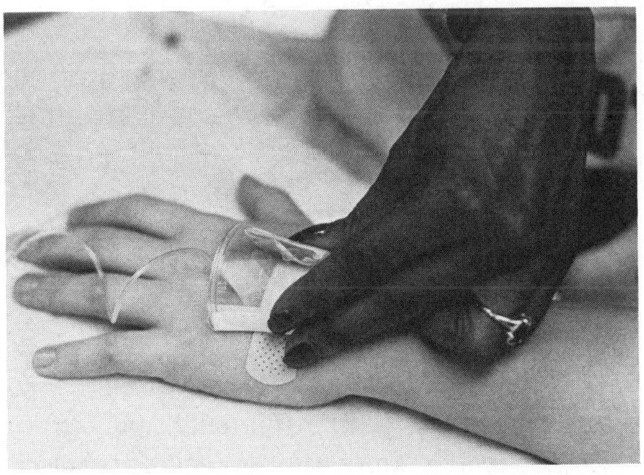

FIG. 7-8 A plastic medicine cup may be split and taped over the intravenous site for added protection.

Because toddlers are both active and curious, all connections must be taped securely and checked frequently. Occasionally, it may be necessary to wrap an elastic bandage lightly around the entire arm and armboard. The disadvantage of this practice is that the bandage must be removed each time the site is checked. Use of diversional therapy works well with this age-group. A variety of playthings may be used to amuse and distract the child. These are often more effective than repeatedly saying no to a child who may be psychologically unable to comply with the nurse's requests.

Preschoolers. Preschool children's fantasies and beliefs in magic present some problems in their care during intravenous therapy. To prepare them for the procedure, children should be allowed to handle the intravenous equipment or some similar equipment. The nurse's explanation of the procedure should be direct and simplified to the child's level. The nurse should reinforce the fact that the procedure is not a punishment.

Preschoolers should be included in simple decision making whenever possible. Their cooperation may be enlisted by involving them in such activities as holding the swab, opening Band-Aids, and helping to apply tape. Assistance in holding the child should be available. Privacy and praise are both important to this age-group. Privacy is a prerequisite for the cooperation of these children, as it helps them to maintain a sense of control over the situation. Praise is also essential in helping them cope with an intrusive procedure of this type. Praise should be given for any efforts to cooperate, not just for complete cooperation. Like the younger age-groups, these children require constant supervision. The intravenous site should be anchored securely and wrapped

FIG. 7-9 The insertion site is taped securely. The patient's name, date, and time of initial infusion are written on the tape.

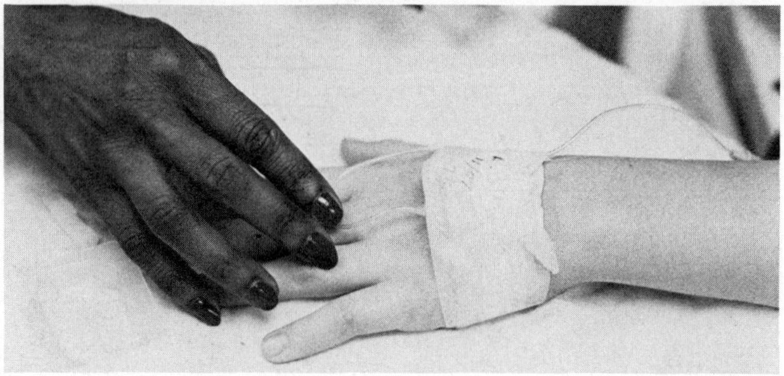

or covered for protection, Figures 7-9 and 7-10. If the child is allowed out of bed, special care must be taken to ensure that the intravenous line is not accidentally dislodged as a result of the child's activities.

School-aged Children. Although school-aged children may place great emphasis on being brave during the intravenous procedure, someone should still be available to assist in holding them still. The staff should anticipate and be accepting of regressive behavior and crying in this age-group. Because of this behavior, the child may not want the parents to be present during the procedure. The child's wishes should be respected. Explanations of the procedure and its rationale should be given to the patient and the family. Both should be taught what activities are permissible and what signs indicate a problem, Figure 7-11. This does not eliminate the need for staff observations. However, it does enhance the child's sense of control over the situation. The use of gowns specially designed to facilitate changes of clothing for the child receiving intravenous therapy may also be helpful, Figure 7-12.

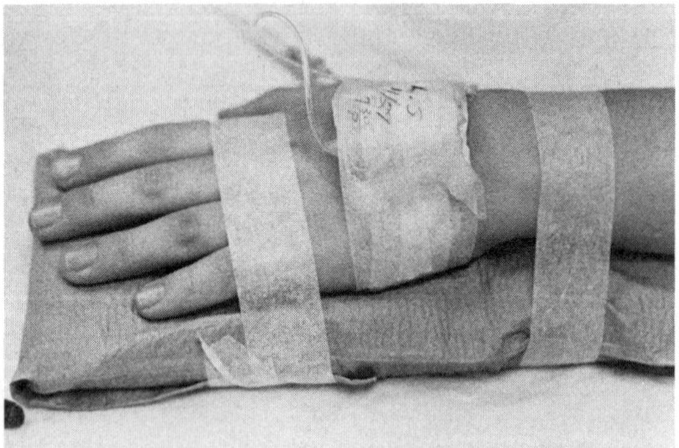

FIG. 7-10 The child's hand may be secured to a covered sandbag. The contour of the sandbag supports the hand while the additional weight reminds the child to be careful.

Adolescents. Adolescents' strong desires for independence add another aspect to their care. They should be told that their independence will be somewhat compromised while they are receiving intravenous therapy. The nursing approach to and explanations offered this age-group are similar to those used for adults. They should be encouraged to help monitor the drip rate, observe for complications, and keep track of intake and output with the staff's supervision. Lack of cooperation is usually related to the adolescent's feelings about parents and authority figures.

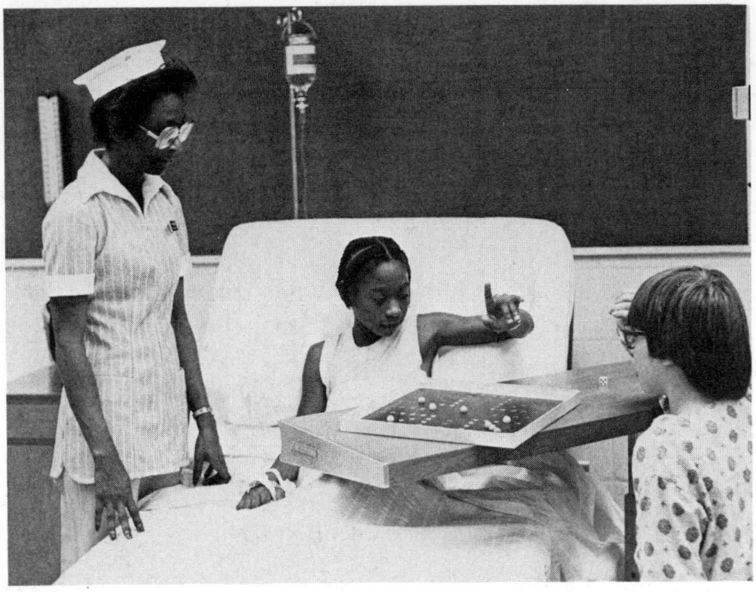

FIG. 7-11 Intravenous therapy should not prevent a patient from continuing activities.

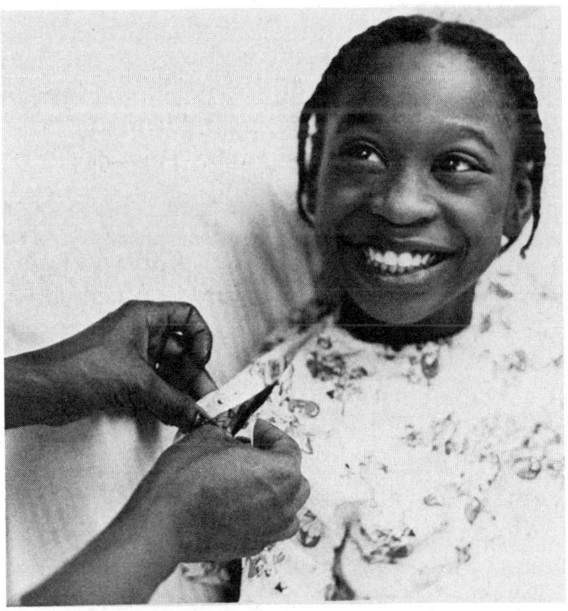

FIG. 7-12 Special gowns have been designed to facilitate the care of patients receiving intravenous therapy.

Estimation of Fluid Requirements

Intravenous therapy is tailored to the specific fluid needs of individual patients. The weight and size of a child, as well as the specific health problem, are considered when calculating fluid needs. Although calculating fluid needs is the physician's responsibility, the nurse should know how it is done.

Fluid needs are closely related to an individual's metabolic rate. The most reliable method of calculating appropriate fluid intake is the calorie expenditure method. With this method, the child's weight in kilograms is recorded. The first 10 kilograms are multiplied by 100 milliliters. The next 10 kilograms are multiplied by 50 milliliters. The remaining kilograms are multiplied by 20 milliliters. The total obtained from adding these amounts together comprises the appropriate twenty-four hour maintenance intake for that particular child. The child with severe fluid deficiencies may need up to one and one-half times this calculation.

This method takes into account the very high percentage of water composition in the tiny infant, as well as the child's decreased fluid requirements per body weight as he or she increases in size. For example, consider the fluid needs of a 14-pound infant. The child's weight is 6.3 kilograms. When that figure is multiplied by 100 milliliters, the result, 630 milliliters, is the child's fluid requirement for twenty-four hours. For an older child weighing 44 pounds (20 kilograms), the first 10 kilograms are multiplied by 100 milliliters which yields 1000 milliliters. The next 10 kilograms are then multiplied by 50 milliliters for a total of 500 milliliters. The total intake for that child should be 1500 milliliters per twenty-four hours.

Administration of Intravenous Therapy

The procedure for administering intravenous therapy varies among different agencies. However, several administration procedures are common to all agencies. The initial order for intravenous therapy is made by the physician who determines the type of solution and the flow rate. Some agencies require that these orders be rewritten at periodic intervals. Others allow the orders to stand until they are changed or discontinued.

A qualified person should perform the venipuncture. Frequently, this is the responsibility of the nurse who has been certified within the agency. This individual selects the size of the needle and the site of puncture. In children, tiny scalp vein or butterfly infusion sets together with a 23- or 25-gauge needle, are preferred. Veins of the hand or forearm are preferred to those in the antecubital space. The superficial veins of the scalp are acceptable sites in infants.

Once the tourniquet is applied, Betadine or another antibacterial preparation is used to cleanse the skin at the venipuncture site. The needle is then inserted and anchored. The size of the needle and the insertion date should be noted on the dressing tape over the intravenous site.

The tubing and the dressing are changed every twenty-four hours. If the intravenous solution is running at a very slow rate and the bag or bottle is not empty within twenty-four hours, it should be changed as well.

The intravenous site should be taped so that the child cannot remove it. Use of restraints should be minimal and will depend on the child's age and ability to cooperate with the therapy.

A volume control chamber, such as Buritrol, may be added to infusion sets between the bag or bottle and the tubing. This chamber contains 50 to 100 milliliters of solution, preventing a greater amount from being infused too rapidly. This device is usually used when an infusion pump is not available. A container of intravenous solution that holds more than 500 milliliters should not be used without a volume control chamber or an infusion pump.

Hyperalimentation Therapy. Special considerations should be made for the child receiving hyperalimentation therapy. The tip of the catheter should be located in the right atrium. The catheter itself is tunneled subcutaneously and sutured at the exit site to prevent it from being dislodged.

The tubing and dressing are changed using strict aseptic technique. The nurse should use alcohol instead of acetone to cleanse the connection sites as acetone causes deterioration of silicone catheters. The hemostats used in changing the tubing should be rubber-shod so that the tubing is not accidentally punctured.

The volume of hyperalimentation fluids is carefully calculated to provide 135 to 150 milliliters of fluid per kilogram of body weight for continuous therapy. The hourly rate must remain within ten percent of the calculated rate in order to reduce the risk of osmotic diuresis or seizures. For this reason, an infusion pump is used.

During hyperalimentation therapy, the daily weight and intake and output of the child are measured carefully. Additionally, the nurse should observe the child frequently for edema and should check the urine periodically for evidence of glycosuria and ketonuria.

MEDICATIONS COMMONLY USED IN CHILDREN

A list of medications commonly used to treat pediatric patients is provided in Table 7-4. Special attention should be directed toward the precautions and the nursing responsibilities relative to each drug.

SUMMARY

The administration of any type of medication carries with it a large measure of responsibility, especially in the treatment of children. The nurse must be familiar with injection sites and administration techniques, as well as the developmental responses of the child.

The ability to calculate the dosage is an important safeguard when children's lives are at stake. It also provides a check system to prevent mathematical errors.

Special considerations apply to hyperalimentation therapy and specific drugs. A knowledge of these considerations enhances the effectiveness and safety of the treatment. Nursing responsibilities include assessment of the child for drug side effects or untoward reactions.

SUGGESTED ACTIVITIES

- Care for a child receiving some type of intravenous or hyperalimentation therapy. Describe the types of solutions used, the calculated flow rate, and the proper use of an infusion pump. Explain how the infusion site can be checked for signs of infiltration.
- Investigate the procedure for administering medications within your assigned agency as stated in the procedure book. Observe how it is carried out on a particular unit. Note especially the correlation of the types and dosages of the medications to the child's age and diagnosis.

DISCUSSION TOPICS

1. Discuss with your class the types of medication errors that can occur and ways in which they can be prevented. Ask the Safety Review Committee within your assigned agency to provide a list of the types of medication errors that have occurred over the past year.
2. Discuss the use of the incident or investigation report in your agency. What is the procedure for its use? What are the legal implications to be considered?

TABLE 7-4 Medications Commonly Used in Pediatrics

Generic Name	Trade Name	Pediatric Dose	Routes of Administration	Special Precautions or Warnings	Nursing Responsibility
Antibacterials					
Amoxicillin	Amoxil Larotid Polymox	20–40 mg/kg in equal, divided doses, q8h	Liquid susp.	Not used in patients with known sensitivity.	Administer doses around the clock. Administer on empty stomach. Observe for hypersensitivity, nausea, vomiting, diarrhea, rash, urticaria, purpura, leukopenia.
Ampicillin	Amcill Alpen Omnipen Penbriten Principen	*Oral:* 50–100 mg/kg in equal, divided doses q6h *IM or IV:* 100–200 mg/kg q6h	PO, IM, IV	May cause agranulocytosis. Use parenteral solutions within one hour of preparation.	Observe for rash, stomatitis, nausea, vomiting, and diarrhea. Administer on an empty stomach.
Cephalexin	Keflex	25–50 mg/kg in divided doses q6h	PO	Possible hypersensitivity to this drug or to penicillins. Contraindicated with renal or hepatic dysfunction.	Observe for rash, diarrhea, pain at injection site, and signs of thrombophlebitis. Evaluate glycosuria with Tes-Tape, or false-positives may result.
Cephalothin sodium	Keflin	40–80 mg/kg/day in divided doses	IM, IV	Same as above	Same as above
Chloramphenicol	Chloromycetin	50–100 mg/kg in divided doses q6h	PO, IV, IM	Contraindicated in patients with bone marrow depression and kidney dysfunction. Restricted to life-threatening infections which cannot be treated by less dangerous drugs.	Observe for rash, diarrhea, and signs of superinfection. Check blood studies weekly. Observe patient for signs of leukopenia.
Disodium carbenicillin	Geopen Pyopen	*IV:* 300–500 mg/kg q4–6h in equal, divided doses *IM:* 50–200 mg/kg q4–6h	IV, IM	High doses may cause bleeding, seizures, vein irritation or pain at injection site. High sodium content may restrict its use in certain conditions. Patients with cephalosporin allergy may react to this drug also.	Observe for hypersensitivity or anaphylaxis. Monitor serum potassium; drug may cause hypokalemia. Monitor venipuncture site for signs of phlebitis.

Erythromycin estolate	Ilosone	*Less than 11.5 kg:* 11 mg/kg q6h *11.5 to 23 kg:* 125 mg/kg q6h *More than 23 kg:* 250–500 mg/kg q6h	Liquid susp.; chewable tablet	Not to be used in patients with pre-existing liver dysfunction or for chronic conditions, such as acne.	Observe for jaundice. Shake oral suspension before use. Store in refrigerator. Administer 1 h before or 2 h after meals (food decreases absorption rate).
Erythromycin ethylsuccinate	E.E.S. Pediamycin	30–50 mg/kg/day in 4–6 equal, divided doses	Same, but buffered	Allergic reactions common.	Observe for skin rashes and urticaria.
Erythromycin stearate	Erythrocin	Same as above	Same as above	Same as above	Same as above
Gentamicin sulfate	Garamycin	*Intrathecal:* 0.5–1.0 mg/day *IM or IV:* 1.0–1.5 mg/kg q8h	IM, IV, intrathecal, cream or ointment	Cautious use in neonates or in patients with impaired renal function.	Observe for ototoxicity and nephrotoxicity. Assess for dizziness, nystagmus, tinnitus, oliguria (include BUN). Maintain adequate I & O. Stop drug on first sign of reaction. Keep patient well-hydrated.
Griseofulvin	Fulvicin Grifulvin-F	11 mg/kg/day in divided doses	PO	Contraindicated in porphyria, liver impairment, and hypersensitivity.	Encourage high fat intake to enhance drug absorption. Observe for photosensitivity, fever, sore throat, and malaise.
Kanamycin sulfate	Kantrex	*IV and IM:* 3–7.5 mg/kg q12h divided doses *Oral:* 12.5 mg/kg q4–6h	PO, IM, IV	Cautious use in patients with impaired kidney function.	Observe for ototoxicity and impaired renal function. Maintain adequate hydration. Record I & O and report decreases.
Sulfamethoxazole	Gantanol	50–60 mg/kg bid; maximum of 75 mg/kg/day	PO	Contraindicated in patients with allergy to sulfa preparations, renal toxicity, or hematologic disorders.	Maintain adequate hydration. Observe for side effects. Obtain blood studies weekly.
Tetracycline hydrochloride	Achromycin Tetracyn	12–25 mg/kg/day in divided doses	PO, IV, IM	Reduced dosage in patients with kidney impairment. Not used in children under 8 years of age because of teeth staining.	Observe for allergic reactions, superinfections, and photosensitivity. Administer on empty stomach. Monitor I & O and evaluate kidney function periodically.

Abbreviation key: mg, milligram; kg, kilogram; q, every; h, hours; IM, intramuscular; IV, intravenously; PO, by mouth; I & O, intake and output; bid, twice daily; tid, three times daily; CNS, central nervous system; HS, at bedtime; PRN, as needed; susp., suspension; GI, gastrointestinal; lb, pound; SC, subcutaneously

(Table continued on following page)

TABLE 7-4 – *Continued*

Generic Name	Trade Name	Pediatric Dose	Routes of Administration	Special Precautions or Warnings	Nursing Responsibility
Anticholinergics					
Atropine sulfate	Same	*Preoperative –IM, IV* 3 kg 0.1 mg/dose 7–9 kg 0.2 mg/dose 12–16 kg 0.3 mg/dose 20–27 kg 0.4 mg/dose *PO*: 0.01 mg/kg; maximum of 0.4 mg/single dose	PO, IM, IV	Can cause respiratory depression and death. Hypersensitivity reaction indicated by urticaria and skin rash.	Observe characteristic flush. Monitor vital signs. Observe for CNS changes and hypersensitivity.
Glycopyrrolate	Robinul	*Preoperative – IM, IV* *Under 2 yr old:* 0.008 mg/kg 2–12 yr old: 0.004 mg/kg	IM, IV	Contraindicated in young children for anticholinergic use for peptic ulcers.	Observe for tachycardia, urinary retention, constipation, blurred vision, and abdominal distention.
Scopolamine hydrobromide	Same	*Preoperative –IM, IV* *6 mo–3 yr old:* 0.1–0.15 mg/dose *3–6 yr old:* 0.15–0.2 mg/dose *6–12 yr old:* 0.2–0.3 mg/dose	IM, IV	Disorientation and delirium; possible respiratory depression. Contraindicated with hepatitis and in patients with asthma.	Monitor vital signs. Observe for tolerance if used for a long period. Administered only in combination with another drug when used for pain relief.
Anticonvulsants					
Phenytoin, sodium	Dilantin	*Under 6 yr old:* 3–8 mg/kg/day *Over 6 yr old:* 100 mg tid	PO, IM, IV	Contraindicated in patients with dermatitis, asthma, renal or liver dysfunction, and heart disease. Effective serum levels 10–20 mcg/mL.	Full effectiveness achieved gradually. Observe for skin rash, jaundice, nystagmus, lack of coordination, hallucinations, and blood dyscrasias. Monitor oral hygiene and gum massage.
Primidone	Mysoline	5–20 mg/kg day	PO	Contraindicated with blood dyscrasias or neurologic dysfunction.	Observe for skin rash, ataxia, hyperexcitability, excessive hair loss, and edema of eyelids and legs.
Trimethadione	Tridione	*Initial dose:* 150–300 mg tid *Maintenance:* 40 mg/kg/day in equal divided doses.	PO	Contraindicated in children on ketogenic diets.	Observe for photosensitivity, increased grand mal seizures and hair loss, and signs of blood dyscrasia.

Valproic acid	Depakene	15 mg/kg, increased weekly by 5–10 mg/kg until seizures are controlled Maximum dose of 30 mg/kg/day	PO	Contraindicated in patients with liver dysfunction. Cautious use in conjunction with other depressants.	Observe for nausea, weight gain, and diplopia. Transient sedation occurs with initial dose. May cause leukopenia, altered bleeding times, and hair loss.
Antiemetics					
Prochlorperazine	Compazine	*Oral and Rectal:* 0.4 mg/kg in 3 to 4 divided doses *IM:* 0.13 mg/kg	PO, IM, rectal	Causes severe drowsiness and ataxia.	Take adequate safety precautions depending on child's age. Observe for untoward reactions such as excitement. Oral preparation may need to be given in 1 to 2 oz of beverage. Observe for extrapyramidal effects and caution parents not to exceed prescribed dose.
Promethazine hydrochloride	Phenergan	0.13 mg/kg in AM, PRN thereafter 0.5 mg/kg may be given hs	IM, IV, PO	Same as above	Take adequate safety precautions depending on child's age. Observe for untoward reactions such as excitement.
Antihistamines					
Brompheniramine maleate	Dimetane	*IM, IV:* 0.5 mg/kg *po:* 1–2 mg/dose q4–6h	PO, IM, IV	CNS depression	Protect from injury secondary to vertigo. Observe for tachycardia.
Chlorpheniramine maleate	Chlor-Trimeton Teldrin	*po:* 1–2 mg/kg tid *IM, IV:* 87.5 mcg/kg 3–4 times/day	PO, IM, IV	May cause drowsiness, tinnitus, dry mouth, and blurred vision.	Observe for drowsiness; protect from injury.
Tripelennamine hydrochloride	Pyribenzamine (PBZ)	5 mg/kg/day in divided doses	PO	Contraindicated in children with GI disorders or with a history of paradoxical response to drugs.	Protect from injury upon ambulation. Administer drug with food.

Abbreviation key: mg, milligram; kg, kilogram; q, every; h, hours; IM, intramuscular; IV, intravenously; PO, by mouth; I & O, intake and output; bid, twice daily; tid, three times daily; CNS, central nervous system; HS, at bedtime; PRN, as needed; susp., suspension; GI, gastrointestinal; lb, pound; SC, subcutaneously

(Table continued on following page)

TABLE 7-4 – *Continued*

Generic Name	Trade Name	Pediatric Dose	Routes of Administration	Special Precautions or Warnings	Nursing Responsibility
Antineoplastics					
Cyclophosphamide	Cytoxan	*Induction: IV:* 2–3 mg/kg × 6 days *Maintenance:* Based on leukocyte count	IV, IM, PO	Causes bone marrow depression, ulcerations of mouth, and gastrointestinal tract, and pulmonary toxicity.	Observe for nausea and vomiting 3 to 4 h after administration. Oral preparations may cause hemorrhagic cystitis. Increase fluid intake by 1 1/2 times normal and check for urinary frequency or burning. Have patient void q2–3h.
Cytosine arabinoside	Cytosar	*Induction:* 0.5–1.0 mg/kg/day up to 2.0 mg/kg/day *Maintenance:* 1 mg/kg/week	IV	May cause severe bone marrow depression, alopecia, neurologic disturbances, cellulitis, liver damage, and kidney damage (from high uric acid levels).	Check mouth for ulcers. Observe for nausea, abdominal distress, vomiting, and rash.
Dactinomycin	Cosmegen	15 μg/kg/day to maximum of 500 μg	IV	May cause severe bone marrow depression, alopecia, neurologic disturbances, dermatitis, and kidney damage (from high uric acid levels).	Check skin for irritations. Observe for nausea and vomiting, diarrhea, and ulcerations of GI tract.
Methotrexate	Amethopterin	*Children:* 2.5–5.0 mg, 3–7 times/week *Infants:* 1.25–2.5 mg	PO, IM, IV, intrathecal	May cause severe bone marrow depression, alopecia, neurologic disturbances, folic acid deficiency, and kidney damage (from high uric acid levels).	Check mouth for ulcers. Observe for nausea, abdominal distress, vomiting, and rash.
Vincristine sulfate	Oncovin	*Induction dose:* 0.05 mg/kg/week *Maximum:* 0.15 mg/week *Maintenance:* 0.05–0.075 mg/kg/week	IV	May cause severe bone marrow depression, alopecia, neurologic disturbances, and kidney damage (from high uric acid levels).	Avoid leakage into tissues. Observe for constipation and buccal ulcerations. Monitor I & O.

Antiparasitics (Anthelmintics)					
Piperazine citrate	Antepar	*Pinworms:* 50–60 mg/kg/day for 7 days; maximum of 3.5 gm *Roundworms:* 75 mg/kg/day for 2 days; maximum of 5.0 gm	PO	Avoid use in patients with nephritis or GI disturbances.	Administer after breakfast. Observe for neurologic disturbances and muscular weakness from overdose.
Pyrantel pamoate	Antiminth	*Single dose:* 11 mg/kg; maximum of 1.0 gm	PO	Use cautiously in patients with any form of liver dysfunction.	No restrictions on food intake. Observe for signs of liver dysfunction.
Pyrvinium pamoate	Povan	*Single dose:* 5 mg/kg *Maximum:* 350 mg	PO	Contact with drug causes bright red staining.	Administer with food or juice. Chewing of tablet should be avoided because of teeth staining.
Barbiturates					
Pentobarbital	Nembutal	*PO:* 2 mg/kg 3 times/day *IM, IV:* 1–2 mg/kg/dose	PO, IM, IV, rectal	Potent CNS depressant. Rapid administration can cause laryngospasm.	Monitor vital signs. Respiratory depression is first sign of overdose. Tissue irritation may develop at injection site.
Phenobarbital	Luminal	*Sedative:* 6 mg/kg/day in 2–3 doses *Anticonvulsant:* 1–6 mg/kg/day	PO, IM, IV	CNS depressant. Contraindicated with hypersensitivity, impaired liver function, or drug dependence.	Observe for skin rashes, jaundice, fever, unusual bleeding, restlessness, or hyperactivity.
Secobarbital sodium	Seconal	*Neonate to 6 mo:* 15–60 mg/dose *6 mo to 3 yr:* 60 mg/dose *3 yr and over:* 60–120 mg/dose	PO, IM, IV	Same as above	Same as above
Bronchodilators					
Cromolyn sodium	Aarane Intal	Over 5 yr old: *Initial dose:* 4 capsules/day (20 mg/capsule) *Maintenance:* lowest possible dose *Under 5 yr old:* not established	Inhaler	Contraindicated in acute disease.	Place gelatin capsule in special inhaler. Observe for wheezing, nasal congestion, cough, and rash.

Abbreviation key: mg, milligram; kg, kilogram; q, every; h, hours; IM, intramuscular; IV, intravenously; PO, by mouth; I & O, intake and output; bid, twice daily; tid, three times daily; CNS, central nervous system; HS, at bedtime; PRN, as needed; susp., suspension; GI, gastrointestinal; lb, pound; SC, subcutaneously

(Table continued on following page)

TABLE 7-4 – *Continued*

Generic Name	Trade Name	Pediatric Dose	Routes of Administration	Special Precautions or Warnings	Nursing Responsibility
Bronchodilators – *Continued*					
Isoproterenol hydrochloride	Isuprel	5–10 mg tid; or qid to 30 mg	Sublingual, PO	Contraindicated with tachycardia and arrhythmias.	Monitor vital signs frequently at the time of initial dose.
Oxtriphylline	Choledyl	*2–12 yr old:* 3.6 mg/kg q6h (100 mg per 60 pounds of body weight)	PO	Small children prone to CNS stimulation	Preferable to give after meals and at bedtime (to prevent nocturnal attacks that are common in children).
Theophylline	Elixophyllin Slo-Phyllin Theolair	2.5 mg/kg q6h in divided doses	PO	Contraindicated with hypertension, diabetes, hyperthyroidism, and ulcers.	Observe for tachycardia, hypertension and irritability. Monitor vital signs.
Metaproterenol	Alupent Metaprel	*Under 60 pounds:* 10 mg tid or qid *Over 60 pounds:* 20 mg tid or qid	PO	Contraindicated with cardiac arrhythmias.	Observe for tremor, nervousness, tachycardia. Monitor blood pressure for changes.
Diuretics					
Chlorothiazide	Diuril	20 mg/kg in divided doses bid	PO	Contraindicated in patients with anuria or sensitivity to sulfa drugs.	Administer with meal to reduce GI upset. Monitor I & O. Observe for hypokalemia. Encourage intake of potassium-rich foods, such as bananas and citrus fruits.
Furosemide	Lasix	*Oral:* 2 mg/kg qd or bid *IM:* 1 mg/kg qd or bid	PO, IM, IV	Contraindicated with oliguria and anuria.	Observe for hypokalemia and hyponatremia. Monitor I & O. Encourage intake of potassium-rich foods.
Hematinics					
Ferrous sulfate	Mol-Iron Feosol Fer-In-Sol	*Under 6 yr old:* 37.5–150 mg/day *6–12 yr old:* 120–600 mg/day in divided doses	PO	Contraindicated with hemosiderosis, hemochromatosis, peptic ulcer, and colitis.	Administer with food to reduce GI upset. Avoid milk products with ingestion as they inhibit absorption. Minimize contact with teeth.
Iron dextran	Imferon	*Less than 3.5 kg:* Maximum of 25 mg *3.5–9.0 kg:* Maximum of 50 mg *9.0–50 kg:* Maximum of 100 mg	IM	Test dose should be administered to check for allergy. Not to be given concurrently with oral iron preparations.	Administer Z-track method. Observe for arthralgia, headache, staining of skin at administration site. Observe for signs of anaphylaxis.

Cardiac Glycosides					
Digitoxin	Crystodigin Purodigin	*Digitalizing Dose:* Divided doses q6 or q8h Newborn: 0.025 mg/kg 2 weeks–1 yr: 0.04–0.045 mg/kg 1–2 yr: 0.04 mg/kg 2 yr or over: 0.02–0.03 mg/kg *Maintenance dose:* 1/10th of digitalizing dose	PO, IM, IV	Dosage must be reduced in children with liver impairment. Two weeks required for elimination of drug after discontinued.	Assess apical rate; withhold if below 90–110 in infants and young children or below 70 in older children. Observe for anorexia, nausea, vomiting, diarrhea, fatigue, weakness, arrhythmias. Monitor serum potassium.
Digoxin	Lanoxin	*Digitalizing Dose:* Divided doses q6 or q8h Newborn 0.04–0.06 mg/kg 1 mo–2 yr: 0.06–0.08 mg/kg 2 yr and over: 0.04–0.06 mg/kg *Maintenance Dose:* Approximately 1/5 to 1/3 of above	PO	Rapid onset of action. Toxicity more common with IV use. Dosage must be reduced in children with renal impairment.	Same as above
		Digitalizing Dose: Divided doses q6 or q8h Newborn: 0.025–0.04 mg/kg 2 weeks–2 yr: 0.035–0.050 mg/kg 2 yr or over: 0.025–0.04 mg/kg *Maintenance Dose:* Approximately 1/5 to 1/3 of above	IV, IM		
Narcotics					
Codeine sulfate	Same	*Analgesic:* 0.5–3.0 mg/kg, 4–6 times per day *Antitussive:* 0.175–0.25 mg/kg 6 times per day	PO, SC, IM	May cause respiratory depression. Contraindicated with head injuries, liver disease, and seizures.	Observe the respiratory status. Watch for nausea, vomiting, pruritus, and weakness.
Meperidine hydrochloride	Demerol	*Analgesic:* 0.5–0.8 mg/kg q4–6h as needed *Preoperatively:* 0.5–1.0 mg/lb	PO, IM	Same as above	Same as above
Morphine sulfate	Same	0.1–0.2 mg/kg; maximum single dose of 15 mg q4–6h as needed	SC, IM (PO not recommended)	Same as above	Same as above. Assess cough reflex and peristaltic action.

Abbreviation key: mg, milligram; kg, kilogram; q, every; h, hours; IM, intramuscular; IV, intravenously; PO, by mouth; I & O, intake and output; bid, twice daily; tid, three times daily; CNS, central nervous system; HS, at bedtime; PRN, as needed; susp., suspension; GI, gastrointestinal; lb, pound; SC, subcutaneously

REVIEW

A. Matching. Match the description in Column I with the site in Column II.

Column I	Column II
1. Child lies prone with toes pointed in	a. Deltoid
2. Injection limited to aqueous preparation of no more than 1/2 cubic centimeter	b. Vastus lateralis
3. Site used in infants to avoid major nerves and blood vessels	c. Posterolateral gluteal

B. Multiple choice. Select the one best answer.

Situation: Janie is a four-year-old girl who was admitted to the hospital with malnutrition and dehydration. She weighs 27 pounds. An intravenous infusion is started immediately.

1. Her weight in kilograms is
   a. 10.5 kilograms.
   b. 12.2 kilograms.
   c. 14.5 kilograms.
   d. 18.0 kilograms.

2. Janie's fluid needs, when calculated according to the calorie expenditure method, would be
   a. 1110 milliliters.
   b. 1350 milliliters.
   c. 1600 milliliters.
   d. 2000 milliliters.

3. Janie is receiving 50 milligrams of Ilosone orally every four hours for an infection. Is this an average dose for this child, based on Clark's rule? (The usual adult dose is 250 milligrams per dose.)
   a. No, my calculations indicate an appropriate dose of 15 milligrams.
   b. No, my calculations indicate an appropriate dose of 25 milligrams.
   c. Yes, my calculations indicate an appropriate dose of 45 milligrams.
   d. Yes, my calculations indicate an appropriate dose of 65 milligrams.

4. When approaching Janie to administer the Ilosone, you should say
   a. "How about taking this, O.K.?"
   b. "Would you like this pink medicine?"
   c. "Here is some pink pop for you to drink."
   d. "Here is your medicine to drink."

5. When Janie fusses about taking her medication, your best response, given the fact that all statements are possible or true, would be
   a. "Take it now and then you can have a popsicle."
   b. "If you don't take it, you won't get better."
   c. "Drink it up so we can look at your picture book."
   d. "If you don't drink it up, Mommy can't stay."

C. Short answer. Briefly respond to the following statements.

1. List the nursing observations that should be made concerning the intravenous infusion site in a child.

2. Describe the special adjustments that must be made regarding the rate of infusion of a hyperalimentation solution.

3. Identify the nursing measures used in administering hyperalimentation therapy that are not necessary with intravenous therapy.

BIBLIOGRAPHY

Albanese, Joseph A. *Nurses' Drug Reference.* New York: McGraw-Hill Book Company, 1979.

Baker, Charles E., Jr. (Publ.) *Physician's Desk Reference.* Oradell, NJ: Medical Economics Company, 1979.

Brandt, P. A., et al. "IM Injections in Children." *American Journal of Nursing,* Vol. 72 (August, 1972), p. 1492.

Chow, Marilyn P., et al. *Handbook of Pediatric Primary Care.* New York: John Wiley and Sons, 1979.

Colley, Rita, and Jeanne Wilson. "Meeting Patients' Nutritional Needs with Hyperalimentation." *Nursing 79,* Vol. 9 (June, 1979), pp. 57–61.

Colley, Rita, and Jeanne Wilson. "Meeting Patients' Nutritional Needs with Hyperalimentation: Providing Hyperalimentation for Infants and Children." *Nursing 79,* Vol. 9 (July, 1979), pp. 50–53.

Guhlow, Linda J., and Janice Kolb. "Pediatric I.V.'s: Special Measures You Must Take." *RN,* Vol. 42 (March, 1979), pp. 40–51.

Hussar, Daniel A. "New Drugs 78/79." *Nursing 79,* Vol. 9 (May, 1979), pp. 32–40.

Kastings, Erwin K., and James R. Boyd. *Facts and Comparisons.* St. Louis: Facts and Comparisons, Inc., 1979.

Kee, Joyce L., and Ann P. Gregory. "The ABC's (and mEqs) of Fluid Balance in Children." *Nursing 74,* Vol. 4 (June, 1974), pp. 28–36.

Millam, Doris A. "How To Insert an I.V." *American Journal of Nursing,* Vol. 79 (July, 1979), pp. 1268–1271.

Reed, Gretchen M. *Regulation of Fluid and Electrolyte Balance.* Philadelphia: W. B. Saunders Company, 1977.

Russell, Helen. *Pediatric Drugs and Nursing Intervention.* New York: McGraw-Hill Book Company, 1980.

Wilson, Jeanne, and Rita Colley. "Meeting Patients' Nutritional Needs with Hyperalimentation." *Nursing 79,* Vol. 9 (August, 1979), pp. 56–63.

Chapter 8

Preoperative and Postoperative Care of Children

OBJECTIVES

Upon completion of this chapter, the student will be able to

- describe the process of preoperative preparation used for the children.
- identify the adaptations of care that are made for children in the recovery room.
- discuss the components of postoperative care and discharge planning.

Surgery is a traumatic situation for well-prepared adults; it is even more traumatic for young children. Nurses involved in the care of pediatric surgical patients must tailor their explanations, care, and equipment to meet the special needs of this population.

PREOPERATIVE PREPARATION

The preparations made prior to a child's surgery may be divided into two phases: remote and immediate. One is dependent on the other. Both are geared to the age and developmental level of the individual child.

Remote Preparation

Remote preparation includes those activities that focus on the identified health problem and the need for its correction. The parents' awareness that their child has strabismus and needs an operation is a good example of initial preparation. The parents may then seek confirmation of this by an ophthalmologist if they have not already consulted one. The child's preparation usually begins with the comments that are made by the parents prior to the first office visit.

Well-intentioned but overprotective parents often convey nonverbal information that is quite disturbing to the child. The concern of the parents exhibited during the office visit and the hushed tones that may be used in discussing the potential surgery contribute to a child's anxiety. Any discussion of the problem or its surgical correction in the presence of the child should be geared to the child's level of understanding. Discussing the corrective procedure and the hospital admission in front of the child using adult terms only multiplies the child's fears and anger and misinterpretation may result.

Overprotective families should be identified as early as possible so that the parents can be assisted in preparing the child for the hospital experience. Often, parents may state or actually believe that the child is too young to understand the information. The nurse should recognize that these parents may be so fearful for the child that they are unable to discuss the problem or procedure with the child or even between themselves.

In the clinic or office setting, parents may be given printed handouts that aid in their explanation of the situation to the child. They may also be told of pertinent storybooks that are available at the local library. These methods help to clarify information for both parents and children.

As a general rule, it is advisable to prepare a child for surgery one day in advance for every year of age. Thus, a two-year-old child needs only two days of advance preparation because of this age-group's poor concept of time and limited ability to comprehend. In contrast, a seven-year-old child would need a week to mull over the idea, to ask questions, and to complete his or her own planning and preparation, Figure 8-1.

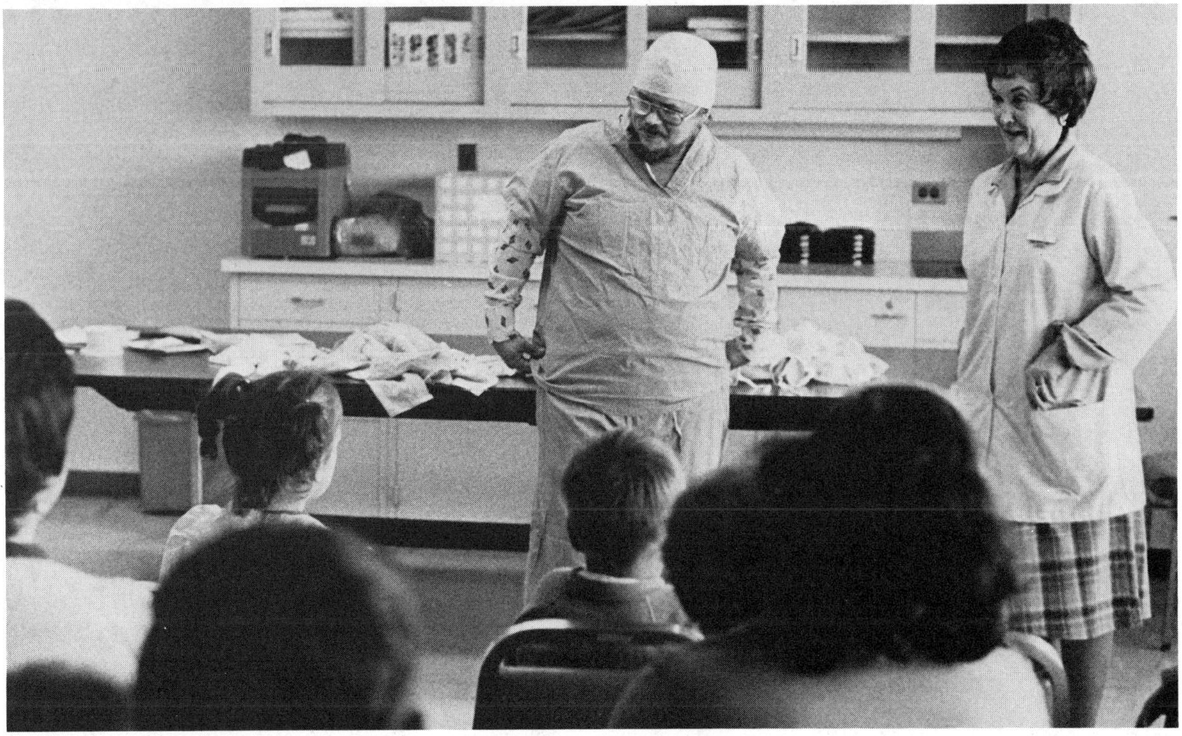

FIG. 8-1 Talking with the surgeon in a group makes the surgeon seem less threatening.

An age-appropriate knowledge of the illness and the reason for the hospitalization should be conveyed to the child. Children with congenital disorders should be told that they were born with the condition and that the doctor knows how to fix it through surgery. The child also should be told that no other part of the body will be operated on, and that neither the child nor the parents are to blame for what has happened. The concept of the surgery as punishment for misbehavior also should be discussed and fears dispelled. Parents and professionals should remind the child that no matter what he or she has done, the surgery is not a punishment. This may be particularly difficult for the child to believe when the surgery to be performed involves the genitalia and the child has been scolded in the past for touching or exploring this area.

Immediate Preparation

The immediate preparation of the child occurs at the time of hospital admission. It involves both clarification of questions or information and certain physical preparation within the hospital setting.

Explanations. While in the strange environment of the hospital, the child is often less fearful of pain than of separation from the parent and from a familiar environment. For instance, the prospects of sharing a room with a stranger instead of sleeping in one's own bed, and using a bedpan instead of the bathroom at home may heighten the child's fear.

Any diagnostic tests to be done prior to surgery, as well as the components of the preoperative routine, should be explained. A brief description of the anesthesia and surgery is necessary to clarify for the child what will be done. Children can be told that they will be put to sleep in a special way by breathing sweet-smelling medicine, and that they will not feel or remember the surgery. The location of the incision should be explained. The child should know whether the area will be covered by a dressing. Likening the dressing to a big Band-Aid may enhance the child's comprehension.

The concept of a special sleep caused by medication should be clarified so the child understands that it is not the same as going to bed. Many children are fearful that they will awaken during the procedure. It is important that they realize that only after the surgery is all over will someone wake them.

Physical Preparation. Physical preparation for the operative procedure usually begins the day prior to the surgery. Preoperative diagnostic testing, such as a complete blood count and urinalysis, is done in all children. Additional tests, such as bleeding and clotting times, typing and cross matching for units of blood, and chest radiographs may be ordered by the physician depending on the type of surgery to be performed.

Food and fluids are routinely withheld for twelve hours prior to the surgery. Depending on the scheduled time of the surgery, the anesthesiologist may reduce this fasting period for young infants, allowing the infant to have liquids until the early morning hours. This prevents excessive fluid depletion.

Special preparation of the skin may be required for children undergoing orthopedic or plastic reconstructive procedures. This may involve giving the child a tub bath with a bacteriostatic agent, or a special washing or "surgical scrub" of a body part. Surgical scrubs must be performed for specific periods of time and with special equipment. The body part is then wrapped in sterile towels. It is important to keep these towels dry as moisture allows organisms to enter from the towel surface.

Preoperative medications may be administered one to two hours before the scheduled surgery. Some children require preoperative medications specific to their condition, such as vitamin K, antibiotics, or cycloplegic drugs (in patients having eye surgery). Other drugs that are used specifically in preoperative patients include analgesics and sedatives, along with anticholinergics, such as Atropine or Robinul, to dry secretions. Because these drugs are used to sedate the child, all care and procedures should be completed prior to their administration. For example, a child who is old enough should be encouraged to void before receiving a sedative injection. Analgesics may be administered rectally in very anxious children so that they are asleep prior to transport to the surgical suite. Children should know whether they will be transported on a stretcher or in their own cribs. Such items as surgical caps, masks, scrub suits, and gloves should be familiar to children from the preadmission program.

POSTOPERATIVE CARE

During surgery, careful attention is directed toward several factors other than the surgical procedure itself. For instance, the child's positioning is considered in order to protect delicate tissues and fragile body parts. The body temperature is monitored using an electronic probe and warmed blankets. Also, the child's fluid balance and blood replacement requirements are calculated carefully according to his or her individual needs. These considerations facilitate the postoperative care of the patient.

Care in the Recovery Room

Family Considerations. Postoperatively, the child is kept in the highly skilled environment of the recovery room until the child recovers from anesthesia, achieves reasonable consciousness, and is found to have stable blood pressure and vital signs, and an adequate airway. Depending on the patient's age, the child's own bed or crib may or may not be used. The presence of a "familiar friend," such as a teddy bear or other toy, is often reassuring to the child upon first arousing from the anesthesia.

In some pediatric centers, parents are prepared in advance for the recovery room experience and are permitted to stay with the child while the child is recovering from the anesthesia. Well-prepared parents are less anxious about their child's condition, and the child is less fearful with the parent present. In the case of an infant, the parents may even be permitted to hold the child.

In hospitals where the procedure is permitted, the parent should visit the recovery room at a quiet time for a brief orientation. This often is provided in the late afternoon on the day prior to the child's surgery. The parent needs to meet the staff member assigned, and be given information regarding the child's appearance under anesthesia, the presence of the airway, and the need for frequent monitoring of vital signs. In addition to the brief orientation the parents should be told that they may be asked to leave the area if an emergency develops. If this happens, parents are told where to wait and are brought back to the recovery area when the crisis has subsided.

If it is known that the child is to be moved from the recovery room to an intensive care unit or to a unit other than the one to which he or she was initially admitted, this information is included in the family's preoperative preparation. Occasionally, the transfer to another unit is unexpected. In this instance, the explanation is the responsibility of the recovery room staff or the physician. It is important that the parents know why the transfer is being made, and they should be helped in reorienting themselves. One parent became quite disoriented and anxious when her son was unexpectedly transferred to the intensive care unit after undergoing closed reduction of a fracture under general anesthesia. She reported that "they wheeled him out of the cast room area and said abruptly, 'We are taking him to intensive care.' I could see him lying on the cart, very pale and still unconscious with the airway in his mouth. My head was spinning with all I thought could have gone wrong. The explanation came some time later and was almost too simple to believe." This mother found out later that the recovery room in the hospital closed after a certain hour and that thereafter all postoperative patients were sent to the intensive care area to recover from anesthesia before being returned to their rooms. A brief explanation at the time the child was transferred would have reduced the parent's anxiety and enhanced her trusting relationship with the staff.

The child, too, should know in advance where he or she will wake up. Children should be told who will be there with them and whether any dressings or other equipment will be used. They should know that they will feel sore in the affected body part, and that they may feel sick and may vomit. If intravenous fluids are administered, their purpose and the equipment used should be explained to the child in terms that are easily understood.

Nursing Care. Recovery room routines include maintenance of a patent airway, monitoring for signs of respiratory obstruction, shock, or hemorrhage, and promotion of the patient's comfort and safety. To maintain a patent airway, the child must be positioned properly and the plastic airway kept in place until the child is responsive. Positioning the child on his side aids in the drainage of secretions or vomitus. Suctioning may also be performed easily with the patient in this position.

Frequent monitoring of vital signs is important in identifying any significant alterations in vital signs and in preventing resultant shock. Initially, vital signs should be checked every fifteen minutes. Recovery room nurses should know the normal range for vital signs in relation to their patient's development so that they can accurately assess any alterations.

The patient's dressing should be checked for signs of blood loss. Small amounts of blood loss in an adult are not a problem. However, because of the smaller circulating volume in children, and depending on the child's size, blood replacement may be required.

Promoting the safety and comfort of a child after surgery involves a consideration of the type of bed used as well as the use of temporary restraints, if necessary. A disoriented child may unthinkingly remove dressings, intravenous needles, or drainage tubes. In some situations, the use of a jacket or wrist restraint may be necessary. However, such restraints should never be substituted for the attention of the nursing staff or the presence of a parent as soon as it is possible.

If the child remains in the recovery room for any length of time or is transferred to the intensive care unit, a number of special concerns arise. Ideally, the child should be prepared for this eventuality through play therapy, hospital tours, and familiarization techniques. Unfortunately, this preparation is not possible in emergency admissions or when unexpected surgical problems dictate a change in the child's level of care.

The disruptive sleep patterns and the continuous monitoring associated with these units are very stressful for children. Normal sleeping patterns, including the usual nap and bedtime routines, should be facilitated whenever possible. Treatments and procedures may need to be reorganized to accommodate such patterns. Normal day-night cycling may be enhanced somewhat by dimming the lights in the unit and reducing the noise level, if possible. In closed units, the door to the patient's room may be shut to exclude noise from the remainder of the unit.

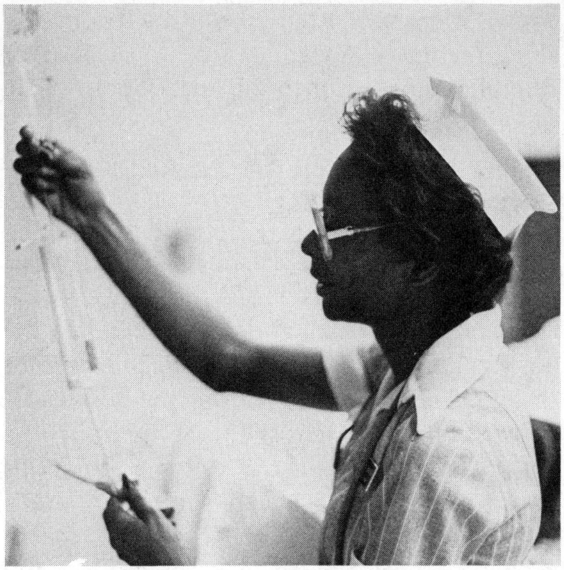

FIG. 8-2 Monitoring intravenous fluid administration is an important part of postoperative care.

Continuing Postoperative Care

The events that follow the surgery should be predictable to both children and parents because of their preoperative preparation. Once the child returns to his or her own room, the assessment of vital signs, surgical dressings, intravenous fluid requirements, and elimination processes continues until there is no further danger of complications, Figure 8-2. The presence of a parent or another significant person greatly eases the child's adjustment in the early postoperative period.

The transition from intravenous fluids to oral fluids may be a gradual one, particularly in the case of abdominal surgery. The child should know what fluids or foods are permitted, with emphasis placed on what is allowed, rather than on what is not allowed. When fluids are restricted, ice chips or popsicles may sometimes be given to relieve thirst. If the child is not permitted anything by mouth, a cold washcloth applied to the child's lips may provide some comfort.

As the child recovers from anesthesia, deep breathing exercises are begun. They may be performed in a number of ways. In an alert child, familiar equipment, such as a balloon or a Ping-Pong ball, may be just as effective as an incentive spirometer. The child's age and condition dictate which method will be most effective.

Pain relief is a priority in children. However, children seldom request anything for pain, fearing a shot. They may even deny pain for this reason. Nurses should evaluate the child's pain and then use their discretion in administering pain medication. Medications may be administered both intramuscularly or orally depending on the assessment of the staff and the needs of the child. If the child is able to tolerate fluids, the oral method is acceptable. In others, the medication may have to be given intramuscularly. In these children, cooperation may often be enlisted by encouraging them to apply an ice cube to the site for several minutes prior to the injection.

PREPARATION FOR DISCHARGE FROM THE HOSPITAL

Preparation for discharge should begin at the time of the admission. At this time, the parent should be told the anticipated length of the hospitalization and the expected outcome of the surgical procedure. During the postoperative period, the parent and, if age permits, the child, should be taught any home-care skills that they will be expected to perform. If dressings must be changed at home, the parent should observe and participate in the daily dressing changes carried out by the nursing staff. Any adaptations for homegoing may be reinforced at that time.

Alterations in the child's activity level may be easier for the family to accept than adjusting to dietary restrictions. Parents should receive such information from the dietitian early in the course of hospitalization so that they can be helped to select appropriate meal plans before the child is discharged. In this way, the change is made gradually, and the parents will not feel quite so overwhelmed by the number of discharge instructions they receive at the last minute.

Discharge from the hospital should be limited to a review of what is expected for home care. If the family has been adequately prepared, no new information should be necessary. Also at this time, the parents should be reminded of any follow-up visits to the clinic or the physician's office. It is often helpful to consult the parents about convenient times for such appointments before the parents leave the hospital. Encouraging the parents to contact their child's primary nurse by telephone or to contact the unit if they have any questions also eases the transition to the home setting. The questions asked are often of minor importance, but the parents need reassurance and clarification of their home care of the child.

SHORT-PROCEDURE UNITS

The terms *day surgery* or *short-stay units* refer to those units developed to care for either adults or children needing minor surgical procedures. The individual is admitted to the unit in the early morning, has the procedure performed, recovers in the unit, and returns home in the late afternoon.

The major advantage for the child is that the period away from the home is brief. All of these children should have the same careful preoperative preparation as a child admitted for a longer hospital stay. The preadmission program is just as important for this child. Much of the reassurance and support in this situation must come from parents or caregivers. They need accurate information themselves so that the child is adequately prepared.

In this situation the parents are responsible for withholding food and fluids from the child after midnight prior to the surgery. Parents then take the child to the admitting office of the hospital in the early morning and the child is admitted to the short-stay unit. All of the routine laboratory work is done prior to this admission. After the surgical procedure is carried out and the child has sufficiently recovered, the parents are allowed to take the child home.

The majority of the preparation and care is the responsibility of the parents in this situation. It is important that they have a contact person to whom questions can be referred both before and after the admission. In some agencies the pediatric nurse practitioner serves this purpose. In other agencies the short-stay staff members provide this.

SUMMARY

The surgical experience can be a positive growth experience for children, or it can be terrifying, depending on their preparation and the support of their parents. The skill of the health care staff in dealing with the child and the parents is crucial to the family's adjustment.

Special adaptations in equipment and care may be necessary in the surgical suite, as well as in the recovery room, when pediatric patients are involved.

Discharge from the hospital should be a well-planned, smooth transition from the protectiveness of the hospital setting to the comfort of familiar home surroundings. The parents, as well as the child, should be prepared to handle whatever home-care activities are required.

SUGGESTED ACTIVITIES

- View two films or read three children's books that deal with hospitalization and surgery in this age-group. How is the information presented? To what age level is it directed? What information is included for the child and what material is directed toward the parents?
- Make arrangements with the supervisor or head nurse to visit the surgical suite in your assigned hospital. What adaptations are made for the pediatric patients requiring surgery?
- Interview the family of a child who recently underwent surgery and was discharged from the hospital. Find out what measures were taken to prepare them for the experience, and determine whether these measures were effective.

DISCUSSION TOPICS

1. Together with your classmates, develop a handout that could be used in the preparation of a seven-year-old child who is scheduled for a myringotomy. Discuss what information could be included for the parents, as well.
2. Sleep deprivation and constant noise levels are characteristic of the intensive care unit setting. Research the effect of prolonged exposure to such conditions and report your findings to the class.

REVIEW

A. Matching. Match the activity in Column I with the appropriate time of the preparation in Column II.

Column I	Column II
1. Surgical scrub	a. Remote preparation
2. Explanation of reason for surgery	b. Immediate preparation
3. Complete blood count	
4. Urinalysis	
5. Preoperative orientation program	
6. Restriction of foods and fluids	

B. Multiple choice. Select the one best answer.

Situation. Jeff is a six-year-old boy who is scheduled for a tonsillectomy in the morning. Use this information to answer questions 1 through 4.

1. Which of the following explanations would best foster Jeff's comprehension of what is going to happen to him?
   a. "You will be put into a deep sleep and the doctor will snip out the infected tissue from your throat. This will keep you from having any more sore throats and will make you better from now on."
   b. "You will be given a medicine for sleep and your tonsils will be removed. Afterward, your throat will be sore so you'll have popsicles to eat. When you are awake and feeling better you'll go home again."
   c. "A doctor will put a mask over your face and give you an anesthetic. While you're unconscious, your tonsils will be cut out. When you wake up, you must not talk or eat solid food for awhile."
   d. "You will be taken on a cart to the operating room, which is a large, bright room filled with a lot of shiny and interesting equipment. The nurse there will talk to you and the doctor will take care of you."

2. Jeff should be told that he cannot have anything to eat or drink after
   a. 8:00 AM.
   b. bedtime.
   c. supper.
   d. midnight.

3. All routines and care should be completed for Jeff
   a. prior to administering the preoperative medication.
   b. immediately after the preoperative preparation.
   c. two hours before the scheduled surgery.
   d. three hours before the scheduled surgery.

4. Jeff confides to you that he is afraid he won't wake up if he is put to sleep for the surgery. Which of the following would be your best response?
   a. "I wouldn't worry about that if I were you."
   b. "Look at Millie over there, she had her tonsils out, and she woke up."
   c. "Tell me why you think you won't wake up."
   d. "Good little boys wake up and I'm sure you're a good little boy."

C. Short answer. Briefly respond to the following statements.

1. Name two priorities for care in the recovery room.
2. List three factors to consider in discharge planning.

BIBLIOGRAPHY

Lubarger, Patricia M. "The Intensive Care Environment: Its Effect on the Child and Parents." *Issues in Comprehensive Pediatric Nursing,* Vol. 3 (October, 1979), pp. 50–57.

Meissner, Judith. "How Can You Improve Care of the Hospitalized Child?" *Nursing 80,* Vol. 10 (October, 1980), pp. 50–51.

Petrillo, Madeline, and Sirgay Sanger. *Emotional Care of Hospitalized Children.* Philadelphia: J. B. Lippincott Company, 1980.

Shufer, Shirley. "Communicating With Young Children: Teaching Via the Play-Discussion Group." *American Journal of Nursing,* Vol. 77 (December, 1977), pp. 1960–1962.

Smith, Elaine C. "Are You Really Communicating?" *American Journal of Nursing,* Vol. 77 (December, 1977), pp. 1966–1968.

Section IV

The Infant

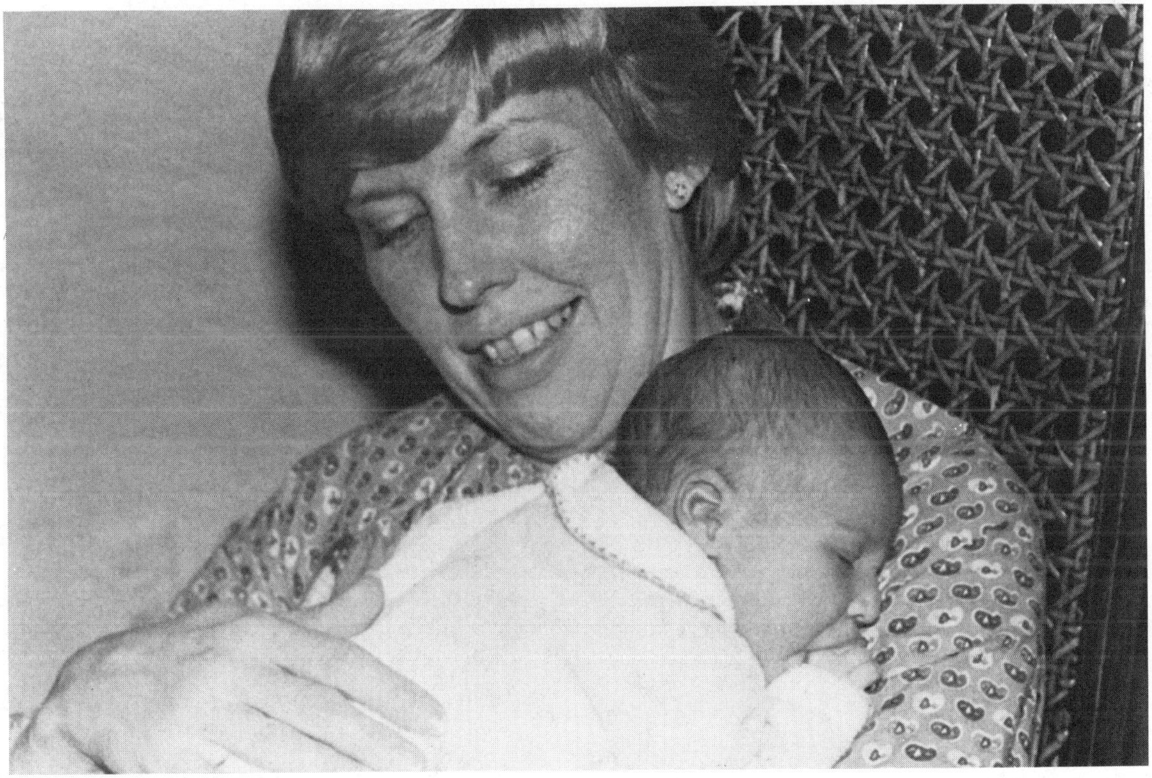

Chapter 9

Growth and Development

OBJECTIVES

Upon completion of this chapter, the student will be able to

- describe the various developmental achievements of infants during the first year of life.
- explain the theories of Piaget and Erikson as they relate to the period of infancy.
- discuss and give examples of the developmental concepts of growth identified for the infant.

The period of infancy is marked by vast changes in physical and emotional development. The infant makes the transition from being a totally dependent, helpless creature to being a semidependent, ambulatory individual within the first year of life. This physical transition is paralleled by a great depth and breadth of emotional growth on the part of both infants and parents.

DEVELOPMENTAL THEORIES

Any discussion of development has as its focus two basic elements: maturation and learning. Maturation refers to the capacity for development that is inherited or genetically transmitted. It is sometimes described as the physical changes that take place in all growing children from the time of conception as a result of internal body processes. Adaptation is the result of the body's accommodation or adjustment to its immediate environment. Learning is the result of life experiences, including training and trial-and-error methods. The true test of learning is evidenced by a change in a child's behavior.

Maturation and learning are closely intertwined and interrelated. For severely retarded individuals, the degree of maturation is limited. Life experiences, no matter how exceptional, have limited meaning to these children. They lack the potential or the capacity for development beyond a certain level. Therefore, learning does not take place.

Erikson's Developmental Theory

Several developmental tasks are deemed appropriate for the period of infancy. Erikson identified the infancy period as one in which the infant develops a sense of trust versus a sense of mistrust, Table 9-1. This sense of trust is the basis for all the relationships that occur during the rest of the child's life. Trust is developed in the infant as a result of the concerned, nurturing, and positive interactions that occur between a loving parent and a receptive child, Figure 9-1. It begins at birth with the bonding process and continues throughout childhood with a profound sensitivity to met and unmet needs.

Infants develop a sense of trust from the sensitive, consistent care that they are given. As their needs are met for food, warmth, and comfort, they develop a trusting attitude toward the world and those about them. The continuous reinforcement of consistently met needs helps the infant develop a sense of confidence or trust which carries over into later life. Infants who are raised in an inconsistent environment in which their needs are only sporadically met may develop a sense of mistrust toward the world and the individuals in it.

Recognition of the receptivity of the child is an important aspect of this process of trust versus mistrust. For instance, a child with brain damage and resultant cerebral palsy may be physically incapable of being receptive to the cuddling of the mother. Likewise, the autistic child may, from the very onset, resist the handling and touching of the parents.

During this period, infants also complete other developmental tasks. They learn a response to a nurturing figure, whether or not it

TABLE 9-1 Erikson's Stages of Development in Children

AGE	STATE	KEY ISSUE
Infancy (0–18 mo)	Trust vs. Mistrust	Testing of significant others' abilities to provide sensitive, consistent care
Toddler (18 mo–3 yr)	Autonomy vs. Shame and Doubt	Testing of child's own ability to separate as well as to relate to others
Preschool (3–5 yr)	Initiative vs. Guilt	Testing of child's ability to compete in relation to others, singly or in a group. Includes conscience formation.
School (5–12 yr)	Industry vs. Inferiority	Developing a mastery of intellectual and technical skills with values expanding to the school and neighborhood
Adolescence (13–19 yr)	Identity vs. Role Diffusion	Developing a sense of personal identity in relation to the peer group, as well as to adults, to form an integrated feeling of unity

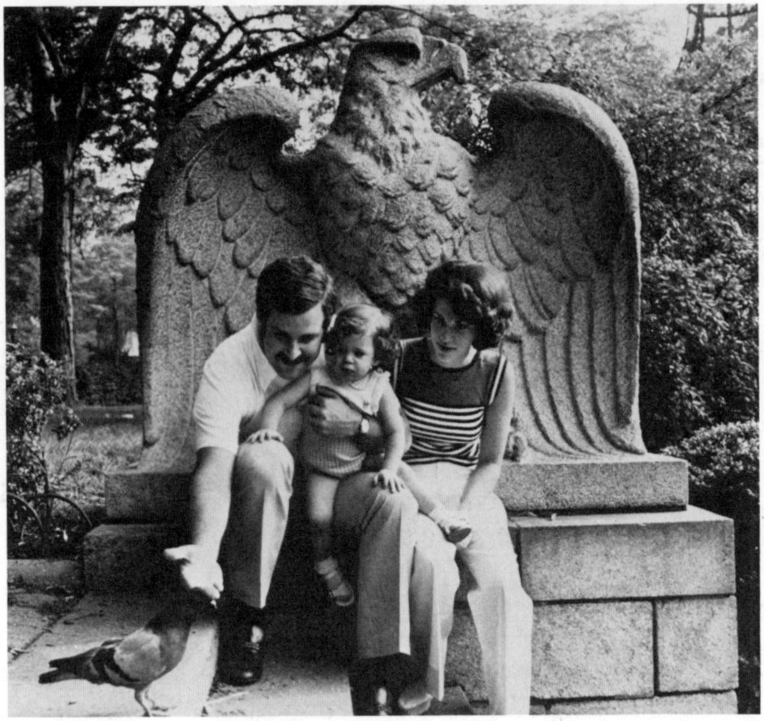

FIG. 9-1 The development of trust is the result of many positive interactions between parents and child. (Courtesy of Gerber Products Company)

is the biologic parent. They also learn attachment to a family group. At the same time, the beginning stages of locomotion are taking place. Infants also learn their name at this time. Vocalization during this period sets the stage for future growth.

Piaget's Developmental Theory

Piaget identified the period of infancy as the stage of sensorimotor coordination, Table 9-2. This period is one in which infants learn responses to the environment. The infant develops a sense of stability of objects over time and space, termed *object constancy* by Piaget. Initially, they respond with reflexes. Gradually, they learn to differentiate objects in the environment and to relate their actions to these objects. Infants explore the world using responses and behavioral patterns that are inherent. An example would be an infant's use of sucking and grasping to explore everything. If the object chosen is too large to be placed in the mouth, the infant attempts to modify the behavior, continuing the exploration by sticking his or her tongue out to taste the object, Figure 9-2. In this adaptation of a previously learned behavior, infants recognize the similarities and differences of the new experience. According to Piaget, this stage of development extends from birth to two years of age. Emphasis is placed on the importance of the interaction between the infant and the environment, as well as the presence of opportunities for exploration.

The nurse should realize that although ages are listed in all of the developmental frameworks, these are only approximations.

TABLE 9-2 Piaget's Stages of Cognitive (Intellectual) Development

STAGE	AGE	DESCRIPTION
Sensorimotor period	Birth to 2 yr	Differentiation of self from objects Development of concept of object constancy (object exists even when not in direct contact) End of stage marked by infant's ability to retain mental images of the object
Preoperational period	2–7 yr	
Preconceptual phase	(2–4 yr)	Egocentric thought Ability to name objects and to use appropriate terms, but inability to recognize relationships between them Inability to distinguish between mental, social, and physical reality
Intuitive phase	(4–7 yr)	Ability to use information to make comparisons based on perceptions Inability to consider all relevant dimensions in a problem
Concrete operations	7–11 yr	Ability to use logic operations, including reversibility (mathematics), classification (organizing objects into a hierarchy), and seriation (organizing a series according to size, weight, etc.)
Formal operations	11–15 yr	Ability to think abstractly and to conceptualize Ability to formulate a hypothesis and test it

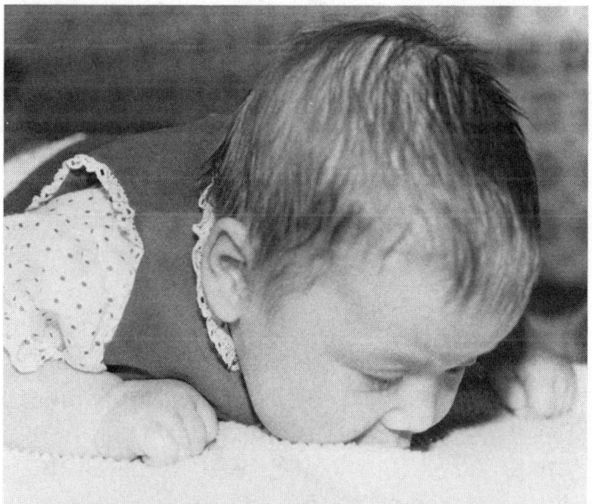

FIG. 9-2 This infant is busy exploring her blanket with her tongue.

Many of the stages overlap and their boundaries are not clear-cut. Some aspects of a given task may be evident earlier than projected; other aspects may persist long into the next stage.

GROWTH RATE

The infancy period is characterized by rapid, purposeful growth. During this period, infants grow in size, but more importantly, they begin to achieve milestones in the areas of motor control and emotional and social responsiveness. The rate of growth and the potential for growth are dependent on many intrinsic and extrinsic factors. Intrinsic factors include those that exist from the time of conception through birth. They include factors such as maternal nutrition; hereditary diseases, such as sickle cell anemia; and circumstantial events, such as oxygen deprivation secondary to a traumatic delivery. Extrinsic factors include all those that relate to influences from the environment. For instance, alterations in the potential for growth occur in children living in environmentally polluted slum areas at a subsistence level. Likewise, nutrition and the occurrence of illness are factors that represent extrinsic influences on the child's ultimate growth.

PRINCIPLES OF GROWTH

In the infancy period, the growth of a child proceeds as it did during fetal life — in a cephalocaudal direction. This is seen rather readily if one compares the motor development skills of a one-month-old infant with those of a six-month-old child. Head control precedes any attempt at assuming a sitting position. Proximal-distal progression aptly describes the direction of muscular development in the infant. Development begins near the trunk and proceeds outward. Control is achieved in an orderly, sequential fashion, Figure 9-3. Muscular control always progresses from general to specific areas. For instance, one may readily observe that children perform gross motor activities, such as stretching an arm out to a toy, before they are able to demonstrate fine motor skills, such as grasping the toy with their fingers.

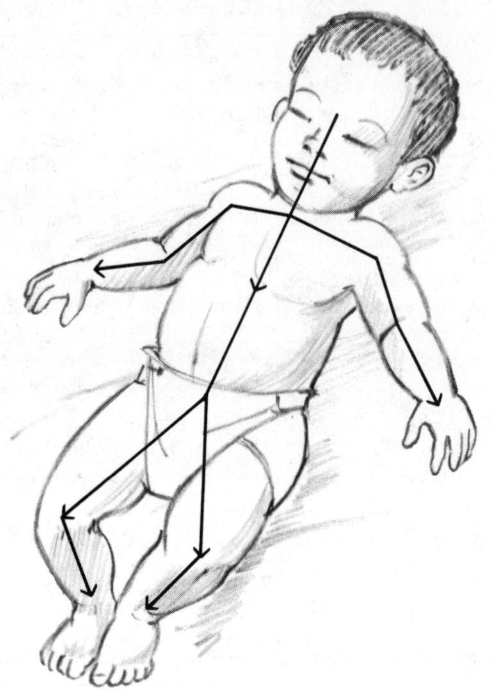

Fig. 9-3 The cephalocaudal and proximal-distal sequences of development

Monthly Achievement Levels

During the first six months of life, the infant gains 5 to 7 ounces of weight per week. This rate may be easy to recall if one remembers that the weight gain is approximately 1 ounce per day "for every day but Sunday." Growth rates are individualized, though, and infants who are small at birth usually exceed this average rate. Conversely, infants who weigh 10 pounds at birth usually gain weight at a rate that is less than this average. Increases in the baby's length parallel increases in weight. The average increase in length amounts to an inch per month during the first six months of life.

One Month of Age. A one-month-old infant has poor muscular control and limited means of communicating pleasure or unhappiness. The infant's motor control is also limited. When placed on the abdomen, the infant lifts the head intermittently, turning it from side to side, but is unable to hold the head upright when placed in a sitting position. The feet or

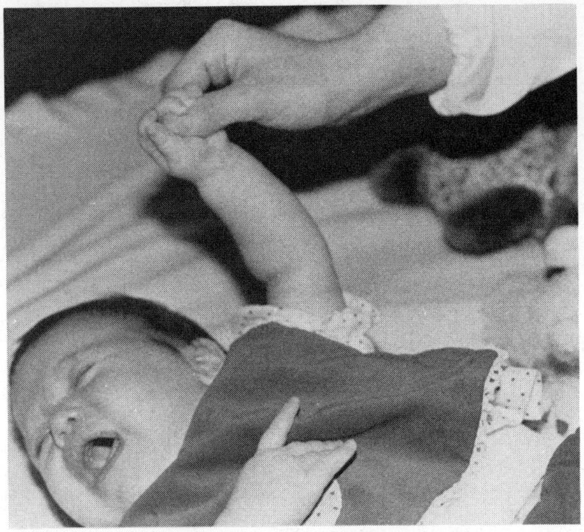

FIG. 9-4 Stimulating the palm of the hand with the thumb elicits the palmar grasp reflex.

legs are used in an uncoordinated fashion to push forward from a hard surface or to make crawling-type movements. The reflexes that are present in one-month-old infants include the protective reflexes of rooting, sucking, swallowing, and blinking. In addition, the palmar grasp reflex is present, Figure 9-4. When the nurse places an object in the infant's hand, the object will be grasped momentarily and then released. The infant's tonic neck reflex is elicited by turning the infant's head to one side. Within seconds, the arm and leg on the same side are extended while the extremities on the opposite side are in flexion. It is often called the fencing position, and is well developed at this age. Moro's reflex or the startle reflex is evident when a loud noise occurs in the infant's room. The infant's extremities extend and then curve inward as in an embrace. The thumb and first finger form a characteristic C position (see Chapter 4, Figure 4-8).

The one-month-old infant takes notice of faces and bright objects. Facial features attracting the infant may resemble a caricature and may not appear to be very human or very detailed. Infants stare indefinitely at objects. Bright colors, such as bright red or yellow, attract the baby's attention easiest. The baby's eyes track an object and follow it to the midline, but the infant will not move the head or turn the body in any way.

Vocalization in one-month-old infants is designed to show dissatisfaction with a situation, such as being wet or hungry. Sometime during this period, infants begin to make small, throaty sounds. Observation of their faces indicates that they cannot identify the source of these noises. Smiles may be frequent and indefinite, or they may be direct responses to persons or pleasure.

Two Months of Age. By two months of age, the infant has learned to respond to specific stimuli. If the infant is placed in the usual position for feeding, attempts to suck or other movements of the mouth signify that the position is recognized. Distinct improvements in motor control occur at this age. For example, the once sagging head of the one-month-old infant is now held erect, Figure 9-5. When lying prone on a firm surface, the infant may raise its head for a short period of time. When placed on its side, the baby may make a quarter turn to lie on its back.

Development during this second month of life builds on earlier bonding behavior. Infants pay attention to the voices of those around them, often smiling in response to friendly faces or familiar voices. Their cries are differentiated according to particular needs — to be fed, changed, held, or cuddled. Waking and sleeping periods become more clearly defined at this time.

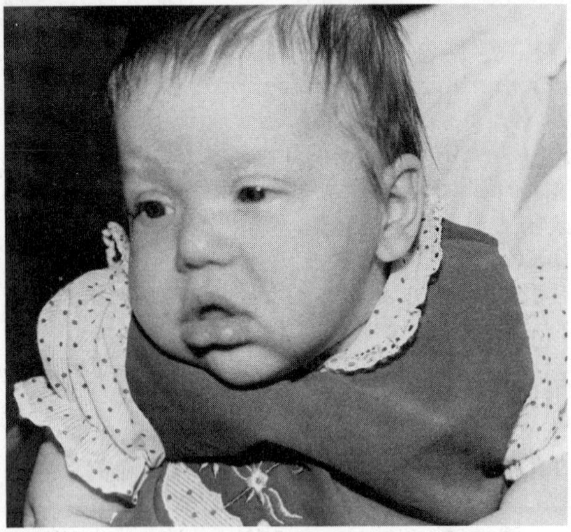

FIG. 9-5 As long as the child's back is adequately supported, a two-month-old infant can hold her head erectly in mid position without wobbling.

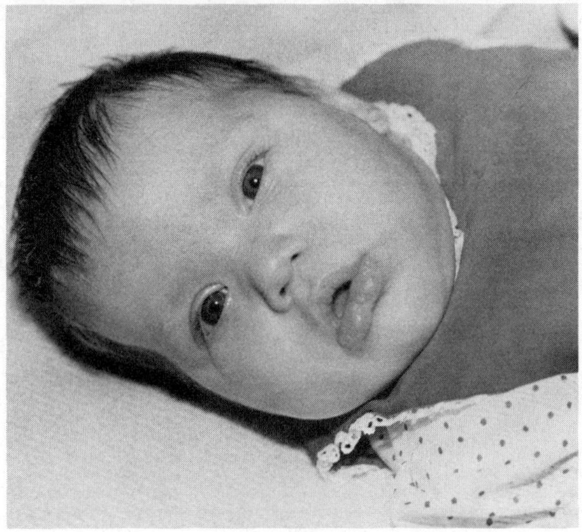

FIG. 9-6 The examiner's smile is rewarded with an intent stare that is typical of three-month-old infants.

Three Months of Age. The personality of the three-month-old infant is more pronounced than before. The little throaty noises now become laughter. The sounds are not only pleasing to parents, but are also obviously pleasant to the child. A special smile is reserved for the sight of familiar faces. In response to a person's smile, the infant will coo, blow bubbles, or simply study the face intently, Figure 9-6.

By three months of age, motor control has extended to the hands. Infants of this age often hold their hands in front of them, staring at them intently. Or, they may play with the hand or fingers. Attempts to reach for objects become evident but actual grasping seldom occurs. The fingers or hands may also be placed in the mouth at will, Figure 9-7.

The infant's vision is more coordinated at this age. Both eyes move together in a coordinated fashion either vertically or hori-

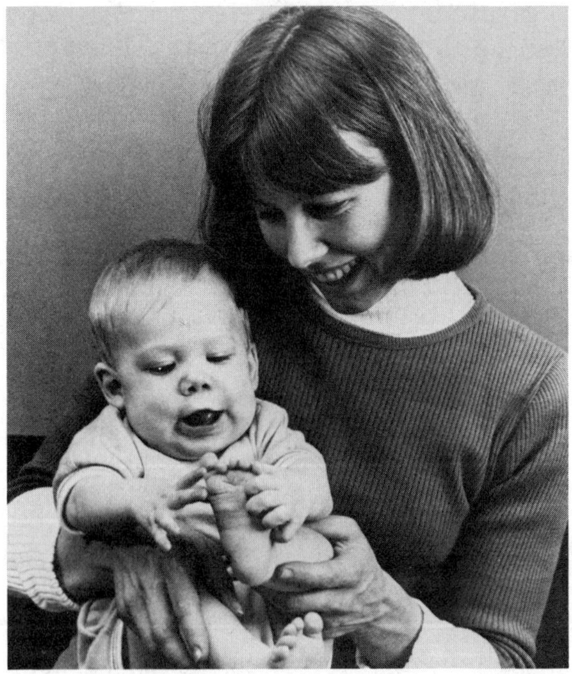

FIG. 9-7 At the age of three months, infants will often place fingers or toes in the mouth. (Courtesy of Gerber Products Company)

zontally to follow a moving object. An object in the marginal field of vision easily attracts attention at this time. In response to the mother's face or to the sound of her voice, the infant makes thrashing movements of the arms and legs to show pleasure or excitement.

Infants who have experienced steady growth up to this point weigh between 12 and 13 pounds. They are about 3 inches longer than they were at birth. The Moro and tonic neck reflexes are gradually fading at this time, and a positive response may not be elicited.

Drooling is noticed in many infants at three months of age or shortly thereafter. This does not mean that teething is starting. It simply means that the infant is producing saliva. Initially, infants will allow it to run out of their mouths until they learn to swallow it.

Four Months of Age. At four months of age, infants' responsiveness to the environment is considerably increased. Their eyes follow moving objects, and they turn their heads toward voices and sounds. They continue to vocalize in a social fashion, demonstrating increasing interest in the family group. This interest is particularly noticeable in the presence of other children.

Muscular coordination is improving in several areas. When four-month-old infants are held in an upright position, they demonstrate good head control. While in the same position, they often extend their legs, partially supporting their own weight. Beginning attempts are made to reach for objects beyond their grasp. Some attempts at rolling over are also made about this time.

Five Months of Age. By the age of five months, infants weigh about 15 pounds, which is roughly twice the birth weight. Exploration of the world takes on new dimensions at this time. The ability to grasp with the whole hand allows the infant to put other objects to the mouth. Anything that can be reached is explored in this fashion. As the object is mouthed, the drooling increases.

Coordination is improving at this stage. As an object is dropped, the infant follows it with the eyes. Displeasure at the loss of a particular toy is vocalized. The child may have enough motor skill at this point to catch a dangling object between two hands. Mobiles are particularly enjoyable to the infant.

Six Months of Age. The rate of growth in six-month-old infants starts to slow. The infant gains about half as much weight during the second six months of life as was gained during the first six months. Approximately 3 to 5 ounces are gained per week. Linear growth slows to 1/2 inch per month. The muscular coordination of six-month-old infants allows sitting momentarily without support. They may even be able to pull themselves up to a sitting position. By this age, rolling over is not limited to half turns. Rather, the infant can now roll completely over onto the stomach and back again, usually with brief pauses in between movements.

Teething begins at about this time. The first of the deciduous teeth to appear are the lower central incisors. Swollen, reddened gums and fussiness may indicate the onset of teething. Because the gums are sore, the baby may refuse to eat or to accept anything by mouth that would touch the area where the teeth are coming through. Cool liquids and chilled teething rings may be soothing to some infants. Topical analgesics also may help. As the infant's resistance is lowered by teething, signs of respiratory infections or diarrhea may be evident.

Seven Months of Age. Seven-month-old infants sit briefly with their weight balanced by leaning forward on the hands. If they are supported somewhat in this position, they can maintain it for about half an hour instead of only several minutes. If they are held in a standing position, they bounce noticeably.

At this age, infants' ability to use their hands indicates further development. They are able to hold small toys, such as blocks, in each hand. They can grasp a toy easily, and will attempt to transfer it from hand to hand. This is done with varying degrees of success, depending on the size of the object.

Speech or vocalization continues to develop and the baby appears to be listening to the sounds made. Displeasure as well as eagerness is vocalized. Also, infants respond to their own names, and demonstrate an awareness of the tone of an adult's voice when it shows displeasure.

Tooth development continues. The upper central incisors appear between the seventh and eighth month. This is a good time to offer cookies or crackers. The biting is satisfying to the infants and their level of coordination is such that they can easily put the food in their mouths. They are also now able to hold their own bottles.

Eight Months of Age. The eighth month brings noticeable changes in the relationship of infants to others. Their strong feelings of affection for and attachment to their family groups are clearly identified. Infants seek their family's attention, hold their arms out to be held, and generally show approval of them. If a stranger approaches, infants become silent and withdrawn. Coy or bashful behavior may be exhibited if they are safe in their mother's lap or arms. Games, such as pat-a-cake or peek-a-boo, make the infant more accepting of the stranger.

Eight-month-old infants are able to sit steadily without support. Finger and thumb apposition makes the handling of objects easier for them than before. Hand-to-hand transfer is quite skillfully executed at this age. Toys may be used to bang on the highchair tray or to make noise in general. Reaching is no longer random, but specific and purposeful.

Nine Months of Age. Nine-month-old infants begin to crawl as a means of locomotion. The term "crawling" refers to the movement effected when infants propel themselves with the abdomen and legs still on the floor, using the arms and shoulders. Some infants progress beyond this maneuver, creeping instead with

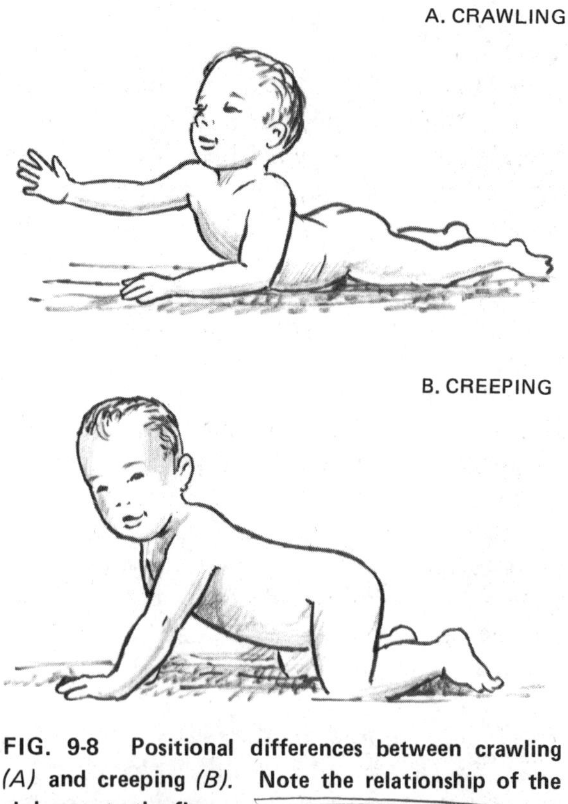

FIG. 9-8 Positional differences between crawling *(A)* and creeping *(B)*. Note the relationship of the abdomen to the floor.

the abdomen raised off the floor, Figure 9-8. Many infants this age stand easily with support.

At nine months of age, infants begin to show some preferences. One of the first is the preference of one hand over the other. If the child has the opportunity to use either hand, one particular hand is used most often.

Vocalizations at this time begin to take on new meaning. Specific sounds assume meaning for the child, and one or two words, such as da-da, may be used. At this age, infants are also aware of strong emotions reflected in speech. Sounds associated with anger or very loud voices cause tears.

Teething has continued in the infant, and at nine months, four teeth are usually evident. The upper lateral incisors are the latest additions.

Ten and Eleven Months of Age. The tenth and eleventh months are marked by continued development of motor skills. Infants are able to sit indefinitely without any support. They make repeated attempts to pull themselves to their feet while holding onto a support. This activity soon progresses to the point at which they are able to stand using only one hand for support. Creeping is the primary means of locomotion; infants travel wherever their curiosity leads. Safety concerns are extremely important in children this age. Infants must be protected from contact with electric cords, plugs, heaters, and other such devices, as well as potentially poisonous substances that may now be within their reach.

Self-feeding skills become evident in this age-group. Infants not only feed themselves finger foods, but they also take time to poke at and examine their food. Parents should provide two spoons at mealtimes to encourage this skill. Whatever their level of skill, infants still find a way to get food into their hair and on their clothes and the adjacent furniture.

Words that are used at this time mimic the normal inflection of an adult. New words are identifiable, not from their sound as the infant makes it, but by the inflection used. Infants this age are very responsive to their own name, turning at the sound of their name being called.

Simple games that can be repeated are a source of great pleasure in the tenth and eleventh months. Singing and hand-clapping are excellent forms of diversion for children this age. Infants demonstrate an understanding of simple commands even though they do not yet use the command words. Appropriate responses to commands may be reinforced by verbalizing the activity for the infant. For example, the parent may encourage the child to help with dressing, asking the child to push his or her foot into the shoes as they are put on.

Twelve Months of Age. At the end of the first year, infants weigh three times their birth weight, or about 21 to 22 pounds. Their linear measurement is about 29 inches. Their metabolic rate slows and their pulse rate is between 100 and 140. The respiratory rate ranges from 20 to 40 respirations per minute.

Motor skills are becoming well developed at this age. Infants are able to walk with assistance, stand momentarily without support, and sit down from a standing position. Their main method of locomotion continues to be creeping.

Fine motor skills are also improving steadily, Figure 9-9. Finger foods are eaten without assistance. The infant is able to roll or throw a ball toward another person, and can imitate the holding of a pencil or crayon to make a mark.

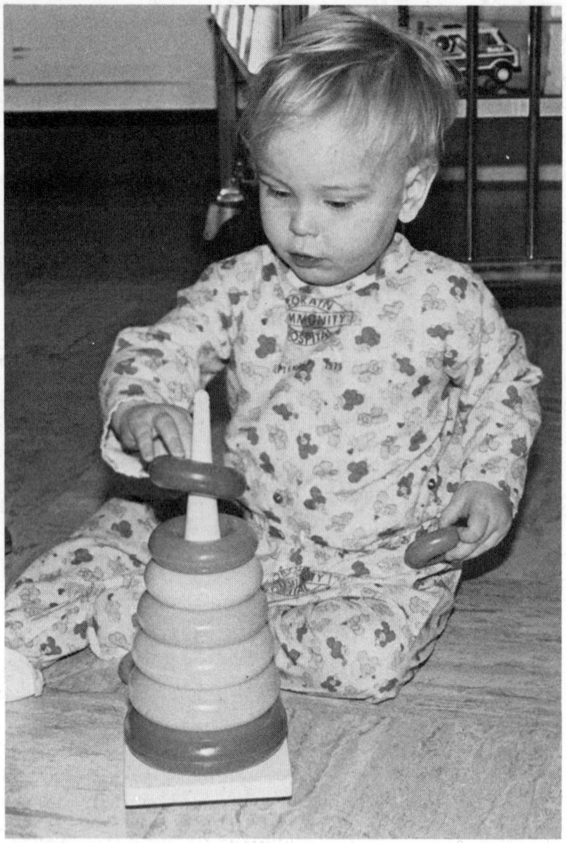

FIG. 9-9 Toys such as this one can improve fine motor skills in the older infant.

Speech is improving, but at a slower rate than before. Most of the child's effort is concentrated on locomotion. By this age, the infant should be able to say about four words. Use of jargon is also evident. Infants this age exhibit strong emotions, and respond to emotions in others. They also vocalize delight at the approval of others.

SUMMARY

Infants progress phenomenally from total dependency at one month of age to limited independence at one year of age. This progression does not mean that the child is grown up, or that the child is like a "little adult." Rather, it means that the infant has developed multiple skills and abilities. One-year-old children are still egocentric and must be so for their needs to be met and for growth to continue.

Nurses should recognize normal growth and development as a sequential pattern that is individualized with each child. They should also be aware that this individuality means that a particular infant may be advanced or delayed in completion of the achievement levels specific to the infant's chronologic age. Knowledge of the various developmental theories aids the nurse in recognizing the tasks that should be accomplished during the infancy period, and how to facilitate their achievement.

SUGGESTED ACTIVITIES

- Observe several infants in a nursery or home setting who are younger than four months of age. Describe the similarities and differences between each. Consider growth, responsiveness, activity, reflexes, and vocalization.
- Care for an infant six months of age or older. Assess the child's developmental ability. Use the Denver Developmental Screening Test if you have access to it and are capable of administering it. Compare the child's abilities with the established norms for children of this age. Share your observations with your group.
- Invite four mothers and/or fathers and their babies to class. Note the similarities and differences in the infants' levels of growth and development. As a group, identify the variations in child-raising practices that may account for the differences. Invite the mothers to contribute to your discussion.

DISCUSSION TOPICS

1. Research the patterns of growth and development in an autistic child. Compare these patterns to those of a normal infant. Discuss your findings with your classmates.

2. Together with your classmates, develop a list of toys or play activities that would facilitate the infant's development during their first year of life. Identify the age at which these toys or activities are most appropriate.

REVIEW

A. Matching. Match the activity in Column I with the age at which it first occurs in Column II.

Column I	Column II
1. Teething	a. 2 months
2. Ability to turn from side to back	b. 4 months
3. Turning of head toward sounds and voices	c. 6 months
4. Good head control in upright position	d. 8 months
5. Noticeable bashfulness with strangers	
6. Weight gain of 3 to 5 ounces per week	
7. Sitting steadily without support	
8. Sucking attempts when placed in feeding position	

B. Multiple choice. Select the one best answer.

1. The developmental theory that focuses on cognitive or intellectual development and describes infancy as a period of sensorimotor organization was developed by
   a. Piaget.
   b. Erikson.
   c. the Denver Developmental Institute.
   d. Freud.

2. The theory that describes infancy as a developmental period of trust versus mistrust was proposed by
   a. Bower.
   b. Piaget.
   c. Rousseau.
   d. Erikson.

3. The theory that recognizes that infants explore their world based on behavioral patterns and responses that are inherent is that of
   a. Piaget.
   b. Gestalt.
   c. Erikson.
   d. Page.

C. Short answer. Briefly respond to the following statements.

1. Describe the cephalocaudal progression of development in infants and give an example.
2. Define proximal-distal progression as it relates to development.

BIBLIOGRAPHY

Caulfield, C. "A Developmental Approach to Hearing Screening in Children." *Pediatric Nursing,* Vol. 4 (March–April, 1978), pp. 39–42.

Chow, Marilyn P., et al. *Handbook of Pediatric Primary Care.* New York: John Wiley and Sons, 1979.

Czarniecki, L. "Developmental Nursing Care: Infant Stimulation for High-Risk Children." *Pediatric Nursing,* Vol. 4 (September–October, 1978), pp. 32–38.

Lands, D. B., et al. "What Do Parents Know About Infant Development?" *Pediatric Nursing,* Vol. 5 (January–February, 1979), pp. 32–36.

Newman, Barbara, and Philip Newman. *Infancy and Childhood: Development and Its Contexts.* New York: John Wiley and Sons, 1978.

Scipien, Gladys M. *Comprehensive Pediatric Nursing.* New York: McGraw-Hill Book Company, 1979.

Tudor, M. "Developmental Screening." *Issues in Comprehensive Pediatric Nursing,* Vol. 2 (July–August, 1977), pp. 1–13.

Chapter 10

Health Care Needs

OBJECTIVES

Upon completion of this chapter, the student will be able to

- describe the immunizations that are appropriate for this age-group.
- identify the purposes of well-baby clinics.
- describe appropriate health care supervision for children of this age.

Infants' health care needs are dependent on their parents' awareness and concern in terms of preventive health care. In the United States, emphasis has traditionally been placed on treatment or acute care. The concept of preventive care has not always been positively received. Health care services to families are often duplicated, fragmented, or designed to meet only isolated needs.

WELL-CHILD CONFERENCES

Well-child conferences (also called well-baby clinics and child-care conferences) are part of the program of supervision developed for young children by public health agencies. These conferences are geared for young rather than older children.

The services provided by these conferences include: health screening and appraisal; special assistance regarding nutrition, dental care, or other areas related to health care; referrals for assistance to other community agencies; and routine immunizations. The aims of each of these services are to maintain a state of wellness in the child and to teach the parent to anticipate development in a positive fashion.

Screening and Appraisal

Health screening and appraisal is an ongoing process in which the parent and child visit the clinic at scheduled intervals. During these sessions, members of the clinic's staff learn about the family directly from the family. The information gathered from the family includes socioeconomic status, cultural background, and the values emphasized in the home setting. The parents, in turn, learn about aspects of growth and development that they may not have considered. By watching the nurse evaluate the child's skill level through a series of tests (such as the Denver Development Screening Test or other health screening tests), parents learn that the child's development may be compared to that of groups of children, rather than merely to the patterns of a sibling.

As the parents become more accepting of the guidance of the health care worker, they are more apt to ask questions and to trust the judgment of the professional. The family views the health care team as persons who are willing to help and to make suggestions in a nonjudgmental way.

Intake Interview. The intake interview with the family covers much of their sociologic background. Information is obtained regarding the home environment, as well as resources in terms of extended family support systems.

The interaction between family members is also noted during these meetings. This observation provides clues to the responsibilities of each member of the group and the patterns of decision making in the home. The influences of culture and the family's religious background are also noted.

Family living patterns are an important aspect of the total life of the child. The rigidity or flexibility with which tasks are carried out strongly influence the functioning of the family members. Exploration of this facet of family living provides clues to the type of information-sharing that should be pursued in the conference setting.

Scheduled Visits. Each conference visit has a similar pattern. At the initial visit for a one-month-old infant, the child is given a complete physical, and information about eating, sleeping, and elimination habits is obtained. Developmental milestones appropriate to the child's age are checked. Also during this visit, parents are encouraged to voice any concerns about the care of the baby. Screening tests such as for phenylketonuria (PKU) may be performed at this time if they were not done in the hospital setting, or if the results were questionable. The nurse offers guidance in the care of the child, focusing on the areas of concern identified by the parents, as well as areas that are age-appropriate.

For the older child of six or eight months, health care guidance focuses on beginning eating habits, foods offered the child, safety concerns, and weaning from the bottle. The physical assessment is not likely to have changed greatly although the developmental achievements appropriate to the child's age have changed. By this time, the parents' concerns have also changed, depending on the growth and behavior of the child.

Special Assistance

In some cases the family may benefit from specialized assistance. For instance, the guidance of a dietitian may be needed in planning a special diet for a child, or routine dental care may have to be arranged for a family on welfare. The dentist or the nutritionist may not attend every clinic session, but each acts as a backup support and information system for the child's parents.

Direct nutritional assistance is usually available for families on welfare. The Women, Infants, and Children (WIC) Nutrition Assistance Program provides monthly packages of food products that are designed to supplement the substandard diet of pregnant women and preschool children on welfare.

Referrals

Referrals are made for acute health care problems and for problems related to social service or those that are not within the realm of health care. Social workers, mental health counselors, or legal aid societies may become involved with the family in this way. Direct referral from the health care professional often helps speed the process.

Immunization Routines

The purpose of immunization is to protect the child against the major communicable diseases. The neonate has passive immunity from the transport in immunoglobulin G of maternal antibodies through the placenta. These antibodies decrease slowly until they completely disappear by fifteen months of age. If infants receive an immunizing agent while the maternal antibodies are still present, the infants will not synthesize adequate amounts of their own immunoglobulin G and will thus remain unprotected against the diseases.

The immunizations recommended for the first year of life include the diphtheria-tetanus-pertussis vaccine. This is given at two, four, and six months of age to provide basic immunization. A booster dose is then administered when the child is eighteen months old, and another booster is given in the preschool period. This is the last dose of the pediatric form. Thereafter, at ten-year intervals, the child should receive the adult form of tetanus-diphtheria. The pertussis is omitted at that time as it no longer poses a threat to the adolescent or young adult, Table 10-1.

Four doses of trivalent oral polio vaccine are given at two, four, and eighteen months, as well as in the preschool period. This is the

TABLE 10-1 Recommended Immunization Schedule for the First Sixteen Years of Life

AGE	TYPE OF IMMUNIZATION
2 months	DTP, TOPV
4 months	DTP, TOPV
6 months	DTP
1 year or older	MR or MMR
18 months	DTP, TOPV
4 to 6 years	DTP, TOPV
14 to 16 years	TD

Abbreviation key: DTP, diphtheria-tetanus-pertussis vaccine; TOPV, trivalent oral poliovirus vaccine; MR or MMR, combined vaccines of measles and rubella or measles, mumps, and rubella; TD, adult-type tetanus-diphtheria toxoid most common form of oral polio virus used for immunization.

The immunizing agents for measles, mumps, and rubella may be given as a combined vaccine. Mumps vaccination may also be administered separately at one year of age, followed by the measles and rubella vaccines at fifteen months.

There are some contraindications that apply to the immunization of children. These include the presence of any type of acute, febrile illness or immunologic deficiency, and current treatment with immunosuppressives. Any child who has received gamma globulin or a blood transfusion six to eight weeks prior to a scheduled immunization should not be immunized because of the high level of passive antibodies.

Nurse's Role

Perhaps the one outstanding result of well-child conferences is the increased confidence of the parents in their ability to cope with a variety of situations. The conferences reinforce parents' knowledge and enhance their ability to deal with their children in a positive and therapeutic fashion.

At each encounter, nurses can aid the parent-child relationship in several ways. The nurse is in a unique position to provide support for the caregiver, recognize both strengths and weaknesses of the family group, supplement or provide education, and make specific recommendations.

Providing support involves praising parents for handling situations well, recognizing and considering parents' suggestions and ideas for care, and allowing parents free expression of their concerns about themselves and their children. Recognition of strengths and weaknesses in the family group involves: identifying the child's primary caregiver when this person is not the parent; establishing specific goals, incorporating input from the family; and maintaining the family's own value system. In educating the family, nurses should remember to provide information in reasonable amounts, using clearly understood language. Specific recommendations made by the nurse should be based on an agreement with the family regarding both the identified problems and the priorities for the child's care.

CONTINUED HEALTH CARE SUPERVISION

The underlying goal of continued health care supervision for the infant is to improve the child's quality of life. To accomplish this, a number of individual aims have been identified. The goals are to prevent disease, immunize against communicable diseases, introduce the child to the routine health care system, aid normal patterns of growth and development, and enhance parent-child interactions.

As mentioned previously, initial screening tests to identify health problems are performed in the hospital setting. Screening is done for phenylketonuria, hypothyroidism, and sometimes for other inborn errors of metabolism. A follow-up screening may be done at the time of the first office visit if there was reason to question the results of any of these tests.

Follow-up visits to the pediatrician involve immunizations, screening for developmental delays, and counseling. Near the end of the first year of life, blood studies to detect anemia are done. The major focuses in counseling at this stage include nutrition, parenting problems, and accident prevention.

Accident Prevention

During this time the infant is helpless and totally dependent on the caregiver. It is important that caregivers be aware of potential hazards and actively prevent accidents or safety hazards. Burns, falls, choking, and motor vehicle accidents are the most common problems in this age-group.

For safe bathing of the infant, the adult must be aware of the temperature of the bath water by careful testing prior to placement of the infant in the tub. Burns may also occur when the parent is handling hot liquids near the infant. Smoking should be avoided near the infant.

Falls can be prevented by holding the infant as care is given. When the child is on a changing table or in an infant seat the restraining strap should be securely fastened. Crib sides should always be fastened securely. If the infant is to be unattended for a few minutes, the infant should be placed in the crib or in a playpen for protection.

Choking and strangulation type accidents can also occur with this age-group. Bottles should never be propped. The parent should be encouraged to hold the child and to burp him or her carefully before putting the infant in the crib. If a pacifier is used, it should not be tied around the infant's neck; it should have a shield at the base to prevent accidental aspiration. Toys should be free of loose parts and should be too large to be swallowed. Crib rails should be no more than 2 3/8 inches apart to prevent the child from becoming caught. Bumper pads should also be securely anchored to the crib rails for an infant.

In the car, the infant should be secured in an approved car seat. An infant should never be left unattended in the car even for a minute. All car doors should be securely locked.

Parental Concerns

The new family initially has many concerns as it clarifies the roles of the individual members. The shift in size from two to three members is important in itself. The change in relationships is significant and parents may have unrealistic expectations of themselves as parents. Participation by both parents in child care and mutual support of each other is desirable. Common attitudes and values related to child care help promote this.

Parents may become overwhelmed at the amount of care needed by the infant in early infancy. The entire cycle of family life evolves around the infant's waking and sleeping patterns. The constant attention needed by the infant may become a source of resentment. Parents need reassurance as well as support during this period. They need to know that the demands of care will decrease as the infant becomes more secure with consistency and growth. Parents need to be encouraged to obtain adequate amounts of rest and to spend some time together away from the infant.

Later in their child's infancy period, the parents should share their feelings and concerns about weaning, toilet training, and discipline. A frank discussion of both parents' attitudes should occur before the child is at that stage. The nurse may assist the parents in identifying common ideas for a positive approach.

Both parents should be aware of the sequence of growth and development during this period. The nurse may discuss this during well-child conferences as a form of anticipatory guidance. Books and pamphlets can be used to reinforce this information. Parenting groups and classes are also very effective in providing support and guidance to parents.

Nutrition

During follow-up visits, parents' concerns often focus on the child's nutritional needs. Parents' perceptions of adequate and proper nutrition for the child may be quite different from the recommendations of the health care team, Table 10-2. For instance, during the first six months of life, food should be provided only in small amounts in order to teach the child how to deal with a semisolid substance on the tongue and also to solidify the parent-child relationship, Figure 10-1.

Nutritional Problems. Some of the nutritional problems that are common in children include

TABLE 10-2 Feeding Recommendations for Infants

Diet	Age	
	0 to 6 months	6 to 12 months
Human Milk	Total diet	Primary nutrition
Supplementation	Iron	Iron
	Fluoride	Fluoride
	Vitamin D	Vitamin D
Formula	Total diet	Primary nutrition
Solid Foods	None	Secondary nutrition
Calories	115–120/kg	100–110/kg

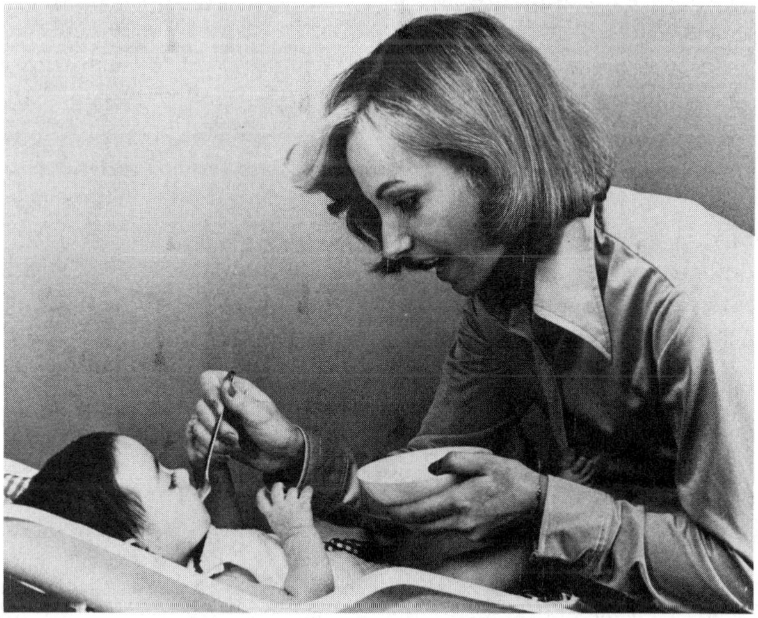

FIG. 10-1 The mother-child interaction that takes place while teaching the infant how to eat solids is more important than the amount of food that is consumed. (Courtesy of Gerber Products Company)

TABLE 10-3 Recommended Daily Allowances for the First Year of Life

Calories	100–120/kg of body weight
Protein	2–4 gm/kg of body weight (6–8% of calories)
Fat	No specific quantity set (30–55% of calories)
Carbohydrates	No specific quantity set (35–55% of calories)
Iron	5–7 mg (1 mg/kg/day up to 15 mg)
Vitamin A	1500 I.U.
Thiamine	0.4–0.5 mg
Riboflavin	0.5–0.8 mg
Niacin	6–7 mg
Vitamin C (ascorbic acid)	30 mg
Vitamin D	400 I.U.

obesity from overnutrition, excessive carbohydrate ingestion, and iron deficiency anemia. All three problems are correctable if recognized.

In past years, great emphasis was placed on what foods the child should be given. As a result, infants were eating larger and larger amounts of a wide variety of foods. According to the American Academy of Pediatrics, the premature addition of solids to the diet may actually contribute to an inadequate diet because carbohydrates are being substituted for quality protein, Table 10-3. Thus, overfeeding of solids predisposes the child to allergies and puts additives such as sugar, salt, flavorings, and colors into the diet.

The potential for obesity is often established in early infancy at the time foods are added to the diet. The addition of large amounts of carbohydrates to the diet raises calorie levels drastically. Insisting that children eat every bit of food at each feeding also may add to this problem. Likewise, continuous use of food as a reward or as solace after an injury establishes a pattern that is difficult to break.

Foods and Feeding Technique. When the infant is first fed solid food, the food of choice is dry rice cereal that is fortified with iron. Rice is chosen because it is least allergenic. After several weeks, bananas and applesauce are added to the diet.

Food should be spooned into the infant's mouth slowly, allowing ample time for the child to get used to the new taste and feel on the tongue. At first, a new parent may think that the infant is trying to spit food out of the mouth. This is actually the retrusion tongue reflex. As children mature, they become better able to cope with food on the tongue and will find it easier to move the food to the back of the mouth for swallowing.

Single-grain cereals are used initially. Wheat is withheld until after six months of age, as are egg whites, even if the infant is already eating the yolk. Orange and citrus juices are also withheld until after six months because of their allergenic potential.

By six months of age, the child should be introduced to junior foods for their coarse consistency. Finger foods should be encouraged as soon as the child's hand-eye coordination improves. Parents should be prepared for the messiness that accompanies the eating of finger foods.

Weaning the child from the bottle to the cup usually begins at about nine to ten months of age, and is completed sometime around the twelfth month or shortly thereafter. The bottle at bedtime is usually the last one replaced by the cup. After the first year, the bottle given at night should contain water rather than juice or milk because of potential problems with cavities.

Weaning the infant from the breast may occur in about the same time span. Some mothers may choose to wean the infant earlier for a variety of reasons, including the mother's inability to produce an adequate milk supply or poor weight gain in the infant. The infant may be weaned to a bottle or to a cup, depending on the child's age and abilities.

Breast-feeding mothers who wish to wean their child should select the nursing period in which the infant seems least interested, substituting either a bottle or a cup. After a few days, the substitution is then made in the same way during another period. The process usually takes two to four weeks as the milk supply decreases. The last feeding is usually readily given up by the infant.

Although breast-feeding or bottle-feeding is being eliminated at this time, parents should maintain close body contact with the infant. The satisfaction the infant derives from this contact should not be eliminated along with the feeding method.

SUMMARY

Preventive health care begins with routine screening tests and immunizations to detect and to prevent diseases. Nutrition is also an important health care consideration. In the preventive health care setting, nurses have a unique opportunity to foster both the child's wellness and positive parenting behavior through assessment, teaching, and support of the family.

SUGGESTED ACTIVITIES

- Participate in the care of a child in a well-child clinic. Observe the areas of assessment and note what tests are performed.
- Complete a nutritional assessment on a nine-month-old infant. Compare the child's diet with current dietary recommendations. Should any alterations be made?

DISCUSSION TOPICS

1. Discuss the parenting problems that may arise at various stages of the infant's development. Describe the nurse's role in supporting families with such problems.
2. Develop a list of foods that are most likely to cause allergies in infants younger than one year of age. Share your findings with the class.

REVIEW

A. Matching. Match the description in Column I with the substance in Column II.

Column I	Column II
1. Withheld until six months of age	a. Water
2. Begun at nine to ten months of age	b. Citrus juice
3. Contents of night bottle at one year of age	c. Weaning from bottle or breast
4. Primary source of nutrition during the first six months	d. Finger foods
5. Encouraged at six months of age	e. Formula or breast milk

B. Multiple choice. Select the one best answer.

1. Routine immunizations during infancy and early childhood include those for
   a. measles, pertussis, scarlet fever, chickenpox, diphtheria, rubella, and tetanus.
   b. pertussis, diphtheria, poliomyelitis, tetanus, measles, rubella, and mumps.
   c. chickenpox, poliomyelitis, measles, diphtheria, typhoid fever, rubella, and possibly, tuberculosis.
   d. tetanus, diphtheria, pertussis, measles, rubella, and chickenpox.

2. Immunizations are withheld in children who have a/an
   a. headache.
   b. acute febrile illness.
   c. upset stomach.
   d. rash.
3. The purpose of well-baby conferences is to
   a. give immunizations.
   b. help the mother.
   c. keep statistics.
   d. provide ongoing health supervision.

C. Short answer. Briefly respond to the following statements.

1. Explain why rice cereal is added first to the infant's diet.
2. Explain why mixed cereals are avoided.
3. List four services provided in well-child conferences.
4. List three ways nurses provide support for parents of infants.

BIBLIOGRAPHY

Committee on Nutrition, American Academy of Pediatrics. "Recommendations for Infant Feeding." *Pediatrics,* Vol. 57 (1976), p. 278.

DeAngelis, Catherine, et al. "Introduction of New Foods Into the Newborn and Infant Diet." *Issues in Comprehensive Pediatric Nursing,* Vol. 2 (January–February, 1977), pp. 22–23.

Food and Nutrition Board. *Recommended Dietary Allowances.* 9th ed. Washington, D.C.: National Academy of Sciences, National Research Council, 1979.

Habersang, Rolf. "Iron and Infant Nutrition." *Issues in Comprehensive Pediatric Nursing,* Vol. 2 (January–February, 1977), pp. 43–49.

Kasanof, David. "New Approach To a Well-Child Care Plan." *Patient Care,* Vol. 8 (October 1, 1974), pp. 69–71.

Kuhn, John G., and Richard G. Fischer. "Vitamins in Pediatrics." *Pediatric Nursing,* Vol. 5 (March–April, 1979), pp. 25–31.

Selekman, Janice. "Immunizations: What's It All About?" *American Journal of Nursing,* Vol. 80 (August, 1980), pp. 1440–1445.

Skinner, Rebecca (ed.). "Preventive Care from Birth to Age 1 Year." *Patient Care,* Vol. 13 (February 15, 1979), pp. 168–178.

Skinner, Rebecca (ed.). "Preventive Care Age 1 Through Adolescence." *Patient Care,* Vol. 13 (April 30, 1979), pp. 201–216.

Chapter 11

Congenital Anomalies

OBJECTIVES

Upon completion of this chapter, the student will be able to

- describe the assessment of an infant with one of the congenital anomalies mentioned in this chapter.
- identify the preoperative and postoperative nursing care activities that are appropriate for children with surgically correctable anomalies.
- identify nursing measures that can assist the parents in accepting a child whose health is less than perfect.

The congenital anomalies discussed in this chapter include those defects that are obvious at birth or shortly after birth. They are conditions for which nursing care must be specialized or adapted to meet the infant's needs.

CONGENITAL HEART DISEASE

The incidence of congenital heart disease is less than one percent of all live births. This amounts to malformations occurring in six or seven infants for every thousand live births. However, congenital heart defects account for 50 percent of the deaths attributed to any type of congenital defect during the perinatal period. The onset of congestive heart failure occurs early in the most severe anomalies, and it is often the cause of death.

Several factors may contribute to the incidence of congenital heart defects. Maternal infections and nutritional disorders in the first trimester of the pregnancy are thought to cause some congenital heart abnormalities. Rubella is responsible for about four percent of such conditions. Heredity also plays a part, although its role is less clear. Similar defects have been observed in siblings. Twenty-five percent of infants with these defects have anomalies involving other biologic systems. Thirty to forty percent of infants with Down's syndrome, for instance, also have cardiac defects.

Nurses should have a basic knowledge of both the development of the fetal heart and the circulatory pathways in order to understand the problems that may arise during the infant's transition to extrauterine life. This knowledge also provides a basis for an understanding of congenital cardiac defects.

Development of the Fetal Heart

Between the second and third weeks of life, the heart is evident in the embryo in the form of a cephalocaudal tube which is anchored at both ends. The center of the tube is flexible enough to grow rapidly and bend. This bending accommodates the changes and differentiation that occur in embryonic structures. By the eighth week, the heart has divided itself into four chambers. Structures that will become the major blood vessels are also identifiable at this time. In the development of the atria, a septum forms from both the cephalic and the caudal end. This septum does not fuse but remains open to form the foramen ovale, a one-way tract that allows blood to flow from the right to the left atria. The truncus arteriosus is the last of the structures to differentiate. It forms the pulmonary artery and the aorta, with the ductus arteriosus coming off the left pulmonary artery.

Fetal Circulation

The main organ for oxygenation of the blood in the fetus is the placenta. Oxygen-rich blood travels from the placenta through the umbilical vein to the liver. A portion of the blood enters the hepatic circulation. The remainder crosses through the ductus venosus and enters the inferior vena cava. The blood travels through the inferior vena cava to the right atrium, crossing through the foramen ovale into the left atrium. From the left atrium, it descends through the bicuspid or mitral valve into the left ventricle, where it passes through the aortic valve and into the aorta. From there, it travels to the head and upper extremities to nourish those structures.

The blood returns to the heart by way of the superior vena cava to make a second circuit through the heart. It enters the right atrium, passes into the right ventricle through the tricuspid valve, and then courses into the pulmonary artery. From the pulmonary artery, it crosses through the ductus arteriosus and into the aorta again to provide oxygenation to the lower extremities. Some of this blood returns to the placenta by way of the hypogastric and umbilical arteries, Figure 11-1.

When reviewing these circulatory pathways, it is important to remember that blood is flowing and mixing in the heart in more than one direction at any given time. Although the lungs are not aerated, a small portion of blood does flow to the lungs to nourish the tissues.

At the time of the neonate's delivery and first breath and upon cutting the umbilical cord, the placenta (which has provided oxygenation until this time) is replaced by the lung. The alveoli expand with respiration, and the resistance to blood flow drops sharply, allowing the blood to enter the lungs for oxygenation. The increase in the pulmonary blood flow and the decrease in pulmonary resistance combine to change the pressures within the right and left sides of the heart. The left-sided pressure

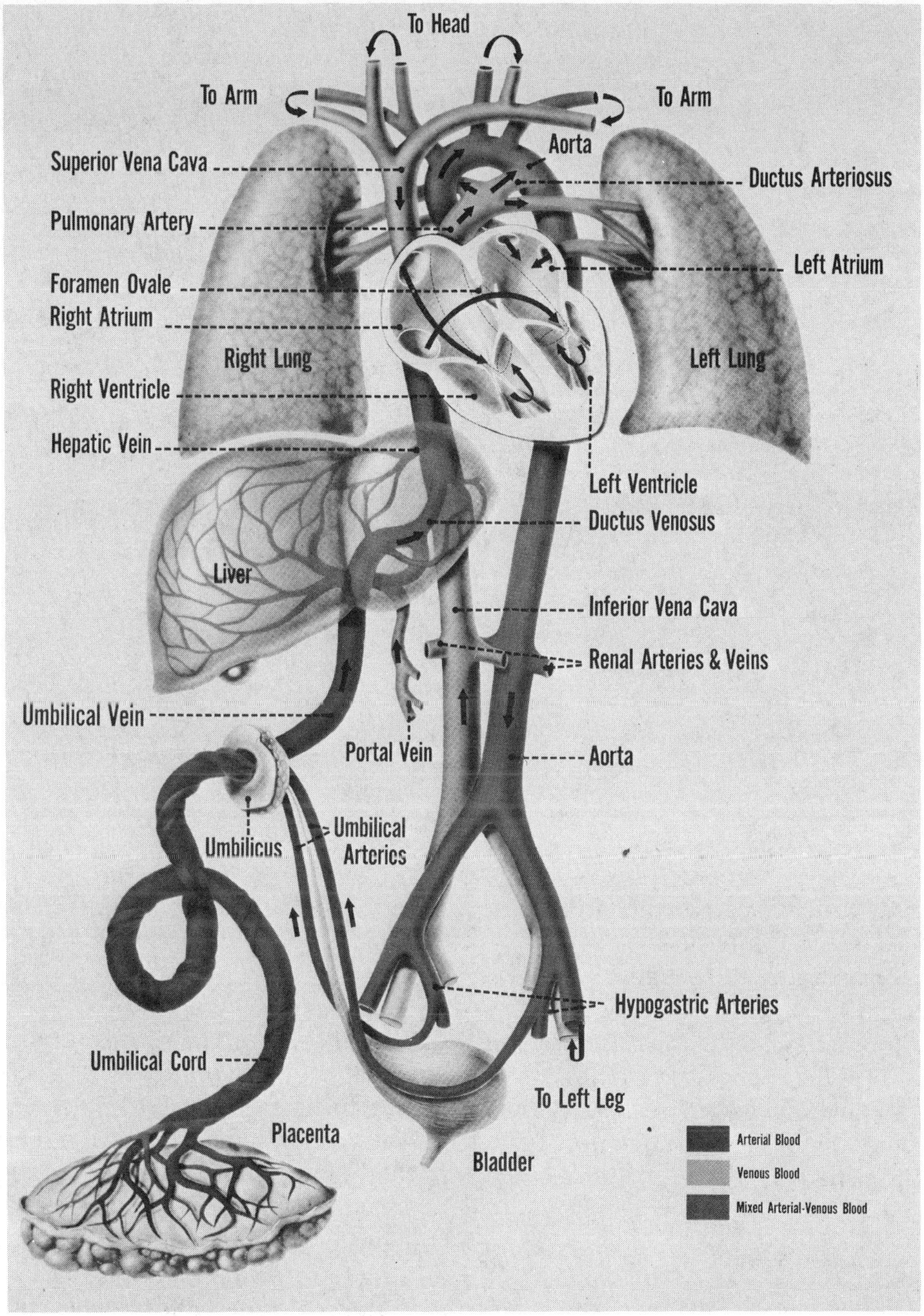

FIG. 11-1 Fetal circulation (Courtesy of Ross Laboratories)

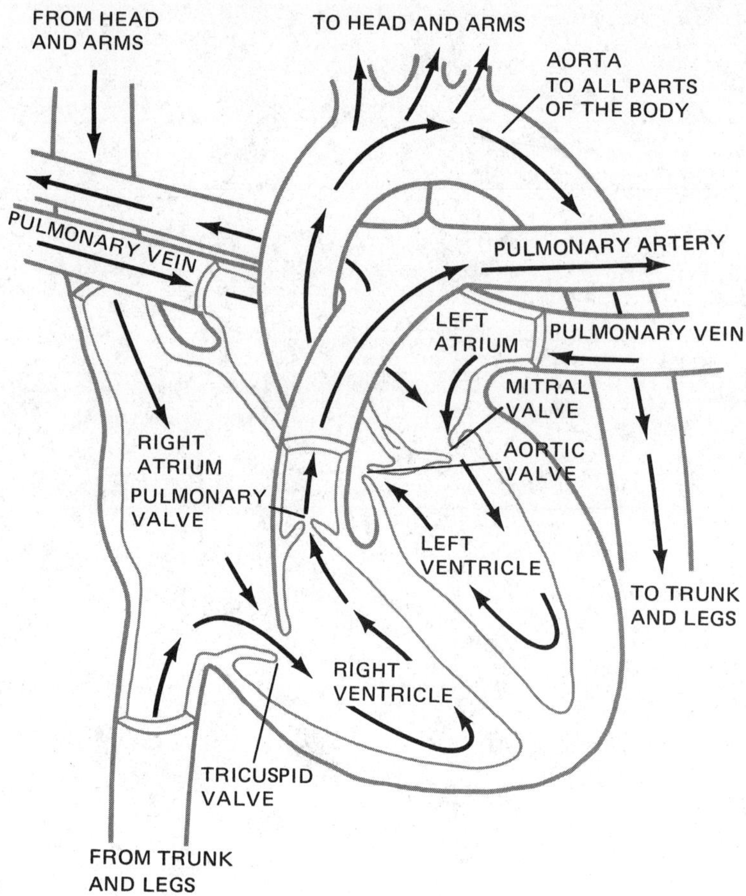

FIG. 11-2 Normal heart circulation

increases markedly, whereas the pressure in the right decreases, Figure 11-2.

The foramen ovale closes gradually because of alterations in oxygen levels as well as pressures in the heart, as does the ductus arteriosus. The function of the hypogastric arteries, umbilical arteries, and ductus venosus ceases when the umbilical cord is cut. They eventually become ligaments.

Cardiovascular Assessment

When assessing an infant or child with possible cardiovascular problems, the following basic information is obtained: blood pressure, peripheral pulse rates, quality of heart sounds, blood studies, and general appearance of the child.

Blood Pressure. The blood pressure is recorded for all children, regardless of age. It is important to use the correct equipment and technique to obtain an accurate reading. The child should be as relaxed as possible. Depending on the child's age, this may be facilitated by allowing the child to handle the equipment for a few minutes before taking a reading. Allowing the young child to remain in the parent's lap during the reading, rather than insisting that the child be in bed or on the examining table, may also be helpful. The blood pressure cuff should cover two-thirds of the child's upper arm. A cuff that is too narrow produces an erroneously high reading. Conversely, one that is too wide produces a misleading low reading.

The blood pressure may also be taken in the leg. To do this, the child lies prone. In order to cover two-thirds of the length of the thigh, the blood pressure cuff should be about 6 millimeters larger than that used to take the blood pressure in the arm. The cuff should be positioned rather high on the thigh. The pulse is then palpated in the popliteal fossa. The systolic pressure is usually higher in the leg than in the arm. Conversely, the diastolic pressure is generally lower than in the arm. In infants younger than one year of age, the systolic pressure in both arm and leg may be equal. In children older than one year of age, the systolic pressure in the leg may be as much as 40 mm Hg higher than in the arm and still be considered within normal limits.

Peripheral Pulses. Assessment of the peripheral pulses should include a determination of the quality, rate, and rhythm of the radial and femoral pulses, as well as of the posterior tibial and dorsalis pedis. A comparison should be made between the quality of the pulses on the left and right sides. The dorsalis pedis and posterior tibial are abnormally strong in infants or children with patent ductus arteriosus. They may be absent in those with coarctation of the aorta. Other factors that may affect the pulse rate include excitement; poor exercise tolerance; endocrine disease, such as hyperthyroidism; toxicity; and fever. An elevated temperature increases the pulse rate about eight to ten beats per minute for every degree of temperature elevation.

Heart Sounds. Any assessment of heart sounds is begun by determining the point of maximal impulse. This impulse is located toward the lower rib margin in the position nearest the axilla, either in the midclavicular line or just left of this, depending on the child's age. It is important to note the quality and intensity of the sounds, as well as their rate and rhythm. The presence of any abnormal sounds should also be noted.

Two heart sounds may be heard in about thirty percent of children because of maximal filling of the ventricles. The first sound is the result of closure of the mitral and tricuspid valves. The second heart sound results from closure of the aortic and pulmonic valves.

Normal sounds that may be heard include friction rubbing, clicks, snapping sounds, and some murmurs. A large percentage of murmurs in children are functional. Murmurs are usually classified according to their timing in the cardiac cycle, as well as their quality, intensity, and duration. Systolic murmurs occur at or after the first heart sound and before the second sound. This is the period in which the ventricles contract as blood is driven into the aorta and the pulmonary artery. Diastolic murmurs, which are more characteristic of heart disease, occur at or after the second sound and before the first sound begins. This is the period during which ventricles are filling and the heart is maximally dilated. The quality of a murmur is described as soft, harsh, blowing, or whistling. The intensity is a grading of the loudness of a murmur from the softest, which is not heard in all positions, to the loudest, which is audible without a stethoscope.

Blood Studies. It is also important to obtain a complete blood count. Is it consistent with the normal values for the age of the child? In the neonate, the normal red blood cell count may be as high as 19 grams with a forty-four to sixty-four percent hematocrit. These same values in a five-year-old child would be inappropriate, and would likely indicate a cardiovascular problem.

General Appearance. Inspection of the child is also important. Does this child show any signs of respiratory distress? Is cyanosis apparent? If it is present, does it improve or worsen with energy expenditure, such as occurs in crying, bottle-feeding, or other activities? Is edema, such as periorbital edema, present in the infant? Is there any clubbing of the fingers or toes? Is there precordial bulging such as that seen with right ventricular enlargement? (An enlarged heart demonstrated on radiography is consistent with several types of heart disease, including congenital heart disease, rheumatic fever, and myocarditis.)

Signs and Symptoms of Heart Disease

The symptoms that are common to both infants and children with congenital heart disease are dyspnea, recurrent respiratory infection, heart murmur, and cyanosis.

Young Infants. In infants younger than one year of age, additional symptoms may be evident. Difficulty with feeding, and stridor or choking spells that occur during feeding, are quite common. Additionally, a pulse rate in a sleeping or resting infant that consistently exceeds two hundred beats per minute is indicative of heart disease. Failure to gain weight is a generalized symptom that may or may not be related to congenital heart disease. Infants with this problem may be too exhausted to consume sufficient calories, or they may rapidly be burning those calories that are consumed because of their high metabolic rate. Cerebrovascular accidents can occur because of the high hematocrit levels. Anoxic attacks are also seen in this age-group.

Older Children. In children older than one year of age, poor physical development is commonly associated with a cardiac defect. Decreased exercise tolerance may also be evident. A squatting posture may be noted in older children with heart disorders. This position reduces the workload of the heart and improves blood flow from the extremities. Clubbing of the fingers and toes may result from decreased oxygenation of the capillaries in the extremities. Elevated blood pressure may be present in children with coarctation of the aorta.

Cyanosis and Congestive Heart Failure. Cyanosis and congestive heart failure are the two major manifestations of cardiac distress in infants. Cyanosis occurs in two-thirds of infants with congenital heart disease. It is not to be confused with acrocyanosis or the peripheral cyanosis in the neonate that clears with increased warmth and activity. The baby's color should be observed carefully in a good light. As fluorescent lights and room color may give erroneous impressions, daylight is preferred for color assessment. The baby's temperature should also be determined. A subnormal temperature causes peripheral vasoconstriction which, in turn, makes the skin of the infant look mottled or marblelike. The effect of crying or increased activity on the infant's color should be observed. An increase in activity exacerbates the cyanosis in children with cardiac problems. Conversely, the color may improve if the child has a respiratory problem. Skin color has various shades of pigmentation and is not always a good indicator of cyanosis. The oral or buccal mucosa should be checked. This gives a better indication of central cyanosis and is not altered by normal shades of pigmentation. Cyanosis is present in any condition that causes shunting of unoxygenated blood from the right side of the heart to the left and into the general circulation.

Those infants who have acyanotic defects often develop congestive heart failure. This condition is prevalent in children with certain disorders, such as patent ductus arteriosus and septal defects, that are accompanied by increased pulmonary vascularity. Initial symptoms include tachypnea, dyspnea, and tachycardia. The symptoms are directly related to the left-to-right shunting that has occurred and the volume overload of the right ventricle. Tachypnea in this population is defined as a respiratory rate of greater than fifty respirations per minute with an infant at rest. Dyspnea may be recognized by flaring nares, expiratory grunts, and retracting of the intercostal muscles. In late cardiac failure when the infant is using the ancillary respiratory muscles, bobbing of the head may be observed on inspiration. Tachycardia is identified as an apical pulse rate of greater than one hundred fifty beats per minute. Other symptoms that may be evident are diaphoresis, hepatomegaly, and edema. Diaphoresis may be diagnosed when perspiration is noted on the head or face during any type of energy expenditure. The edema may be most prominent in the facial and periorbital areas, but it may also be generalized. Nurses should observe the child carefully for any of these symptoms on a regular basis.

General Nursing Care. Positioning of the infant is very important. The infant's head should be elevated in a semi-Fowler's position. This may be achieved by using an infant seat or by elevating the head end of the mattress board in the incubator. To maintain the position, a small, rolled towel is placed under the infant's knees. Infants who are cyanotic or recurrently anoxic should be placed on their abdomens in a knee-chest position.

Oxygen therapy may be administered in a number of ways. The infant may be placed in an incubator, or a mask, tent, or hood may be used. Because the cyanosis is a result of a congenital heart defect, the appearance of the infant does not improve significantly with the use of oxygen.

Oral feedings or fluids are not administered to these infants until a physician has performed an evaluation. The potential for regurgitation and aspiration is high and should thus be avoided. These infants also become easily exhausted by oral feedings. In the interest of conserving the infant's energy, tube feedings are used.

Assisting Parents

Because many infants with heart defects are diagnosed at birth or during their stay in the newborn nursery, particular emphasis must be placed on the process of maternal and infant bonding. Parents must have the opportunity to see their child and to have those factors that are causes for concern, such as the baby's color and any difficulty in breathing, pointed out to them. At the same time, all the normal features of the child should also be noted. Parents should have as much contact as possible with the infant, particularly if the child is to be transferred to a regional center for care. The parents are thus given time to ask questions and to cope with the problem in a realistic fashion. They should be told where the child will be transferred, who will be responsible for their child's care, and how to contact either the hospital or that individual to obtain information regarding the infant. Parents are usually very anxious during this time. Therefore, information should be repeated several times and also be written out so the parents can refer to it when needed. Informed written consent should be obtained by the physician for any necessary procedures. Children with suspected congenital heart defects routinely undergo a history and physical assessment, a complete blood count, x-ray studies, an electrocardiogram, and a cardiac catheterization in order to confirm or exclude the diagnosis. Additionally, echocardiograms or phonocardiograms may be done in some children.

Cardiac Catheterization

Since these children routinely undergo cardiac catheterization, nurses must know how to care for them when they return to the unit. Frequent vital signs are performed in all such children for a period of twenty-four to forty-eight hours. When measuring vital signs, the nurse should be especially alert to any sign of bradycardia. This is a particularly ominous sign as it often is accompanied by hypotension and hypoxia and may precede cardiac arrest.

Pulses are evaluated in the extremities, with special attention given any sign of arterial thrombosis, the most common complication. Signs of this complication include coolness of the skin to touch, mottling of the skin, weakened pulse, and absence of response to blanching.

The pressure dressing should be checked frequently for any sign of bleeding. The nurse should also feel underneath the infant or child as the use of the femoral site for the cardiac catheterization in a small infant may cause blood to seep along the inguinal area. In this case, the blood would not be readily seen on the surface dressings.

Intake and output should be monitored carefully after the cardiac catheterization. Fluid balance is always a concern. After the procedure, an untoward reaction to the dye used in the procedure is an added concern. In particular, the first voiding is checked for hematuria. Hematuria may be a response to presence of the dye or it may be the first sign of renal failure.

Preoperative Preparation

General preoperative preparation is the same as for any other surgery. However, some special considerations must be made for children with heart conditions, depending on their age, as well as for their families. Parents of infants and toddlers should be told what to expect in terms of what will be done, where the child will be, and how they may participate in the child's care. It is advantageous if this information is provided in a small group setting of two or more sets of parents. This approach frequently establishes a supportive network among the parents that may continue throughout the hospitalization.

When preschool or school-aged children are to undergo heart surgery, they and their parents must be adequately informed. It may be beneficial to conduct this session in a small group setting as well, but with children of the same developmental age. Small amounts of information should be presented over several short sessions rather than all at once, as children cannot absorb large amounts of information at one setting. Their behavior will indicate whether they have lost interest in the presentation. The most common evidence of too much stress or too much information for the child is movement away from the group or disruptive behavior.

Children of this age-group should visit the intensive care area to which they will be transferred after surgery. Meeting some of the staff members may also be helpful. Opportunities to practice coughing and deep breathing with a chest splint, to be in an oxygen or mist tent, or to use a nasal cannula help to familiarize this child with postoperative activities.

All children who are candidates for heart surgery should be protected from infection during the preoperative period. Their room assignment, their contact with other patients, particularly older ones, and the persons with whom they are allowed to visit should be monitored. Since their tolerance for active participation is limited, the nurse must schedule activities to provide the maximal amount of rest for the child. Conservation of energy is important, and yet these children should not be made to feel isolated from other children because of their physical limitations.

Operative Procedures

Operative procedures for congenital heart defects may be divided into two types: palliative and corrective. The purpose of palliative procedures is to improve the oxygenation of tissues through the alteration of abnormal circulatory pathways. Palliative procedures are closed cardiac procedures. Corrective procedures are open-heart procedures that require cardiopulmonary bypass techniques for the maintenance of circulation during the operation.

Surgery for Cyanotic Defects. Two congenital heart defects have cyanosis as the major feature. These are transposition of the great vessels and tetralogy of Fallot. (Fallo-)

Transposition of the Great Vessels. In transposition of the great vessels, the positions of the aorta and the pulmonary arteries are reversed. They arise from the wrong side of the heart, Figure 11-3. The infant cannot survive without the presence of other defects, such as a ventricular septal defect or a patent ductus arteriosus. These additional defects provide a mixing of the oxygenated and unoxygenated blood. The greater the mixing that occurs, the less cyanotic the infant will be.

Palliative correction of this condition involves one of several procedures. The Glenn procedure involves anastomosis of the right pulmonary artery to the superior vena cava. The Blalock-Hanlon procedure creates an artificial atrial septal defect. Following both of these procedures, the infant's head must be elevated to decrease edema in the head and neck area. The nurse should also assess the function of the infant's right lung. The infant should be checked frequently for cyanosis above the nipple line as this indicates pooling of blood in the pulmonary artery.

The open-heart procedure for correction of transposition of the great vessels is called the Mustard procedure. A new atrial septum is created by using a baffle constructed of pericardium. This redirects the oxygenated blood into the general circulation and the unoxygenated blood into the pulmonary circuit.

Tetralogy of Fallot. Tetralogy of Fallot consists of four major defects. These are right ventricular hypertrophy, pulmonary stenosis, a ventricular septal defect, and dextraposition or overriding of the aorta. The major difficulty

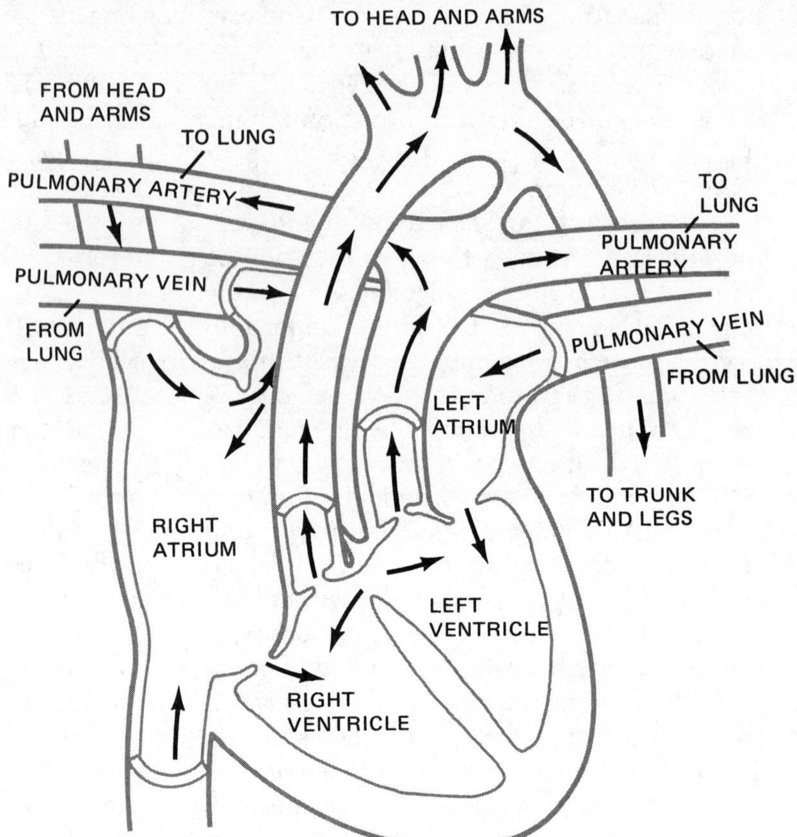

FIG. 11-3 Transposition of the great vessels

in this condition is the obstruction to flow in the right ventricle. Pulmonary stenosis, which may or may not involve the valve itself, increases the pressure in the right ventricle. As the pressure rises, a right-to-left shunting occurs through the ventricular septal defect, and unoxygenated blood passes into the general circulation as it mixes with the blood in the left ventricle, Figure 11-4.

The degree of cyanosis in children with this defect is dependent on the amount of blood that is shunted. The infant may have minimal cyanosis when resting, but cyanosis may increase upon increased energy expenditure. As the child grows, the cyanosis may be intermittent at first. Gradually, it will increase in frequency until it persists continuously, with variations in degrees occurring only with activity. Clubbing of fingers and toes, a squatting posture, and anoxic attacks may be among the symptoms.

The palliative procedures that are undertaken to improve oxygenation include Pott's procedure, which is a side-to-side anastomosis between the ascending aorta and the pulmonary artery. Another is the Blalock-Taussig

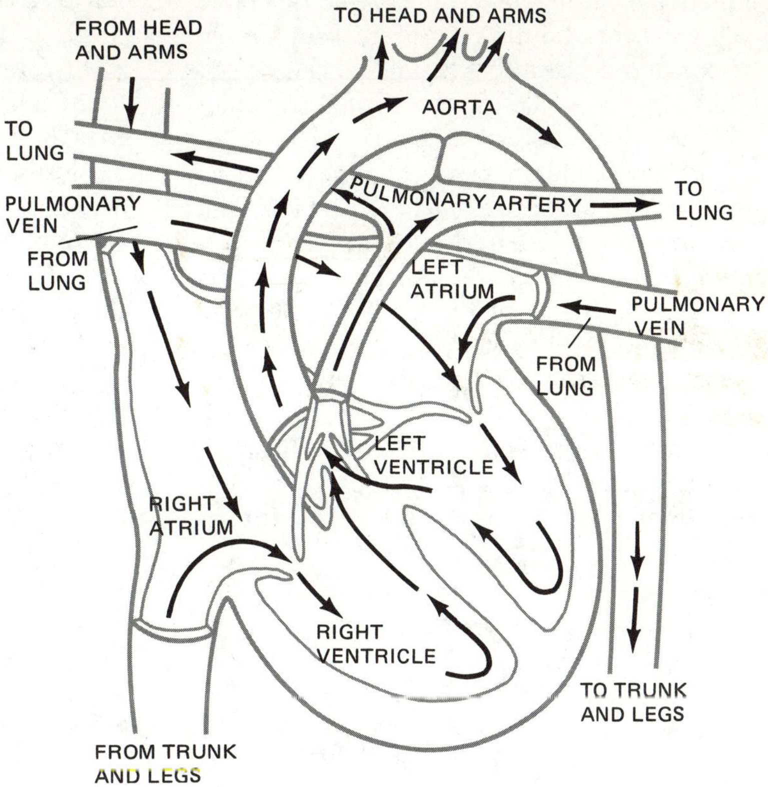

FIG. 11-4 Tetralogy of Fallot

procedure, which is an anastomosis between the subclavian and pulmonary arteries.

Postoperatively, the nurse must observe the child carefully for signs of congestive heart failure, arrhythmias, and hemorrhage. Congestive failure occurs more commonly with the Pott's procedure.

The open-heart procedure is usually performed in older children. Prior to placing the child on cardiopulmonary bypass, any previous shunts must be repaired or closed. The correction involves closure of the ventricular septal defect and opening of the pulmonary stenosis.

Surgery for Acyanotic Defects. The remainder of the congenital heart defects are classified as acyanotic. In these infants and children, the defect causes left-to-right shunting and excess blood volume coursing through the pulmonary circuit. The result is a high incidence of congestive heart failure.

Patent Ductus Arteriosus. Patent ductus arteriosus is the best example of an acyanotic heart defect. The ductus arteriosus begins closing shortly after birth. Complete closure may take several weeks. Because the retrograde blood flow from the aorta through the ductus is minimal, the closure is considered to be functional during that time. A considerable volume of blood flows into the pulmonary artery and again into the lungs, Figure 11-5. The larger the ductus, the earlier the child shows signs of congestive failure.

Many children with this defect have minimal symptoms except for a characteristic murmur. It is referred to as a "machinery murmur" because its continuous hum is evident through all phases of the cardiac cycle. The murmur may be heard most easily at the upper left sternal border at the midclavicular line.

The corrective procedure involves ligation of the ductus arteriosus. Postoperative complications that may occur include the formation of an aneurysm at the site of the repair, as well as damage to the phrenic nerve.

Coarctation of the Aorta. Coarctation of the aorta is a stenosis or narrowing of the aorta that occurs near the site of the ductus arteriosus, Figure 11-6. Characteristic findings include hypertension in the upper extremities and hypotension in the lower extremities. Assessment of the child's pulse will support these findings as the pulses in the lower extremities will be weak or entirely absent.

The surgical procedure to correct this defect is an aortic resection with an end-to-end anastomosis. The time of surgery depends on the degree of hypertension. The defect is most commonly corrected between the third and tenth year of age. Nursing responsibilities

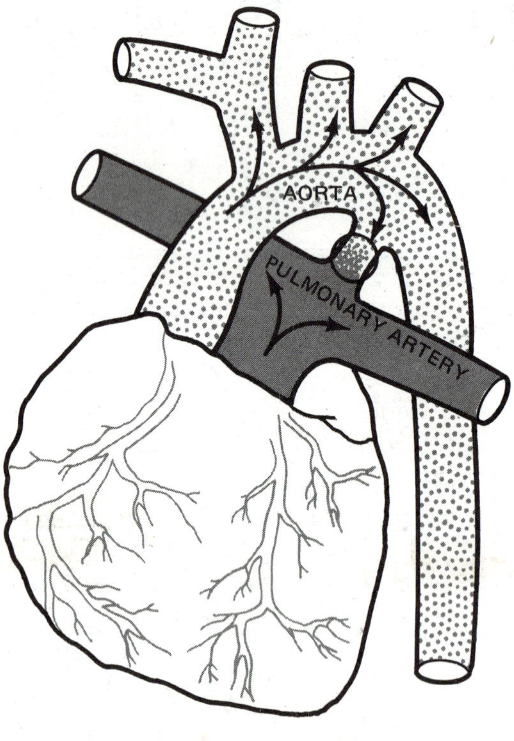

FIG. 11-5 Patent ductus arteriosus

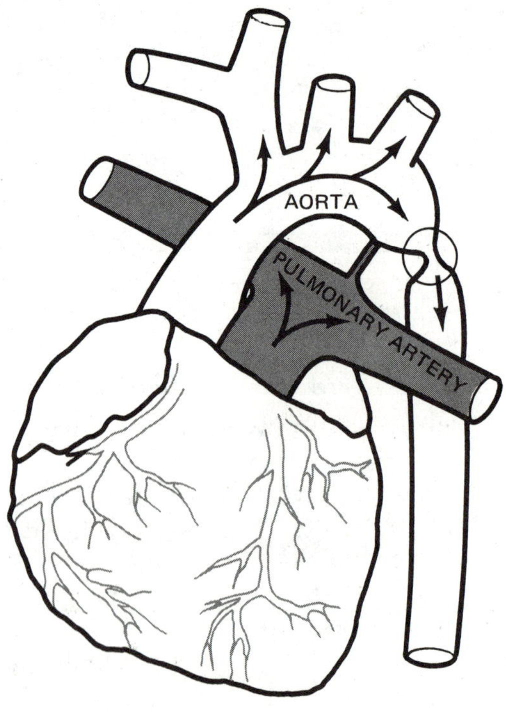

FIG. 11-6 Coarctation of the aorta

include an assessment for altered blood pressures. A sudden drop in blood pressure occurs following the procedure. Pedal pulses should be assessed carefully, as thrombus formation can occur. One complication is known as the postcoarctation syndrome. It is characterized by severe abdominal pain caused by increased blood flow to the organs within the abdomen and to the lower extremities.

Atrial and Ventricular Septal Defects. Atrial and ventricular septal defects, if small, may be heralded by few symptoms in the pediatric age-group. With these defects, left-to-right shunting of blood occurs and the pulmonary circuit becomes overloaded, Figures 11-7 and 11-8. Symptoms in affected children may include recurrent respiratory infections that are more evident with fatigue or overexertion. These children do have audible murmurs. Spontaneous closure of small defects occurs in some children over a period of years. For this reason, treatment is conservative. In children with large defects, signs of congestive failure develop early in infancy.

Surgical correction involves simple suturing for the smaller defects and grafting for the

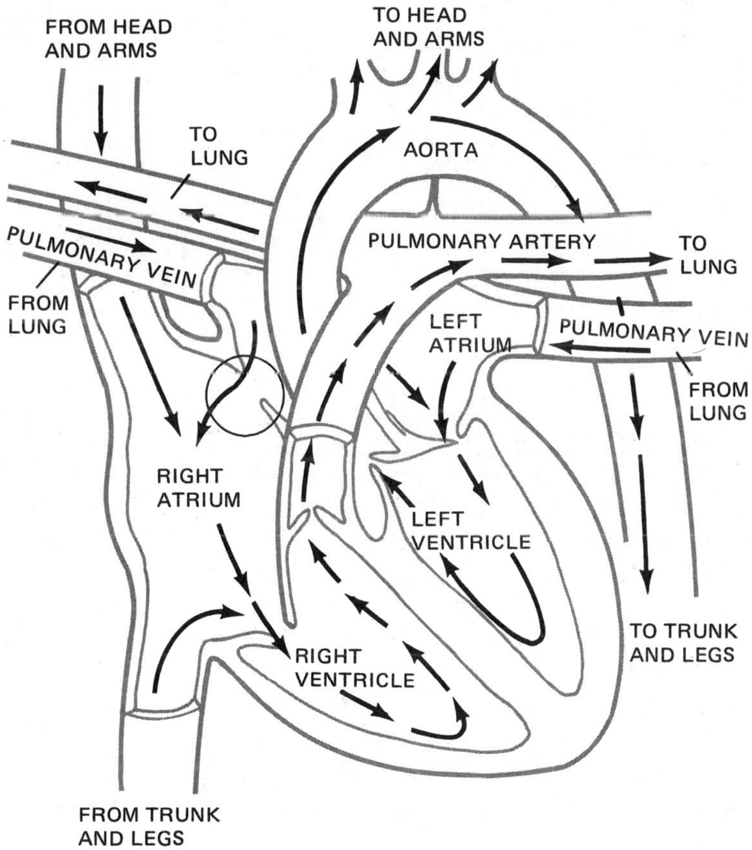

FIG. 11-7 Atrial septal defect

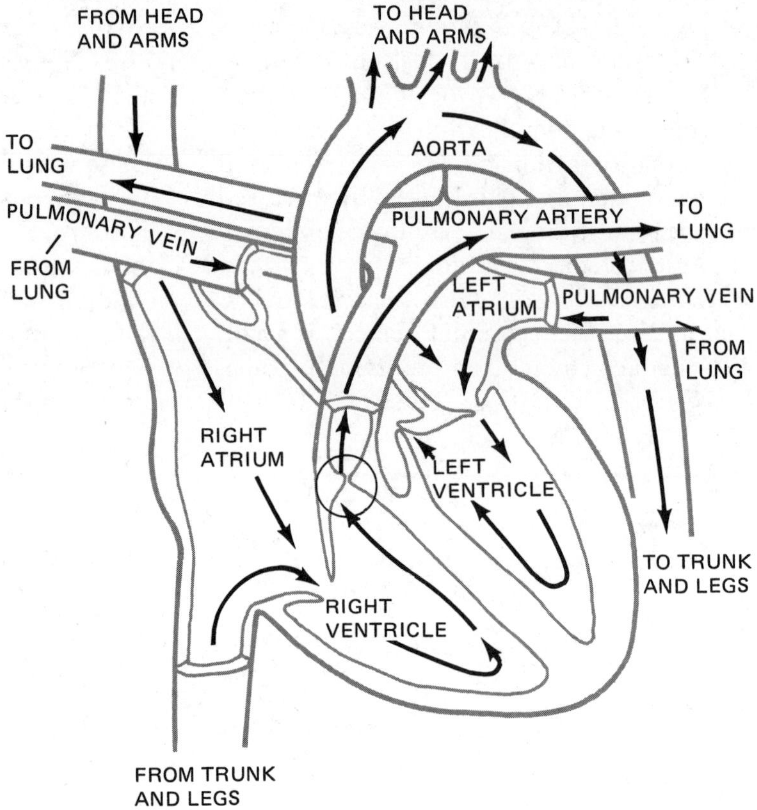

11-9 Pulmonary stenosis
FIG. ~~11-8 Ventricular septal defect~~

larger procedures. Nursing responsibilities include observing the child for pulmonary edema, arrhythmias (which may indicate the need for a pacemaker), and hypotension, which may be life-threatening.

Pulmonary and Aortic Stenosis. Pulmonary and aortic stenosis are two other examples of acyanotic heart defects. Both are obstructions of outflow from one of the ventricles, Figures 11-9 and 11-10. In some instances, the defect is mild, with few symptoms except for a loud murmur. The more severe defects cause congestive heart failure relatively early in life. Exertional dyspnea and decreased exercise tolerance may occur with pulmonary stenosis in later childhood or early adolescence.

Surgical correction involves valvotomy to separate the fused cusps. Nursing responsibilities include observation of the child for hemorrhage and cardiac tamponade, which may occur twenty-four to forty-eight hours postoperatively. Symptoms include air hunger, distended neck veins, narrow pulse pressure, and muffled heart sounds.

Postoperative Nursing Care

Children who have undergone heart surgery are transported to an intensive care area postoperatively. They have multiple indwelling catheters in place. A line for central venous pressure monitoring and a line into the

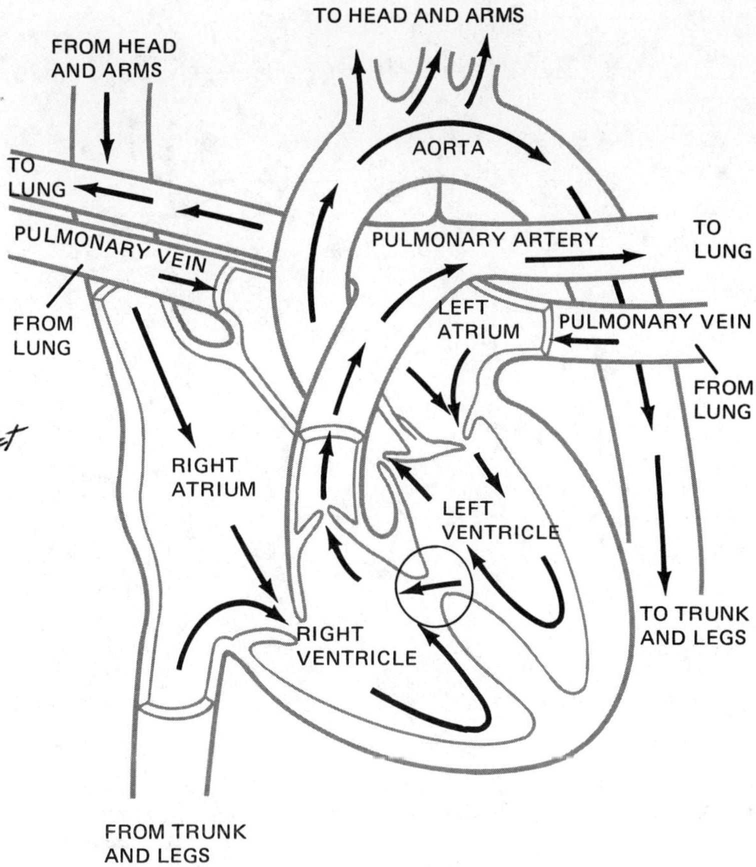

FIG. ~~11-9 Pulmonary stenosis~~ 11-8 Ventricular Septal Defect

pulmonary artery and left atrium are also present. A Foley catheter is in place to facilitate output measurements. One or two thoracotomy tubes are in place and are connected to water-seal drainage. If one of the potential complications of the surgery is arrhythmias, the child may also have an epicardial pacing wire in place to prevent heart block.

Vital Signs. The postoperative care of these children is similar to that given all children who have had surgery. Vital signs are monitored carefully. Immediately after the surgery, the infant or child is placed on a hypothermia blanket with a rectal probe in place to monitor and maintain body temperature. Body temperature is usually subnormal after surgery. An incubator is used to provide warmth as well as oxygenation in very small infants.

Airway Maintenance. Maintenance of a clear airway is a nursing priority for these children. Any sign of respiratory distress should be noted, including stridor, tracheal edema, and tachypnea. Children who are old enough to cooperate are encouraged to do deep breathing exercises and to cough and change position regularly.

Intake and Output. Fluid intake and output should be monitored carefully. All fluids should be administered via microdrip tubing, usually with the assistance of an intravenous

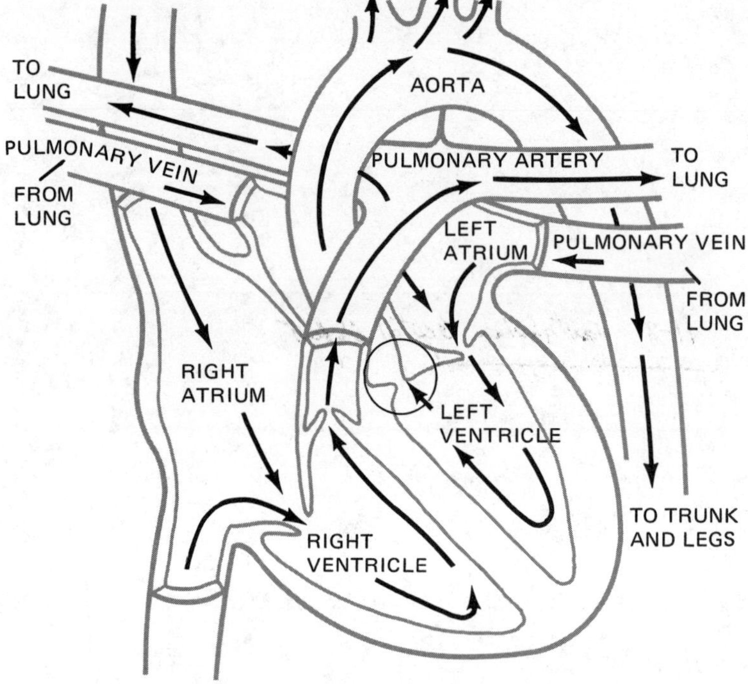

FIG. 11-10 Aortic stenosis

pump. Output is monitored by a urinometer. The child's output should be maintained at 1 milliliter per kilogram of body weight per hour.

Cyanosis. Careful observations are made to detect cyanosis of these children. The color and appearance of the nailbeds upon blanching and of the buccal mucosa are noted. Initially, the child receives oxygen with the aid of an incubator or oxygen tent. A nasal cannula may be used in older children, but this is less common.

Thoracotomy Tubes. The nurse also has specific responsibilities related to the care of patients with thoracotomy tubes in place. When the child arrives on the unit, the nurse should mark the level of drainage in the bottle and note the appearance of the drainage. Fluctuations in the waterseal apparatus as the child breathes should also be noted. The bottles are maintained at a specified level below the chest. The tubing should be kept free of kinks and should be long enough to allow the child some freedom of movement. Hourly milking of the tubing is necessary to clear blood clots or serum that may clog the tube. Drainage is recorded hourly as a part of the patient's output record.

Two large hemostats are kept at the bedside in case of emergency. They should be placed on the tubing in alternate directions as close to the chest wall as possible. They must be used immediately if the bottle breaks or if the child has symptoms of pneumothorax.

Continued Care. As the child improves, he or she is moved out of the intensive care area and allowed to increase activities. During this time, it is important for the nurse to recognize regressive behavior on the part of the child as his or her means of coping with the stress of the hospitalization. A play therapist or a child-life worker, as well as the nurse, can encourage the child in an honest expression of feeling through play.

At the time of discharge, activity restrictions may be minimal. Parents may have some difficulty accepting the relaxed restrictions and may tend to overprotect the child. This is a problem that the health team should explore with the parents so they can work through their feelings.

CLEFT LIP AND PALATE

A cleft lip and palate may occur either separately or in combination. Both represent a congenital failure of two parts to fuse during uterine life. The problem occurs during the fifth to the tenth week of embryonic or fetal life. Each defect by itself occurs in varying degrees of severity, Figures 11-11 and 11-12. The cleft lip may be so slight that mere notching of the vermilion border of the lip is the only sign of the defect. It may also be so severe that the fissure extends bilaterally into the nares, leaving a minimal amount of upper lip tissue. The severity of a cleft palate can range from a fissure in the uvula to complete extension of the cleft along the length of the palate and into the alveolar ridge.

Attitudes of Parents and Caregivers

Cleft defects are both visible and upsetting to parents expecting a perfect child. Their anger, disappointment, and fear soon give way to strong feelings of guilt. Nurses can provide the parents with support, comfort, and accurate information. Parents should be told what must be done to correct the defect, who can do it, and how they can cope with the baby's care in the interim.

Anger, tears, and many questions are normal parts of the process of adjustment, and the nurse should provide support and reassurance during this time. Once the physician has explained correction of the defect to the parents, the parents must be given adequate time to assimilate the information and to pose questions about their own concerns.

During this time, the parents need support in facing relatives and friends who may come to see the baby. The nurse can facilitate a positive response and approach by treating the infant as a normal infant. Parents may need to be encouraged to cuddle and handle this infant in order to achieve secure bonding.

Parents should be informed that cleft corrections are usually performed in several stages, depending on the extent of the defect. They should also be told that the child's appearance will improve gradually, rather than all at once after the first surgical procedure. Members of the cleft palate team often keep photographs of individual children which document the gradually improving appearance of the child. These photographs may be shared with the parents.

Later, the parents' attendance at the cleft lip and palate clinic will expose them to other parents who have faced the same problems. They may derive needed support from this as

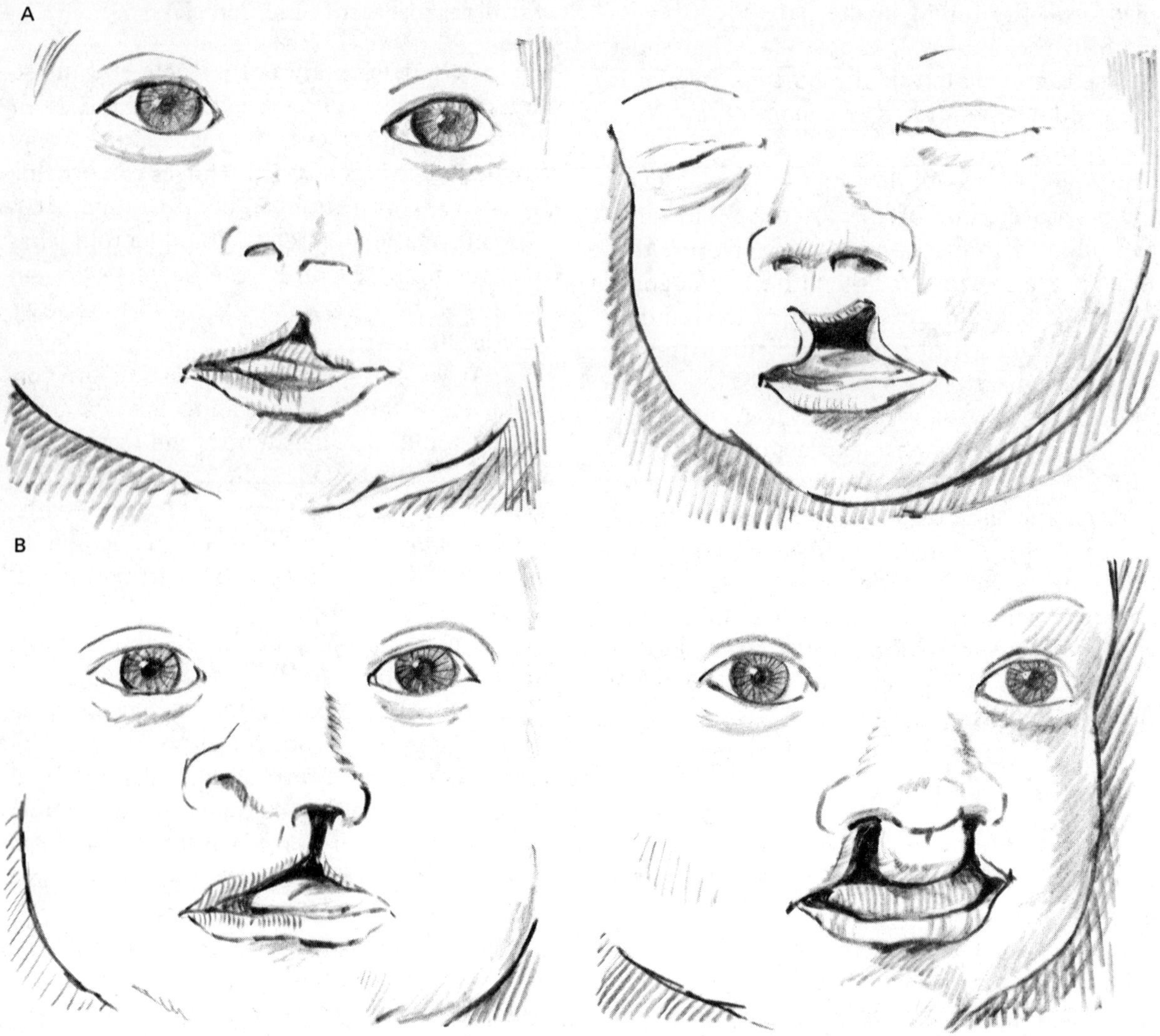

FIG. 11-11 Varying degrees of severity of clefts of the lip. *A)* Incomplete clefts of the lip – unilateral (left) and bilateral (right). *B)* Complete clefts of the lip – unilateral (left) and bilateral (right).

well as from seeing the improved appearances of other children following surgical correction. In some facilities, the clinic may also sponsor a parent support group which assists these parents from the time of the infant's birth.

Feeding Difficulties

Infants with a cleft lip or palate have feeding problems from the onset. Their inability to suck is a source of frustration. They generally have a good appetite but fuss or cry because

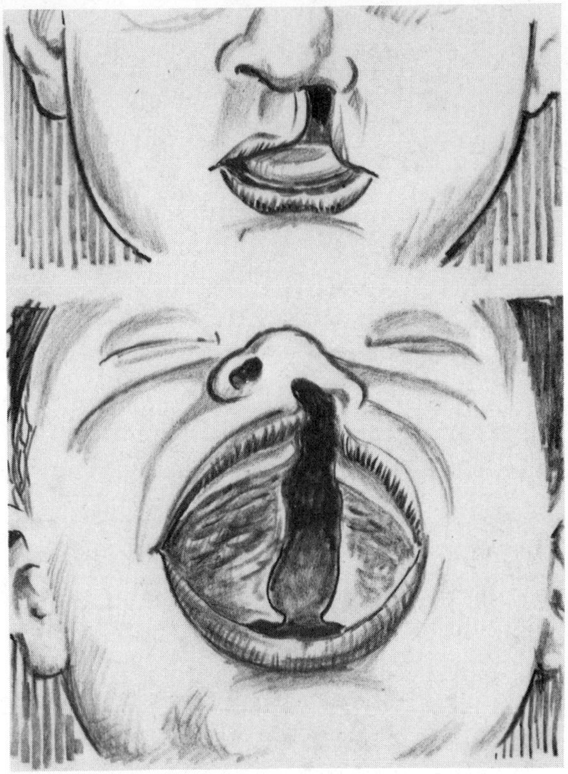

FIG. 11-12 Unilateral complete cleft lip and palate

of the meager amount obtained when attempts are made to feed them. These babies also have larger amounts of mucus than normal, and those with palatal defects may regurgitate fluids through the nose.

Infants may be fed with special feeders, such as duck-billed nipples or Brecht feeders. Alternatively, they may be fed with soft, cross-cut nipples or disposable plastic nursers, such as a Beniflex. They may also be breast-fed if the mother had planned to nurse the baby. The breast tissue occludes the cleft nicely. The method of choice for these infants is the one which provides the greatest amount of milk or formula for them with the least amount of effort on the part of the infant.

Infants with cleft palates or lips should be held in a sitting or upright position for feedings in order to reduce the risk of aspiration. If a plastic, controllable feeder is used, it is best to direct the flow of formula to the side, rather than directly in the midline. The baby should be burped frequently during the feeding because of the large amount of air that is swallowed. After the feeding, the infant should be kept in an infant seat or upright for twenty to thirty minutes to prevent any aspiration of the milk or formula. A small amount of water should be offered after each feeding to rinse the mouth.

Cleft Lip Repair

Surgical correction of a cleft lip, or cheiloplasty, is carried out when the child weighs between six and ten pounds. Some surgeons delay the procedure until the infant is eight to ten weeks of age. The infant must have at least a ten-gram hemoglobin. The major criteria that dictate the time of surgery are the amount of available tissue for the repair, the attitude of the parents toward the child, and the degree of difficulty in feeding. Parents need time to bond with the infant and to adjust to the infant's problem. The later the correction, the more positive the parents will be in recognizing the degree of improvement seen in the child. This is a very important consideration because parental attitudes last for a lifetime.

Preoperative Care. Preoperatively, the infant is admitted several days prior to the surgery. During this time, the infant is fed with a rubber-tipped syringe or medicine dropper by squirt-

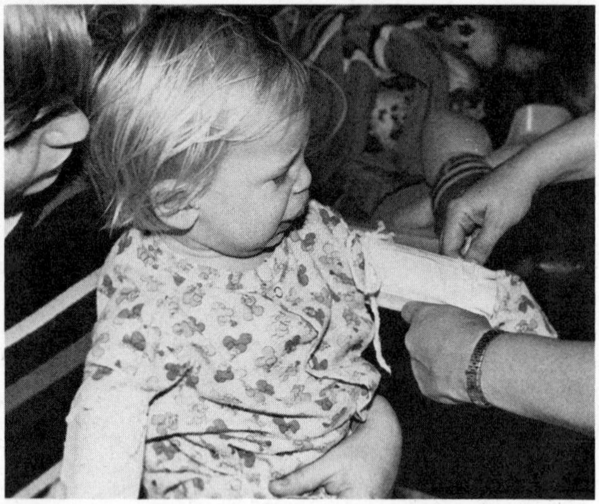

FIG. 11-13 **Restraints should be removed every two hours to check the skin condition underneath. They are then reapplied.**

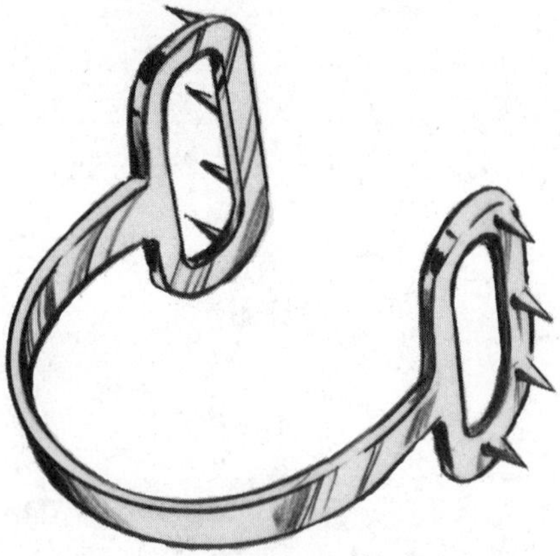

FIG. 11-14 A Logan bow is used to protect the suture line after repair of a cleft lip.

ing small amounts of formula or breast milk into the baby's mouth. Use of elbow restraints may be initiated at this time so that the child may become accustomed to them. The restraints are removed every two hours to check the skin, Figure 11-13. It is also helpful if the infant is positioned on the side or back to sleep, as these are the prescribed positions after the surgery.

Immediately prior to the surgery, the infant is immobilized on a papoose board after being sedated. The lip is marked carefully and the area is infiltrated with a local anesthetic such as lidocaine and epinephrine. Older children may be given thiopental rectally. Immediately after the surgery, a Logan bow is attached to the child's cheeks with adhesive tape to prevent any tension on the suture line, Figure 11-14.

Postoperative Care. Postoperatively, large amounts of mucus may be present in the mouth

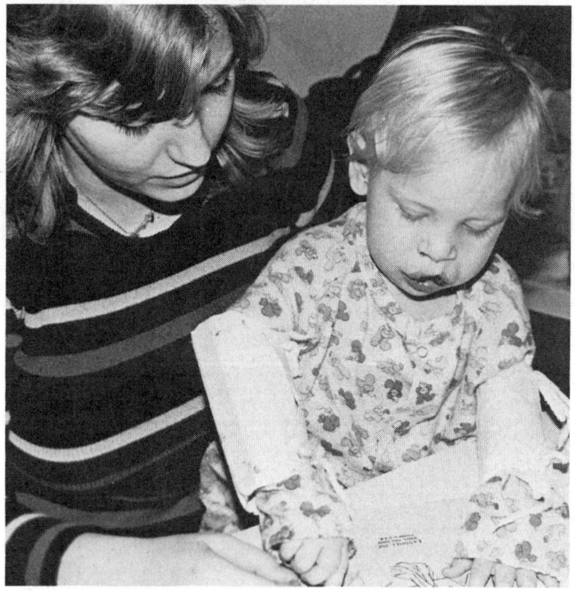

FIG. 11-15 Properly applied elbow restraints should not limit the child's activities.

and pharynx. Gentle suctioning may be required to remove the mucus. A side-lying position is necessary at this point. A croupette may be used to provide additional humidity.

If it is properly placed, the Logan bow will prevent the child from rubbing the face in the sheets or otherwise traumatizing the surgical correction. Elbow restraints keep little hands and fingers out of the mouth and away from the incision, Figure 11-15.

Feedings begin with the squirting of clear liquids into the mouth with a syringe. The child must not suck on the syringe as this produces tension on the suture line. Feedings are routinely followed by rinsing the mouth with water as before.

Suture care involves cleansing of the suture line to prevent crusting and resultant scarring. The incision is cleansed with hydrogen peroxide three to four times daily using cotton-tipped applicators, Figure 11-16. An antibacterial ointment is usually applied after the cleansing. At this time, the Logan bow should be checked to ensure that it is secure.

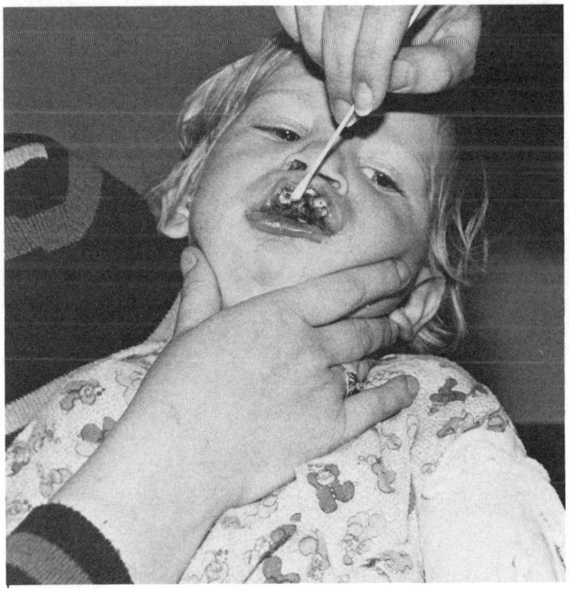

FIG. 11-16 Postoperative cleansing is performed three or four times each day using cotton applicators, hydrogen peroxide, and normal saline.

The postoperative period is rather traumatic for infants who have undergone a cleft lip repair, particularly if comfort is sought from thumbsucking. Both thumbsucking and crying cause tension on the suture line and must be avoided. Slight sedation is often used in these children. Frequent holding and rocking, as well as frequent diaper changes and the presence of loving parents reduces crying significantly. Positioning the infant in a baby seat may also be helpful for diversion.

Long-Term Considerations. Surgical correction may have to be completed in stages, even if only a single defect is involved. Moreover, cleft lip repairs may require revision at some point. The flattened side of the nares, for instance, will have to be realigned surgically sometime after the initial repair, Figure 11-17.

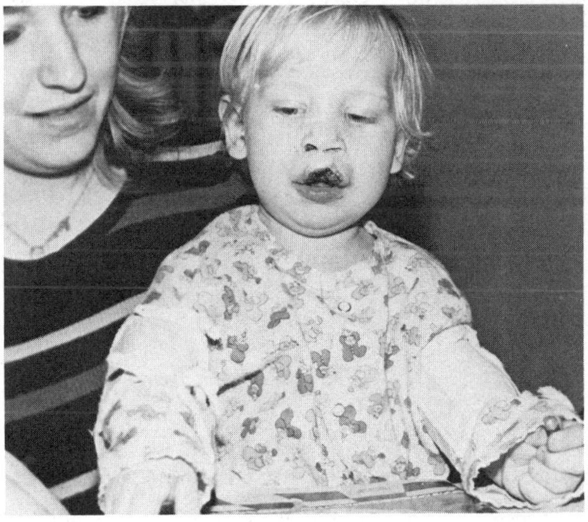

FIG. 11-17 Future corrective surgery will be needed to reshape this child's flattened left nares following completion of the palate and lip repairs.

The type of correction is dependent on the extent of the anomaly.

Cleft Palate Repair

Similar problems and care practices apply to children with cleft palates. The repair of the palate is carried out later than that of the lip, usually when the child is about eighteen months old. The time is dependent on the extent of the anomaly and the process of growth. When large areas of the palate are involved, the repair may be done in several stages.

Preoperative and Postoperative Care. Preoperative care for children undergoing a cleft palate repair is much the same as for those scheduled for cleft lip repairs. In the immediate postoperative period, children who have undergone surgical repair should be placed on their abdomen to facilitate drainage of mucus. The use of elbow restraints is necessary to prevent the child from placing anything, including the thumb, into the mouth. The child can easily drink from a cup, so feeding is less difficult. Mouth care is performed several times a day. This may simply consist of rinsing the mouth carefully with water after feedings. The child should not resume a regular diet until three to four weeks have elapsed.

Long-Term Considerations. The long-term care of these children involves not only the surgical correction of the anomaly, but other concerns for dental care and speech and hearing problems. For instance, dental or orthodontic treatment may be indicated in the case of missing or malpositioned teeth in the alveolar ridge. It also may be indicated to provide temporary occlusion of the palate prior to surgery.

Speech therapists may assist the child in many ways. The child may be making beginning speech sounds long before the palate is closed. These sounds are usually grossly distorted. Disturbances in the nerve supply to the palate may also be present. Correction of the resultant problems with articulation in speech may require special help.

The nurse's responsibility throughout the care of these children includes teaching the parents as much as possible about their child's care, supporting the parents in their parenting skills and home care of the child, and administering appropriate care during the period of the child's hospitalization. In many agencies, a nurse practitioner is a member of the team that initially evaluates the child and can assist with continuity and follow-up after hospitalization.

HYDROCEPHALUS

Hydrocephalus refers to an enlargement of the head caused by a problem with the spinal fluid. In order for hydrocephalus to occur, spinal fluid may be produced in abnormally large quantities; it may be inadequately absorbed, leading to an increase in volume, or an obstruction to its normal flow may be present. The terms noncommunicating and communicating refer to the location of the obstruction. In the noncommunicating type, the obstruction is within the ventricular system. This prevents the fluid from leaving the ventricles to reach the subarachnoid space. The term *communicating* refers to the free flow of fluid between the ventricles and the subarachnoid space. This is the most common type and includes abnormal reabsorption of the fluid in the subarachnoid space.

Assessment

In a normal child, spinal fluid is formed in the choroid plexus that is located in each of the lateral ventricles. The fluid then passes through the foramina of Monro and into the third ventricle. It leaves this ventricle by way of the aqueduct of Sylvius. The fluid then enters the fourth ventricle. It exits laterally through the foramina of Luschka and at the midline through the foramen of Magendie. It then flows into the cisterna magna and finally into the subarachnoid space.

The aqueduct of Sylvius is a common site of obstruction and, when associated with myelomeningocele, the condition is referred to as the Arnold-Chiari malformation. In some children, the fourth ventricle never develops. This is called a Dandy-Walker malformation. This condition can exist singly or in combination with other defects of the nervous system, such as meningocele.

The head of a hydrocephalic child may be greatly enlarged at birth, necessitating a cesarean section rather than a vaginal delivery. In other infants, the first sign of hydrocephalus is the presence of bulging fontanelles. The forehead is prominent. As the head size increases, the scalp stretches and the veins become increasingly dilated. The orbital plate of the eyes is depressed. This depression causes the eyeballs to be pushed down and forward. Because the sclera is very evident over the eye, this sign is known as the sunset sign. With increasing head size, the forehead becomes even more prominent. The head appears to be very heavy and unstable on the infant's tiny neck. Upon percussion of the skull, a distinctive "cracked-pot" sign, or Macewen's sign, is noted. This is an abnormally resonant note that is heard because of the separation of the suture lines.

If the hydrocephalus is allowed to progress, additional signs become evident. The infant develops a shrill, high-pitched cry. Vomiting occurs rather easily. Difficulties with sucking and swallowing make feeding and the maintenance of adequate hydration problematic. As the spinal fluid accumulates, the pressure exerted on the cerebral cortex eventually destroys it. Seizures, coma, and death may ensue.

The diagnostic procedure of choice is computerized axial tomography, or CAT scanning. The infant must be sedated for the procedure to ensure absolute stillness. Other invasive diagnostic procedures that might be required include ventriculography, pneumoencephalography, arteriography, and echoencephalography. Additionally, transillumination may be used to view the abnormal accumulation of spinal fluid. This is accomplished with the use of a flashlight equipped with a special rubber cup around the end. With the child's room darkened, the lighted flashlight is held to the side of the child's head; this maneuver causes the spinal fluid to glow. When a specimen of spinal fluid is desired, a ventricular tap is usually preferred to a lumbar puncture because of the decreased risk to the child.

Preoperative Care

Preoperatively, the nursing care of a hydrocephalic child involves daily head measurements, assessment of the tenseness of the fontanelles, observations for increased intracranial pressure, and seizure precautions. The routine aspects of this child's nursing care often present the greatest challenge. The size of the head frequently requires some adaptation on the part of the nurse when feeding or holding the infant. The head and neck must be protected and well supported at all times. As the head size enlarges, this will become increasingly difficult, and the assistance of another nurse may be needed to lift the infant.

The infant should be held for feedings, as should all infants. The nurse must balance the child comfortably in the arms so that the head and neck are protected. Use of a foam pad under the infant's neck and head may facilitate handling, as may a chair with arm rests. Feedings should be scheduled around the diagnostic procedures. Excess handling immediately before or after a feeding often causes vomiting in this infant. Small, frequent feedings may be easiest for the child to tolerate. Everything that is consumed is recorded carefully on the intake and output record.

Skin care is another aspect of routine care that deserves special attention in hydrocephalic infants. The increased size and weight of the head predispose these infants to pressure injuries and skin breakdown. The skin should be inspected carefully each day for any signs of irritation or redness. Use of a piece of lamb's wool or a gel-type float pad may be necessary to prevent such deterioration.

Surgical Correction

The operative procedure undertaken to correct hydrocephalus is referred to as a shunt. A polyethylene catheter is placed in the ventricle and secured. A one-way valve facilitates the flow of the cerebrospinal fluid. One of the most commonly used valves is a Spitz-Holter valve which is usually anchored under the skin behind the ear over the mastoid process. The distal portion of the shunt is located in the right atrium or in the peritoneal cavity, Figure 11-18. It may also be secured in any of the vessels leading to the right atrium. Ideally, the shunt should be inserted within the first few days of life in order to decrease the risk of infection.

Postoperative Care

Postoperative care should include all of the care activities of the preoperative period, as well as some additional responsibilities. Signs of increased intracranial pressure indicate plugging or obstruction of the shunt and should be reported. These signs include irritability, vomiting, altered vital signs, and increasing head size. The nurse may also be responsible for routine pumping of the valve a prescribed number of times a day. The child should be positioned on the side opposite the surgical repair. The head is not elevated in order to prevent an overly rapid reduction of fluid in the ventricles.

Infection is a major concern in these infants. They are usually maintained on prophylactic antibiotics to reduce the risk of meningeal infection. The nurse should observe carefully for any signs of infection, including irritability, vomiting, and reduced fluid intake. Additionally the fontanelles may increase in tenseness or show signs of bulging in the absence of crying.

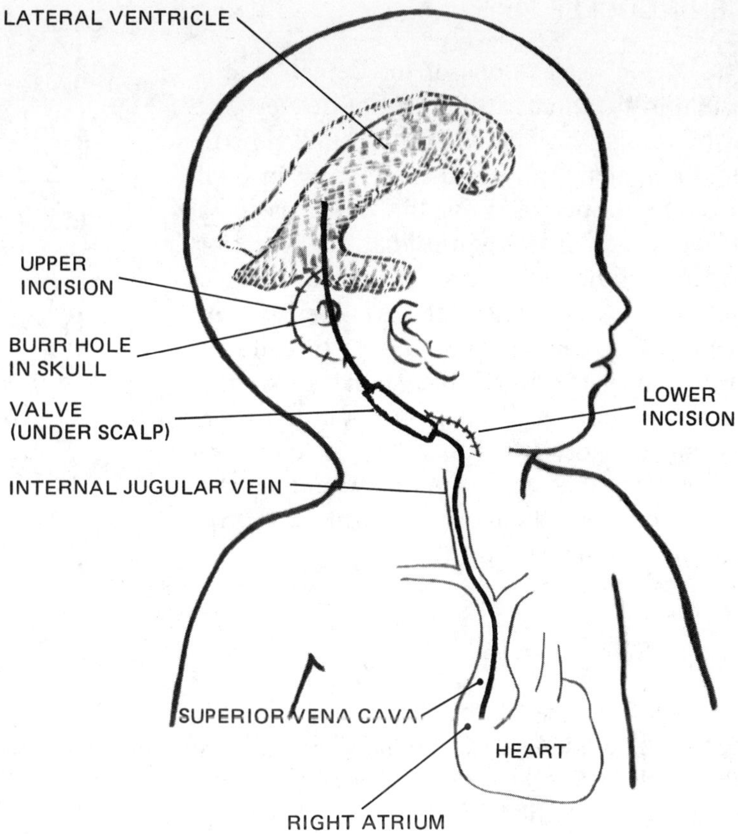

FIG. 11-18 A ventriculoatrial shunt drains spinal fluid via a one-way valve located over the mastoid process.

Postoperatively, as well as preoperatively, the parents should be included in the infant's care as much as possible. All care practices should be explained to them and they should be given ample opportunities to ask questions of the staff members. If the infant has been moved from the newborn nursery to a pediatric unit, it is important to facilitate the bonding process in any way possible. The parents' disappointment in their less than perfect child should be accepted as normal.

Part of the discharge planning for this family includes teaching the parent to recognize the signs of increased intracranial pressure that indicate dislodging of the shunt. Parents should be told that this can happen normally as a part of the growth process, and that the child will be returning to the hospital periodically for a revision of the shunt. Parents should be encouraged to treat the child as a normal child. No activity restrictions are imposed on older children with hydrocephalus except for the avoidance of contact sports. The family may be referred to crippled children's services for financial assistance for the surgery or to the hospital social services department when necessary.

MENINGOCELE

Meningocele is one of the defects that is visible in the infant at the time of delivery. It is the result of a failure of the neural tube to close completely; it occurs very early in fetal life. The proper term for this defect is spina bifida cystica. This signifies that the posterior portions of the spinous processes are not joined and there is herniation of a saclike mass of meninges containing spinal fluid. In children in whom portions of the spinal cord and nerves are also involved in the sac, the term myelomeningocele is used. Either of these defects can occur at any point along the spinal cord, but the most common area is the lumbosacral region, Figure 11-19.

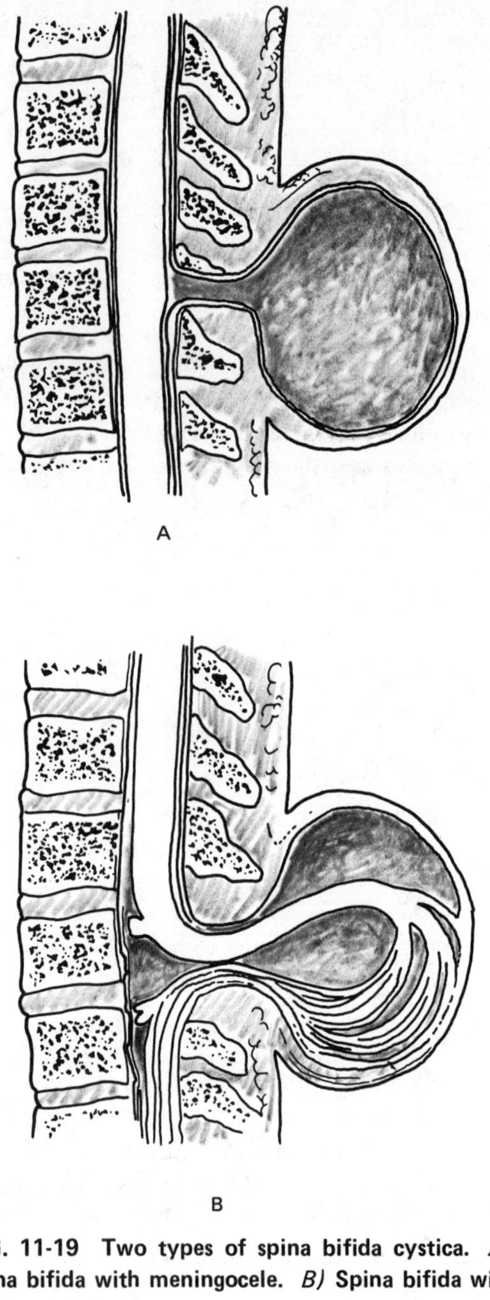

Nursing Care

Nursing care of the infant with myelomeningocele involves routine newborn care as well as observation for other anomalies. Additionally, the location of the sac and the presence of spinal cord and nerve roots within it indicate the need for a complete neurologic assessment to determine the child's functional capabilities.

Care of the Meningeal Sac. The sac itself must be protected from trauma, infection, and drying. The infant is placed in an incubator so that the body temperature can be maintained without covers or clothing. This reduces the risk of irritation of the meningeal sac. The sac is kept moist by using a frequently changed dressing of normal saline and, in some instances, an antibiotic preparation. Surgical closure of the sac is often accomplished within the first twenty-four to forty-eight hours of life to reduce the risk of infection. If repair of the defect is to be delayed, the sac is exposed to the air. A protective foam cushion with a large hole cut in the center to accommodate the sac is anchored on the back with nonadhesive tape. A large plastic bubble may also be used to protect the sac. This also aids in preventing fecal contamination of the site.

Bowel and Bladder Dysfunction. Children with a meningocele will have varying degrees of bowel and bladder dysfunction, depending on the level of the lesion. The infant should be evaluated routinely for distention of the bladder, and for fecal impaction. The infant's sphincter control, although not yet voluntary, must be evaluated. Many of these children have bladder dysfunction and, ultimately, renal damage because of the interrupted nerve pathways to the bladder. Typical symptoms include incontinence, infection, and ureteral reflux. Urine may be expressed manually using Crede's maneuver, which involves applying pressure on the abdomen over the bladder. Eventually, bladder drainage may be effected through an indwelling catheter or through an external drainage device. In children for whom these modalities are ineffective, a surgical form of urinary diversion, such as an ileal conduit or a ureterostomy, may be necessary.

Orthopedic Anomalies. Orthopedic problems may also exist in this infant. Many have flexion deformities and hip dislocations. These children demonstrate spasticity above and flaccidity below the level of the lesion. Infants should lie prone with their legs in abduction in order to prevent further deformities. Absence of sensation and the loss of position sense create long-term problems for these children. Any time the child is found to have a swollen extremity that is warm to the touch, a fracture should be considered until it is ruled out by x-ray studies. Osteoporosis may also create difficulties although healing occurs normally. Braces may be used to promote mobility. When a fracture is diagnosed, the continuous use of braces has been shown to be as effective as traction or casting.

Feeding and Skin Care. Another aspect of care that should be considered is feeding of the child. Preoperatively, the child may be held in any position that does not put pressure on the sac, Figure 11-20. Feedings should be given slowly and should be accompanied by frequent bubbling of the infant.

Skin care should be scrupulous in order to prevent breakdown or infection. Along with skin care, passive range of motion is carried out on all joints which the infant cannot spontaneously move.

Operative Procedure and Postoperative Care

Surgical repair of meningocele defects does not involve removal of the sac, but rather covering of it. It is frequently necessary to do skin grafting to effect a closure.

Postoperatively, the child will be in a prone position and the head may be positioned slightly lower than the buttocks. This is to reduce the stress on the suture lines. The dressing over the sac should be kept clean and dry and free of any contamination. The infant should be placed in an incubator or Isolette to

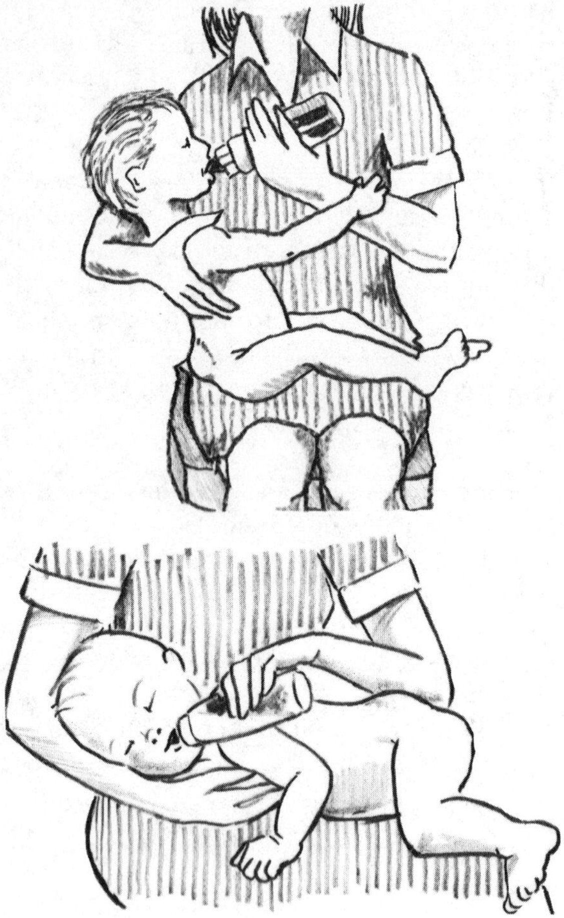

FIG. 11-20 Positions for feeding the infant with spina bifida cystica

maintain good temperature control. Vital signs should be checked frequently. An assessment for increased intracranial pressure should also be performed periodically. Fluids are administered intravenously at first. The nurse is responsible for maintaining the desired drip rate and for diagnosing fluid overloads if they occur.

Once the infant is allowed fluids by mouth, small amounts are given with the infant's head turned to the side. The nurse should check with the physician regarding the slight raising of the infant's head for feedings.

During this postoperative period, careful monitoring of intake and output should continue. Assessment for skin breakdown is also important, and the head, as well as other parts of the infant's body, should be checked regularly.

Working with the Families

The long-term goals for children with meningocele defects are correction of as many defects as possible and achievement of maximal control of the functions of the other systems. Attainment of these goals requires a multidisciplinary effort over a long period of time. Parents should understand what is wrong with the child and what can be done to correct it. Parents often need group counseling. Their involvement in team meetings and conferences regarding their child should be actively sought. Emotional problems are common in these families because of the social isolation caused by the care of the child, as well as the long-term economic hardships.

Caregivers should be taught how they can facilitate developmental achievements in the child. The guidelines used for teaching are the achievements of a normal child at a comparable age level. First, parents are instructed to encourage the infant to hold the head erect and to strengthen the neck muscles. Parents are taught the value of daily, gentle, passive range-of-motion exercises in maintaining joint function. They should also be able to recognize problems that require notification of the physician. Information, such as the fact that surgical covering of the sac does not eliminate the underlying permanent nerve damage, should be shared with the parents.

Regular and consistent follow-up by a treatment team is important for both the parents and the child in order to preserve the highest functional level for the child. Lack of bowel and bladder control, lack of sensory stimuli in the lower extremities, and immobility are all major long-term problems faced by the child and parents.

ORTHOPEDIC ANOMALIES

Deformities of the Foot

Deformities of the foot in the newborn are readily apparent. These deformities can be corrected easily if treatment is begun early, preferably within the first few days or weeks of life.

Talipes Equinovarus. Infants with talipes equinovarus, or clubfoot, have a deformity that includes forefoot adduction and supination, inversion of the heel, and fixed plantar flexion of the heel. This deformity is not positional as can be demonstrated by attempting to turn the child's foot into normal alignment.

Unilateral talipes equinovarus is more commonly seen than its bilateral form, Figure 11-21. Its incidence in males is twice that in females. Occasionally, it is inherited as an autosomal recessive disorder. The parents may confirm a history of the defect in their family. More commonly, it is embryologic in origin. It occurs two or three times for each 1000 births. Ten percent of these infants have other neuromuscular defects.

Assessment. On assessment, the nurse notes that the entire foot is inverted, the heel drawn up, and the forefoot adducted. Commonly, a deep transverse crease is present on

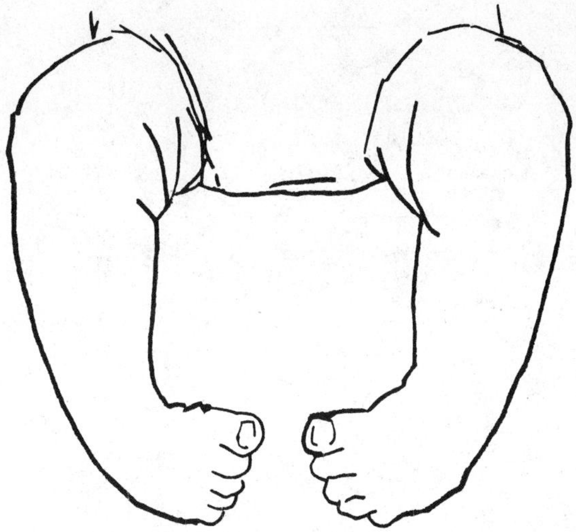

FIG. 11-21 Anterior view of bilateral talipes equinovarus.

the sole of the foot. Any attempt to manipulate the foot into a normal position is met with resistance. The foot is not flexible and cannot be corrected passively because of the involvement of joints, anomalous insertion of ligaments and tendons, and bony changes.

Treatment. Correction begins as early as possible with the use of plaster or plastic casts. A long leg cast is used with the knee in right angle flexion. In children younger than three months of age, the casts are changed every week to ten days to allow for the growth of the child. For children three to six months of age, the cast is usually changed every ten days. Children older than six months of age should have the cast changed every two weeks. These intervals are approximate, and ultimately depend on the child's rate of growth. The deformity is corrected in stages rather than all at once in order to prevent the development of a "rocker-bottom" foot. Treatment is continued until full correction has been achieved. The final

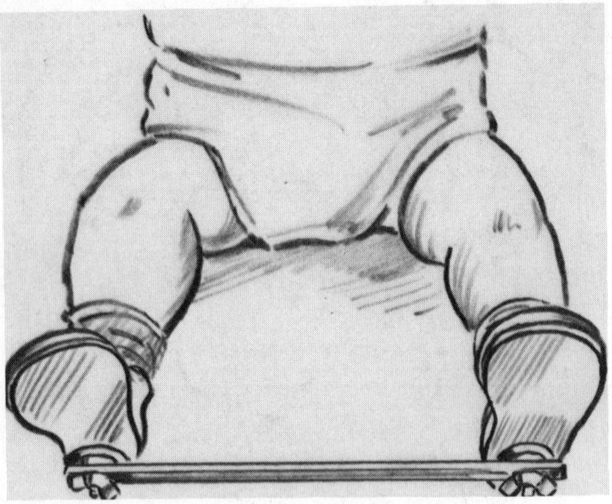

FIG. 11-22 Denis Browne splint

casting position is maintained for four to eight weeks.

After casting has been completed, the child may wear a Denis Browne splint at night and during naps. The splint is a 12- to 16-inch metal bar that is attached to the bottom of the child's shoes to maintain the position of the feet, Figure 11-22. It is used predominantly in children who are not yet bearing weight. It is designed to prevent the child's corrected foot from reverting to the original position. Without the splint, the infant's sleeping position might contribute to the original problem. Infants frequently sleep in a knee-chest position or in a fetal position with their toes pointed inward. Pinning the child's diaper to the sheet or taping the heels of the shoes together will prevent this.

If the child is already walking, a similar device, called a Brachman skate, may be used. High top reverse last shoes may be worn during the day with splints at night.

If the child's feet cannot be corrected by casting and splinting, or if they revert to the original position, surgical correction may be necessary. Surgical corrections in children younger than ten years involve only repair of soft tissue structures. This is because sufficient ossification of the bones has not yet taken place. A procedure that lengthens and transplants the tendons is the most common.

Metatarsus Varus and Valgus. Among the forefoot deviations that may be seen in infants are metatarsus varus and valgus. Metatarsus varus is medial deviation of the forefoot and is the more common of the two. Metatarsus valgus is lateral deviation of the forefoot. Manipulation and exercise may be all that is required for treatment. The regimen of care may dictate that the nurse or parent manipulate the foot ten times with each diaper change. With internal rotation, the Denis Browne splint may be used.

Another method of correction involves the use of a foam block that is strapped between the child's knees. The heels of the child's shoes are then attached, with the forefoot rolled outward. In older children, the Brachman skate or the Becker twister cable, may be used to effect the correction. The Becker type of brace consists of a pelvic band and cables that are attached to the shoes. The apparatus is worn twenty-four hours a day.

Nursing Care. The nursing care of children with foot deformities includes assisting with the initial assessment, teaching the parent how to care for the child wearing casts or braces, and encouraging the parents to persist in the treatment and follow-up for the child. In teaching the parents, the nurse should encourage them to observe the older child as he or she sits and plays or watches television. Many children assume a tailor's position or sit on their legs with their toes pointed inward. Parents should suggest alternative positions so that the child does not reverse the correction achieved.

If frequent cast applications are required in infants or young children, it may help to withhold the child's bottle until the time of the cast application. The child is then less apt to squirm and wriggle during the procedure. Since many casts are thinly applied, nurses may suggest that the cast be soaked off. Using a cast-cutter to cut off the cast may frighten the infant. A cup of vinegar added to the bath water helps to soften the cast so that it can be removed easily.

Congenital Dislocation of the Hip

The condition commonly referred to as congenital dislocation of the hip appears in several forms. It may occur as a dysplasia, a subluxation, or a luxation of the normal ball-and-socket joint of the hip. In dysplasia, the acetabular roof slants upward. The capsule of the hip is large, allowing the femoral head to displace. In subluxation, the head of the femur is already partially displaced, the acetabulum is shallow, and the ligaments are stretched. In luxation, the femoral head is located above the rim of the acetabulum and the tendons are markedly stretched and elongated. Children with untreated dysplasia may progress to a more severe anomaly, particularly with the onset of weight-bearing.

Hip dysplasia is more common in females, infants born in a breech position, and those with metatarsus varus deformities. Bilateral dysplasia may occur, but the unilateral form is the most common.

Assessment. All infants should be assessed for hip dislocation while in the newborn nursery. To do so, the infant is placed in a supine position and the hips and knees are flexed. The nurse then grasps the infant's knee with the thumb on the medial aspect of the thigh and the forefinger against the greater trochanter. As the leg is gently abducted, a jerk or click may be felt as the head of the femur crosses the acetabular rim. This is Ortolani's sign, or the "sign of the jerk," and is considered diagnostic. Other early signs that indicate dysplasia include asymmetric skin folds in the thigh and gluteal area and limited abduction of the affected side, Figure 11-23. In the case of dislocation, additional symptoms may include shortening of the affected leg, prominence and elevation of the greater trochanter, broadening of the perineum, and telescoping of the affected hip. Shortening of the affected leg, also called Allis' sign, is demonstrated by placing the child in a supine position with the hips and knees flexed and the feet on a flat surface. The knee on the affected side will be visibly lower than that on the normal side because of the movement of the femoral head above the level of the acetabulum, Figure 11-24.

Other later signs may be evident in children older than one year of age who have been walking with an uncorrected hip dysplasia. These include flattening of the buttock on the affected side, scoliosis and lordosis, a painless limp characterized by lurching toward the affected side, adduction and flexion contractures of the affected side, and a positive

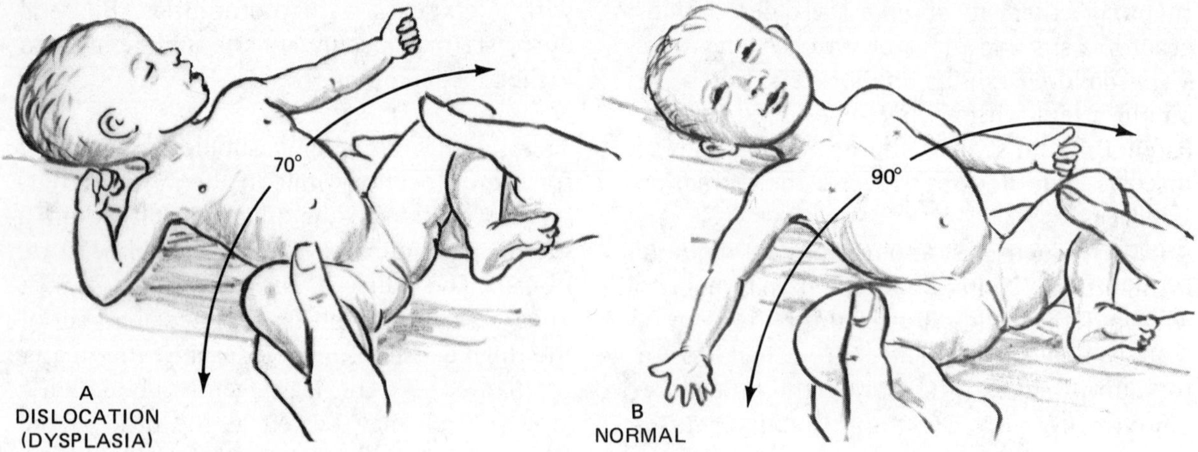

FIG. 11-23 *A)* Limited abduction of the hip in an infant with congenital dislocation of the hip *B)* Normal abduction

Trendelenburg sign. The Trendelenburg sign is seen when the child stands on the affected leg and raises the normal leg. The pelvis will tilt noticeably toward the unaffected side. A waddling gait may also be evident in older children with bilateral dislocations.

Treatment. The earlier the treatment is started, the less time it takes, and the more effective the correction. Treatment is aimed at preventing further dislocation and promoting normal joint formation. Initially, in the small infant, the hips are maintained in a position of abduction. This may be accomplished with the use of triple diapers, a Frejka pillow splint, a Pavlik harness, or a Von Rosen splint. All of these devices will keep the hips in 90-degree flexion and will allow the legs to fall into abduction. A frog-leg position can be maintained in a cast but it does not allow active movement of the legs. The duration of treatment may range from two

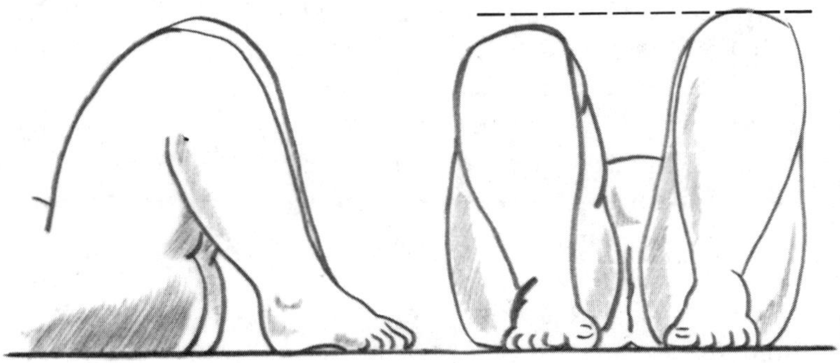

FIG. 11-24 Shortening of the knee on the affected side is visible when the hips and knees are flexed and the feet are firmly on the examining table.

months in the neonate to a full year in the older infant.

Older children, particularly those in whom a hip is dislocated, require traction prior to the application of a cast. This is usually skeletal traction; the legs are gradually abducted over a period of time. Traction is especially necessary when the muscles and tendons have contracted in order to accommodate the child's abnormal position. Traction is then followed by a closed reduction and application of a hip spica cast. Immobilization in a hip spica cast continues for a period of eight to twelve weeks, depending on the progression of healing.

In some children, it is necessary to correct the problem surgically. Corrective surgery is usually performed in those whose problem is not identified in infancy. The procedures, such as a Salter osteotomy, a Colonna arthroplasty, or a Shelf operation, are all designed to improve both the stability and the functioning of the affected hip. These open reductions are followed by a cast application.

Nursing Care. Nurses should know the proper application of splints for the early treatment of hip dysplasia. All of the devices maintain the hips in 90-degree flexion. All have a bib or harness that is positioned over the shoulders to aid in maintaining this position. Buckles or Velcro closures also help to maintain the position. The nurse should know exactly how securely these closures are to be fastened, especially considering the frequency of diaper changes in this age group.

Neurovascular assessments should be performed in children with hip dysplasia since pressure may be exerted on nerves and blood vessels if splints are inappropriately applied. These devices are usually worn twenty-four hours a day with removal being permitted only for bathing and diaper changes. The nurse should reinforce this regimen with the parents. If the child is to wear the splint for less than twenty-four hours a day, the order should state this specifically. The parents should be encouraged to handle this baby and care for it like any other child its age. Initially, the nurse may need to assist the parents in adapting care practices to the needs of the child.

The care of children in traction, whether it be skin or skeletal traction, relates primarily to the immobilization imposed. It is imperative that the nurse maintain the child in proper alignment, recognize the developmental needs of the child, and continue to assess the child's neurovascular status. During this period of immobilization, additional nutritional needs may be identified and elimination problems caused by the position must be addressed. Diversional therapy geared to the child's age and developmental level may be provided by the parents, the nurse, or a child-life worker.

Following the cast application, the nurse's concerns focus on drying the cast, protecting the perineal area, reducing skin irritation at the cast edges, and preparing the child and the parents for discharge. All of these nursing activities are discussed in detail in Chapter 25.

SUMMARY

Each of the congenital anomalies presented in this chapter is visible at birth or shortly thereafter. Because of this, significant adjustments are required on the part of the family. The perfect child the parents anticipated is suddenly not a reality, and the parents must cope with their shock, grief, and guilt before they can accept their child.

The nurse must be knowledgeable about these conditions so that information may be shared with the parents in a therapeutic and realistic fashion. The nurse's attitudes and feelings toward the child are reflected in the care that is delivered. Parents should be given a positive role model to follow in caring for their child.

SUGGESTED ACTIVITIES

- Observe an infant with a congenital anomaly. Make a list of all the attractive features of the child. On the opposite side of the page, list the obvious characteristics of the anomaly. Share this information with a group of students who have completed a similar study of other children.
- Talk with several parents of handicapped children. Ask the parents to share their experiences and feelings related to the infant's birth. Identify for your student group what forms of assistance the parents found most helpful.
- Make arrangements for your group to tour a regional care center for neonates. Observe the types of care given to various infants. Note the amount and type of parent participation you observe.

DISCUSSION TOPICS

1. Research the possible or probable causes that have been identified for various congenital anomalies. Discuss their implications in terms of prenatal care and genetic counseling.
2. Compile a list of agencies in your area that may be able to provide assistance to children with congenital defects and their families. Together with your classmates, determine the type of assistance each offers.

REVIEW

A. Matching. Match the major sign or symptom in Column I with the corresponding anomaly in Column II.

Column I	Column II
1. Acyanotic heart disease	a. Hydrocephalus
2. Limited abduction of hip	b. Myelomeningocele
3. Excessive production of spinal fluid	c. Tetralogy of Fallot
4. Incomplete fusion of the facial bones	d. Patent ductus arteriosus
5. Protruding sac containing nerve roots	e. Congenital hip dysplasia
6. Cyanotic heart disease	f. Cleft palate

B. Multiple choice. Select the one best answer.

1. Bobby is a newborn infant with a unilateral cleft lip and palate. Before repair of the lip and palate defects, the physician will probably order the baby to be fed by
   a. tube feedings.
   b. intravenous fluids.
   c. metal spout cup.
   d. rubber-tipped medicine dropper.
2. Of the following measures, which would be effective in minimizing Bobby's crying postoperatively?
   1. Changing his diapers immediately after wetting or soiling
   2. Administering formula slowly and in several small feedings
   3. Changing his position and performing passive arm exercises frequently
   4. Providing additional cuddling, rocking, or other pleasurable stimuli
   5. Arranging for his parents to assist in his care

   a. 1 and 2
   b. 3 and 4
   c. 1, 2, 3 and 4
   d. 1, 2, 3, 4 and 5

3. Prevention of crusting of Bobby's incision is particularly important in the prevention of
   a. hypopigmentation.
   b. scarring.
   c. pain.
   d. infection.

4. Brenda, a five-year-old girl with a congenital heart defect, is admitted to your unit. As you take the ordered blood pressures on both upper and lower extremities, you notice a fifty point difference between the right arm and the right leg. Given this information, which one of the following conditions would you suspect?
   a. Subaortic stenosis
   b. Patent ductus arteriosus
   c. Coarctation of the aorta
   d. Mitral stenosis

5. The observation of a child with congenital heart defects should include an assessment for central cyanosis. This would be best indicated by
   a. the skin color.
   b. the oral mucosa.
   c. the nail beds.
   d. the apical rate.

6. Which of the following signs might lead you to suspect that an infant has congenital dislocation of the hip?
   1. Limited abduction of one of the thighs
   2. Shortening of one leg
   3. Apparent deformity of the head of the femur on the affected side
   4. Extra gluteal folds on the affected side
   5. Lengthening of the leg on the affected side
      a. 1, 2 and 4
      b. 1, 4 and 5
      c. 2, 4 and 5
      d. 2, 3 and 5

C. Short answer. Briefly respond to the following statements.

1. List the nursing responsibilities in the care of a patient who has water-seal drainage.
2. Describe the purpose of the Frejka pillow splint.
3. List the observations to be made following a cardiac catheterization

BIBLIOGRAPHY

Berkowitz, Samuel. *The Road to Normalcy for the Cleft Lip and Palate Child.* Evansville, IN: Mead Johnson Company, 1972.

Berkowitz, Samuel. *Steps in Habilitation for the Cleft Lip and Palate Child.* Evansville, IN: Mead Johnson Company, 1972.

Bernardo, Marie L. "When Your Caseload Includes a Hydrocephalic Child." *Pediatric Nursing,* Vol. 5 No. 3 (May–June, 1979), pp. 27–29.

Bliven, Floyd E., et al. "Help for the Child with a Foot Problem." *Journal of Patient Care,* Vol. 7 No. 17 (September 1, 1973), pp. 128–148.

Braney, Mary Louise. "The Child with Hydrocephalus." *American Journal of Nursing,* Vol. 73 (May, 1973), pp. 828–830.

Clark, Jane. "Kelly – An Infant with Heart Defects." *American Journal of Nursing,* Vol. 77 (November, 1977), pp. 1823–1827.

DePasso, Sherrilyn. "Positioning Infants with Myelomeningocele." *American Journal of Nursing,* Vol. 74 (September, 1974), pp. 1658–1660.

Eilert, Robert E. "Foot Care for the Very Young Patient." *Journal of Patient Care,* Vol. 13 No. 9 (May 15, 1979), pp. 108–140.

Gildes, Joan K. "Congenital Cardiac Defects: Pre and Postoperative Nursing Care." *American Journal of Nursing,* Vol. 78 (February, 1978), pp. 273–278.

Gillion, Janet E. "Behavior of Newborns with Cardiac Distress." *American Journal of Nursing,* Vol. 73 (February, 1973), pp. 254–255.

Henderson, Marcia L., and Diane M. Synhorst. "Bladder and Bowel Management in the Child with Myelomeningocele." *Pediatric Nursing,* Vol. 3 No. 5 (September–October, 1977), pp. 24–31.

Irwin, Eleanor C., and Betty J. McWilliams. "Play Therapy for Children with Cleft Palates." *Children Today,* Vol. 3 No. 3 (May–June, 1974), pp. 18–22.

Lane, Phyllis. "Home Care of a Toddler in a Spica Cast." *American Journal of Nursing,* Vol. 71 (November, 1971), pp. 2141–2143.

Posey, Ruth. "Creative Nursing Care of Babies with Heart Disease." *Nursing 74,* Vol. 4 (October, 1974), pp. 40–45.

Reif, Kerry. "A Heart Makes You Live." *American Journal of Nursing,* Vol. 72 (June, 1972), pp. 1085–1086.

Roberts, Florence B. "The Child With Heart Disease." *American Journal of Nursing,* Vol. 72 (June, 1972), pp. 1080–1084.

Sacksteder, Sara, et al. "Common Congenital Cardiac Defects." *American Journal of Nursing,* Vol. 78 (February, 1978), pp. 266–272.

Sacksteder, Sara. "Embryology and Fetal Circulation." *American Journal of Nursing,* Vol. 78 (February, 1978), pp. 262–265.

Shor, Vivian Z. "Congenital Cardiac Defects: Assessment and Case Finding." *American Journal of Nursing,* Vol. 78 (February, 1978), pp. 256–261.

Tesler, Mary, and Carol Hardgrove. "Cardiac Catheterization: Preparing the Child." *American Journal of Nursing,* Vol. 73 (January, 1973), pp. 80–82.

Vigliarolo, Diane. "Managing Bowel Incontinence in Children with Meningomyelocele." *American Journal of Nursing,* Vol. 80 (January, 1980), pp. 105–107.

Warren, Freda M. "Getting a Quick Reading on an Infant's Blood Pressure." *Nursing 75,* Vol. 5 (April, 1975), pp. 13–14.

Wise, Doreen. "Crisis Intervention Before Cardiac Surgery." *American Journal of Nursing,* Vol. 75 (August, 1975), pp. 1316–1317.

Weinberg, Arim D., et al. "Respiratory Rate: Forgotten Clue in the Early Detection of Congenital Heart Disease." *Pediatric Nursing,* Vol. 3 No. 3 (May–June, 1977), pp. 38–41.

Chapter 12

Endocrine and Metabolic Defects

OBJECTIVES

Upon completion of this chapter, the student will be able to

- describe the assessment of a child with an endocrine or metabolic problem.
- differentiate between the types of diagnostic testing used for endocrine or metabolic conditions.
- identify the nursing approaches used with a child having an endocrine or metabolic problem.
- identify appropriate dietary adaptations for the child with an endocrine or metabolic condition.

Endocrine disorders and metabolic defects are manifested by a wide range of symptoms and disease processes in the infant. If all the problems that could occur were to be listed, the listing would be phenomenal. The incidence of *enzymopathies* (the metabolic defects caused by the absence of an enzyme) has been increasing rapidly since the beginning of the 1900s when the first cases were identified. Included in this chapter are three such disorders that affect protein, carbohydrate, or fat metabolism. The endocrine problems that are presented are those that affect the pituitary gland, the thyroid, and the adrenal glands. All are evident within the first year of life.

PHENYLKETONURIA

Phenylketonuria (PKU) is an autosomal recessive defect in which the enzyme phenylalanine hydroxylase is not manufactured by the liver. It results in the accumulation of high blood levels of phenylalanine and its metabolic derivatives. A compensatory mechanism partially metabolizes some of this phenylalanine, excreting it in the urine in the abnormal forms of phenylpyruvic acid, phenylacetic acid, and

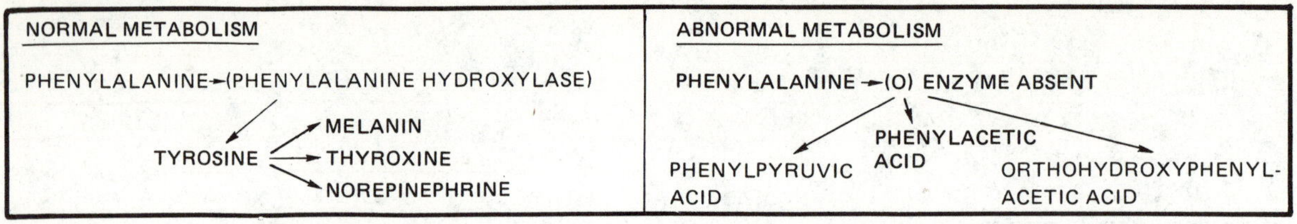

FIG. 12-1 Normal and abnormal phenylalanine metabolism

orthohydroxyphenylacetic acid, Figure 12-1. The excessively high levels of phenylalanine in the blood are toxic to both brain and nervous system tissues.

Phenylalanine, as one of the essential amino acids, is available in abundance in the protein fraction of foods. It is needed for normal growth and development. Excessive amounts, however, cause severe mental retardation unless dietary control is effected.

Normally, phenylalanine is converted to tyrosine by the enzyme phenylalanine hydroxylase. Tyrosine is a component of pigment in the body, as well as of some hormones. The absence of pigment in affected children led to the association of a fair complexion, pale irises, and often, chronic eczema with the condition.

Diagnosis

In 1934, when the disease was initially identified, the characteristic reaction of the urine with ferric chloride, producing a green color, was noted. This was the effect of the high levels of phenylpyruvic acid being excreted. The original diagnostic tests were done on the urine in the diaper or on filter paper saturated with urine. The urine had a distinctive musty or barnlike odor caused by the phenylacetic acid.

Currently, a number of blood tests can accurately determine phenylalanine levels. One of these is the Guthrie test. Normally, in full-term infants, phenylalanine levels range from 1.2 to 3.5 milligrams per 100 milliliters of serum. In affected infants, after a twenty-four-hour period during which either breast milk or formula is ingested, the level is usually about three to four times greater than normal. Because its incidence is 1 in 10,000 live births, most states mandate testing of all neonates.

Treatment

Affected children are placed on phenylalanine-restricted diets that are adjusted on the basis of the blood levels of phenylalanine. Lofenalac or Phenyl-free formulas are the basis of the diet. These formulas are composed of fats, carbohydrates, and the essential amino acids, but their phenylalanine levels are extremely low. In Lofenalac, for example, the amount of phenylalanine is 0.4 percent as compared with 5.0 percent level that is found in natural food proteins. When mixed with water in a ratio of one level measure of powder to two ounces of water, it provides the standard twenty calories per ounce. It is easiest to mix by making a paste with a small amount of the water and then adding the remainder of the water. A blender may also be used.

Since 1977, another preparation, made of synthetic amino acids, has also been available under the name of Product 3229. It is phenylalanine-free and can be mixed with powdered orange drink mixes or carob powder for a more palatable preparation for older children.

In addition to the formula, the child is gradually started on baby foods and then table foods. The diet, determined by a nutritionist or dietitian is calculated according to the child's growth needs and blood levels of phenylalanine. An exchange system, similar to the food exchanges in a diabetic diet, is used. One exchange is equivalent to 15 milligrams of phenylalanine. A child is allowed fifteen to twenty-five exchanges, Table 12-1.

During the early months of treatment, the infant may be given a challenge test. This involves removing the child from the restricted diet and feeding a standard formula for a period of three days. During this time, daily blood levels of phenylalanine are determined. Elevated blood levels confirm the diagnosis. Usually, the parents will also describe an irritable, hyperactive, screaming baby whose behavior is far different from that demonstrated while the restricted diet was being fed.

TABLE 12-1 Phenylalanine Food Exchanges

	AMOUNTS	EXCHANGES
Vegetables		
Beans, green, cooked	1/2 cup	3
Strained, baby	1-1/2 tbsp	1
Carrots, cooked	1/4 cup	1
Strained, baby	3 tbsp	1
Cucumber, raw	1/3 medium	1
Potato, baked	1 medium	8
Potato, French fried, thin	24 2-inch long	4
Fruits		
Apple	1 small	1
Applesauce, strained	10 tbsp	1
Orange	1 small	3
Orange juice, fresh	1 1/2 oz	1
Pears, canned	2 halves	1
Strained, baby	10 tbsp	1
Breads and Cereals		
Cracker, saltines	1	1
Corn Flakes	1/3 cup	2
Enriched wheat flour	1 tbsp	3
Oatmeal, cooked	1/3 cup	6
Baby cereal, dry	1 tbsp	1

Nursing Implications

Nurses must monitor the scheduling of blood tests in the nursery setting for any infant. It is imperative that blood tests for phenylalanine levels be delayed until the infant is fed milk or formula for a minimum of twenty-four hours. Infants who are difficult to feed because of mucous secretions and who are placed on glucose water instead of formula for a period of time should not have blood studies performed at this time, or the studies should be repeated two weeks after discharge of the infant from the hospital. The same holds true for breast-fed infants. Because the volume of breast milk becomes established gradually, the infant may not initially consume enough breast milk over a twenty-four-hour period to elevate the phenylalanine level abnormally.

Knowledge of available sources of help for parents of children with PKU is important. Clinics that deal routinely with such children can offer a supportive atmosphere for the family. They can help the family adjust to and cope with the problem as well as provide an opportunity for affected families to share their experiences. Support may be derived from something as simple as a recipe exchange that meets the adapted low-protein requirements of the child's diet.

Clinic visits are initially scheduled weekly, and then tapered to a monthly schedule. Assessment at the time of the visit will include a physical examination, an assessment of the child's development, and blood studies to determine any dietary adjustments that should be made. If the same nurse, nutritionist, and other members of the health team initially provide the support for the family, improved continuity of information will result. Written information on dietary adjustments and low-protein recipes may be helpful to the families. Additionally, the family may be informed that *Low Protein Cookery for Phenylketonuria* is available from the University of Wisconsin Press.

Genetic counseling is a priority for these families. Parents should know that they are both carriers of PKU. This may reduce their respective burdens of guilt for the child's hereditary problem. They should also know that the risk factor in any subsequent pregnancy is one in four. A professional counselor may become involved with the family initially to help them adjust to the problem.

Long-Term Considerations

A federally funded research project is being conducted to determine when a child with PKU may safely be removed from the restricted diet. Dietary restrictions have been lifted for some children in the project at the age of six years. Others may remain on the diet until the age of twelve years. Children are evaluated while both on the diet and off the diet. Phenylalanine levels, intelligence quotients (IQs), and electroencephalograms are used in the assessment. The rationale for discontinuing the diet at the age of six years or shortly thereafter is that the major portion of brain development has occurred by this time. Some European studies indicate that children who are taken off the diet exhibit decreased IQ scores, electroencephalographic abnormalities, and behavioral changes comparable to learning disabilities.

The age at which the disorder is identified, and the time the treatment is started, and the family's compliance to the regimen are important. Dietary control must be initiated prior to three months of age, preferably by two months of age, in order to prevent irreparable damage. Maternal PKU may also cause fetal retardation if dietary restrictions are not observed. Unless the mother with PKU adheres to a low-phenylalanine diet during pregnancy, the fetus will be exposed to unduly high levels of phenylalanine and its metabolites. This may lead to damage of the nervous system tissue.

GALACTOSEMIA

Galactosemia is a hereditary condition that is carried by an autosomal recessive gene. It involves a defect in carbohydrate metabolism. An infant's formula or breast milk contains lactose, which is broken down into glucose and galactose. Galactosemic infants are unable to metabolize the galactose, which accumulates in the tissues as galactose-1-phosphate, Figure 12-2. The enzyme that is lacking in this condition is called uridyl transferase.

Because of the enzyme deficiency, the galactose-1-phosphate accumulates in the liver and brain, causing both cirrhosis and mental retardation. Symptoms include jaundice, an enlarged liver, feeding difficulties with resultant poor weight gain, irritability, lethargy, vomiting, hypoglycemia, and cataract formation. Death may eventually result from liver failure.

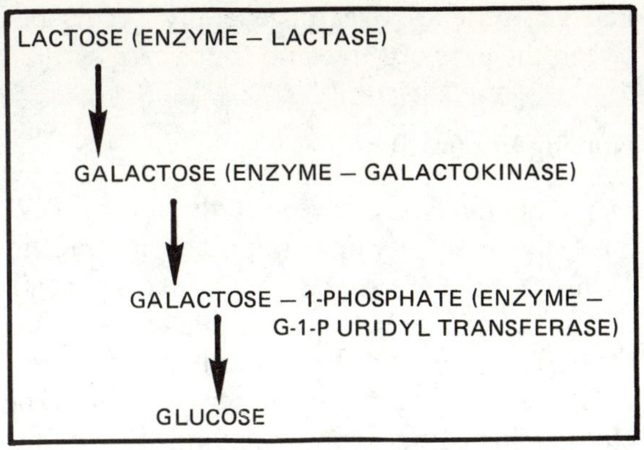

FIG. 12-2 Normal lactose metabolism. The absence of any of the enzymes can cause a form of the disease. The most serious and classic form occurs in the absence of uridyl transferease.

Diagnosis

To diagnose the infant's problem, a galactose tolerance test can be done, but the resultant high levels of the toxic substance can cause severe hypoglycemia and seizures. Alternatively, the presence of galactose-1-phosphate in the red blood cells is considered to be diagnostic, and may be determined by routine blood studies.

Treatment

Treatment for this condition involves the use of a milk-free diet since a defect of lactose or milk sugar metabolism is involved. Foods that are contraindicated for affected children include all forms of milk, cheese, butter, products containing nonfat milk solids, organ meats, chocolate, peas, beets, and lima beans. Medications, particularly syrups or suspensions, should be checked to identify the sweetening agent as it may be lactose. The formula that is usually given is Nutramigen. Pro-Sobee or some of the other soybean preparations may not be as well tolerated as Nutramigen as they contain a small amount of a substance which ultimately is metabolized into galactose.

Dietary compliance can be monitored easily by observing whether the child begins to gain weight and whether vomiting and diarrhea stop. Hypoglycemic symptoms also disappear. At first, the blood sugar level may be within normal range, but much of this is galactose instead of glucose. The normal level after dietary control is derived from the presence of glucose.

Nursing Implications

A nutritionist, as well as the nursing staff, may assist in reinforcing dietary teaching for the family. The health care team must be perceptive in identifying the parents' concerns early and in helping them to work through their feelings about the problem as well as the actual management of the infant's care.

During the diagnostic period in the hospital, the nurse should point out to the family any noticeable improvements. For instance, the nurse may cite a decrease in symptoms and an improvement in the baby's disposition. Later, as the infant's growth and development progress, even if only slightly, these improvements should be pointed out to the parents.

In addition to the identification of improvements, parents may benefit from the nurse's reassurance and reinforcement of their parenting skills. They may have cared for an irritable, fussy, sick baby since birth and may be uncertain as to how to approach their more normal baby. The nurse assigned to the care of this infant should support the parents by answering questions, providing assistance, and acting as a role model in the handling of this infant.

TAY-SACHS DISEASE

Tay-Sachs disease is one of a group of diseases called sphingolipidoses. The disease is a degeneration of the central nervous system that occurs as a result of progressive, intracellular accumulations of excessive amounts of a sphingolipid called ganglioside GM_2. The infant lacks the normal enzyme hexosaminidase A.

The disease was identified over one hundred years ago and first described by an ophthalmologist (Tay) and a neurologist (Sachs). The disease is an autosomal recessive trait and is seen most commonly in Jewish families of Eastern European origin. In the population of Ashkenazi Jews in the United States, the incidence is one in twenty-five carriers.

Diagnosis

Infants with Tay-Sachs disease are normal in appearance at birth. Their development is also normal until about four or five months of age when a noticeable slowing of development occurs. The infant then begins to regress.

Three stages of the disease are identifiable. The child is usually diagnosed during the first stage. At this time, the infant is flaccid, reflexes are hyperactive, and he or she is startled easily. The infant also appears to have difficulty fixating an object with the eyes. When the eyes are examined, a distinguishing cherry-red spot in the macula, and optic atrophy are evident. In the second stage, signs of central nervous system degeneration are apparent, including blindness, a high-pitched cry, increased reflexes, spasticity, and decerebrate posturing. Stage three is characterized by enlargement of the head, severe weight loss, seizures, and loss of protective reflexes, such as the swallowing and gag reflexes. Death generally occurs between the ages of three and four years.

Nursing Implications

The nursing care of children with Tay-Sachs disease is very demanding considering the fatal nature of the disease. Comfort is a major feature of the care. Because of the child's increased reflexes and the possibility of seizures, it is important to reduce external stimuli, including light and sound. Moving slowly and handling the child gently and deliberately with good support to the body parts are essential.

As the child's disease progresses, the ability to swallow is lost. Frequent choking on feedings may signify the onset of this problem. When it does, a gavage tube for feeding is inserted. Pressure sores and skin breakdown are hazards that are secondary to the child's inability to move about. Frequent turning and assessment of skin integrity are routine care practices. Because of the increasing size of the head, pressure sores may occur on the ears or head, depending on the child's positioning. Foam mattresses or gel pads may be helpful in addition to the frequent turning.

Genetic counseling is necessary for the parents. The risk factor for each subsequent pregnancy is one in four births. Amniocentesis performed between the sixteenth and twenty-second week of the pregnancy can determine the presence or absence of hexosaminidase A.

Young Jewish people with an Eastern European background and nonJewish persons of Eastern European extraction should consider undergoing a screening test designed to detect carriers. Persons or families affected by the disease should be told about the National Tay-Sachs Foundation which has been in existence since 1955.

CONGENITAL HYPOTHYROIDISM

Cretinism, or the lack of thyroid hormone, is often difficult to detect in newborn infants. Individual signs are nonspecific. However, collectively, the most common signs may be used as a screening tool to identify those infants who need blood studies to determine their thyroxine levels, Figure 12-3.

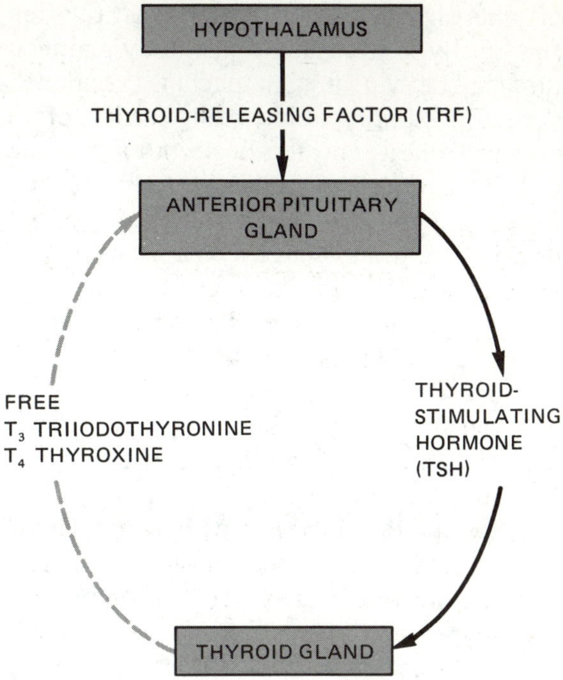

FIG. 12-3 Normal thyroid feedback mechanism

Signs and Symptoms

The most common signs of congenital hypothyroidism identified in the neonate include

- inactivity in utero
- postdatism, or a gestational term of greater than forty-two weeks
- large body mass or a weight of more than 4 kilograms
- an unusually large posterior fontanelle
- hypothermia, respiratory distress, or hypoactivity
- peripheral cyanosis despite adequate oxygenation
- intervals of more than twenty hours between stooling
- the presence of abdominal distention or vomiting
- poor feeding patterns
- unexplained icterus or jaundice lasting for more than three days
- edema

Any combination of these symptoms indicates the need for screening in the nursery situation. Because of the high incidence of the disease (one in five thousand live births) and because retardation can be prevented, the nurse should be alert to such symptom combinations.

As the infant grows, manifestations of the disease become more obvious. Feeding problems increase, with the infant sleeping through feedings and demonstrating no interest in eating. As time goes on, the tongue may be in the way, choking spells may occur, and respiratory difficulties may be evident. The infant cries infrequently and sleeps a great deal. When questioned, mothers often describe such infants as "good babies" because they do not fuss and seldom awaken during the night. Other signs that become evident with time include obstinate constipation, dry and scaly skin, coarse brittle hair, and poor muscle tone.

When assessing children with congenital hypothyroidism, the nurse will note a number of other signs as well. The vital signs are often abnormally low. A subnormal body temperature may be evident upon touching the infant's skin. The stunting of physical growth is often evident to health professionals, but not to the child's family. The child's extremities and fingers are unusually short and the hands are broad. The head is large with a wide anterior fontanelle. Dentition is delayed beyond the normal age, and those teeth that have erupted decay easily. The neck appears to be short and unusually thick because of fat deposits between the neck and shoulders. The muscles are hypotonic and the infant is markedly delayed in motor development.

Retardation increases with aging. Therefore, it is important to identify the disease and institute treatment early for this preventable form of retardation. Best results are achieved when thyroid hormone therapy is begun before two to three months of age.

Definitive Diagnosis

Serum levels of T_3 (triiodothyronine) and T_4 (thyroxine) are determined in order to confirm or rule out congenital hypothyroidism. The tests are specific for the assessment of thyroid functioning.

Other diagnostic tests may include a complete blood count, which will usually show anemia. Radiographs may be taken of the hands to determine the child's bone age. As the child grows, the discrepancy between chronologic age and bone age becomes markedly increased if the condition is left untreated.

Nursing Implications

The major nursing responsibility is early assessment and recognition of signs of the disease and developmental delays. If any possibility of depressed thyroid function exists, infants should always be screened in the newborn nursery.

Once the condition has been diagnosed and the infant treated with thyroxine, the nurse should emphasize to the parents the necessity for lifelong use of the medication. Parents should also be told to watch for specific side effects that would indicate that too much or too little of the hormone is being administered.

The dosage of thyroxine is increased gradually until tissue saturation is reached and the therapeutic dose has been achieved. Adjustments will be made in the dose to accommodate increases in growth, particularly during the rapid growth spurt of adolescence.

While the infant is hospitalized for regulation of the initial dose of medication, a developmental screening test is performed to determine the infant's functional level. The nurse should then share the results with the parents, explaining what types of activities may help to improve skills and abilities. Specific, concrete suggestions regarding the type of activities and the sequence in which they should be used are most helpful to the parents.

Affected infants should return to the clinic or hospital setting periodically for tests to determine the effectiveness of the thyroxine and for adjustments of dosage if necessary. During these visits, the developmental skills of the child are again assessed and his or her progress documented.

Parental Care

The initial problem usually described by parents is difficulty with feeding. They may describe the problems they have encountered in trying to feed a baby who chokes easily, who prefers to sleep, and whose tongue may protrude slightly. They should be instructed to feed the baby slowly while he or she is in a sitting position in order to reduce the chance of choking. The infant should also be burped frequently. Use of a soft nipple may make feeding easier as the infant does not have to work as hard to obtain the formula and thus is less apt to give up on eating and go back to sleep. Tilting the infant's chin upward slightly also may help to maintain the tongue's proper position.

Developing a routine for the infant is imperative. Parents should know that these infants will not develop a schedule on their own until they are well regulated on thyroid medication. At first, their activities are depressed, and parents must establish a routine for waking, sleeping, and all other necessary activities.

In developing a routine, the importance of using external stimuli should be emphasized. These infants have lost a period of time in growth and development which must be compensated for. They should be exposed to sights, sounds, and gentle activities. Parents should stimulate the infant to cry periodically, as well as to change position. The use of an infant seat or a backpack is invaluable in keeping the baby with the mother and exposing the infant to sights and sounds, including the mother's voice, as daily activities are performed.

Placing mobiles, pictures, music boxes, or a radio near the infant's crib provides both diversion and stimulation. Other children in the family can be encouraged to play pat-a-cake or peek-a-boo with the infant. Older children may become involved in the infant's care by taking him or her for a walk in the stroller, either in the house or outside when the weather is pleasant.

During this period, the parents should observe the infant for any signs of overdosage. The physician should be contacted if the infant shows signs of excess irritability, fever, diarrhea, tachycardia, or disturbed sleep patterns.

Initial improvement in the infant should be obvious to the parents. If it is not, the nurse should identify for them the changes in the infant's eating and sleeping habits, and the improvements in the condition of the skin and temperature, as well as in the level of alertness. As the child's developmental level is reevaluated at follow-up visits, the parents should receive reinforcement of all they have achieved with the infant, as well as concrete suggestions for activities that must be continued to improve the infant's skills.

PITUITARY SYNDROMES

The pituitary syndromes that are of concern in infants are those that directly alter growth. Two of these pituitary disorders are pituitary dwarfism and cerebral gigantism. Each reflects the action of the anterior pituitary gland and its oversecretion or undersecretion of the growth hormone, or somatotropin, Figure 12-4.

Pituitary Dwarfism

The growth deficit of children with pituitary dwarfism is not evident at birth, but becomes obvious by the end of the first year of life. When the height and weight of the child are consistently plotted on a growth chart, it eventually becomes evident that the rate of growth has slowed markedly or has even stopped.

Assessment of affected infants reveals normal developmental abilities. Physically,

Secreted Hormone	Affected Organ
Growth hormone (somatotropin)	Bones and soft tissues
Thyroid-stimulating hormone (thyrotropin)	Thyroid
Adrenocorticotropic hormone (ACTH)	Adrenal cortex
Gonadotropic hormones	
Luteinizing hormone (LH)	Ovary
Follicle-stimulating hormone (FSH)	Ovary
Interstitial cell stimulating hormone (ICSH)	Testes
Prolactin	Mammary glands

FIG. 12-4 Normal function of the anterior pituitary gland

the child has a small, rounded head, prominent eyes, and small but well-proportioned extremities. In children older than one year of age, the fontanelles are open and the bones of the cranium are noticeably thin, providing evidence of osteoporosis.

Diagnosis. The diagnostic evaluation of infants in whom pituitary dwarfism is suspected includes x-ray studies to rule out the presence of a causative tumor, determination of hormone levels, and an assessment of bone age.

Radiographs. Radiographs of certain portions of the skeletal system, such as the hand, elbow, shoulder, foot, knee, and hip, may be performed to assess skeletal maturity, as well as to mark interruptions in growth and altered nutritional status. Changes in the shape and contour of a bone, as well as its degree of ossification, are noted by the radiologist and are used as an accurate determination of age in these children, Figure 12-5.

Levels of growth hormone are also evaluated. Growth hormone levels rise after a period of deep sleep, as well as after a brief period of exercise that is strenuous enough to cause breathlessness. As exercise is difficult to achieve for a young infant, an intravenous infusion is started so that a blood sample may be drawn after a period of sleep without disturbing the infant.

Evaluation of Growth Patterns. The child's growth pattern from the time of birth is carefully evaluated. Results are then used to determine whether the problem is one of consistent delays in the growth cycle or of sudden cessation of growth. If the growth pattern is consistently delayed from the time of birth, a lack of pituitary functioning is likely to be the cause. Conversely, a normal growth pattern that is suddenly disrupted at a certain age suggests that a tumor or nutritional impairment is responsible.

When an evaluation of bone age is done, the degree of ossification is correlated with the actual linear growth or height of the child. In pituitary dwarfism, both of these measurements are inconsistent with the child's chronologic age.

In the process of evaluating a child, the linear measurements are taken. The nurse should be as accurate as possible in determining both single measurements and serial measurements. These are then plotted on a growth curve for the child. It is important to remember that growth charts for infants from zero to thirty-six months of age are standardized for linear measurements to be taken with the child in a supine position. Growth charts for children two to eighteen years of age are standardized on the basis of measurement in the upright or standing position. The differences between supine and standing measurements are slight, but in children with this condition, they may be quite significant.

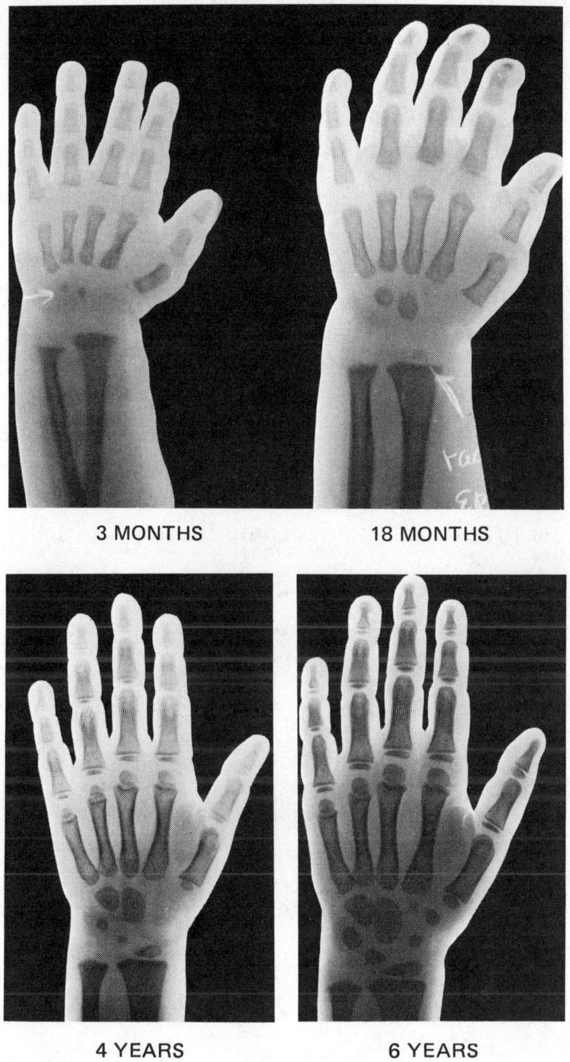

FIG. 12-5 Serial radiographs of a child's left hand at the ages of three months, 18 months, four years, and six years. Note the marked changes in the wrist. The hand is considered to be a primary growth indicator after six months.

Treatment. The treatment of this condition depends on the identified cause. If a tumor of the anterior pituitary gland is the causative factor, the tumor is removed. If a low level of growth hormone is the cause, then medication is supplied.

The supply of human growth hormone is very scarce. (One pituitary gland at autopsy supplies about 5 milligrams of the hormone.) Therefore children who are being treated for pituitary dwarfism are usually linked with research projects conducted by endocrine clinics at major medical centers. These children may need as much as one to two IU of the hormone three times a week. In some of the clinics, growth hormone is administered together with fluoxymesterone (Halotestin) for a synergistic effect. Only one unit of the growth hormone is given daily for twelve to thirty-six days. This regimen, when repeated four times a year, has resulted in normal growth as well as decreased cost. When the child achieves a height of five feet, the growth clinic program is discontinued.

Pituitary Gigantism

Although children with pituitary gigantism are within the normal range of growth at birth, they are above the ninetieth percentile by the end of their first year of life. Some may be above the ninety-seventh percentile at this point. This accelerated growth pattern may continue for a number of years before it is recognized as a problem. Plotting the child's growth patterns on a chart and noting any signs of precocious puberty may lead to detection of the condition.

Diagnostic evaluations are aimed at detecting the cause of the abnormal growth. Pituitary tumors may be responsible for oversecretion of growth hormones resulting in gigantism. The child's height and weight are proportionately large, which may be caused by the oversecretion of growth hormone prior to epiphyseal closure. Osseous maturation is consistently advanced in these children but does correlate with the child's linear growth. In the case of a tumor, those children whose fontanelles have closed may also show signs of increased intracranial pressure and headaches. The tumor may be removed surgically or destroyed by radiation. In those cases in which oversecretion of growth hormone or somatotropin is the cause of the problem, the treatment involves administering small doses of androgens. This allows the epiphyses to close gradually and limits the degree of growth possible.

For families affected by gigantism, counseling may be necessary. The child often has difficulty coping with the consequences of excess size and frequent comparisons with the peer group. Expectations for the performance of this child are frequently geared to the child's size rather than to chronologic age or developmental abilities.

CONGENITAL ADRENAL HYPERPLASIA

The primary adrenal disorder in infancy is congenital adrenal hyperplasia, also referred to as the adrenogenital syndrome. A defective enzyme system that inhibits the production of cortisol by the adrenal cortex is involved. Continued stimulation of the adrenal cortex by the secretion of ACTH from the pituitary gland causes the hyperplasia. The excess cortisol precursors then become androgens, Figure 12-6.

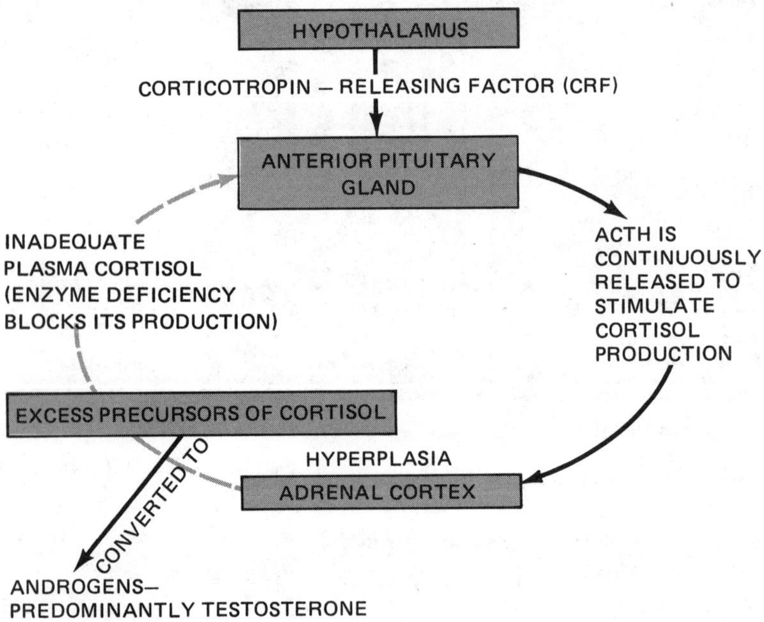

FIG. 12-6 Abnormal adrenal function is operant in congenital adrenal hyperplasia.

The problem is not recognized at birth in male infants because no physical abnormality is visible. In female infants, however, a question of sexual identity arises. These infants have been bombarded in utero with testosterone from about the tenth to the twelfth week. As a result, the female genitalia are ambiguous, or masculinized. The clitoris is disproportionately large. The labia are fused and resemble a scrotum with normal rugae. The urethral opening may be located at any point within this area. These infants are frequently identified as male infants with cryptorchidism.

In affected infants, whether male or female, the additional abnormality of a salt-loss trait may be present. This condition may go unrecognized. The infant has symptoms of anorexia, vomiting, diarrhea, weight loss, and extreme dehydration. Any restriction of either fluids or salt causes collapse. This condition occurs in about one-third of all the children with adrenogenital syndrome.

Diagnosis

A number of diagnostic tests are used to document the child's condition. These tests include a thorough history and physical examination, twenty-four-hour urine collections, and, in the case of an infant with ambiguous genitalia, endoscopic examinations and chromosomal studies.

The history should include a careful detailing of developmental achievements, as well as any height and weight measurements recorded by the parents. Male children with this syndrome are larger than average and usually achieve a level of skill that is above average. Physical examination may reveal signs of precocious puberty developing in the toddler or preschooler.

The twenty-four-hour urine collection is designed to detect the presence of 17-hydroxyketosteroids which are the urinary metabolites of androgen. The urine is also tested for pregnanetriol. This metabolite indicates the level of production of 17-hydroxyprogesterone, which is elevated when cortisol levels are decreased. The urine is also checked for the amount of aldosterone secretion. This value is decreased in children with the salt-loss trait.

In female children with ambiguous genitalia, a buccal scraping is done to determine the presence of Barr bodies, the sex chromatin material. These Barr bodies are present in female children and absent in male children. A urethrovaginogram or an endoscopic examination is also performed to determine whether the cervix and the uterus are present, as well as whether the vagina has a common opening with the urethra, Figure 12-7.

Treatment

Treatment of the child with this syndrome involves the administration of cortisol to slow the oversecretion of ACTH by the pituitary gland and to arrest the adrenal hyperplasia. The dose of the drug is based on the results of the twenty-four-hour urine collections, the growth rate of the child, and his or her bone age. The cortisol dose is 15 to 20 milligrams per square meter. The total is divided into three doses, with one-half the daily dose being administered in the evening to stimulate the normal fluctuation of blood levels. Cortisol therapy is continued for the remainder of the child's life.

When ill, the child may be unable to manufacture additional cortisol to cope with the stress. During minor illnesses, the dose is doubled. In the case of a major illness, the

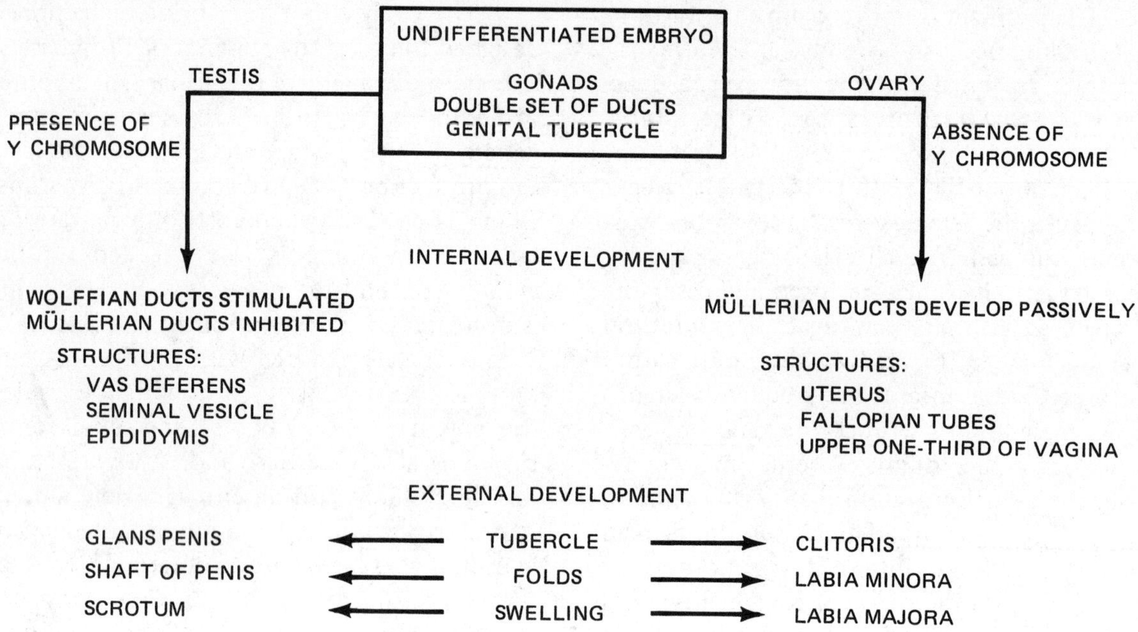

FIG. 12-7 Commonalities in the genital development of males and females

daily dose is tripled. Administration of this excessively large dose should be maintained only for the duration of the health crisis.

In those children with the salt-loss phenomenon, mineralocorticoids and additional dietary salt are added to the therapeutic regimen. Fludrocortisone acetate (Florinef Acetate) is one of the oral preparations that are available. Doca acetate is an injectable preparation that is given either intramuscularly or in pellets as a subcutaneous implant that lasts nine months to a year.

Surgical correction in infants with ambiguous genitalia should be undertaken prior to eighteen months of age as the child's gender role becomes well established after that time. Plastic reconstruction of the genitalia, as well as clitoridectomy, may be done in several stages, but usually not until the child is six months of age.

Nursing Implications

The nurse may be involved in the initial identification of this condition. The syndrome should be suspected in any infant in the delivery room or the nursery with questionable genitalia. Infants with undescended testes should also be examined carefully and an analysis of sex chromatin material done.

The nurse should be alert to any subsequent hospitalization of this same child for questionable pyloric stenosis or formula intolerance. Persistent vomiting or diarrhea causes loss of extracellular fluids and severe dehydration. The frequency of this problem, as well as the severity of the illness, should raise the possibility of the salt-losing form of the syndrome.

During the child's hospitalization, the nurse is involved in the collection of the urine specimens. It is very important that even small amounts of urine not be lost. The accuracy of the twenty-four-hour urine collection is dependent on the precision of the collection, as well as the method of analysis. Urine specimens are usually kept refrigerated during the collection period.

Another nursing responsibility is the determination of vital signs on a routine basis. Blood pressure measurements must be taken routinely on these children. Some children have a form of the disease that causes hypertension; others do not. Careful recording of blood pressure values and a knowledge of normal values for the child's age are important. The child's temperature should be taken on a regular basis in order to detect beginning signs of infection. If the temperature is elevated, the child's dose of cortisol should be increased to allow him or her to cope with the infection.

The nursing staff should also assess the child carefully for signs of acute adrenal insufficiency. This condition is characterized by apparent acute illness, unresponsiveness, and often, vomiting. Its rapid onset and severity indicate the need for additional cortisol. Parents should be taught to recognize these signs in the home situation, and should know how to administer cortisone by injection. Acute adrenal insufficiency is life-threatening to children with an endocrine or metabolic problem. The parents should have an emergency kit available, as well as medications and specific instructions for their use.

An assessment of bone age and a twenty-four-hour urine collection, are done every few months. It is important that the nurse reinforce the necessity of follow-up to the parents. The parents should know that these tests are done so that the child will achieve maximal growth. The financial burden of this condition is one reason parents, without realizing the risks, may prolong the intervals between the clinic visits.

Identification with a bracelet or Medic-Alert tag is mandatory in these children. The child's school should also be informed of the problem. The teacher should know that any sign of sudden weakness or illness in the child should not be ignored, but should be treated.

The child's attitude toward the medication regimen, the frequent injections, and the illness itself will be a reflection of the attitude of those around him. As these children grow older, they should learn about their problem, as well as how to take care of themselves.

SUMMARY

Children with endocrine or metabolic disorders have in common a serious alteration of an essential substance that is necessary for normal growth. The child with PKU has an enzyme deficiency that allows metabolites to accumulate and destroy brain tissue. Galactosemia and Tay-Sachs disease ultimately create the same problem. The child with cretinism is missing the substance necessary for normal growth and functioning, as is the child with hypopituitarism. Conversely, children in whom oversecretion of either growth hormone or ACTH occurs have in their systems too much of a normal substance.

A primary nursing responsibility in the care of children with any of these problems is initial recognition of the disorder. Careful assessment of the child's pattern of growth and development compared with the norms established for other children of the same age is important and helps to identify some of these conditions. Parents require a great deal of support, as well as education, so that they learn how to cope with the child's problem in a home situation. Dietary control of some of the conditions requires a firm commitment on the part of the family to that child's well-being. Consistent ongoing adaptations of care are crucial in all of these conditions.

SUGGESTED ACTIVITIES

- Ask a nurse clinician from a growth or endocrine clinic to talk to your group. Find out how the children are referred to the clinic, what the criteria are for attending the clinic, and what is done for the children.
- Care for a child with an endocrine or a metabolism disorder. Ask the parents how they identified the problem and in what way they have altered this child's home care. Find out who helped them most in coping with the child's problem.

DISCUSSION TOPICS

1. With your group, make a list of foods that would comprise a typical twenty-four-hour intake. Identify which foods would be eliminated if you had phenylketonuria. Which foods would be eliminated if you had galactosemia? Discuss ways in which the nurse can help parents and children cope with these dietary restrictions.
2. As a nurse, you know that the male or female gender of a child is established by the age of two and a half years. Discuss the activities in the home that help reinforce either a male or female self-concept. Share examples from either your own childhood or that of your children.

REVIEW

A. Matching. Match the disease in Column I with the missing enzyme or hormone in Column II.

Column I	Column II
1. Phenylketonuria	a. Hexosaminidase A
2. Cretinism	b. Somatotropin
3. Galactosemia	c. Thyroxine
4. Hypopituitary dwarfism	d. Phenylalanine hydroxylase
5. Tay-Sachs disease	e. Uridyl transferase

B. Multiple choice. Select the one best answer.

1. When assessing Brett, a nine-month-old infant with cerebral gigantism, you would expect his
   a. weight to be double his birth weight.
   b. length to be slightly above average.
   c. weight and length to be in the fiftieth percentile.
   d. weight and length to be between the ninetieth and ninety-seventh percentiles.

2. Brett is producing excess amounts of
   a. thyroid-stimulating hormone.
   b. adrenocorticotropic hormone.
   c. somatotropic hormone.
   d. antidiuretic hormone.

3. Deanna, a four-month-old infant, has cretinism. The clinical manifestations of cretinism that may be recognized in her are
   a. feeding problems, noisy respirations, lethargy, subnormal temperature, and obstinate constipation.
   b. irritability, frequent crying spells, a voracious appetite, and rapid respirations.
   c. nausea, vomiting, diarrhea, tachycardia, and inspiratory stridor.
   d. hyperactive reflexes, tachycardia, poor eating patterns, and advanced motor development.

4. The nursing care of Deanna should include
   1. feeding her carefully to prevent choking.
   2. stimulating her to cry and to change her position.
   3. administering Lanoxin as ordered.
   4. observing her for signs of toxicity from thyroxine.
   5. providing a quiet, nonstimulating environment.
      a. 1 only
      b. 2 and 3
      c. 1, 3, and 5
      d. 1, 2, and 4

5. Justin is a six-month-old, blue-eyed blond with PKU. Which of the following menus is appropriate for Justin's breakfast?
   a. Apple juice
      Scrambled eggs
      Plain oatmeal
      Lofenalac
   b. Orange juice
      Rice cereal with whole milk
      Strained plums
      Lofenalac
   c. Apple juice
      Egg yolk
      Strained peaches
      Lofenalac
   d. Orange juice
      Plain oatmeal
      Strained plums
      Lofenalac
6. The diet that is required to prevent permanent brain damage in children with phenylketonuria is
   a. low in phenylalanine.
   b. high in phenylalanine.
   c. low in pyruvic acid.
   d. high in phenylacetic acid.
7. In order to prevent permanent damage from phenylketonuria, the special diet must be given to the infant
   a. within the first week of life.
   b. before three months of age.
   c. before six months of age.
   d. before the end of the first year.

C. Short answer. Briefly respond to the following statements.

1. List three nursing responsibilities when teaching the parents of a six-month-old infant with recently diagnosed cretinism.
2. Describe three physical findings that might prompt the nurse to question an infant's sex assignment.

BIBLIOGRAPHY

Burnett, Joanne. "Congenital Adrenal Hyperplasia: A Boy With CAH." *American Journal of Nursing,* Vol. 80 (July, 1980), pp. 1304–1305.

Burnett, Joanne. "Congenital Adrenal Hyperplasia: Nursing Interactions." *American Journal of Nursing,* Vol. 80 (July, 1980), pp. 1309–1311.

Burnett, Joanne. "Congenital Adrenal Hyperplasia: The Syndrome." *American Journal of Nursing,* Vol. 80 (July, 1980), pp. 1306–1308.

Elliott, Diane D. "Adrenocortical Insufficiency – A Self-Instruction Unit." *American Journal of Nursing,* Vol. 74 (June, 1974), pp. 1115–1129.

Krause, Marie V., and L. Kathleen Mahan. *Food, Nutritions and Diet Therapy.* Philadelphia: W. B. Saunders Company, 1979.

Lessick, Mira L. "Genetic Counseling of Families with Endocrine Disorders." *Issues in Comprehensive Pediatric Nursing,* Vol. 4 (April, 1980), pp. 27–40.

Reyzer, Nancy. "Diagnosis: PKU." *American Journal of Nursing,* Vol. 79 (November, 1979), pp. 1895–1898.

Tilkian, Sarko M., and Mary B. Conover. *Clinical Implications of Laboratory Tests.* St. Louis: C. V. Mosby Company, 1975.

Vaughan, V. C., et al. *Nelson's Textbook of Pediatrics,* 11th ed. Philadelphia: W. B. Saunders Company, 1979.

Chapter 13

Other Health Care Problems

OBJECTIVES

Upon completion of this chapter, the student will be able to

- describe the abnormal conditions that occur in infants.
- identify the measures that are used to prevent anemia and febrile convulsions.
- describe the assessment of and nursing care for a child with cerebral palsy and Hirschsprung's disease.

Many abnormal conditions can occur in the infancy period, ranging from correctable anemia to the sudden infant death syndrome. The nurse should know the appropriate methods for assessment and early detection of such conditions in children. (Note: refer to Chapter 24 for a discussion of meningitis and other communicable diseases.)

IRON DEFICIENCY ANEMIA

The most common cause of nutritional anemia in children is a diet that is inadequate in iron. In newborn infants, iron is contained only in the circulating hemoglobin. Therefore, it is important that a pregnant woman's intake of iron be adequate during the last two to three months of the pregnancy.

Signs and Symptoms

At birth, the infant's hemoglobin ranges from 16 to 22 grams. During the first two to three months of life, the hemoglobin concentration decreases to 11.4 to 12.2 grams. In the process, much of the iron, or heme, portion is reclaimed and stored by the liver. A diet that is inadequate in iron results in decreased hemoglobin formation. The result is hypochromic red blood cells which may be seen in the laboratory when hemoglobin is not synthesized. Additionally, these cells are usually decreased in size, or microcytic. In premature infants, the problem of decreased hemoglobin production may be complicated further by decreased blood production and immature liver function.

Treatment

The American Academy of Pediatrics recommends that the diet of normal infants provide 1 milligram per kilogram of elemental iron per day up to a maximum of 15 milligrams per day. This recommendation is for children three months of age and older. For low-birth-weight infants and those with a poor iron endowment, 2 milligrams of iron per kilogram per day is the recommended regimen beginning at two months of age.

Nursing Responsibilities

The nurse's primary role lies in identifying those children with anemia, as well as those with potential problems. Children with anemia should be treated. Preventive measures and intake guidelines should be shared with their parents, Figure 13-1.

HYPERTROPHIC PYLORIC STENOSIS

Pyloric stenosis is a condition caused by narrowing or obstruction of the pyloric canal between the stomach and the duodenum, Figure 13-2. The circular muscle of the pylorus becomes hypertrophied, inflamed, and edematous, initially causing mild vomiting and then more severe, projectile emesis. It occurs in

Adequate Iron Intake = 2 to 3 Servings Daily

IRON-RICH FOODS*

Liver	Dried peas and beans	Greens (beet greens, spinach, collards, kale, turnip greens)	Dried fruits (prunes raisins, dates, apricots, peaches)
All kinds of meat	Asparagus	Molasses	Plums, purple
Fish	Broccoli		Berries
Eggs	Brussels sprouts		
Peanut butter			

*Potatoes, whole grains, and enriched bread and cereals also provide some iron.

FOODS THAT INCREASE IRON UTILIZATION BY THE BODY*
(Foods Rich in Vitamin C)

Oranges	Papayas	Greens (beet greens, dandelion greens, kale, mustard greens, spinach, turnip greens)	Green pepper
Grapefruit	Asparagus	Cauliflower	Tomato
Tangerines	Broccoli		Turnip
Cantaloupe	Brussels sprouts		Okra
Strawberries	Cabbage, raw		

*Other raw fruit and raw vegetables, as well as freshly cooked potatoes, provide some vitamin C.

FIG. 13-1 Foods that provide iron or that enhance its utilization by the body

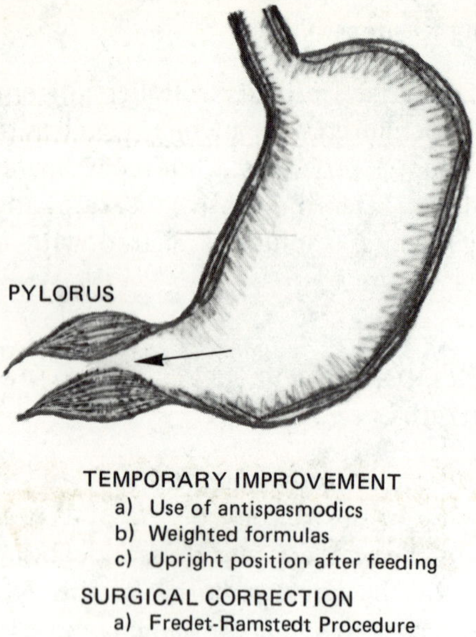

FIG. 13-2 Hypertrophic pyloric stenosis

about five of one thousand live births, usually in male infants.

Signs and Symptoms

Mild symptoms, usually regurgitation of the feeding, may be exhibited in the second or third week of life. As this pattern continues, the infant loses weight. Signs of dehydration, such as poor skin turgor, sunken eyeballs, lethargy, and loss of subcutaneous fat, will appear. The child resembles failure-to-thrive infants. As the vomiting continues, it becomes increasingly projectile, often projecting several feet away from the baby, depending on the infant's position.

Diagnosis

On physical examination, a hard, nontender mass is palpable in the epigastric area. In some infants, the peristaltic waves may be visible, moving from the left side of the abdomen to the right.

Diagnostic procedures include an upper gastrointestinal series. A delayed gastric emptying time and a tiny, threadlike pyloric opening are characteristic. Laboratory studies reveal decreased levels of chloride, potassium, and sodium. On examination of the vomitus, no trace of bile is found.

Treatment

Surgical correction of this condition is warranted. The Fredet-Ramstedt procedure is used. The muscle is split to the submucus layer parallel to the lumen.

Nursing Responsibilities

Preoperative nursing care may involve feeding the child in an upright position with thickened formula following the administration of antispasmodics. Frequently, the child is refed after emesis. Postoperatively, the infant is allowed clear liquids in small amounts initially. The amount is gradually increased until the normal formula feeding pattern is resumed. Postoperatively, the infant should be kept upright for approximately thirty minutes after feeding. This is done to prevent emesis secondary to the edema around the operative site.

FEBRILE CONVULSIONS

Seizures caused by a rapid rise in body temperature occur most commonly in the infancy and toddler periods. They usually occur at the beginning of an illness when the rise of temperature may go unnoticed until the actual seizure occurs. The seizures usually last less than five minutes and subside spontaneously. The risk of a recurrence is greater in children with a family history of seizures as well as in those who have the first seizure at a very early age.

Treatment

Measures to reduce temperature should be instituted immediately. In those children with recurrent seizures related to temperature, prophylactic phenobarbital may be ordered by the physician. Aspirin and acetominophen may both be ordered for this child. The aspirin is administered at ten-two-six, while the acetominophen is given at twelve-four-eight.

Nursing Responsibilities

Nursing care involves acute measures to control the seizure and subsequent intervention to lower the child's temperature. Because febrile convulsions tend to recur in some individuals, the parents should be taught how to control elevations in temperature as a preventive technique. These seizures do not have any bearing on epileptic seizures that may occur later in life.

HIRSCHSPRUNG'S DISEASE

Hirschsprung's disease, or aganglionic megacolon, is an obstructive problem caused by the absence of the parasympathetic ganglion nerve cells. It results in a lack of peristalsis or motility in the intestinal tract. The disorder can either be acute or chronic, depending on the size of the intestinal segment involved. This familial defect occurs four times more often in males than in females. The most common site of involvement is the rectosigmoid colon.

Signs and Symptoms

The lack of peristalsis associated with this disease allows fecal contents and gas to accumulate, causing dilatation of the bowel. Emptying of the bowel is further inhibited by the failure of the rectal sphincter to relax. Symptoms seen in the neonate may include failure to pass meconium, emesis containing bile, and progressive abdominal distention. In older infants, a history of explosive watery stools, fever, and prostration is common. These are signs of enterocolitis, which may be fatal in these children as it leads to bowel perforation and shock. A chronic pattern of severe constipation with hard, pelletlike, foul-smelling stools and severe abdominal distention is typical in older children. All children with this disease appear to be poorly nourished.

Diagnosis

Diagnostic evaluation includes a barium enema, which will confirm the dilation of the proximal colon and the aganglionic distal segment. Biopsy of the aganglionic portion shows an absence of nerve endings.

Treatment

Conservative management of this disease involves colonic lavage, as this infant is unable to evacuate the contents of the colon. The solution of choice is an isotonic electrolyte. Alternatively, skim milk may be used. Use of plain water is contraindicated as it may cause water intoxication because of the large amount absorbed through the increased surface area. The catheter should be carefully inserted and the appropriate amount of solution measured. Vigorous insertion of the catheter may cause perforation of the bowel. Colonic lavage is performed daily unless irritability, abdominal distention, and poor feeding dictate more frequent treatment.

Surgical correction of Hirschsprung's disease involves the creation of a temporary double-barrel colostomy to allow decompression of the bowel. This colostomy is maintained until the infant is close to one year old and weighs about twenty pounds. Then, corrective surgery involving an abdominoperineal pull-through is undertaken. The operation of choice is either a Soave or Duhamel procedure.

Nursing Responsibilities

Postoperative care for children with Hirschsprung's disease includes initial care of the colostomy with careful attention to the fluid and electrolyte balance. The irregularity and frequency of the infant's stools are quite different from the adult. The character and frequency of the stools must be noted by the nurse and later by the parents. An increased number of liquid stools may indicate a need for increases in the fluid intake to prevent dehydration.

The careful fitting of the colostomy bag is very important in the young child. Several different types of appliances may have to be tried before a satisfactory one is found. Both Hollister Company and Coloplast Company have pediatric sizes and equipment available. A nurse specializing in enterostomal therapy may be especially helpful both to the staff and the family in this situation.

The skin surrounding the colostomy is very susceptible to irritation and breakdown. It must be cleansed gently and protected from drainage coming from the adjacent stoma. A thin layer of cream or ointment containing zinc oxide may be applied to protect the skin surface. Frequent checking to be sure the appliance is intact and adhering also protects the adjacent skin.

Older children undergoing surgical treatment are maintained on a low-residue diet. Depending on the age of the child, even a temporary colostomy may be emotionally traumatic. The toddler may benefit from playing with a doll having an appliance and dressings similar to what the child will have after surgery. The preschool child can benefit from the same type of play, but in addition needs to hear that he or she did not cause the problem. Any participation in dressing changes is beneficial.

After the corrective procedure, the child's perineum should be protected from pressure. A sterile pad should be kept underneath the child in order to absorb the bloody mucus and drainage. No diaper is used. The child is usually positioned with the hips and knees flexed to reduce tension on the abdominal muscles. The postoperative diet should exclude any type of laxative food. Problems with distention may recur in these children, but are likely to be related to the one centimeter of defective bowel that was left intact to provide good sphincter control. If ordered, a small catheter inserted into the rectum rapidly relieves this distention. Postoperatively, the child is observed carefully for signs of infection, distention, and leakage at the site of the anastomosis.

SUDDEN INFANT DEATH SYNDROME

Sudden infant death syndrome (SIDS), or crib death as it is sometimes called, occurs in sleeping infants from one week to one year of age. No sounds of distress are made by the infant. A previous history of a slight upper respiratory infection that would be insufficient to cause death may be cited by the parents. These infants are most commonly low-birth-weight infants and male.

On autopsy, petechiae are usually present in the thorax. The frothy fluid present in the nose and mouth is suggestive of pulmonary edema. Special studies conducted at the Cleveland

Clinic suggest that an abnormality in the infant's brain stem may be involved in the syndrome.

Because the infant is often found in the crib with blankets nearby, many parents assume that the infant has smothered or that the vomitus on the face suggests aspiration. Neither theory is correct; the exact cause of the syndrome is unknown at this time.

The incidence of SIDS is higher in the winter months and in those infants with a slight upper respiratory infection. It also occurs more often in higher density living areas. It is for these reasons that some researchers feel a virus acts as a trigger mechanism for infants already at risk.

More attention at this time is being directed to those infants who are considered "near-miss" for sudden infant death syndrome. These infants have stopped breathing and have been resuscitated by prompt intervention. The nurse directly involved in the care of this infant must demonstrate a great deal of empathy and support for this family under stress. A detailed nursing history aids the family in describing what happened and in airing their feelings of stress. The history also provides the nurse with an opportunity to correct misinformation.

During the hospitalization, the prompt response of the nurse to the apnea alarm, assessment of the infant, and gentle stimulation aid the parents in adjusting to the homegoing care of the infant. The nurse is responsible for documenting any apneic episodes, administration of theophylline or other ordered medications, and resuscitation if necessary.

Apnea monitoring in the home is not done for every child. The monitors are often difficult for families to operate and cause a great deal of psychologic stress. These factors and the cost limit their uses in the home.

Nursing responsibilities in relation to the parent who has already lost a child to SIDS usually occur in the emergency room setting. The parents exhibit an intense grief reaction because of the infant's death.

Parents require a great deal of support in coping with the grief and guilt that follows the sudden death of their infant. The stress of the parent may be increased further by the presence of the police, the coroner, and by the required autopsy. Even though this syndrome may be explained to the parents at the time, and health care workers may be available to give support, the parents may be too distraught to absorb the information. Parents may also tend to overprotect other children in the family as a result of the death of their infant. The most effective support for parents often comes from other parents who are members of the local SIDS organization.

CEREBRAL PALSY

The term cerebral palsy designates a group of nonprogressive neurologic conditions that affect the motor cortex, the basal ganglia, or the cerebellum. The disease may be divided into three major forms: spastic, athetoid, and ataxic.

Classification

Spastic cerebral palsy is the most common type, occurring in about seventy-five percent of the cases. It affects the pyramidal tract and the cerebral cortex. Children with this form of the disease have hyperactive reflexes and exaggerated stretch reflexes, or involvement of the voluntary control of the limb muscles.

The athetoid form involves the basal ganglia. The resultant abnormal movements are more common in the upper extremities, are writhing in nature, and disappear during sleep. They may be increased by emotional tension. This form of the disease occurs in about twenty percent of the cases.

The ataxic form is the least common, occurring in only two percent of the cases. Affected children have disturbances of balance, lack of coordination of the upper extremities, hypoactive reflexes, horizontal nystagmus, and minimal movement of the lower extremities. These disorders are related to damage to the cerebellum itself.

All forms of cerebral palsy are the result of trauma to the nervous system that occurs in the perinatal period. Any factor that causes anoxia in the mother or the fetus may cause cerebral palsy, as may trauma or certain infections in the mother, Table 13-1.

Initially, the care of the child should involve a comprehensive evaluation with a long-term plan for intervention. Periodic reassessment of the child should be done by the health care team. Continuity of care provides maximal gains for the child as well as a greater degree of education and support for the parents.

TABLE 13-1 Causes of Cerebral Palsy

Maternal Conditions
Anoxia
Hemorrhage
Blood incompatibilities (Rh and ABO)
Rubella
Cytomegalovirus disease
Toxoplasmosis
Radiation of any type
Fetal Conditions
Anoxia from any source
Maternal anesthesia
Placenta previa or placenta abruptio
Prolonged labor
Kernicterus from hyperbilirubinemia
Cerebral trauma during delivery
Infections of the central nervous system

Nursing Responsibilities

Early signs of cerebral palsy include difficulties with sucking and swallowing, seizures, excess irritability, and abnormal reflexes. As the child grows, the abnormal motor development, persistent abnormal reflexes, and delayed speech become more evident. The child may also have mental retardation. The major care problems associated with this disease when it is detected early include maintaining the child's nutritional status, performing the activities of daily living, and expanding the child's exposure to the environment.

The nutritional status may be improved by measures that increase the child's ability to suck, chew, and swallow. Placing glucose on the nipple of a bottle or on a pacifier gives the infant incentive to put his or her lips on the nipple. Stimulating the lips with the nipple may also help. Infants who hyperextend themselves when an attempt is made to hold them should be positioned on their abdomens with their heads extended for feedings. As these children grow, they should be encouraged to use their tongues. Placing something sticky and adherent, like peanut butter, on the tongue prompts the child to try to get it off the tongue. This, in turn, promotes tongue mobility. The skills of chewing, sucking, and swallowing must be achieved in order for speech to occur.

Range of motion exercises are used to maintain joint motion in children with cerebral palsy. These maneuvers should be done slowly and firmly so that the spasticity is not increased by the action. All motor movements with this child should be slow and gentle. Moreover, bathing should always be with warm water to reduce the possibility of shivering and a resultant spastic response.

The child's exposure to the environment should be like that of any normal child. This requires some thought on the part of the parents, as well as some adaptation of equipment. Change of position is crucial to prevent skin breakdown even though the child often prefers a supine position.

With older children, communication may create real problems. If the child is unable to speak, assistive devices, such as the Bliss symbol board or picture cards, should be used to enhance the child's ability.

Cerebral palsy is a lifelong and complex problem. Parents need a great deal of support and assistance, especially initially. This support, as well as suggestions for care, may be largely derived from the local chapters of the United Cerebral Palsy Association.

ECZEMA

Eczema, or infantile eczema as it is often called, is a persistent or chronic skin disorder that occurs in children. It is an allergic response, but it also has a hereditary component and is magnified by emotional stress.

Signs and Symptoms

Eczematous lesions occur in the moist folds of the elbows, knees, and neck, and on the face itself. During an acute attack, the lesions spread, and may cover most of the child's body surface. The individual lesions are tiny vesicles that are situated on a reddened, itchy base. As the vesicles rupture, the oozing secretions dry and form crusts over the area.

Between attacks, the area of skin eruption continues to be red, scaly, and very dry. Over the years, and as a result of repeated irritation and scratching, the skin darkens. The skin may become thick and leatherlike, a characteristic properly referred to as lichenification.

Because of the pruritis during an acute attack, the child scratches or rubs the lesions until they rupture. The raw surfaces become covered with a thick, yellow, sticky exudate. The weeping, oozing areas continue to spread. Continued scratching and skin irritation may result in bacterial infection. Depending on the depth of the infectious process, scarring may also occur.

Children with eczema are usually very irritable and fretful. On closer examination, lymphadenopathy and a low-grade fever may be present. In some children, splenomegaly may also occur. The acute phase of eczema occurs more commonly in the winter months and is seldom seen in children younger than four months of age. This age limitation is thought to be a result of the low level of immunoglobulin E in these children, as it plays a part in hypersensitivity responses.

Treatment

The treatment of eczema is directed toward two distinct goals. The first is determining the allergens. The second involves alleviating the acute phase of the disease.

Identification of the allergens begins with a careful and thorough history. Dietary allergens are most common in infants and toddlers. Some of the most common dietary allergens are cow's milk, egg whites, grains such as wheat, and some fruits (particularly oranges).

An elimination diet may be selected for the child. This restricts intake of the most common of the allergenic foods. In infants, this may mean substituting soybean-based formula for cow's milk formula. This diet is also low in carbohydrates and fats.

Inhalants may also cause eczema. Environmental precautions include dust-proofing the child's room by eliminating items that collect dust, and avoiding the use of aerosols, sprays, and powders. It is particularly important to avoid using powder on small infants because the inhaled particles may cause respiratory problems.

Nursing Care

In the nursing care of the child with eczema, emphasis should be placed on relief of the inflammatory process, prevention of secondary infection, and protection of healthy tissue from further damage, Table 13-2. Pruritis is one of the major signs of the eczema. Intervention should be aimed at preventing increased circulation to the areas of the lesions, as this reduces the pruritis. Appropriate measures include bathing the child with tepid water, blotting the skin dry, avoiding friction from clothing, and using a minimum of cotton clothing. Elbow restraints or some type of mitt may be required to prevent the child from scratching. The child should be observed carefully when these restraints are used, as other ways of scratching may be found, such as rubbing the face against the sheets or using the shoulder to rub the side of a cheek. Colloid or starch baths may be administered to reduce inflammation. Wet dressings may be used to aid in crust removal in smaller areas. Antipruritics and corticosteroids may also be used to relieve the inflammation.

Secondary infection may be prevented in a number of ways. One method is simply to prevent scratching. The child's nails may be trimmed to reduce the potential for damage. Frequent washing of the child's hands reduces the bacterial count and may prevent organisms from being introduced. Exposure to other children with bacterial infections should be

TABLE 13-2 Nursing Care of the Child with Eczema

To reduce itching:
Avoid all known allergens
Maintain a cool environment
Trim child's fingernails
Provide light clothing (cotton or synthetic blends)
Provide safe toys
Keep wet dressings cool rather than warm
Apply medication gently, without rubbing
Administer analgesics or sedatives as needed
Avoid excess soap on normal skin
Avoid foods that cause flushing, such as condiments and hot drinks
Use mittens, if necessary, to cover the child's hands to prevent scratching
To prevent crust formations:
Check the diaper area frequently and expose it to air
Provide tub baths and dressings as ordered
Remove medications gently before reapplying
Provide increased protein in the diet if oozing is excessive
To protect healthy skin:
Pat the skin dry after bathing
Cover healthy skin with a non-water soluble protector if it is adjacent to wet dressings
Prevent scratching of healthy skin
Prevent exposure of the child to other children with infections
Provide diversion

carefully avoided. For this reason, children with eczema are seldom treated in a hospital setting. The potential for and exposure to bacterial infections are much greater in a hospital environment.

Education of the parents and improvement of the parent-child interaction may be a difficult objective for the nurse to achieve. The education of the parent must include a knowledge of the allergy and of the substances that have caused it, as well as of the planned method of treatment. Parents should be taught how to prevent or control the allergic response. Certainly, parents can effect certain environmental controls at home. The parents should know what they can realistically achieve.

Improvement of the parent-child interaction may take a considerable amount of time and effort. The continuing stress of an irritable, unhappy child can disrupt this interaction. Some parents may be upset by the appearance of the oozing crusted lesions on the child. The burden of care and treatments is often delegated to one individual. Parents may have strong feelings of rejection toward both the child and the illness. The nurse may detect avoidance, rejection, or overprotectiveness toward the child. In any situation, the child is usually aware of these strong feelings and reacts to them. When working with the parents, the nurse should recognize their feelings and give them an opportunity to discuss them openly. Recognition of these feelings facilitates the establishment of a supportive and constructive relationship. The nurse may help the family explore effective ways to cope with the treatments and the child's overall behavior. Reinforcement should also be provided for the positive parenting skills displayed by the parents. If ineffective parenting techniques are observed, the nurse can offer alternatives and, in some situations, act as a role model.

INTUSSUSCEPTION

Intussusception is an invagination or telescoping of one portion of the intestines into an adjacent section causing intestinal obstruction. The most common site is at the ileocecal valve with a portion of the ileum telescoping into the cecum. This condition is most common between three months and two years of age and has a higher incidence in males. It is seen more often in those children with celiac disease and cystic fibrosis, as well as those children with abdominal injuries, itestinal polyps, and Meckel's diverticulum.

This condition becomes apparent when a normal, healthy child develops a sudden onset of acute abdominal pain. The child demonstrates this with the typical screaming cry and by drawing the knees up on the abdomen. During this initial period the child may have a normal brown stool. At first, the episodes of pain occur at intervals rather than continuously. As they recur, the child may also exhibit vomiting. With the progression of the problem the child becomes listless and may pass stools containing only blood and mucus. These are the characteristic "currant jelly" stools seen with intussusception. Fever, prostration, and peritonitis may occur if treatment is not sought in this acute emergency.

Inspection of the child's abdomen reveals it to be tender and distended. Gentle palpation of the upper right quadrant usually reveals an elongated mass, while the lower quadrant feels devoid of contents. This is referred to as Dance's sign. The diagnosis is usually confirmed when a barium enema is done on the child. The barium enema may correct the intussusception because of the pressure exerted by the barium. If this is not effective, a surgical correction is carried out. This involves manual reduction of the telescoped portion and sometimes resection depending on the amount of damage done and the period of time since the onset of the symptoms.

Nursing responsibilities involve recognition of this potentially life-threatening emergency. The history given by the parents and the obvious signs are quite consistent. Explanations are given to the parents regarding the barium enema and its expected outcome as well as the possibility of surgery.

Monitoring vital signs, observing symptoms, and withholding food and fluids are important aspects of this child's care during the preoperative period. Postoperatively, the nurse should continue to assess the child for potential intussusception. The potential for recurrence is greatest in the first days postoperatively.

SUMMARY

Health alterations that occur in the infancy period range from mild to severe. Anemia and pyloric stenosis, for instance, are correctable conditions that are associated with a relatively short period of stress for the parents. Conversely, for the parents of the child with megacolon or cerebral palsy, the problem continues indefinitely. A great deal of assistance and support are needed in order for parents to cope with the ongoing care of these children. Infant crib death is a sudden and fatal syndrome. The families of these infants also require emotional support to work through their feelings. The role of the nurse in all these conditions involves careful assessment to aid in the identification of the care problem, skillful nursing care during the acute phase, and parent support and education throughout.

SUGGESTED ACTIVITIES

- Report to the class on the types of communication boards available for children and adults with speech impairments. If possible, provide a display of such devices.
- Visit your local chapter of the United Cerebral Palsy Association. Determine what services are provided. Obtain some samples of their educational materials and share them with your class.
- Make a list of the types of food and clothing that should be avoided by a child with eczema.

DISCUSSION TOPICS

1. Contact the local chapter of the National Sudden Infant Death Foundation. Find out what services are provided and the types of available literature. If possible, ask a speaker to present this to your class. Discuss ways in which nurses and family members can provide support to the parents and other siblings.
2. Research the various types of assistive devices that are available to help children with the normal activities of daily living. A physical or occupational therapist working with handicapped children would be a good resource person for this information. Share your findings with your class.

REVIEW

A. Matching. Match the description in Column I with the disease in Column II.

Column I	Column II
1. Hyperplasia of the pylorus	a. Sudden infant death syndrome
2. Lack of ganglia in the rectosigmoid area	b. Pyloric stenosis
3. Nonprogressive neurologic defect of the cerebral cortex	c. Hirschsprung's disease
4. Apnea-associated disease	d. Cerebral palsy

B. Multiple choice. Select the one best answer.

1. Billy is a four-week-old infant who was admitted to the hospital with a history of weight loss from vomiting. The adjective projectile might be used to describe the
   a. forceful contraction of the abdomen.
   b. nonforceful expelling of food from the stomach.
   c. rhythmic contractions of the abdomen that precede forceful defecations.
   d. forceful expulsion of the stomach contents.
2. The vomitus of an infant with pyloric stenosis is the color of the formula and does not contain bile because the
   a. obstruction is above the opening of the common bile duct.
   b. liver does not secrete bile since its functioning is impaired.
   c. obstruction at the cardiac sphincter prevents the flow of bile to the stomach.
   d. stenosis of the common bile duct prevents bile from flowing properly.
3. Before speech sounds may be taught to a child with cerebral palsy, which of the following reflexes must be well established?
   a. Blinking, coughing, and sneezing reflexes
   b. Moro and tonic neck reflexes
   c. Tonic neck and coughing reflexes
   d. Chewing, sucking, and swallowing reflexes
4. One type of cerebral palsy is called athetoid. Athetosis is characterized by
   a. a disturbance of the sense of balance and posture.
   b. fine tremors or muscular movements that occur in regular patterns.
   c. involuntary or excess movements that interfere with normal precision.
   d. tension in certain muscle groups that restricts movement.

C. Short answer. Briefly respond to the following statements.

1. Name three iron-rich foods that are suitable for a six-month-old infant.
2. List two types of surgery for a child with Hirschsprung's disease.

BIBLIOGRAPHY

Beckwith, J. Bruce, et al. "When An Infant Dies Without Cause." *Patient Care,* Vol. 12 (March 15, 1978), pp. 216–232.

Brown, Marie Scott. "How To Tell If a Baby has Cerebral Palsy . . . And What to Tell His Parents When He Does." *Nursing 79,* Vol. 9 (May, 1979), pp. 88–91.

Cohen, Stephen. "Skin Rashes in Infants and Children." *American Journal of Nursing,* Vol. 78 (June, 1978), pp. 1041–1072.

Crelin, Edmund S., et al. "Can the Cause of SIDS Be This Simple?" *Patient Care,* Vol. 12 (March, 1978), pp. 234–240.

Favorito, John, et al. "Apnea Monitoring to Prevent SIDS." *American Journal of Nursing,* Vol. 79 (January, 1979), pp. 101–104.

Habersang, Rolf, and Alice Marsh. "Iron and Infant Nutrition." *Issues in Comprehensive Pediatric Nursing,* Vol. 2 (January-February, 1977), pp. 43–49.

Hawley, Donna, and Diane W. Reiser. "Reducing Muscle Spasms in a Child With Cerebral Palsy." *American Journal of Nursing,* Vol. 78 (July, 1978), pp. 1214–1215.

Jones, Katherine M. "Love and Lavage." *Nursing 78,* Vol. 8 (July, 1978), pp. 32–39.

Sinnott, Frank, et al. "Cerebral Palsy: From Suspicion to Therapy." *Patient Care,* Vol. 12 (October 30, 1978), pp. 156–192.

Spenner, Dorothy. "When the Baby Is Sick and the Mother's Concerns Are Ignored." *American Journal of Nursing,* Vol. 80 (December, 1980), pp. 2222–2224.

Wachowiak, Kathleen D. "Sudden Infant Death Syndrome: What You Can Do To Help the Family." *RN,* Vol. 41 (February, 1978), p. 4649.

Section V

The Toddler

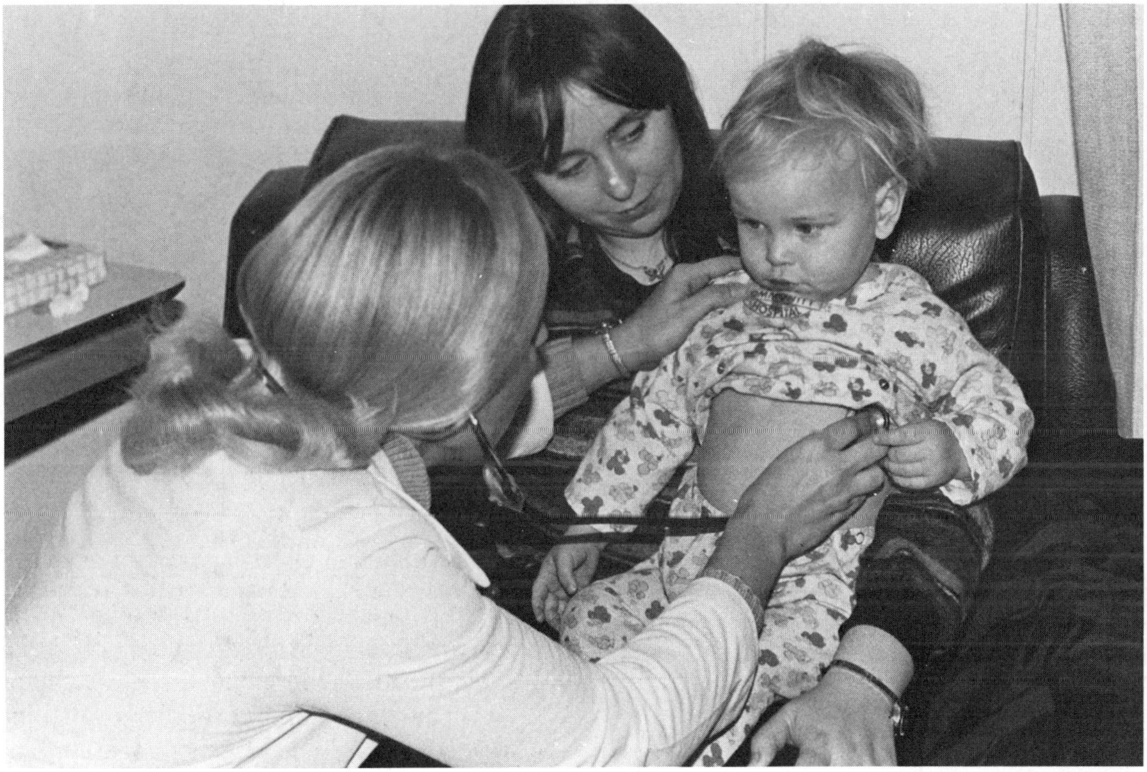

Chapter 14
Growth and Development

OBJECTIVES

Upon completion of this chapter, the student will be able to

- describe the physical development that occurs during the toddler period.
- compare the developmental tasks for toddlers identified by Erikson with those identified by Piaget.
- explain the application of developmental tasks to the care of toddlers in the hospital setting.

The toddler stage of growth and development extends from one to three years of age. It is marked by a slowing of physical growth and a rapid increase in motor skills and communication ability.

DEVELOPMENTAL TASKS

The developmental tasks of the toddler period have two major foci: motor skill development and relationships with others. Among the motor skills learned during this stage are walking and talking. Additionally, control of elimination becomes just as important a task as the manipulation of play materials and the use of parallel play. Each is another step in the development of skills that provide a building block for future development of the child.

The basis for the toddler's relationship with others is the development of autonomy or independence. With the realization that they are totally separate individuals, toddlers begin to differentiate themselves from other people and things. For instance, they tolerate temporary separations from their mothers during this period. They begin to see themselves in a new light, seeking the approval of the important people in their lives. This reflected appraisal helps develop a beginning self-concept of "I am good" or "I can do it." Obedience to simple commands is part of this interaction with others. The control of unacceptable emotional impulses is also learned during the toddler period. Temper tantrums or the urge to bite others in anger, evident in the early part of this period, becomes less evident as the child approaches the preschool years.

Erikson's Sense of Autonomy

As described by Erikson, the period of toddlerhood is the stage of autonomy. During this time, the toddler develops a sense of autonomy versus a sense of shame and doubt. Building on the trusting relationships of infancy and the knowledge of their environment, toddlers begin to perceive themselves as separate human beings.

This progression involves a transition from the dependent, submissive infant to the toddler who revolts against the surroundings and attempts to manipulate the environment to suit personal whims. The sense of shame and doubt arises when the child maintains dependency rather than testing his or her own potential. Shame or loss of self-esteem becomes a factor when the toddler resists the urge to revolt against the will and restrictions of the parent. The unlimited capacity to control people and things in the environment because of overpermissive parents evokes fear in the toddler, who realizes his or her limitations. These children may later become compulsive about controlling.

Some authors refer to the autonomy of the toddler as a graded independence. This takes into account the setting of limits and structure by the adult for the toddler. The consistency with which limit-setting and discipline are imposed has a bearing on the ability of the toddler to function at maximal capacity and yet develop an awareness of acceptable and nonacceptable behavior.

Piaget's Cognitive Development

Piaget considers the beginning of the toddler stage to be a continuation of the sensorimotor phase of the infant. During this period, which roughly extends from twelve to twenty-four months of age, children learn to differentiate themselves from objects, developing both an increased awareness of object permanence and the beginnings of memory. Other developmental milestones identified in the latter part of the first year include a sense of egocentricity, the organization of thought, and a beginning sense of time.

Observation of the activities of a child documents this behavioral development rather readily. Initially, for instance, the child will hunt for an object in one location only. Later, the child will look in several hiding places, even opening doors or drawers in the search. Thought organization is demonstrated by the child's ritualistic behavior, the ability to play in a parallel fashion, the concept of ownership of objects, and the references to self. A developing sense of time is evident when the child responds appropriately to "in a minute" or to the announcement of mealtime.

During the latter half of the toddler period, Piaget describes children as being in a stage of preoperational or preconceptual thought. During this time, children internalize mental images for both objects and actions. The objects which, in infancy, were handled in exploration are, in the toddler stage, transformed into symbols. The various means by which objects or events may be represented include

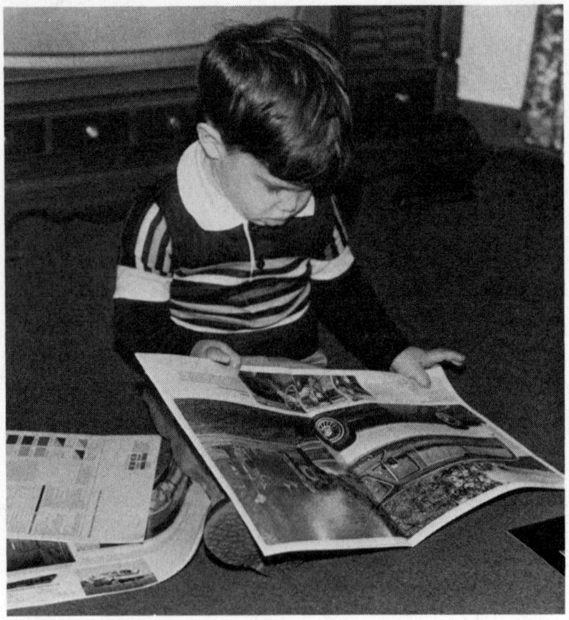

FIG. 14-1 This toddler is imitating the way his father studies advertisements for new cars.

mental images, imitation, symbolic play, symbolic drawing, and language, Figure 14-1.

The imitation skills of toddlers are apparent in their vocalization of animal sounds. These skills are also evident in their realistic imitation of an angry mother or father, using not only the same words but also the same voice inflections. The use of symbolic play allows the child to participate in events which could not otherwise occur. For instance, through symbols, children may pretend that they are playing in the sandbox when they are actually confined to the house on a rainy day. Such symbolic play serves to expand their environment through pretending.

The increased language ability of toddlers is recognized in their use of prepositions, such as over, under, above, and below, which convey directions. The use of verbs is marked by the past tense. The use of the possessive term "mine" increases during this period. The toddler is likely to use a pronoun, often "meself," to refer to himself or herself and to emphasize whose wishes should be acknowledged.

PHYSICAL DEVELOPMENT

The growth of the toddler is a continuation of the decelerated growth pattern that marks the end of the infancy period. The increase in weight is about four to six pounds per year. The average one-year-old child weighs 22.5 pounds. By age two, young boys generally weigh between 27 and 28 pounds. The normal range of weight for boys this age is 23 to 32 pounds. By age three, young boys usually weigh about 32 pounds, with the norm ranging from 27 to 38 pounds. Young girls of the same age generally weigh two pounds less than boys, both in average weight and in the normal range of weight.

A similar deceleration occurs in linear growth during this period. The yearly increase approximates three inches per year. At the age of two years, the normal range for boys is 32 to 37 inches, with the average being 34.5 inches. By the age of three years, the average height is 38 inches, with the normal range being 36 to 40 inches. Linear measurements in girls are generally one-half inch less than they are for boys, both for the normal range and the average height for each age.

Individual children set their own growth rate and set of norms for development. The nurse should record serial measurements of height and weight, as well as head circumference, on a standardized growth chart. Only in this fashion can growth patterns be identified as consistent or inconsistent. For instance, the effects of a prolonged illness may first be noted from the growth chart as the child drops from the fiftieth percentile to a lower range. Distinct pathologic growth patterns may also be identified earlier with these standardized recordings.

Body Contour and Proportion

Unique changes in body contour and proportion are evident in the toddler. The arms and legs lengthen noticeably as ossification and growth occur in the epiphyseal centers of the long bones. Conversely, the rate of growth of the head and trunk decreases. The child's increased ability to walk which improves the strength of the abdominal muscles also brings about a change. The lumbar lordosis and the protuberant abdomen that are typical of the early part of the toddler stage disappear as the child approaches the preschool period.

Development of the Large and Small Muscles

The activities of the child are used as parameters of growth. Both large muscle coordination and small muscle development are necessary for the child to achieve the tasks of the toddler period. Indications of large muscle development include the ability to walk unassisted. This activity is usually mastered by the age of eighteen months. The speed with which the child walks increases progressively, enabling the child to run by the age of two years. Toddlers are also capable of maintaining their balance while picking up objects that are lying on the floor. By three years of age, large muscle development has progressed sufficiently to allow the child to ride a tricycle, Figure 14-2, walk up and down stairs using a handrail, and kick a large ball forward.

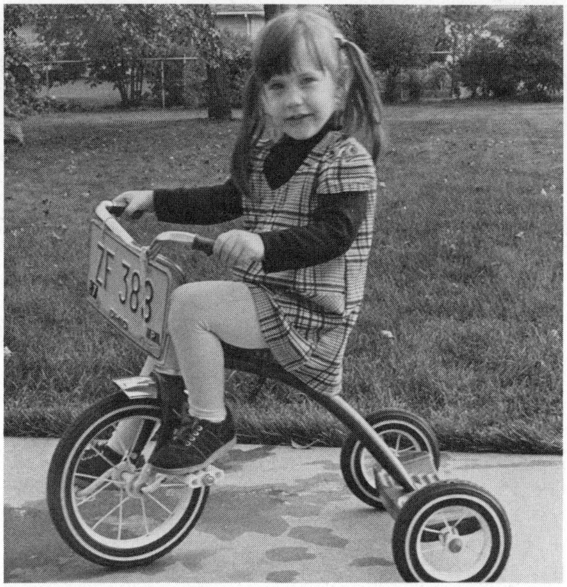

FIG. 14-2 This child shows pride in her newfound skill – riding a tricycle.

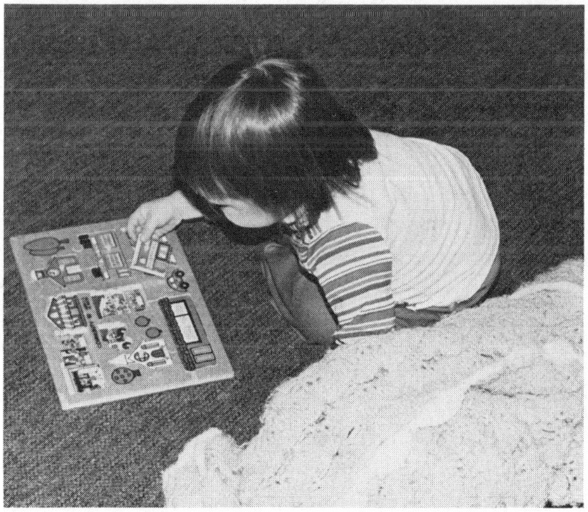

FIG. 14-3 Small muscle development is enhanced by playing with picture puzzles.

Small muscle development during this period is primarily evident in the skill with which the hands are used, Figure 14-3. Scribbling is

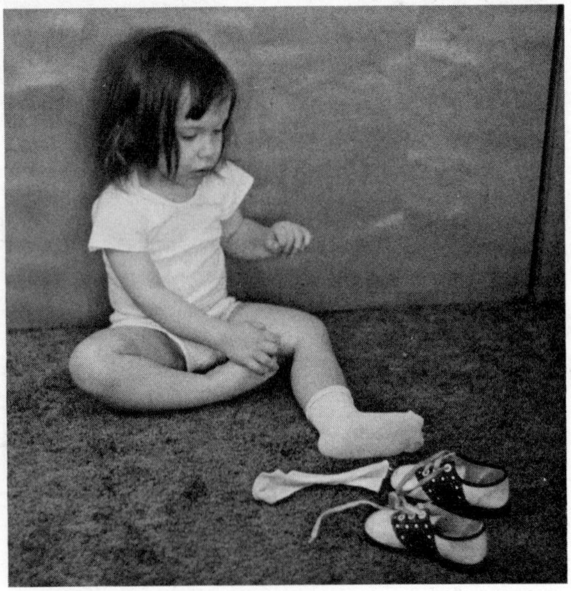

FIG. 14-4 At this age, removing a sock is much easier than putting it on.

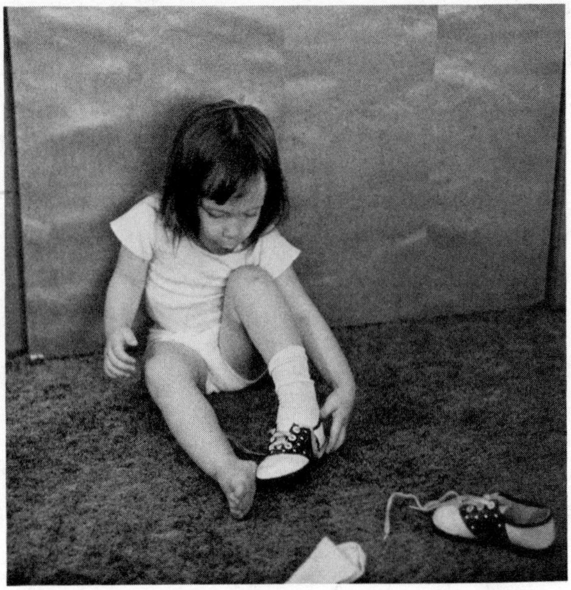

FIG. 14-5 Getting one's heel into a shoe requires a great deal of concentration for a young child.

the most common demonstration of this skill in very young children. In eighteen-month-old children, scribbling is likely to take place with or without benefit of paper. The edges of the paper do not constitute a boundary for children this age as they do for two-year-old children. By two years of age, the toddler is able to copy a vertical line and can build a tower of four cubes. Moreover, two-year-old toddlers should be able to use a spoon to feed themselves with minimal spillage. By three years of age, their writing ability has expanded to the copying of circles and the naming of the scribbles and doodles on the paper. By the age of three years, they are able to build a tower of blocks that is at least eight cubes high. Also at this age, a fork substituted for the spoon is used correctly. The toddler's dressing skills include the ability to fasten buttons and to remove clothing, Figures 14-4 and 14-5.

Special Senses

The visual acuity of toddlers changes gradually. Normally, they are farsighted or hyperopic. The clearest vision for these children occurs at a distance of six feet. The use of relatively large objects improves their visual imagery. During this period, the strength and equality of the eye muscles should be assessed. Strabismus may occur as an occasional phenomenon in some children, but should not be a recurrent pattern in a given child. If strabismus occurs repeatedly or persists, the child should be referred for an evaluation by an ophthalmologist.

The toddler's sense of hearing is fully matured. An assessment of hearing acuity should be performed on a serial basis to detect any early changes. Children in this age-group often suffer from pharyngitis which may develop into otitis media. A single infection that is adequately treated should create no long-term problems. However, a series of infections may cause a hearing deficit. Decreased or altered communication skills are also reasons for audiometric studies.

Dentition

At the start of the toddler period, six to eight teeth have erupted. These include the upper and lower central and lateral incisors. During the toddler period, the cuspids and molars erupt. By the age of two and a half years, the process of dentition for the deciduous teeth is completed.

At the time of eruption of the earliest teeth, consideration should be given to cleaning the teeth. The parents should be taught to clean the child's teeth with a soft, moist cloth on a regular basis. The use of a toothbrush should be delayed until twelve to eighteen months of age. Vigorous brushing should be avoided as it may injure the delicate gingival tissues of the child's mouth. Toothpaste is used very sparingly, if at all, as the child is likely to eat it. Visits to the dentist should begin around the age of two years. Parents should be present during these examinations.

Fluoride protects both deciduous and permanent teeth. In many areas, fluoride is available through the water supply and fluoride supplements are not required. Small amounts of water to rinse the mouth and provide fluoride may be offered to the child after meals or snacks. In those areas where it is not generally available, fluoride may have to be supplemented on a daily basis. The recommended amount of fluoride from infancy to the age of ten years ranges from 0.03 milligram per kilogram to 0.06 milligram per kilogram.

Bottle-mouth syndrome also interferes with proper dentition. The toddler who continues to take a bedtime bottle is at great risk for serious dental caries. The sugar content of the ingested liquid pools around the back teeth, particularly the maxillary incisors, destroying the enamel and dentine. Weaning the child from the night bottle or substituting plain water prevents this problem. Otherwise, reconstructive dentistry and the application of stainless steel crowns may be required later to correct the damage from bottle-mouth syndrome. Parents should remember that neither the bottle nor the breast should be used as a substitute for comfort measures for the child.

TOILET TRAINING

The accomplishment that is most commonly identified with the toddler period is toilet training. It signals the end of diapers, at least in the daytime, and a movement toward greater independence for the child. The process of toilet training is commonly marked by a major power struggle within the family.

Grandparents, aunts, uncles, and neighbors may exert undue influence on this process. Parents may be assailed by the question "Is he out of diapers yet?" from the time the infant is six months old. This intense pressure, if exerted on a young or first-time parent, may, in turn, be transferred to the child. Unfortunately, the readiness of the child for this activity may not even be considered by the adults involved.

Nurses involved in the anticipatory guidance of parents of young children should discuss the issue of toilet training early enough to avert or defuse some of the pressure from relatives. The parents will need time to sort out their own attitudes and feelings about the process. They should also know what clues signal the child's readiness for toilet training.

Finally, they must be able to encourage the child without forcing or pressuring compliance.

In considering this stage of their child's development, parents should know that toilet training is not possible until myelination of the spinal cord is complete. When this occurs, the child is able to walk well and sphincter control is developed. Voluntary sphincter control occurs between the ages of eighteen and twenty-four months. This physiologic development must be paralleled by some positive psychological factors as well. The child must be willing to hold on, as well as to let go, in an effort to please the parent figure rather than to achieve self-pleasure. The ability to recognize the urge to void is as important as the ability to communicate this urge to the parent. This recognition may be somewhat easier in bowel training than in bladder training as the urge is usually stronger and occurs more regularly for a bowel movement. These factors account for the child's ability to control bowel functions earlier than bladder functions.

The nurse may offer several suggestions to the parents regarding toilet training. First, the potty chair should be located in the bathroom and identified as belonging to the child. It should be a comfortable height for the child so that the feet are securely on the floor when the child is seated, Figure 14-6. Initially, the child should be encouraged to sit on the potty chair fully clothed. After the toddler demonstrates a willingness to sit on it fully clothed, he or she should then be encouraged to sit on it with diapers off in the conventional fashion. At this time, the child should be urged, but not ordered, to use the toilet appropriately. At some point after the child is comfortable with this routine, training pants may be substituted for the diapers, Figure 14-7. Parents should recognize the child's pride in the accom-

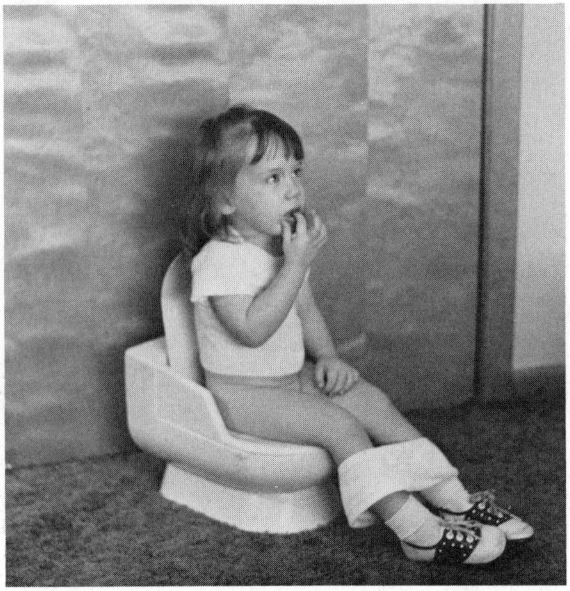

FIG. 14-6 During toilet training, the child should be taught to sit properly on the potty chair. The chair should be at a comfortable height for the child.

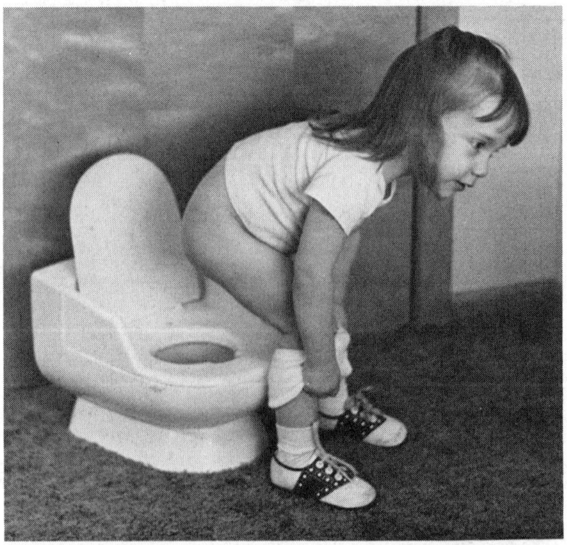

FIG. 14-7 The ease with which training pants may be removed facilitates the child's use of the potty chair.

plishment and should instill a feeling of self-confidence through praise. Accidents that occur after this period of training should be de-emphasized and positive behavioral patterns reinforced. Initially, many children are capable of staying dry during the daytime but not during periods of sleep. Control is seldom as good when the child is under stress from changes in the family or the environment as it is in normal situations. Parents should make allowances for the child during such times without decreasing the child's sense of confidence.

EMOTIONAL AND SOCIAL DEVELOPMENT

Toddlers have a very egocentric view of their environment. They see themselves as the center of the world. Indeed, they may be the center of a particular family, but the total family does not revolve around their thoughts and ideas. Toddlers have no concept of another individual's thoughts or ideas being different from their own.

This perception has an interesting effect on communications with toddlers. If they feel that everyone is thinking exactly as they are, they will not feel a need to verbalize their thoughts. For toddlers, the events that occur in a given household become intertwined with their thoughts, and they take both credit and blame for events over which they actually have no control.

Inanimate objects in the environment also take on inappropriate qualities in the child's mind. For example, chairs, tables, and pictures appear lifelike to toddlers and may be viewed as a source of problems. If, for instance, the toddler falls off a chair as a result of sitting too close to the edge, he or she is likely to blame the chair as the cause for tipping. Toddlers may also avoid certain rooms where the pictures are thought to be looking at them. This animism and magical thinking persist into the early preschool years.

Language Development

The use of recognizable words first occurs around one year of age, or at the beginning of the toddler period. At the onset of this stage, the child's vocabulary consists of about ten words. By the time the child is eighteen months of age, the child's vocabulary has increased to about fifty words. The rate of increase over the next six months is dramatic. The child achieves a vocabulary of about 200 words by the age of two years. Combining two words to make simple sentences may also be noted. Many of these words are the names of familiar objects or body parts, or have been used in simple commands to the child.

By the age of two and a half years, references to self are made with pronouns. Toddlers are usually able to repeat two or three numbers and to use prepositions. Their vocabulary has increased to around 450 words. By the age of three years, some of the toddler's experiences may be told to others, plural forms are evident in speech, and questions are asked. As understanding usually precedes verbal usage, the child's vocabulary may be quite extensive.

Language skills are dependent on the encouragement given to the child by the family group. Reading to the child, pointing out pictures, and listening to what the child says all contribute to communication skills. The toddler should be an active participant in the process of communication rather than a passive observer. Separation of the child from the home environment, such as occurs with hospitalization, may cause serious disruptions in the child's language development.

Development of skills in this area may be enhanced by parental awareness. Children mimic the speech patterns of the adults with whom they come in contact. For this reason, baby talk and nontraditional structure should be avoided. Talking with toddlers provides an opportunity for them to improve their language skills. Dialogues may be enhanced by questions and answers, as well as by simple games. Pretend games encourage not only speech but also the child's use of imagination.

Play Activities

Play is a normal part of the development of a child, whether in the home or in the hospital setting. For this reason, appropriate play activities should not be denied but should be encouraged and promoted. Play is called the work of the child. As such, it facilitates not only learning, but also coping mechanisms for the stresses and strains of one's world.

Moreover, play allows mastery of both gross and fine motor skills which further enhances physical development. Experimentation and resultant learning also take place through appropriate play activities. All feelings may be expressed in play activities without fear of repercussions from the adults in the environment. One only needs to spend a brief time in a playroom with a group of toddlers to see the gamut of feelings expressed through play activities. Language skills are also enhanced.

Play is divided into four distinct types, depending on the developmental age of the child. These include: solitary, parallel, cooperative, and team or group play. Solitary play may be observed in the infancy period as the infant touches and mouths a toy, oblivious to anyone in the immediate surroundings. By the age of two years, parallel play is observed. For example, toddlers often play at washing dishes alongside other toddlers of the same age doing the exact same thing. Generally, there is little or no interaction between these children except to defend either the possessions or the territory when necessary.

The child's progression to the preschool period heralds the onset of cooperative play. The child is able to participate in games with others, taking turns is accepted, and skills are better developed. The activities involved in group play allow children to act out what they are, as well as to fantasize about what they might like to be.

School-aged children are most often involved in team or group play activities. Normally, this is a period of extensive rule-learning, which is reflected in board games such as Monopoly and team sports such as soccer, baseball, and football. The focus on rules and playing fairly allows the child to function, yet encourages the control of socially unacceptable impulses. Play in this school-age period provides the groundwork for the self-restraint that is necessary in life. Later in life, these codes of conduct are internalized.

Behavioral Responses

A wide range of behavioral problems can occur during the toddler stage of development. Every child is unique, expressing individuality in their own ways. Both parents and nurses should recognize the basis for various behavioral patterns. This will allow them to deal with the child appropriately.

Temper Tantrums. Impulsive behavior, best illustrated by temper tantrums, is a function of the toddler's attempts to control the environment, and his or her resultant frustration when this control is thwarted by an adult for reasons of safety or other social considerations. The increased independence of toddlers is accompanied by the restriction of many activities. The toddler soon begins to test the limits of these restrictions.

Even though toddlers are advanced in terms of motor skills, their reasoning ability and communication skills are minimal. They wish to please their parents, but also wish to please themselves, Figure 14-8. Their behavior is often modeled after the behavior of others which receives approval. Consistent limit-setting on the part of the adults in the environment allows the child to internalize the appropriate social behaviors and to learn impulse control.

Inconsistency teaches the child that the parents are unreliable and that they do not mean what they say. This encourages the child to test the limits that have been set by the adult. Temper tantrums are an excellent controlling mechanism used by the toddler. They are generally used selectively, as the child quickly learns that tantrums are ignored in the home setting and are given undue attention in the supermarket or shopping mall when others are present. The child thus learns to use this method of control very selectively in the presence of a nonfamily audience.

Children learn self-control when their parents agree on specific restrictions and standards of behavior and enforce these consistently, regardless of the environment. This enforcement within a hospital setting may be difficult for the parents. Their concern over the child's illness or hospitalization and their own anxieties in the foreign environment of the hospital tend to foster permissiveness and inconsistency. The temper tantrum of a hospitalized child and the unexpected appeasement by the parent serves to heighten the child's feelings of insecurity. The nurse can help by encouraging the parents to ignore the child's behavior, by reducing the environmental stimuli, and by praising the child when he or she regains control.

Reduction of external stimuli can be achieved by closing the door to the child's

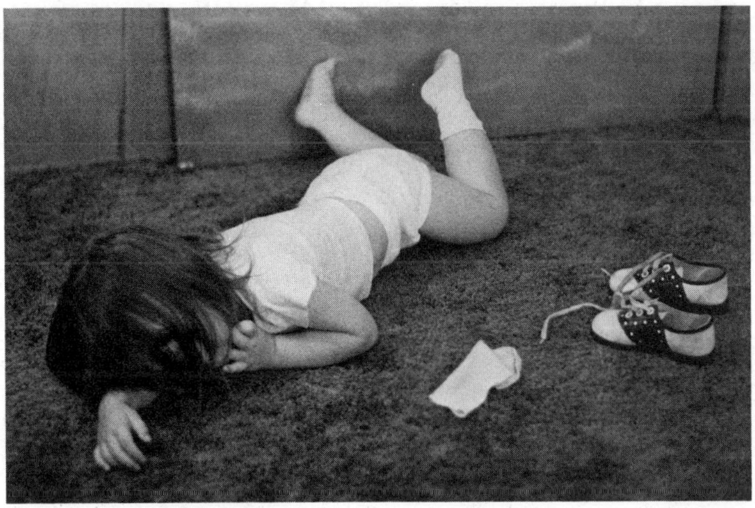

FIG. 14-8 Frustration can often evoke a tantrum. For this child, putting the fingers in the mouth provides some comfort.

room, turning off the television, and dimming the lights. If the child is in the playroom, he or she should be picked up unceremoniously and taken back to the room. Expressions of anger, raised voices, and threats only prolong the child's lack of control. Meeting the child's demands by providing the object desired does not usually help the situation, but only reinforces negative behavior.

Once the tantrum is over, the child should be reassured of the parents' love and concern. If the parents are not present, the nurse should provide the positive support. For those parents who are unable or unwilling to assume this role, the nurse may serve as a role model for the proper approach to the child.

Some preventive techniques may be used to neutralize the situation that might provoke a temper tantrum. Tantrums frequently occur when a child is overly tired, hungry, or forced to change an activity level abruptly. Periods of quiet play should follow active play to allow the child to wind down before naps and bedtime. Being rocked on mother's lap, listening to a story, or playing quietly in the bathtub are all effective means of changing the pace to make bedtimes more acceptable. Anticipating the stress of fatigue and hunger by removing the child gently from the environment or distracting him or her with another activity can also serve to defuse tantrums.

Ritualistic Behavior. Ritualistic behavior in toddlers is an attempt to control both their environment and their own behavior. The rituals are an exaggeration of normal concerns and the fear of possible harm. The enforcement of an exact routine makes life predictable and thus enhances the sense of security these children seek. By maintaining a routine, they also protect themselves from the unpredictable behavior that occurs when their impulses control the situation. The routine can thus prevent the punishment that follows the impulsive behavior.

Ritualism involves all the activities of daily living, but it is most obvious at mealtime and bedtime. At the family dinner table, the child will sit in exactly the same seat with the dishes and utensils arranged the identical way each time. At bedtime, the familiar snack is often followed by brushing one's teeth, being tucked into bed with the same toy or doll, and hearing a standard phrase, such as "Goodnight, Jimmy; see you in the morning," after the parent's hug and kiss.

In the hospital setting, the child's bedtime and mealtime rituals should be identified at the time of admission. It is important to the well-being of the child to maintain as many of these routines as possible. The presence of a parent in the hospital helps to preserve the child's rituals. In the parents' absence, the responsibility for maintaining these rituals is that of the nurse who is assigned to the child's care.

Negativism. Negativism in the hospital setting may, in part, be a response to the insecurity of abandoned rituals. It is another manifestation of the toddler's search for power and the ability to control others. As children progress through infancy assuming greater independence, parents set limitations and restrictions on their activities. Many of these restrictions are heralded by the word "no," used both as a warning and as a direction, Figure 14-9. Seldom is the child given a legitimate choice, and questions such as "would you like a cookie – yes?" are rarely so positively stated.

As toddlers begin to realize that their behavior and activities are controlled by the par-

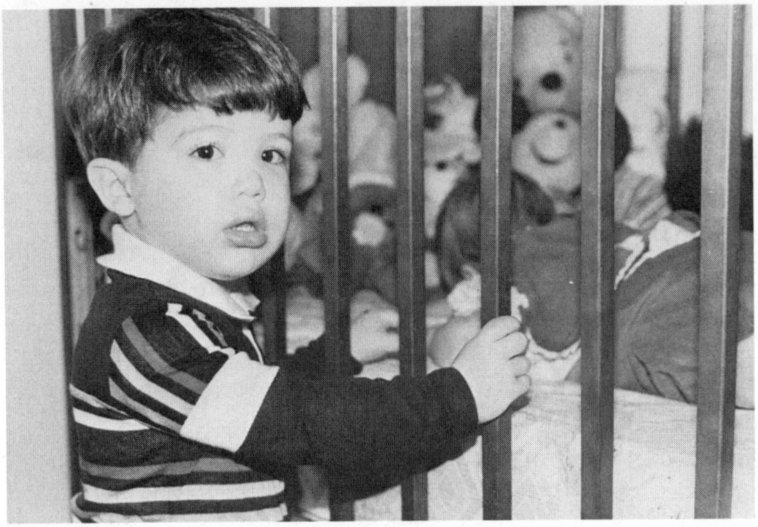

FIG. 14-9 Toddlers often test the limitations imposed on them, even if a "no" is expected. As this child reaches for his little sister, he turns to his parents to gauge their approval or disapproval.

ent through the use of the word "no," they begin to use the word with the parent in an attempt to exert their own control. The word itself has multiple meanings for children. They may or may not be recognized by the parent or the caregiver. The meanings range from "don't interrupt me" to an actual refusal to do something. Many times, the toddler will use the term "no" in response to a request by the parent, but a few seconds later will do just what was requested. It is simply one more way of asserting independence.

In the process of caring for the child, it is important to remember that the child should be given some legitimate choices. On a simple scale, this assists the child in making choices. It also gives the toddler a sense of control. The choices should be comparable and legitimate. There should be no effort to influence the child either way. For children in the hospital setting, choices in small matters permit them to cope with the many aspects of hospitalization over which they have no control, such as medications, meals, and diagnostic procedures.

Parents and nurses should remember that consistency is important in this aspect of limit-setting. What the child was not permitted to touch yesterday he or she should not be allowed to touch today. Allowing the child a brief period of transition from one activity to another tends to reduce the negativism that may arise when instant conformity is demanded from a toddler who is engrossed in his or her own thoughts and activities. Stubborn opposition to the toddler's defiance only aggravates the situation. The child may be helped to comply with a request by a gentle, tactful approach that avoids the negativism. Praising the child for cooperation, for instance, is a more positive approach than any discipline for negativism. Positive recognition of the child's efforts provides increased incentive to please the parent. Negativism is often very short-lived if it is accepted as just another step in the growth toward independence.

Separation Anxiety. Toddlers are still affected by separation anxiety, but to a lesser degree than are infants. As toddlers increase their independence, tolerating brief separations from their parents, they also learn that the parents do come back to them. Going to bed alone in a room each night reinforces this concept just as being left in the care of a grandmother or a babysitter does.

Toddlers are usually less fearful of strangers when their parents are present. Without the parents, toddlers' behavior may be passive, regressive, or may reflect the very real fear and anger that they feel. Brief separations do not cause any real harm to the child so long as the parents reinforce their love and concern for the child when they are together. Long-term hospitalizations, divorce, or the death of a parent are not as easily handled. Ideally, the toddler should be prepared for such events if they occur. In actuality, the remaining parent is often overprotective of the child because of his or her own anxiety.

In the hospital setting, the nurse should encourage the parents to be honest about their leave-taking. Nurses not only should support the child during this period, but if another member of the family is not available, they should also reinforce the fact that the parents will return. Encouraging the child to keep some visible reminder of the parent – a picture, handkerchief, or some other personal item – often helps this toddler to deal with the separation effectively. The love and concern of the parent for the child should be reinforced, both during the separation and upon the parents' return.

ACCULTURATION

The process of acculturation, or the acceptance of the values and standards of a given culture, begins in the toddler period. Children are not isolated from the particular culture but are molded into it from the very earliest age. Their behavior reflects the limits that are considered to be acceptable within that culture.

The influences of a culture include the elements of race, religion, national origin, and economic status, as well as the interaction and relationships within a given family group. These influences have a bearing on the child's responses to life situations. Some cultural influences are more easily identified than others, depending on the geographic and educational isolation of a particular group. Other cultures influencing a given family group may be a blend of more than one culture.

The practices and behavioral expectations of a cultural group are unique to that group. It is important for health care workers to recognize the living patterns and values of the family with whom they are working. Behavior that is acceptable in the child's culture may not be considered acceptable in the nurse's culture. This may lead to the display of judgmental attitudes or behavior by the nurse, which may affect the quality of health care delivered.

SUMMARY

The toddler period of growth is one in which the child's physical growth slows while the motor skills and language skills advance rapidly. Erikson calls it the stage of autonomy versus shame and doubt. Piaget describes this period of cognitive development in terms of object permanence and memory development. The special senses are developing during this period and dentition is completed. All activities of the child are influenced by the particular culture in which he or she grows up.

Problems may arise as a result of the toddler's increasing assertiveness. This assertiveness is reflected in negativism, ritualistic behavior, and temper tantrums. Separation anxiety, though not as strong as in infancy, is still in evidence. Toilet training and discipline may or may not present difficulties, depending on parental attitudes and the consistency of the guidelines imposed.

SUGGESTED ACTIVITIES

- Care for a toddler in the hospital setting. Assess the child's level of motor skills and development. Observe the child's interaction with the parent, noting particularly any examples of ritualism and negativism and how they are handled. Share your observations with your group.
- Observe play activities in the playroom of a hospital or day care center. Note the ages of the children involved and the various types of play in which they are engaged. Share with your group the types of play materials that are available and the skills that may be enhanced by each.

DISCUSSION TOPICS

1. Ask the mothers of three hospitalized toddlers to visit your group. Find out how they prepared their child for the hospitalization process. Ask them to share information about their child's response to the hospital environment, noting in particular any rituals that were maintained, any negativism that was displayed, and the manner in which they were able to cope with the child.
2. In your discussion group, identify play activities that could be used with a hospitalized toddler in a body cast, one in traction, and one who is ambulatory. Consider the activities that are appropriate for their age, as well as those that would allow them to express their feelings regarding the hospitalization.

REVIEW

A. Matching. Match the developmental task in Column I with the theorist in Column II.

Column I	Column II
b 1. Internalizing mental images	a. Erikson
b 2. Using symbolic play	b. Piaget
a 3. Tolerating separation from mother	
a 4. Attempting to control individuals in the environment	
b 5. Imitating the behavior of others	

B. Multiple Choice. Select the one best answer.

1. Toddlers usually establish ritualistic behavior patterns to
   a. manipulate or control adults and family members.
   b. establish learning patterns for future use.
   c. feel secure despite the changes and inconsistencies of their world.
   d. reestablish their sense of identity.
2. The earliest form of *peer* play activity is
   a. solitary play.
   b. parallel play.
   c. cooperative play.
   d. team play.
3. The motor development of a three-year-old child is sufficient to permit him to
   a. feed himself using a knife and a fork.
   b. spread butter and jam on his toast with a knife.
   c. pare an apple.
   d. pour milk into a glass.
4. By the age of eighteen months, language development usually includes
   a. a vocabulary of approximately fifty words.
   b. a vocabulary of one or two distinguishable words.
   c. a vocabulary of ten to twenty words.
   d. the ability to form a five-word sentence.

5. Which of the following best describes the toddler's probable behavior in play activities?
   a. Plays alongside, but not with, peers
   b. Usually prefers group play with other toddlers
   c. Enjoys playing hopscotch with an older child
   d. Chooses only a child of the same age and sex for a playmate

C. Short answer. Briefly respond to the following statements.

1. List three approaches that would facilitate the care of a hospitalized toddler.
2. List three ways in which dental health can be promoted in the toddler.

BIBLIOGRAPHY

Elkind, David, and Irving B. Weiner. *Development of the Child.* New York: John Wiley and Sons, Inc., 1978.

Hester, Nancy. "Discipline and the Nurse Clinician's Role." *Issues in Comprehensive Pediatric Nursing,* Vol. 1 (November–December, 1976), pp. 11–18.

Hilliard, Asa G. "Respecting the Child's Culture." *Children Today,* Vol. 8 (January–February, 1979), pp. 21–23.

Isler, Charlotte. "The Fine Art of Handling a Hospitalized Child." *RN,* Vol. 41 (March, 1978), pp. 41–45.

Johnson, Nancy. "Teaching Dental Health to Children." *Pediatric Nursing,* Vol. 4 (March–April, 1978), pp. 20–23.

Newman, Barbara M., and Philip R. Newman. *Infancy and Childhood: Development and Its Contexts.* New York: John Wiley and Sons, Inc., 1978.

Rainey, Susan K., and Edward R. Christophersen. "Behavioral Pediatrics: The Role of the Nurse Clinician." *Issues in Comprehensive Pediatric Nursing,* Vol. 1 (November–December, 1976), pp. 19–28.

Scipien, Gladys M., et al. *Comprehensive Pediatric Nursing.* New York: McGraw-Hill Book Company, 1979.

Slattery, Jill. "Dental Health in Children." *American Journal of Nursing,* Vol. 76 (July, 1976), pp. 1159–1161.

Stephens, K. S. "A Toddler's Separation Anxiety." *American Journal of Nursing,* Vol. 73 (September, 1973), pp. 1553–1555.

Chapter 15

Health Care Needs

OBJECTIVES

Upon completion of this chapter, the student will be able to

- describe the feeding methods for and the nutritional needs of this age-group.
- identify the routine immunizations that are administered during the toddler period.
- list several safety precautions for the prevention of accidents in the toddler stage.

The health care needs of the toddler include nutrition, safety, and on-going health supervision. As such, they are closely intertwined with the developmental level of the child. The nurse must be knowledgeable about the health care needs in order to provide anticipatory guidance to parents and caregivers. The problems encountered in these areas are preventable if the parents have been prepared to deal with them.

NUTRITION

The quality, quantity, and consistency of foods are important considerations when approaching any aspect of nutrition with a toddler. Although their growth rate has slowed considerably by this stage, toddlers undergo distinct changes in their activity levels. Their diet should provide the necessary nutrients for adequate growth and tissue repair and a sufficient amount of calories for their activity level, as well as pleasure and satisfaction from eating.

Recommended Dietary Allowances

Guidelines for evaluating the adequacy of the components of a given diet may be obtained from the Recommended Dietary Allowances (RDA) established by the Food and Nutrition Board of the National Academy of Sciences. These guidelines are averages based on large groups of people and the available scientific knowledge to date. These are the same guidelines that are used for evaluating the quality of nutritional assistance programs.

Most toddlers need about 1300 calories per day. The normal range for any given child is from 900 to 1600 calories per day based on the child's energy needs. An exact amount is difficult to determine as the physical activity levels of children vary widely. A relative state of healthiness, as well as steady increases in growth indicated by the height and weight grids, are the primary guidelines for judging dietary adequacy.

Caloric intake is divided into protein, fat, and carbohydrate intake according to percentages. The proportion should be approximately fifty to sixty percent carbohydrates, twenty-five to thirty-five percent fats and ten to fifteen percent (or the remainder) proteins. Protein intake, which is so necessary in this age-group, must meet growth as well as maintenance needs in a form that contains all of the essential amino acids. The established requirement is 1.8 grams of protein per kilogram of body weight. The ratio of calories to proteins is then 55 to 1, Figure 15-1.

The type of protein available to the child should be of high quality. Milk, meat, and eggs are the major sources of protein in a child's diet. Other sources that provide smaller amounts of protein include breads, cereals, fruits, and vegetables. Emphasis should be placed on the quality of the protein source rather than on the quantity of protein foods the child consumes.

Vitamin and Mineral Supplements

Water-soluble vitamins B and C are essential parts of the toddler's diet. An adequate diet provides the toddler with 45 milligrams (mg) of vitamin C per day. This amount represents an increase over previously established levels as a result of new information. Requirements for the various B vitamins remain the same. See Appendix I for additional information.

The requirements for the fat-soluble vitamins has not changed. However, the labeling of some of the requirements has been altered. Vitamin A is now expressed in micrograms (μg)

Calorie Range for Toddlers:	900 to 1600 calories per day
Protein Requirements for Toddlers:	1.8 Gm per kg of body weight
Ratio of Calories to Proteins:	55:1

Case Example: Eddie is 2 1/2 years of age. He weighs 33 pounds. His protein and calorie needs may be calculated as follows:

33 lb ÷ 2.2	= 15 kg of weight
15 kg X 1.8 Gm of protein	= 27 Gm of protein
27 Gm X 55 calories	= 1485 calories per day

FIG. 15-1 Calculation of protein requirements and total caloric intake for toddlers

VITAMINS	
Fat-Soluble	
A	400 μg retinol equivalents
D	10 μg cholecalciferol
E	5 μg alpha-tocopherol
Water-Soluble	
C	45 mg
Thiamine	0.7 mg
Riboflavin	0.8 mg
Niacin	9.0 mg
B_6	0.9 mg
Folacin	100 μg
B_{12}	2.0 μg
MINERALS	
Calcium	800 mg
Phosphorus	800 mg
Magnesium	150 mg
Iron	15 mg
Zinc	10 mg
Iodine	70 μg

FIG. 15-2 Vitamin and mineral needs of the toddler

of retinol equivalents (RE) rather than in international units. Vitamin D is expressed as micrograms of cholecalciferol. Ten micrograms are the equivalent of 400 IU of Vitamin D. Vitamin E is now expressed as micrograms of alpha-tocopherol, Figure 15-2.

Iron must often be supplemented in a toddler's diet to maintain adequate levels. Iron itself, depending on the type, has a variable absorption rate. Absorption is dependent on the amount of ascorbic acid and meat ingested at the same time. The food choices for a given meal may thus significantly affect the amount of usable iron available. Large amounts of milk and dairy products decrease the absorption rate of iron when ingested at the same time.

The use of a vitamin or mineral supplement in toddlers should be based on the adequacy of the diet itself. If the child is ill and needs the additional supplement, or if the diet is inadequate, a supplement should be used. These supplements should never take the place of the food products themselves. Constipation may be a side effect of the supplements that contain iron.

Eating Patterns

The eating habits of individuals are established over a lifetime, beginning in infancy. Food requirements for toddlers are much less than those for older children. The best approximation is to give the toddler one tablespoon of each type of food served at a given meal for each year of the child's age. Hence, a two-year-old child would be given two tablespoons each of meat, potatoes, and vegetables.

The choice of foods for the child depends on the family menu. However, some guidelines are appropriate. Children of this age like to be able to recognize particular foods and thus prefer simple foods without gravies or cream sauces. Finger foods are well-liked and may be handled easily by the child. Raw vegetables cut in bite-sized pieces are generally better accepted than are cooked vegetables. Because of their pleasant taste, both fresh and dried fruits are usually well-liked.

Meats are usually the least liked by the toddler. This is because of the effort required to chew the food. Ground meat is better accepted and may be prepared in a number of ways for variety. Tender meats should be cut in small pieces and consumed as finger foods. Other sources of quality protein include eggs, cheese, fish, and peanut butter.

Highly seasoned foods are usually disliked by toddlers. Their taste buds may be more sensitive than those of an adult, and they react to the strength of the flavors. Limiting spices, particularly salt, may improve the child's acceptance of the food.

Food preferences are realistic expressions of the child's likes and dislikes. They should be accepted by the parents as a normal part of the development of eating patterns. They are not a deliberate attempt to be negative unless mealtimes have already taken on the character of a battleground between parent and child. Disliked foods or refusals to eat certain foods should be ignored whenever possible. The child will not starve because one meal is omitted. Children who have a marked preference for a given food should be offered that food every day at every meal as long as other foods are not excluded. The novelty soon fades and the reappearance of the same item at every meal soon loses its appeal for the toddler.

Most children prefer to eat more often than the standard meal pattern of three meals per day. Nutritional snacks between meals may be offered. Snacks that are high in protein such as cheese, yogurt, peanut butter, and hard-boiled eggs, are good choices. Fresh fruit and juices are also appropriate. Snacks such as potato chips, candy, sodas, and doughnuts should be avoided because of their high carbohydrate content, their tendency to cause tooth decay, and their low nutrient value.

Ideally, mealtimes should be pleasant interludes in the toddler's day. Behavior of the child should not be an issue. Parents should understand that some children are dawdlers, whereas others are rapid eaters. The youngest child is often expected to behave beyond his or her developmental level. Spilled milk or dropped utensils should not be treated as major disasters. Allowing overly active children to leave the table for a few minutes between the main course and dessert may help them to settle down enough to finish the remainder of the meal.

A child's interest in foods may be encouraged in a number of ways. Creating visual appeal by serving colorful foods and using attractive serving pieces may be helpful. Providing children with their own plate and cup decorated with a nursery rhyme figure may be all that is needed. Allowing toddlers to help select items from the supermarket also stimulates interest in the meal. The child may then help to prepare the item for the meal. For instance, the child may toss the salad with a parent's help, or decide where a certain dish is placed on the table.

Eating Patterns During Illness

Children who are ill may use food to convey their feelings about all that is happening to them. Their appetite may not be at its usual level, and the foods offered may not be those they prefer. Short periods of inadequate intake do not present major problems. However, children who have a prolonged illness or those who are acutely ill for a long period are at great risk for nutritional deficiencies.

Ill children should be encouraged to eat whatever they are able to at regular mealtimes. Toddlers may or may not allow the parent or another adult to feed them. Their wishes should be respected. If they do not eat particular items, substitutes should be offered to compensate for the nutritional difference. For instance, breakfast of bacon, eggs, toast, and juice may not be appealing to the child initially, but a sandwich made of bacon, eggs, and toast may be more acceptable. Substitution of eggnog for the juice may also meet with greater acceptance.

Small feedings of easily tolerated foods are easiest for sick children to accept. They should be encouraged to eat when they feel like eating, particularly if nausea is a problem. Liquid nutritional supplements may be offered to children who are unable to consume an adequate amount of food because of their illness.

In the hospital setting, children may refuse to eat because they are angry with their parents for their hospitalization. Food may also be used in an attempt to control the parents or to reassert control within the hospital setting where the child has little control. Children also frequently experience a degree of disappointment and anger at themselves. They often believe that they are the cause of the hospitalization. Regression in eating habits may also be evident during hospitalization.

Need for Nutritional Assistance

Many young children who enter the health care system for routine care need nutritional assistance. This may involve assessment and counseling, or actual assistance through any of the various programs available to families. Children who should receive such assistance include those who are extremely underweight or overweight. Toddlers with acute or chronic illnesses that directly interfere with nutritional intake should routinely be given nutritional assistance. Other children may require assistance because of socioeconomic factors that interfere with good nutrition and present health problems only after long-term deprivation.

This latter group may need financial assistance through various programs, as well as education and advice regarding the wise use and choice of foods. Stretching a fixed income over the costs of housing, utilities, and other living costs frequently leaves little for food purchases. What money is available should be used with discretion to maintain the family group in an optimal nutritional state.

When identifying families with problems, the physical setting of the home must be considered. It is important to know the facilities that are available for food preparation, the ease of access to a safe water supply, the presence or absence of refrigeration, and the proximity of stores or food markets in the area.

Cultural values and behavior influence both the acceptance and the preparation of many food substances. They also influence the feeding patterns of the young child. Culture also influences the family's acceptance of assistance in the form of food stamps or other types of local, state, and federal assistance.

Programs that are available to help these families include the food stamp program; the Women, Infants, and Children Supplemental Feeding Program (WIC Program); the National School Lunch Program; the National School Breakfast Program (available in some areas); and the milk and snack programs available through Head Start, day care centers, and some schools on a year-round basis.

The food stamp program provides free or reduced-price stamps to families who qualify for various types of welfare assistance. The intent is to stretch the food dollar for those who need aid. Only food items may be purchased with the stamps. Qualification of individual families is based on an assessment of actual assets, as well as of their necessary expenditures for housing, utilities, and medical care.

The WIC Program, in contrast, provides direct aid in the form of food packages that are available to pregnant women and to preschool children five years of age or younger. Qualification is based on the need for free or reduced-cost health care, as well as nutritional needs. This program operates through the local health clinics in economically deprived areas.

The National School Lunch Program provides free or reduced-cost lunches to families meeting certain income guidelines. Type-A School Lunch programs provide one-third of the child's nutritional needs. They do not in any way assist other family members, but they are designed to help meet the nutritional needs of school-aged children.

Other programs that provide breakfast, milk, and snacks are not available in every location. In the areas in which they do operate, though, they effectively supplement the limited diet of a given family. Nurses should be aware of the nutritional programs that are available for children in the area so that they can make appropriate referrals either to an agency or, in the hospital setting, to the social service staff.

The greatest problem with nutritional assistance is that many families do not recognize the need for help. Many consider their primary problem to be economic. They often rate nutrition and health care as low-priority needs, provided acute illness is not a factor. If the child does become ill and the problem is related to poor nutrition, then the focus may change and nutrition may come to be viewed as the ultimate cure-all. Advertising in the media, unfortunately, often presents this same image.

SAFETY NEEDS

Accident prevention is an important aspect of the care of toddlers. The full impact of accidents may not be realized until one recognizes that accidents are the major causes of death in children ages one to fifteen years. In recent studies, the rate of accidents requiring emergency room visits for children between the ages of one and five years was 48.1 per 1000. These statistics do not include automobile accidents or accidents involving animals. More than two-thirds of these injuries occurred within the child's home.

Children of this age-group are at great risk for accidents. They are busy exploring the environment, using all their senses. Their inquisitive natures and lack of judgment combine to create a potentially dangerous situation. An absolute necessity for intervention is the presence of at least one caring adult or responsible older sibling who can anticipate the child's explorations or intervene effectively at the time of the potential incident. Young children must be protected from such situations as they lack the judgment necessary to avoid accidents. Older children can be educated to avoid dangerous situations. Consistent discipline on the part of the parents also reinforces what situations the child must avoid. Ongoing safety education of the child is a responsibility of the parent.

Safety in the Home

Toxic Substances. Poisoning from ingestion of toxic substances ranks high on the list of accidents that take place within the home. Children of the toddler age-group continue to explore the environment using their mouths. Through trial and error, a container may be opened, a drawer emptied of pills, or a plant divested of its leaves. The toddler's ability to climb also is a factor in these explorations, Figure 15-3. The medications that were secure in the top cupboard during the infancy period are no longer safe with a toddler in the area.

Nurses should teach parents or responsible individuals in the family to keep all toxic substances, whether drugs or chemicals, in locked cupboards. All medications should be

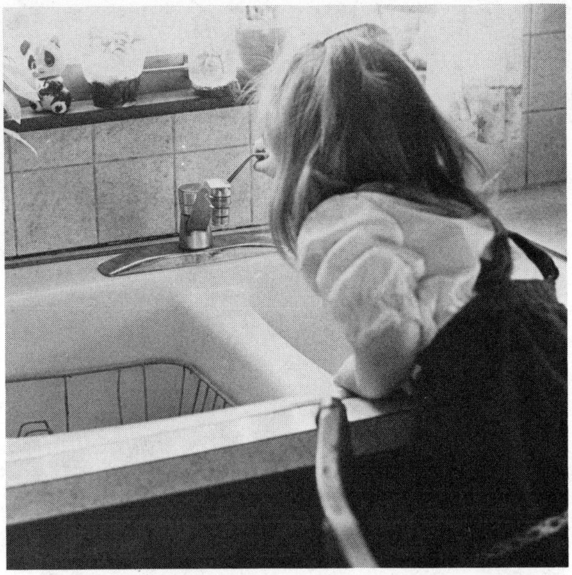

FIG. 15-3 Toddlers often climb to reach forbidden articles. The child who can reach the faucet may also be able to reach the plants on the windowsill, and some houseplants are poisonous.

treated as such and should never be referred to as candy. Child-proof lids on containers should be replaced securely. All toxic substances should be kept in the original container. Containers for corrosive substances should be rinsed thoroughly before being discarded.

Aspiration. Aspiration of foreign substances and food items is another hazard for children in this age-group. Toddlers may be able to chew well, but they may still have problems with hard objects, such as candy, or large chunks of meat. Inedible objects, such as marbles, coins, small parts of toys, and other substances are often put in the mouth. Any of these objects may be aspirated, causing partial or complete airway obstruction.

An initial attempt should be made to remove the foreign body from the child's mouth without forcing it deeper into the airway. If this is unsuccessful, the Heimlich maneuver is often effective in dislodging such objects. The victim is grasped from behind with the rescuer's hands clenched together over the lower chest. The chest is then compressed with a quick, upward thrust. This maneuver may need to be repeated to dislodge the item. The amount of compression used will also depend on the size of the child. Abdominal compression may cause laceration of the liver. Objects that are deep within the respiratory tract may have to be removed through bronchoscopy. **Caution: Children should never be slapped on the back while in an upright position as this will lodge the object even deeper in the airway.**

Falls. Falls are a frequent hazard for the young explorer in the home setting. Prevention of falls may involve the use of gates to block the child's use of the stairway except when supervised. Screens and windows should be secured with a lock. Doors that allow access to outside porches or other areas should also be secured with a child-proof lock.

Burns. Burns are another major hazard to toddlers. A variety of sources for burns exist within the home. Certainly, the kitchen is the area in the home with the greatest potential for danger. For instance, scalds may occur when a child pulls the cord of an electric coffeepot, causing the contents to spill over him. Additionally, the handles of pots and pans located on the stove may be an open invitation for the young child who is trying to imitate the cooking activities of the parents, Figure 15-4. Moreover, burner controls that are located on the front of the range may be easy to reach and turn, posing the additional risk of igniting the child's clothing as well as burning

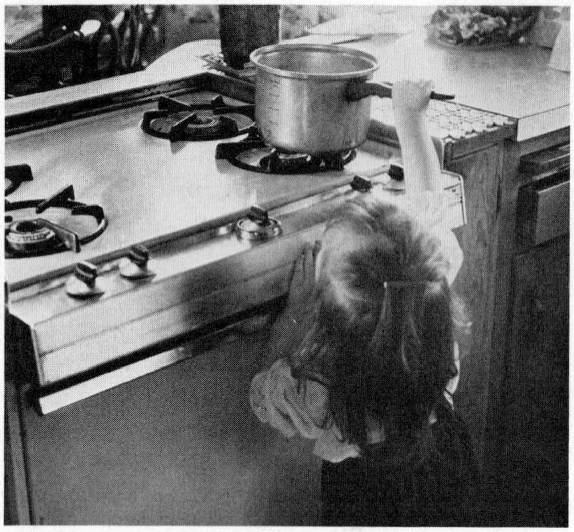

FIG. 15-4 The incorrect placement of a pot handle can cause a disaster.

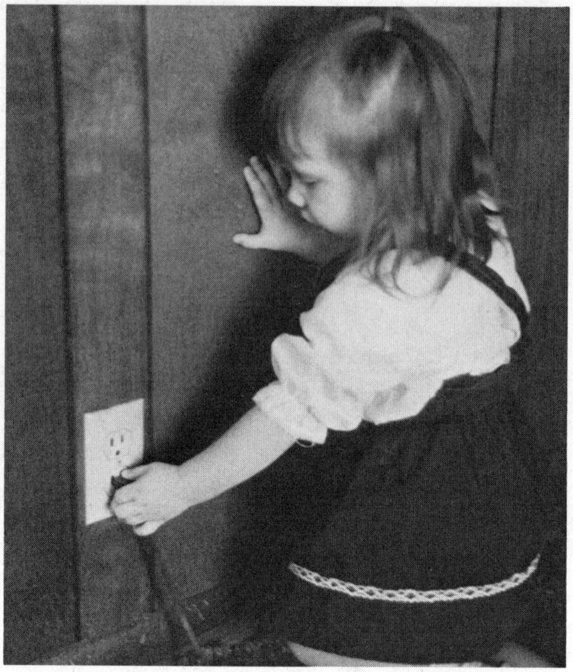

FIG. 15-5 This child should not have been permitted to touch the electrical cord. Moreover, the upper outlet should have a protective cap on it.

the hands. To eliminate such hazards, pots should be placed on back burners with their handles out of reach, electrical cords should be kept out of the child's reach, and the child should be supervised carefully when in the kitchen.

Other hazards that can cause burns include electrical outlets. In the course of their explorations, toddlers may be tempted to insert a metal object, such as a key, nail file, or hair clip, into an unguarded outlet, causing injury. Younger toddlers may bite or chew electrical cords, thereby risking severe injury as the moisture in the mouth serves as a good conductor of electricity. These hazards may be avoided by placing heavy furniture in front of outlets, or by placing a protective plug into unused outlets, Figure 15-5.

Another common type of thermal injury in this age-group is caused by scalds from overly hot water in a bathtub. Children can fall into the tub, turn the hot water on themselves, or in the case of abuse, may deliberately be placed in the tub. The temperature of the water must always be checked before placing the child in the tub. The child should never be permitted to manipulate the faucets in the tub. Lowering the temperature of the hot water tank to 120° may also be effective. Scalds can still occur at this temperature, but a longer period of exposure is necessary for this to occur. Children must be carefully supervised while bathing, Figure 15-6.

Burn injuries can also result from contact with fireplaces, radiators, or small objects, such as candles and cigarettes. A guard can be placed in front of fireplaces and radiators to minimize the potential risk to the child. The open flame of a candle should be well out of a

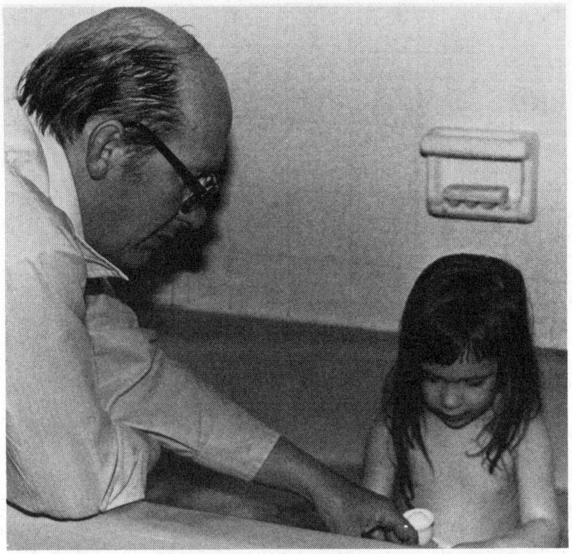

FIG. 15-6 Parents must be vigilant to protect children from burns or falls while bathing.

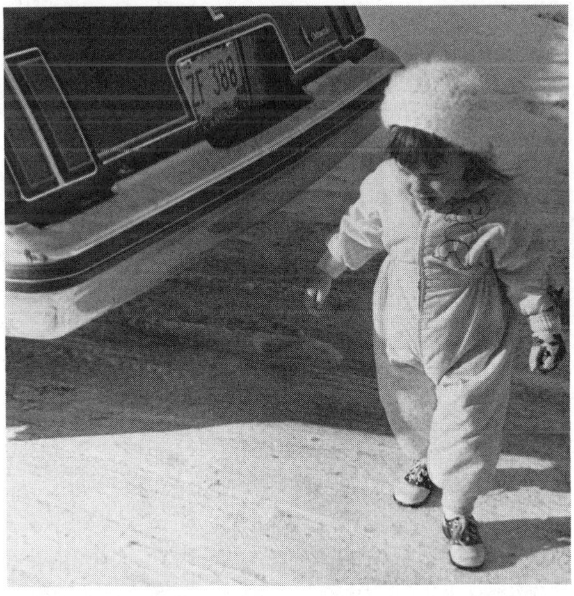

FIG. 15-7 Because of their height, toddlers may easily be obscured from the driver's view.

child's reach and away from any combustible items for the protection of everyone in the home. Cigarettes should not be left burning in ashtrays where a young child might have access to them. A young child held in the arms of a person who is smoking can be burned accidentally or exposed to toxic inhalants.

Other Trauma. Other objects in the environment may also cause trauma in toddlers. Sharp objects, such as knives and scissors, are inappropriate items for toddlers to play with and should be kept out of their reach. Eventually, as children grow older, they may be taught both how to use these devices and how to carry them with the point directed downward. Pencils and lollipop sticks can also cause serious injuries. The child should be seated when eating a lollipop or making a drawing. Allowing a child to walk or run with these objects increases the possibility of a fall, which could result in perforation of the inside of the mouth or of other areas of the body.

Safety Outside the Home

Deaths from motor vehicles outrank all other types of accidental injuries in this age-group. Injuries may be sustained either as a passenger or as a pedestrian. The toddler's motor skills permit walking, running, and climbing. Seldom does the child make a distinction between the yard and the street if chasing a ball or riding a tricycle. In addition, leaves or snow may further obscure the boundaries of the yard and street. The toddler's small size is also a disadvantage, as he or she may not be visible to a driver who is backing a car out of a driveway, Figure 15-7.

As a passenger, the child may be a victim of an accident, as well as the cause of it. Any child who is unrestrained and thus able to move about freely inside the car may be a source of distraction to the adult driver. Even a momentary lapse of the driver's attention to the road may be sufficient to cause an accident. Moreover, in the event that the driver anticipates an accident situation, the unrestrained child may not be able to be adequately shielded or held secure. If an accident does occur, or if the brakes must be applied sharply, the body of the unrestrained child may become a projectile that may be pitched toward the windshield or another hazardous part of the car's interior.

Car Restraints. Infants and toddlers who weigh less than 40 pounds should be restrained in a properly tested seat equipped with a safety harness or a protective shield to anchor them. In the event of an accident, seats equipped with harnesses allow the crushing impact of an accident to be distributed over a large body area. Infant car seats should face the rear of the car. All seats should be anchored properly according to the manufacturer's directions. Children weighing more than 40 pounds can be secured using a safety harness that crosses both shoulders and passes through the crotch. This restraint device has an anchoring strap that must be applied securely. The child, in an appropriate restraint device, should be placed in the rear seat of the auto whenever possible.

Parents may demonstrate real concern over the health of their children, yet fail to secure them in the car when transporting them. Parents may not realize how vulnerable the child actually is in an accident situation. Emphasis in teaching should be placed on prevention. Since this child is likely to imitate adult behavior, the example the parents set is also important.

Two groups that provide up-to-date information on car safety are the Physicians for Automotive Safety (PAS) in New Jersey and Action for Child Transportation Safety (ACTS). The transportation group is an affiliated group composed of citizens.

Safety in the Hospital

The need for safety in the hospital setting cannot be underestimated. Toddlers require close supervision and protection. In some situations, restraints may be necessary for the child's safety. Their use should be as limited as possible.

Restraints should never be used as a substitute for the presence of a parent or a caring member of the staff. Moreover, they should never be used for punishment, and should be applied so that no physical injury to the child can occur. The child's position should be changed frequently and the restraints removed periodically. The rationale for the use of any restraint should be explained carefully to the parents.

Restraints that can be applied directly to children include safety belts and jacket, and elbow, wrist, and ankle restraints.

Jacket restraints may be used to keep a child flat in bed, to maintain a sitting position, or to keep the child in a wheelchair. Elbow, wrist, and ankle restraints are rigid devices that do not permit the child to bend the joint. They are commonly used after certain surgical procedures.

An additional type of restraint may also be used for toddlers. This type is a net that is applied to the crib to prevent the child from

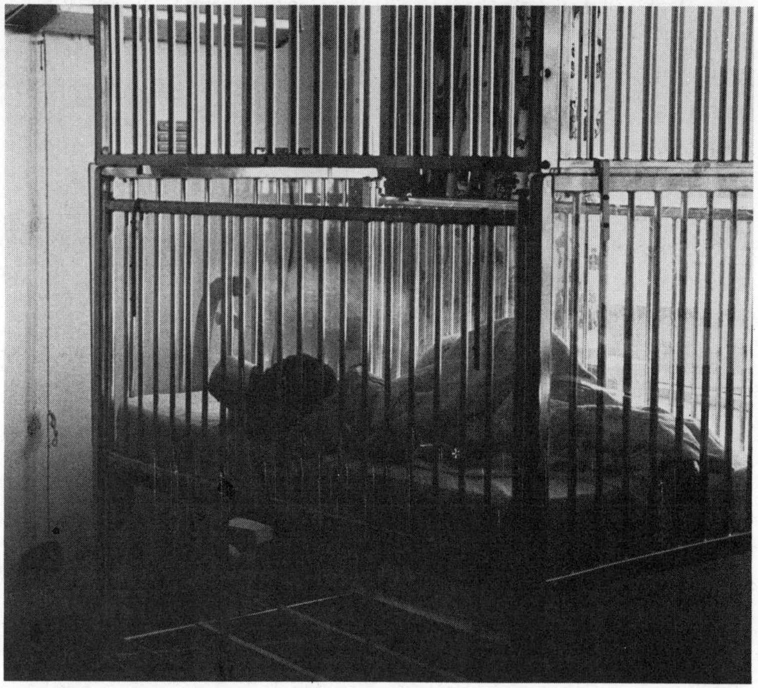

FIG. 15-8 The crib cage allows the child free movement within the crib, as well as ample headroom.

climbing over the siderails or becoming injured in a fall. The net is fastened to the bed frame inside the lower portion of the siderails so that the child can be removed rapidly from the crib in case of an emergency. Alternatively, an acrylic bubble top for the crib may also be used for this purpose. In some hospitals, both the nets and the bubble tops are being replaced by cage cribs that are large enough to allow the child to ambulate easily and safely, Figure 15-8.

GENERAL HEALTH CARE PRACTICES

Routine health care and supervision is important at every age. During the toddler period, the child should be in the care of a physician or a participant in a well-child clinic. Care focuses on the assessment of normal development, the identification of real or potential problems, and the provision of counseling or anticipatory guidance for the parents.

Assessment of the toddler's development, as compared to the established norms for age, is carried out through the use of standardized testing. The most commonly used test is the Denver Developmental Screening Test (DDST). It provides information on the child's personal-social skills, language level, and fine and gross motor abilities.

Parental counseling regarding the physical care of the toddler involves the provision of information about nutrition, dental care, toilet training, and accident prevention. As the child approaches the preschool years, the focus of the counseling may shift to problems with sleep and contacts with other children, either through neighbors or a preschool group.

Immunizations that should be given during the toddler period include those for measles, mumps, and rubella. These are usually administered as a combined vaccine at fifteen months of age. Immunizations are not given earlier because of the possibility of maternal antibodies remaining in the child's circulation, the presence of which would reduce the effectiveness of the immunization. Effectiveness approaches ninety-five percent if this time framework is followed. At eighteen months of age, the child is given a booster vaccination for DPT and TOPV.

Diagnostic testing, which may also be a part of the routine screening, includes a determination of hemoglobin and hematocrit levels and a urinalysis. Testing for abnormal lead absorption may also be done in those children considered to be at risk for lead poisoning.

SUMMARY

The health needs of the toddler comprise two major areas of concern: nutrition and accident prevention. The period is marked by a transition from the total dependency of infancy to the independence and increased skill level of the three-year-old child.

The toddler requires careful nourishment to meet growth needs adequately, as well as to provide sufficient calories to compensate for energy expenditures. Accident prevention is crucial to the survival of toddlers as they lack the judgment necessary to avoid hazardous situations.

Routine health care of the toddler includes developmental screening, as well as anticipatory guidance for the parent. During this period, the initial immunization program is usually completed. Dental care is also initiated in this age-group.

SUGGESTED ACTIVITIES

- Observe toddlers during mealtime in the pediatric unit. What types of foods are most commonly accepted? How is the child encouraged to eat? What substitutions are made for the child who refuses the food?
- Investigate the types of car seats that are available in local stores. What limitations or restrictions are identified by the manufacturer for the various types? What is the cost of purchase?

DISCUSSION TOPICS

1. Arrange for a pediatric nurse practitioner from the local health department's well-child clinic to explain the program to your class. Discuss the availability of nutritional assistance programs in the area. Inquire about safety education programs for the parents of young children.
2. Discuss the kinds of nutritional snacks that might be prepared for a toddler who is ill but who has no dietary restrictions. Determine the relative protein, carbohydrate and fat content of these snacks.
3. Work with other class members to develop a teaching plan for informing parents about the safety needs of the toddler. Use a checklist format so that each item may be identified when it is discussed with the parent.

REVIEW

A. Matching. Match the provision in Column I with the program in Column II.

Column I	Column II
1. Provides milk and nutritional snacks to children enrolled in Head Start programs	a. Welfare Food Stamp Program
2. Provides one-third of a school-aged child's nutritional needs	b. WIC Program
3. Provides food packages to pregnant women and to children who are five years of age or younger	c. School Lunch Program
4. Offers reduced-price stamps that may only be used to purchase food	d. Breakfast, milk, and snack programs

B. Multiple choice. Select the one best answer.

1. Jimmy is a two-year-old child who weighs 28 pounds. An average amount of calories for him to consume each day would be
   a. 800. c. 2000.
   b. 1300. d. 2500.
2. The daily protein requirement for Jimmy would be
   a. 1.0 gram per kilogram of body weight.
   b. 1.5 grams per kilogram of body weight.
   c. 1.8 grams per kilogram of body weight.
   d. 2.2 grams per kilogram of body weight.
3. Iron may have to be supplemented in Jimmy's diet because
   a. it has a variable absorption rate, depending on the foods that are consumed at the same time.
   b. he may not like the taste of iron and may refuse it.
   c. he, like other children his age, seldom consumes an adequate amount of iron in his diet.
   d. the liver is unable to store iron at his age.
4. A guideline for the amount of food that should be offered to Jimmy at one meal is
   a. one-half cup each of meat, potatoes, and vegetables.
   b. one cup of meat and one-half cup each of potatoes and vegetables.
   c. one teaspoon of each food item per year of age.
   d. one tablespoon of each food item per year of age.
5. Jimmy's immunizations for measles, mumps, and rubella were completed at fifteen months of age. The reason they were not given earlier is that
   a. Jimmy may have had an allergic reaction to the vaccine.
   b. circulating maternal antibodies can neutralize the effect of the vaccine.
   c. children do not form antibodies to these substances until they reach the toddler period.
   d. immunizations do not have to be completed until the child is ready to enter school.

C. Short answer. Briefly respond to the following statements.

1. List three safety precautions that should be implemented in the kitchen when a toddler is part of the family group.
2. Describe the rationale for keeping toddlers in a safety harness or a child-safe car seat.
3. List two approaches that may be used to encourage the hospitalized child to eat.

BIBLIOGRAPHY

Chow, Marilyn P. *Handbook of Pediatric Primary Care.* New York: John Wiley and Sons, Inc., 1979.

Cooney, C. Ernest, and Susan Kummerow. "Childsafe: When Children Travel by Car." *Children Today,* Vol. 6 (July–August, 1977), pp. 11–15.

Davis, Rene Clark. "Prevention of Childhood Accidents Through Safety Education." *Issues in Comprehensive Pediatric Nursing,* Vol. 1 (May, 1977), pp. 57–72.

Dwyer, Johanna T. "Family Nutrition and the Health Care Team." *Issues in Comprehensive Pediatric Nursing,* Vol. 1 (April, 1977), pp. 1–22.

Krause, Marie V., and L. Kathleen Mahan. *Food, Nutrition, and Diet Therapy.* Philadelphia: W. B. Saunders Company, 1979.

National Dairy Council. "Recommended Dietary Allowances (Revised 1980)." *Dairy Council Digest,* Vol. 51 (March–April, 1980), pp. 7–12.

Suitor, Carol W., and Merrily F. Hunter. *Nutrition: Principles and Application in Health Promotion.* Philadelphia: J. B. Lippincott Company, 1980.

Wills, Betty B. "Food Becomes Fun for Children." *American Journal of Nursing,* Vol. 78 (December, 1978), pp. 2082–2085.

Chapter 16

Accidents and Poisoning

OBJECTIVES

Upon completion of this chapter, the student will be able to

- describe the type of accidents that are likely to occur in this age-group.
- list several aspects of parental education that aid in accident prevention.
- identify four nursing measures that are used in caring for a child with burns.

Problems with safety and the resulting accidents can occur in any age-group. However, toddlers are at greater risk of involvement than other age-groups. Their interest in exploring and their newfound mobility contribute immensely to this problem. Anticipation of their curiosity and setting of limits in the environment help to reduce the potential for accidents. However, this in itself may not be enough; both parents and nurses may find themselves in the midst of an accident situation.

BURNS

Pediatric burn centers have established that the mean age of children with burns from hot liquids is four years of age. The mean age for burns from flames is eight years. Burns occur at a rate of one for every four to five minutes. They usually occur in the home and in the younger age-groups, and their incidence is directly related to the adequacy or inadequacy of adult supervision.

Classification of Burns

Burns in both children and adults are classified in a number of ways. They may be classified according to the cause, the extent of the burn injury, or the depth.

Cause. Burns may be the result of thermal, chemical, electrical, or irradiation exposure. Thermal burns from flames, hot liquids, steam, or grease are the most common types seen in pediatric patients.

Extent. The extent of the burn refers to the amount of the total body surface area involved. In assessing the extent of a burned area in children, it is important to remember that this varies dramatically with the age-group of the child. The greatest differences are seen in the percentages for the head, the thigh, and the leg from infancy through adolescence, Figure 16-1. The Rule of Nines, commonly applied to burns in the adult population, is not applicable to children.

Depth. The depth of the burn is classified according to degrees or thickness. When differentiating according to degrees, first-, second-, and third-degree designations are used. First-degree burns refer to burns that involve only the epidermis which is reddened, has no blisters or edema, and will blanch in response to pressure. Second-degree burns are those which involve the dermal layer, which appears to be wet and has thick-walled blisters. Third-degree burns involve the dermal layer, the subcutaneous tissue, and underlying structures, such as muscle and bone. These burns produce a dry, charred, or opaque-white appearance, markedly reduced pain sensitivity, few, if any, blisters, and no blanching response to pressure.

When burns are classified according to thickness, it is best to describe the patient's responses to sensation, the configuration of the blisters, and the color and texture of the skin. In partial-thickness burns, sensation is normal with increased sensitivity to pain and temperature. In contrast, full-thickness burns cause anesthesia as a result of the destruction of nerve endings. The blisters formed as a result of partial-thickness burns are large and thick-walled, and increase in size. Few blisters, if any, are formed in full-thickness burns. Those few that do form are thin-walled, break easily, and do not change in size. The skin color associated with a partial-thickness burn is

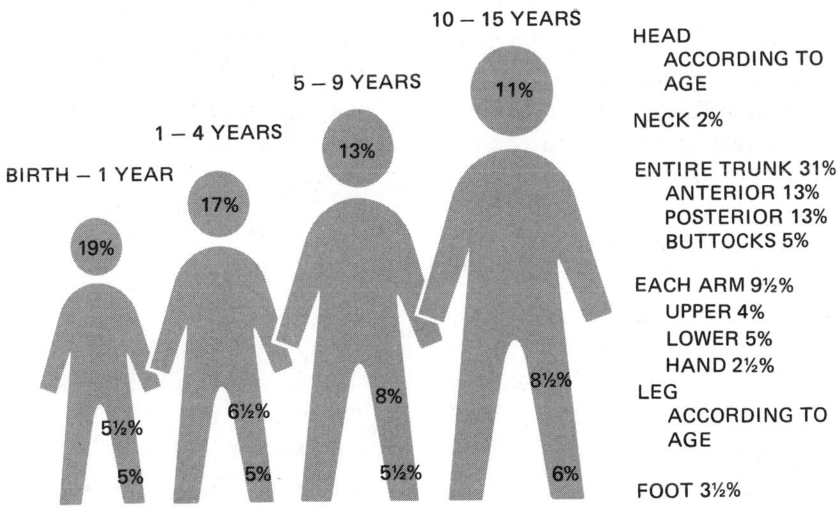

red, with blanching and refilling clearly evident. Conversely, the skin is white, brown, or black in full-thickness burns, and blanching is absent. Skin that is normal or slightly firm in texture is typical of partial-thickness burns, whereas a firm or leatherlike skin texture is indicative of full-thickness burns.

Assessment of Burn Injuries

An assessment of the burned area is done by the physician and the nurse upon admission of the child. This information is marked on a body figure outline. A reassessment is done twenty-four hours later. The outline chart should be revamped at that time. The extent of the total burn injury may not be immediately apparent. The criteria for hospitalization of a burned child may vary slightly, depending on whether admission to a local hospital or to a central burn unit is being considered. Children younger than four years of age; those with burns involving greater than ten percent of the total body surface area; those with burns of the face, hands, or perineum; and those with other illnesses or health problems are generally admitted for in-hospital treatment. Transfer to a regional burn center is dependent on the availability of local treatment facilities; the extent of the burn; the presence of other injuries, particularly those that compromise the respiratory system; and the possibility of a lengthy period of hospitalization and rehabilitation.

The immediate care administered by witnesses of the accident or by parents influences the depth and extent of the burn. In the case of an injury due to flames, the flames should be smothered as rapidly as possible by wrapping the child in a blanket, rug, or other similar material, and rolling the child on the ground to smother the flames. Removal of all pieces of clothing is important as otherwise the clothing may continue to smolder, causing additional harm. This is particularly true of synthetic fabrics which can melt, forming a superheated, adherent dressing. Immersion in cool water reduces both the extent and the depth of damage. Ice packs, which are sometimes used, create an additional hazard — that of freezing the tissues around the burn — thereby destroying viable tissue with cold rather than heat. The principle of cooling also applies to those burns caused by hot liquids. **Caution: Rapid cooling of large areas of the body surface can cause hypothermia, as well as cardiac arrhythmias.**

The child is subsequently covered with a clean cloth or a sheet and transported to a health care facility. No home remedies or sprays should be applied to the burn surface.

The history that is taken during the assessment period should include when and how the burn actually occurred. Parents are encouraged to share as many details about the incident as are known. In the process of describing when and how the burn occurred, the parent may also be able to offer some clues as to the likelihood of additional injuries. It is important to obtain a description of the first aid measures that were applied prior to transport of the child. The child's past history with regard to tetanus prophylaxis and health problems, such as allergies or renal disease, should also be obtained.

Treatment During the Acute Phase

The immediate treatment in the care center is aimed at stabilizing the child and preventing shock from fluid loss. Hypovolemic shock generally occurs twelve to twenty hours after the injury. During this time, massive fluid shifts from the plasma and intravascular compartment to the extravascular compartment occur.

These shifts are primarily caused by increased capillary permeability. The fluid shifts can create problems since increases in blood viscosity and hypercoagulability of the blood can cause the microcirculation to become static. This in turn, can cause a decrease in cardiac workload with possible circulatory failure. Acidosis and reduced renal blood flow may be additional problems.

Medical treatment includes fluid replacement, correction of the metabolic acidosis, and a reduction of the blood viscosity. Prompt replacement of fluids in a volume sufficient to correct deficiencies is necessary to prevent death within the first few days after the injury. Both sodium and water are utilized in fluid replacement, as they are needed in sizeable amounts to repair the injured tissues, depending on the extent and depth of the burn.

Fluid Administration

The amount of fluids replaced is dependent on the size of the child. In small children, the proportion of water composition is greater in relation to total body size. Their physical immaturity, poor tolerance to decreased fluid volume, and altered electrolyte levels add to their risk factor. In very young children, the integumentary system is particularly thin, and thus is susceptible to deep and destructive burn injury. Kidney function is variable and dysfunction may lead to problems of overload or dehydration.

Calculation of appropriate fluid replacement may be accomplished by a number of different methods. The methods that are most commonly used include the Brooke formula, which is based on body weight expressed in kilograms, Figure 16-2, and a formula that is based on total body surface area. Both calculations involve a colloid solution, such as plasma or a plasma expander. The amount of fluid is based on the number of hours that have elapsed since the burn injury. The greatest amount of fluid is administered within the first eight hours after the burn. This initial period is often referred to as the period of resuscitation. Over the next sixteen hours, the fluid amount is reduced as the child's condition stabilizes.

All fluids are administered intravenously and are initiated in the immediate postburn period. The cannula that is used should be large enough to accommodate the colloid solutions.

COLLOID (plasma or plasma expander)
0.5 mL X body weight in kg X percentage of burn

ELECTROLYTE (preferably, lactated Ringer's solution)
1.5 mL X body weight in kg X percentage of burn

GLUCOSE (dextrose–5% in water)

Newborn to 2 years	150 mL/kg of body weight
2 to 5 years	100 mL/kg of body weight
5 to 8 years	75 mL/kg of body weight
8 to 12 years	50 mL/kg of body weight

Guidelines for Administration: Burns estimated at over 30% are calculated at the 30% level. One-half of the fluid calculation is administered in the first 8 hours. The remainder of the fluids are given over the next 16 hours. On the second day of resuscitation, one-half the amount of colloid and electrolyte calculated is used for the 24-hour period.

FIG. 16-2 Brooke formula for fluid replacement in children

For accuracy, a fluid pump is used. More than one intravenous site may be used initially in order to prevent hypovolemic shock.

The effectiveness of the fluid administration is monitored by an assessment of urinary output, as well as of cardiac function. At the onset of fluid treatment, a Foley catheter which is connected to a urinometer is inserted into the bladder and continuous drainage collection is begun. The urinometer allows hourly monitoring of the urinary output. Fluid therapy is maintained at a rate sufficient to produce a urinary output of 1.0 to 1.5 milliliters per kilogram of body weight per hour. Such regulation prevents congestion of the renal tubules secondary to the excess amounts of pigment and uric acid generated by the destruction of cells. The urine is also monitored for glucose, acetone, pH, and specific gravity levels, as well as for the presence of blood.

6-11-81

Additional Emergency Measures

NPO Initially, children admitted for burns are not permitted to ingest anything by mouth. Paralytic ileus is a common problem in the first forty-eight hours postburn. To prevent vomiting and its attendant risk of electrolyte imbalance, as well as aspiration, a nasogastric tube is inserted and connected to low suction. When bowel sounds resume, the tube is removed. The child is permitted only sips of water initially. Subsequently, the child is given clear liquids. Eventually, a high-calorie, high-protein diet is instituted.

Medications for pain relief are given intravenously at first. The absorption rate for intramuscular medications is erratic and can result in cumulative doses that are toxic. Small amounts of intravenous morphine sulfate (0.05 milligram per kilogram) diluted in normal saline are administered slowly over a period of three to five minutes. This relieves pain and reduces apprehension. The extreme restlessness that may be observed in children with burns is often the result of hypovolemia and hypoxia rather than of pain.

Tetanus prophylaxis may be initiated in nonimmunized or inadequately protected children. Tetanus is always a threat to patients with large amounts of necrotic tissue. A precise history of the child's immunizations is crucial. On the basis of this history, the child may be given a booster dose of tetanus toxoid. In nonimmunized children, hyperimmune tetanus globulin is administered. Antibiotics are not used unless a specific indication of infection is present. Hypersensitivity and the development of drug resistance are realistic concerns.

Care of the Wound

Care of the wound is undertaken only after measures have been initiated to control hypovolemic shock.

Cleansing. Cleansing of the burn with large amounts of normal saline is then begun. In some burn units, the wound is cleansed with a solution composed of 1 liter of normal saline, 250 milliliters of hydrogen peroxide, and 15 milliliters of Dreft. The surface of the fresh burn is considered to be sterile, or free of pathogens. In children with burns involving large areas of the body, the entire body may be bathed in a tub of water to which a solution of antiseptic and germicidal povidone-iodine has been added. This method is not used in children with a history of skin sensitivity to iodine preparations.

Hair and Fingernails. The hair is shaved from areas adjacent to the burn wound. In the case of scalp or facial burns, the head may be shaved. Shaving is extended just to the edges of the burn to remove a potential source of contamination. The child's fingernails are also trimmed at this time.

Debridement. Debridement of the skin is accomplished prior to the application of any topical preparations. Any loose, necrotic tissue is removed by either the physician or the nurses on the burn unit, using sterile scissors and a hemostat. Large, thick-walled blisters are not incised at this time as they provide a sterile protective covering for the undamaged dermal layer. Once cleansing of the wound is completed, photographs of the burned area are usually taken for future reference.

Dressings. Burns may be treated using either an open or a closed method of wound dressing. The open method involves the application of a topical preparation without the use of surface dressings. The advantage of this method is clear visibility of the wound, as well as the ease with which passive exercises may be carried out in order to maintain joint mobility. With this method, cleansing of the burn site and reapplication of the topical ointment are accomplished with the least amount of discomfort for the patient. Frequent reapplication of the topical preparation is necessary.

The closed method involves the use of dressings over the topical medication. This method has several drawbacks. Occlusive dressings interfere with the child's temperature-regulating mechanism. They also increase heat loss. The closed dressing method involves the use of moist dressings that are resaturated every few hours. Heat is lost by evaporation of the water from the dressings, particularly when silver nitrate is used.

Topical Preparations. The three preparations, most commonly used for the treatment of burns include silver nitrate solution, mafenide acetate or Sulfamylon cream, and silver sulfadiazine or Silvadene cream.

Silver Nitrate Solution. A 0.5 percent solution of silver nitrate is used in the closed method. It is effective against most organisms, nonallergenic and inexpensive. Silver nitrate solution cannot penetrate burn eschar and thus must be applied as soon as possible to the fresh burn wound before organisms begin to grow. It can be used over both grafted areas and donor sites.

Silver nitrate in a warmed solution is used to saturate gauze pads that cover the entire burned area. The dressings are held in place with loosely applied rolls of stretchable gauze, or Kerlex. The dressings are resaturated every two hours. The outermost dressings are applied dry. To prevent loss of heat, the child is covered with blankets. These blankets are checked frequently to make certain that the outermost coverings remain dry. Once the child's fluid shifts are stabilized, an Ace bandage or stockinette may be used to keep the dressings in place. A major disadvantage of the silver nitrate dressings is the leeching of electrolytes such as sodium, chloride, potassium, and calcium from the burn wound. It is less often used in children because of the electrolyte problems. Another, less significant disadvantage is the dark-brown or black staining of anything that comes into contact with the silver nitrate solution. This staining may be upsetting to children if they are not forewarned.

Mafenide Acetate. Sulfamylon cream, or mafenide acetate, was developed after World

War II by the army's burn units. For greatest effectiveness, it is used in a strength of ten percent with the open method of wound dressing. It has a bacteriostatic effect that combats a wide variety of organisms including pseudomonas and it effectively penetrates burn eschar. It must be reapplied at twelve-hour intervals. Its major disadvantages are the stinging or burning sensation that persists for twenty to thirty minutes after its application to partial-thickness burns and the metabolic acidosis caused by its absorption by the body. The stinging sensation may be reduced by refrigerating the ointment. However, because of these disadvantages, it is often used only in the beginning of the treatment period when an eschar is present. It is never used with an occlusive dressing because of skin maceration and dermatitis.

Silver Sulfadiazine. Silvadene cream, or silver sulfadiazine, is also an effective topical treatment for burns. It is used in a strength of one percent and is applied to the burn surface in a layer that is about 1/8 inch thick. If the closed method is used, a layer of fine mesh gauze is applied directly on top of the cream. Additional dressings are then applied to cover the site. The open method of wound dressing is preferred as exposure of this medication to the air enhances its efficacy.

The major advantage of this preparation is its effectiveness against bacteria, such as pseudomonas organisms. It does not cause acidosis or electrolyte abnormalities. Its major disadvantage is that the individual may become sensitized to sulfa preparations. Silvadene is able to penetrate burn eschar somewhat, but is not as effective as Sulfamylon in doing so. It is contraindicated in neonates because of possible kernicterus from sulfa preparations. Leukopenia may also occur in some patients.

Eschar. Removal or incision of eschar is done by the physician to hasten wound healing and to prepare the skin for grafting. In children, removal of full-thickness eschar should be done prior to the application of a temporary graft. If the eschar is compromising respiratory function, as it might in circumferential wounds of the chest, it may be incised in a gridlike pattern. If it is constricting distal blood flow or compromising the underlying tissue perfusion of the extremities, longitudinal incisions may be made. Primary excision of eschar is always performed with the aid of general anesthesia.

Grafts

Several types of skin grafts are available for use in burn victims, Tables 16-1 and 16-2.

Temporary Grafts. A number of different types of temporary grafts may be used to cover the wound surface and to prepare it for permanent grafting. A homograft, or allograft, involves skin that is taken from a human donor. Cadaveric skin is also used for this type of graft. A heterograft, or xenograft, is composed of skin taken from an animal, most commonly from a pig. Fresh or frozen porcine skin dressings may also be used for the temporary graft. Human amnion is also used as a vapor barrier or a skin substitute in children only.

Temporary grafts, regardless of the type used effect a temporary closure or biologic dressing of the burn wound. They also result in a marked reduction in heat and fluid loss as well as pain since previously exposed nerve endings are protected. These temporary coverings improve the vascular bed and help prepare the site for a permanent graft, or an autograft, of the patient's own skin. The temporary grafts

TABLE 16-1 Classification of Grafts According to Permanence

TEMPORARY GRAFTS
1. Allografts (homografts) — Tissues for grafting are obtained from members of the same species (human). Living donors, preferably middle-aged individuals, may be used, as may cadaveric donors.
2. Xenografts (heterografts) — Tissues for grafting are obtained from a different species (animal). Porcine skin (pig skin) is most commonly used and is available commercially in both fresh and frozen forms.
PERMANENT GRAFTS
1. Autografts — Tissues for grafting are obtained from undamaged areas of the child's body.
2. Isografts — Tissues for grafting are obtained from histologically compatible donors. A twin or sibling generally provides the best tissue match.

may be applied only two or three times before rejection of the foreign protein occurs.

Permanent Grafts. The permanent graft is a split-thickness autograft that is cut with a dermatome from a usable portion of the child's own body. The piece of skin may be notched in many places to allow the graft to expand to several times its original size. The graft is laid on the burn site. No sutures are used to hold it in place, but small pieces of paper tape may anchor it temporarily. The graft is then covered with a sterile dressing. If the graft is over a joint or a moveable area, a posterior splint may be applied to maintain a specific position.

During the first few days after grafting, the nurse is responsible for "rolling" the graft site. This process involves the use of a sterile cotton-tipped applicator which is held parallel to the skin of the graft. Starting at the center of the graft and moving outward, the applicator is rolled to remove the serum between the graft and the burn site. This enhances the adherence of the graft to the wound. Careful observation of the appearance of the wound and any drainage is also important. Expandable mesh grafts do not require rolling as the serous drainage seeps through the open areas without reducing the contact between the graft and the tissue bed.

The donor site is covered in surgery by a layer of nylon Adaptic gauze. The donor site is not covered with a dressing so as to allow easy observation. The gauze covering is not removed, but is allowed to dry and to slough

TABLE 16-2 Classification of Grafts According to Thickness or Size

SPLIT-THICKNESS GRAFTS
1. Composed of the epidermis and part of the dermal layer
2. The various types include full-sheet, postage-stamp, mesh, lace, and slit grafts. (Only full-sheet grafts provide a desirable cosmetic appearance.)
FULL-THICKNESS GRAFTS
1. Composed of the epidermis and part of the dermal layer
2. This type of graft is used less often as the site cannot be reharvested as can that of split-thickness grafts.

spontaneously, usually in about a week. Afterward, topical lanolin may be applied to this site to keep it soft.

Long-term Care. Long-term protection of the graft site involves protection from trauma. This area is particularly vulnerable to damage and can be completely destroyed. One of the most commonly overlooked causes of damage is the sun. The graft site should be protected from exposure to the sun for a minimum of six months and preferably for a year. The cosmetic appearance of the graft may also be a long-term concern. Mesh grafts or pinch grafts are often rough or irregular in contour. Their configuration may have to be corrected with plastic surgery at a later time.

Nursing Responsibilities

The care given to the child is directly related to the phase of the burn injury. The care given during the acute or resuscitative period, which usually continues for the first forty-eight hours postburn or until the fluid shifts have stabilized, is distinctly different from the care given during the second period. This second period is called the phase of management or the repair phase, which directly precedes permanent grafting. The last phase is the rehabilitative phase, which extends from the time of permanent grafting to the time at which the patient achieves complete recovery. This phase includes any plastic reconstruction that takes place.

Environment. During the acute phase, the environment of the child is a concern. It is necessary to protect the child from undue exposure to outside organisms, so protective or reverse isolation should be effected. The number of individuals coming in contact with the child should be restricted. The wearing of sterile gloves, mask, cap, and gown is required when in the child's room. During this time, parents and visitors are assisted in carrying out the sterile technique. Generally, no more than three people are permitted in the room at any one time.

The child's room is also a concern in terms of comfort for the patient. Normally, the skin provides a vapor barrier and controls body temperature for the individual. When burns occur, both heat loss and energy expenditure are major problems unless the environment is controlled for temperature and humidity. The temperature should be set at 80°F to 85°F for comfort. Higher temperatures may be achieved by using a head cradle or a similar device. The humidity within the room is maintained at a level as high as ninety-five percent. The controlling factors for both heat and humidity are the child's comfort, if he or she is old enough to verbalize this, and the absence of shivering. This massive heat and vapor loss subsides when a temporary or permanent graft or skin covers the burn site.

Fluid Therapy. In assessing the effectiveness of fluid therapy, the status of the cardiovascular system and renal function must be evaluated. All of the considerations that usually apply to intravenous therapy in children also apply to burn patients, but there are some additional concerns in the latter. The intravenous rate should be calculated according to the output of the child. Ideally, the hourly output is maintained at 10 to 30 milliliters depending on the child's age. Assessment of the intravenous therapy, as well as of the child's output, is done every one-half to one hour during the acute phase. The child should produce one milliliter of urine for every kilogram of weight per hour.

Signs of thirst, dry mucous membranes, decreased output, elevated temperature, increased pulse, or increases in the specific gravity level of the urine indicate dehydration. The presence of any of these indicates the need for a change in the flow rate of the intravenous fluids. The child should also be observed for any signs of metabolic acidosis, such as a change in the level of consciousness, or a period of disorientation that worsens progressively. Nausea, vomiting, abdominal pain, or headache may indicate acidosis. Kussmaul's respirations, elevated blood levels of pCO_2, and increased blood pH levels are distinct indications of this problem.

Output is critically important in assessing the child's status. Careful hourly evaluations of the urine should include an observation of its color, an analysis of its specific gravity, and a measurement of the amount. Concentrations in excess of 1.020 to 1.030 indicate progressive hemoconcentration. A deepening color indicates increasingly large amounts of sediment that can obstruct the renal tubules. The position of the drainage tubing should also be noted each time, and any kinks or obstructions to urine flow removed.

Pulmonary Assessment. An awareness of the possibility of pulmonary complications should trigger a careful assessment right from the time of admission, Figure 16-3. Pulmonary complications may be related to thermal coagulation of the tracheobronchial tree. The most common cause, however, is the inhalation of irritating products of combustion. In a home fire, for example, the child is exposed to the residue and large particles of many synthetic substances that have burned. The inhalation of these irritants causes tracheobronchitis and resultant respiratory distress if left untreated.

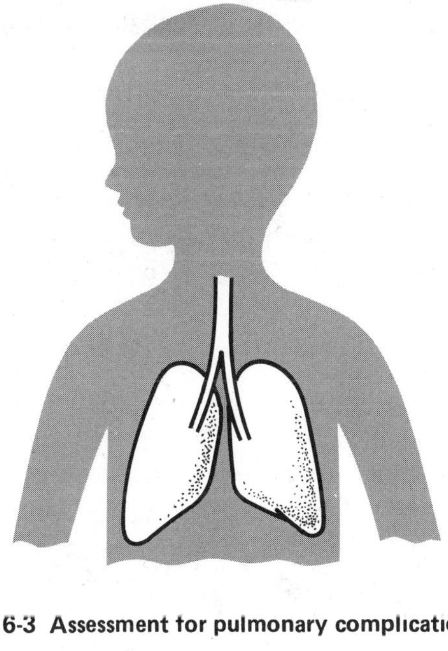

FIG. 16-3 Assessment for pulmonary complications

Various signs which should be recognized on admission indicate respiratory complications. These signs include blackened or singed nasal hairs, darkened rims of the nares without adjacent facial burns, black particles or blood in the sputum, a dry, hacking cough, and rapid respirations.

Respiratory distress is generally evident eighteen to thirty-six hours postburn. Children with burns of the chest, neck, and facial areas are at high risk for the development of pulmonary complications. Many of these children are intubated at the time of admission. In addition to ensuring a patent airway, intubation also allows easy removal of secretions by suctioning. Tracheostomies are performed selectively as they add to the trauma and may create further difficulties with healing.

Pulmonary assessment should include an evaluation of the rate, depth, and quality of respirations, as well as of the equality of chest excursion and the presence or absence of rales. The child should be encouraged to cough and breathe deeply every two hours. This is especially helpful in removing debris from the lungs.

Signs of hoarseness in the child indicate the beginning of a critical upper airway obstruction. Many children with minor respiratory problems on admission benefit from the use of a mist tent or an ultrasonic nebulizer to provide soothing moisture. Suctioning should be minimized, but used when necessary to reduce trauma to the overly irritated mucosa.

Infection. Prevention of infection is an ongoing process for the burned child, Table 16-3. Observation of the burn wound upon each dressing change or topical application is mandatory. The dressing procedure is carried out under aseptic conditions. Once the wound has been cleansed either topically or by placing the child in a Hubbard tank, the surface of the burn must be re-covered with dressings or topical preparations within twenty to thirty minutes. This minimizes the possibility of colonization with airborne organisms. Another potential site for the introduction of organisms is the intravenous site. In addition to checking the infusion and the drip rates, the site should be checked for tenderness, pain, or redness that is indicative of thrombophlebitis. If the dressing procedure is carried out while the child is in bed, the linens should be changed immediately after the dressing procedure. This minimizes the possibility of external contamination of the dressings by moisture or high droplet concentrations of organisms.

Dressing Changes, Debridement, and Grafts. During dressing changes, the nurse should be gentle but thorough. External dressings are removed prior to placing a child in a Hubbard tank. The child is encouraged to assist in removing the outer dressings, as well as those that are removed while in the tank. This enhances the child's sense of control over a difficult procedure.

In some cases, a temporary graft is used to debride the wound. In these situations, the graft is removed and reapplied every few days until the debridement is completed and the tissue bed is readied for the permanent graft to be applied. Rejection of the graft occurs slowly at first. With increased grafting, it occurs more rapidly. Removal of temporary grafts within a few days delays this process.

Comfort Measures. Discomfort to the child may be reduced in a number of ways. Analgesics should be administered at least one-half hour prior to the tub baths or dressing changes. The tub room should be warmed prior to remov-

TABLE 16-3 Measures for the Prevention of Infection in Burn Patients

ENVIRONMENTAL CONTROLS

Implement reverse isolation appropriately.

Limit the number of persons in the room to three at any one time.

Arrange for the room to be cleaned daily with a disinfectant.

Schedule the cleaning of the room for a time when the child is absent from the room.

Remove soiled dressings and linen from the environment as soon as possible.

PATIENT CARE

Maintain strict asepsis during dressing changes.

Maintain the sterility of all items that come in direct contact with the child.

Observe the burn site for any signs of infection each time the dressing is changed.

Prevent contamination from and possible infection in other areas of the body by:

- performing frequent mouth care
- using antibacterial soaps on unburned skin regions
- carefully cleansing the perineal area after voiding and stooling
- treating the catheter with an antibacterial preparation every shift
- cleaning and trimming of patient's nails as needed

Carefully monitor the intravenous site by:

- observing the site for irritation or inflammation
- changing the dressing and applying an antibacterial agent
- changing the intravenous tubing every 24 hours

Assess the patient for any signs of systemic infection, as indicated by:

- a sudden increase in temperature, pulse, or respiration rate
- chilling or diaphoresis
- sudden changes in the level of activity or alertness
- increased irritability, especially in young children

ing either the clothing or the dressings of the child. The temperature of the water should remain constant throughout the procedure. This reduces the incidence of chilling and resultant shivering in an attempt to maintain the body temperature. Warmed, sterile bath blankets are used to pat the child dry. Dressings should be applied immediately, taking care to place them properly the first time. Repeated removal and reapplication of the dressings to a burn site cause increased pain, as does shifting them on the granulating wound surface.

Body Image

The difficulties children have with their altered body image depend both on their developmental age at the time of the injury and their life experiences to date. Infants, for instance, have limited knowledge and no concept of separateness from parental figures. However, as infants become toddlers, a concept of separateness is acquired, as is the ability to distinguish their body parts from those of others. Children learn this through exploration of their own bodies and through exploration of objects within the environment. The boundaries of their bodies are not clearly defined at this point, though, and toddlers consider their hair, fingernails, and body discharges to be integral parts of themselves.

Preschoolers have a more clearly defined body image, but tend to focus strongly on the genital area, which may increase their feelings of guilt. School-aged children have an even more specific image of their bodies that is related to the similarities and differences of body parts. Young school-aged children view the skin as a surface covering that holds the blood, muscles, and bones inside, much as Raggedy Ann's cloth covering keeps her stuffing in place. As children approach adolescence with its accompanying sexual characteristics, they begin to view their bodies as others do. Adjustment to normal physical changes occupies much of the adolescent's time. Impairments or imperfections of a minor nature may temporarily be viewed by the adolescent as catastrophes until the task of adjustment is completed.

Effect on Care. When caring for any child with a burn, the developmental concepts of body image take on added importance. Injuries involving a particular area, as well as the dressings applied to that area, alter the child's ability to use that body part. The degree of emotional energy invested in that body part strongly influences the child's feelings. In toddlers, for instance, a great deal of stress is likely to be generated by shaving the head or trimming the nails. During dressing changes, this child is often upset by the debridement of damaged skin, as well as by the sight of any drainage on the dressings. It is important to allow toddlers to participate in wound care as much as possible. Improvements in healing, as well as any increase in ability to function, should repeatedly be pointed out to the child. During the initial care phase when a catheter is placed in the urinary bladder, the child should be told that this means of elimination is desirable and that he or she is not wetting the bed. In children who were toilet trained prior to the burn incident, burns of the perineal area are upsetting, and may be misunderstood as a form of punishment for bed-wetting or bowel or bladder accidents. In the case of an abused child, burns may have been one of the punishments used during the toilet training period.

The level of understanding in preschool children is more extensive than in toddlers, and explanations may evoke more questions in this age-group. These children should be reassured that their blood and bones will not fall out even though a sizeable portion of their body may be burned. At this age, children have also developed a concept of certain body parts that are mentionable and others that are unmentionable. This concept is related to past experiences and to what they consider to be public and private body regions. The nurse should emphasize that all areas of the body are good, clean, and acceptable regardless of their location. This should be emphasized particularly for the genital area, which the child may consider to be dirty, repulsive, or bad. A burn that extends to the genitalia is often associated with strong feelings of guilt related to pleasurable explorations of the area. The burn itself may be viewed by the preschooler as repulsive, regardless of its site. The child may tend to focus on negative thoughts which may be reinforced further by visitors who make faces or who refuse to look at the injured sites when the child offers them for view.

School-aged children and adolescents understand more about the functioning of the body than younger children, but they also seek a greater degree of perfection. The young girl who is very proud of her flawless complexion, especially when her peers all have acne, may be devastated by burns, particularly if they are facial. Such emotional investment dictates the degree of value assigned to the loss. The primary focus for young persons is not so much what they think about the injury, but what their peers will think and say and do. Negative feelings about the burn site, even after grafting, may be so strong that young individuals may feel that they are totally unacceptable to others. Therefore, the provision of ongoing peer support throughout hospitalization is just as crucial for this age-group as is good nursing care. Helping the child to focus daily on gains rather than losses in both healing and functional ability is a priority of care.

Nutrition

At the onset of acute burn treatment, a nasogastric tube that is connected to low suction is inserted. Once peristalsis has returned and the risk of paralytic ileus has diminished, oral feedings are begun. The feedings usually start about forty-eight to seventy-two hours after the initial injury. The feedings may include oral hyperalimentation solutions, as well as regular foods offered to the child at the usual intervals. The advantage of offering the child regular food is that the orientation to the routine of eating is maintained. Often, only a few spoonfuls of food are consumed, but even this small amount adds to the child's caloric intake.

Immediately postinjury, in the absence of protein intake, the child's body begins to utilize protein for glucose. This is evident in the burn patient at the end of the first week, when the excretion rate of nitrogen is generally twice the normal rate. During that first week, the child retains little of the protein ingested. During the following weeks, the metabolic rate increases in direct proportion to the depth and extent of the burn.

The diet that is provided to burn victims has a high protein, caloric, and vitamin content. It is calculated according to the child's preburn or immediately postburn weight, taking into account the percentage of the burn injury. The initial intake of foods by children is usually limited, so between-meal supplements are often high-protein beverages. Vitamin and iron supplements are also important. The intake of vitamin C, for instance, should be increased by five to ten times the recommended daily allowance. Iron is also essential, as iron depletion in tissues interferes with successful skin grafting.

In children with extensive burns who are unable to consume an adequate intake orally, other methods may be used. Tube feedings may provide either partial or complete dietary assistance. If the child is maintained on oral intake partially supplemented by tube feedings, the two types of feedings are scheduled so that they do not interfere with each other. Aspiration of the gastric contents is done to confirm that the stomach does not contain more than 50 cubic centimeters prior to the feeding. This practice prevents problems of overload and reduces the risks of vomiting and aspiration. The aspirated gastric contents are not removed and discarded but are reinstilled after measurement. Further losses of electrolytes are thereby avoided. Total parenteral nutrition may also be provided in the form of hyperalimentation. The nursing responsibilities related to this form of treatment are discussed in an earlier section on intravenous therapy.

One gastrointestinal complication that may occur in burn patients in response to stress is Curling's ulcer. It can occur without any significant inflammatory reaction. Nursing observations should include an assessment of the condition and color of any emesis, particularly hematemesis and "coffee ground" emesis. Other signs of the condition include poor food tolerance, abdominal distention, and epigastric pain. The character and consistency of the stools should also be noted. Melena, as well as tarry stools, are significant.

Working With Parents

In working with the parents of a burned child, the nurse should reflect a supportive attitude, a demonstrated concern for both parents and child, and a high level of skill. The supportive attitude is essential from the beginning to help distraught parents cope with the injury of their child. During the initial phase of acute care, the parents and child are usually separated. A nurse or health care worker who is knowledgeable about burn care should spend as much time as possible with the parents to support them and to provide information on the measures that are being taken to help the child. In this way, when the parents are reunited with the child, they are prepared for what they will see and what treatments have been instituted.

The nurse should help the parents adjust to looking directly at the child, as well as to holding and touching him or her. This may be particularly difficult if the parents are overwhelmed with feelings of guilt. Their feelings of responsibility for the injury should be recognized and discussed prior to their reunion with the child. Whether or not these feelings are justified, they are both real and overwhelming for many parents.

The parents' sense of control in the situation may be enhanced by knowledge. Treatment routines should be explained to the parents, and they should be taught what to do and how to help during dressing changes. They should also be taught and encouraged to be supportive to the child. The parents should be prepared to accept the child's feelings of anger and resentment, while coping with their own strong feelings of guilt. Activities that help to maintain the child's normal developmental level may also be delegated to the parents.

Parents and staff often learn together how to cope with the child's reaction to painful treatments and procedures. They should try to teach the child how to maintain control, yet the child's need to cry during painful procedures should be accepted. It is important to remember that the child frequently perceives the treatments as a form of punishment for real or imagined wrongdoing. The child whose burns were caused by a scalding tub of water can hardly be expected to view the tub treatments and dressing changes in a positive manner, or at least without apprehension and fear.

As soon as possible after the injury, the parents and staff should personalize the child's care in as many ways as possible. Every opportunity should be taken to make the child feel that his or her appearance is improving and is becoming increasingly acceptable to others. Clothing from home may facilitate this feeling for some children. For others, a special hairdo or hair ribbons may help improve the child's self-image. The message that should be conveyed to others is that, even with a burn, the child is special and unique in his or her individuality.

ACCIDENTAL POISONING

Toddlers are aggressive explorers of their environment. Their explorations are an outgrowth of the patterns previously set in infancy, when objects or substances were placed in the mouth for tasting. So many pleasurable experiences have resulted from this tasting in the past that the toddler is often eager for more of the same type of experiences. The bright package on the supermarket shelf that was appealing to the child in infancy has the same appeal during the toddler stage. The only difference is that the toddler has the motor skills to open the package or bottle of detergent or cleaner, and hence, the capacity to ingest contents.

Circumstances of Poisoning

The circumstances involved in poisoning accidents may appear to be unique at first. However, all such incidents have remarkable similarities that may be emphasized in educating parents. For instance, the child's environment may be unsafe because of the storage of multiple toxic substances in easily accessible places. Moreover, toxic substances may be stored in open containers or in cups, bottles, or cans that previously were used for foodstuffs. The toxic products that are most often ingested by children are listed in Table 16-4.

Inadequate supervision of the toddler contributes significantly to the incidence of accidents. For instance, an irritable, hungry child who may be inadequately supervised just prior to the supper hour is a likely candidate for the ingestion of a toxic substance.

Although toddlers are somewhat independent because of their acquired skills, they lack the judgment necessary to keep themselves out of trouble. They are unable, for example, to distinguish between the bottle of red pop that was offered earlier and the bottle of red furniture polish that they found in the cupboard. The availability of harmful substances that resemble harmless ones has increased dramatically.

Parental stress also has a bearing on accidental poisoning. The parent who is preoccupied with economic concerns or with preparing

TABLE 16-4 Categories of Toxic Products Commonly Ingested by Children

Soaps, detergents, and cleaners Includes such items as automatic dishwasher detergent, drain and toilet bowl cleaners, and caustic soaps
Plants Includes indoor and outdoor plant materials whose toxicities range from nontoxic (such as the African violet) to highly toxic (such as castor beans)
Vitamins and minerals Includes ordinary multiple vitamins as well as the newer megavitamins and high-iron preparations
Aspirin Includes all aspirin and aspirinlike products

a meal on time may not be appropriately attentive to an active toddler.

The presence or absence of the parent may also be significant. A young babysitter or an older sibling may not be as keenly aware of the child's developmental skills as is the parent, and accident situations that would normally be anticipated and prevented by the parent might go unchecked. Again, inadequate supervision, whether by the parent or another individual, is a prime contributing factor to accidental poisonings.

The day of the week and time of day may also be significant factors in the potential accident situation. Poisonings are less likely to occur on weekends, for instance, as more individuals are generally present in the home to observe the child. The highest percentage of poisonings occurs near the end of the week in the predinner hours (4 to 6 PM). Just as children learn that they can investigate more freely when their mother receives a telephone call, they also learn that her preoccupation with dinner preparations affords them freer access to many items and places that are usually forbidden at other times.

Poisoning Reporting and Initial Care Measures

Frequently, the poisoning incident is first reported by a frantic parent who calls a hospital emergency room, a poison control center, or a neighbor to say that "Susie took something that I think is poisonous" or "Johnnie ate some pills out of my purse." It is first necessary to calm the caller so that an accurate description of the incident can be elicited.

Known Substances. The first priority is to find out what substance was ingested, if known, as well as the amount that was ingested. The parent should be asked to read the product label and to describe the packaging. The ingested substance may have been found near the child. It is also important to obtain information regarding any other substances found in the immediate vicinity. More than one substance may have been ingested by the child.

An approximation of the amount ingested should be made. An estimation of the amount may be expressed in such terms as "one or two mouthfuls." In preschool children, each mouthful is about equal to 4 to 5 milliliters. Children can usually consume more of a liquid than they can of a granular or powdered substance. The type of container also may limit the amount ingested. A bottle with a small mouth or an aerosol pump container generally permits only a limited amount to be consumed.

The information on the label often helps to determine the toxicity of the substance. Products that are highly toxic must, by law, be accompanied by identifiable warnings on the label, Table 16-5. They also carry antidote information on the label. Even a statement such as "call a physician immediately" provides a clue to the substance's level of toxicity. However, if the substance was previously transferred to an inappropriate container, this information may not be available. If there are specific antidote directions on the label, the parent should follow these and then transport the child to the nearest emergency room.

If ingestion of a toxic substance is suspected or has definitely occurred, the child and the container(s), should be transported to the nearest emergency care center. The parent should be advised against giving the child any kind of home remedy or large amounts of liquid. These can actually enhance the absorp-

TABLE 16-5 The Relative Toxicity of Various Poisonous Substances (All are marked "Keep out of reach of children.")

MILDLY TOXIC TO NONTOXIC	
Substance:	Cosmetics, bubble bath, shaving lotions, lubricants, and perfumes
Warning label:	"Caution" (Additional instructions may be included.)
Toxic amount:	30 to 500 mL
MODERATELY TOXIC	
Substance:	Soaps, cleansers, bleaches, and disinfectants
Warning label:	"Warning" (Additional instructions are included.)
Toxic amount:	5 to 30 mL
SEVERELY TOXIC	
Substance:	Corrosives, petroleum substances, lye, pesticides, waxes, and furniture polishes
Warning label:	"Danger — Poison" "Call Physician Immediately" Antidote instructions included on the label
Toxic amount:	0.5 to 5 mL

tion of the substance, or may cause vomiting of corrosive substances or other dangerous side effects. For example, attempts to neutralize alkali substances with fruit juices or vinegar can have disastrous results. The neutralization process involves a chemical reaction that produces heat which, in turn, increases burn damage. Likewise, the neutralization of an acid with sodium bicarbonate is also dangerous, as this causes large amounts of carbon dioxide to be released. This can perforate the child's stomach. All home remedies delay the initiation of more effective treatments and may increase the damage to the child.

Unidentified Substances. In the case of an unidentified substance, the parent should be asked to review the events that preceded ingestion of the substance. Important clues may be found by reviewing what the adult or parent was handling immediately prior to the incident. The child may have observed the parent taking medication. Older children may have given aspirin to a younger child. Playing "doctor" or "hospital" is often the impetus for administering a foul-tasting substance to a younger child.

Observation of the area in which the child was playing may elicit other clues. Identifying what substances are within reach of the toddler may also be helpful. Other items in the environment that are adjacent to the area of play should also be noted. Mother's purse or father's shaving equipment may be overlooked as clues to the identity of the ingested substance.

Emergency Care

In the treatment center, whether it be a doctor's office or the emergency room, a decision on treatment must be made as rapidly as possible. If vomiting is to be induced, 15 cubic centimeters of Ipecac Syrup is given orally, followed by 6 to 8 ounces of clear liquids. Emesis occurs in most children within fifteen to twenty minutes. The dose may be repeated one time if emesis is not successfully induced. As an alternative, apomorphine may be admininistered subcutaneously in a dose of 0.07 milligram per kilogram per dose. It causes emesis within two to three minutes. However, it may be contraindicated in cases of ingestion of antihistamines, barbiturates, salicylates, and carbon monoxide poisoning which cause respiratory depression. Narcotic antagonists may be administered to counteract its depressant action.

Caution: It is important for any child receiving an emetic to be kept ambulating or in a high Fowler's position in order to reduce the risk of aspiration when vomiting occurs. Once the vomiting begins in a young child, it may be advantageous to place the child across the nurse's lap so that the head is lower than the hips. A specimen of the vomitus is saved for a toxicologic analysis.

Emesis is contraindicated in children who have ingested a corrosive substance. Gastric lavage is used instead. Before beginning lavage, however, one should determine whether the child's protective reflexes are functioning. If they are not, the child should be intubated before proceeding. The gastric tube that is passed should be large enough to handle the volume involved.

Once the substance has been recovered, activated charcoal is often instilled. Its relative effectiveness may be determined by the length of time elapsed since the poison was ingested. It is most effective when used within thirty minutes. Its absorptive ability is inhibited by the presence of food. The most effective dose is eight to ten times the amount of substance ingested. Activated charcoal will not remove the portion of the substance that has already been absorbed into the tissue. It is important for the emetic to be allowed to work before administering the activated charcoal. Other methods of breaking the contact with the offending substance or enhancing the excretion rate of the ingested substance are also available.

Substances may also be inhaled or absorbed through the skin, although ingestion is the most common means of poisoning in children. If a substance has been inhaled, removing the child from the environment breaks the child's contact with it, but it will not effectively remove the substance from the child's body. This child requires supportive measures of care.

When a toxic substance is absorbed through the skin, the child should be washed with copious amounts of running water. All clothing should be removed promptly, as it often absorbs the substance, thereby prolonging the contact of the toxic substance with the skin.

Cathartics may be administered to speed the transit of the substance through the gastrointestinal tract. Other methods of treatment generally precede their administration. This is intended to enhance the excretion of the portion of the substance that has already left the stomach.

Diuretics may be administered if the poisonous substance is excreted through the kidneys. This prevents reabsorption of the substance in the renal tubules. Osmotic diuretics may be administered intravenously as well. The disadvantage associated with their use is the possibility of fluid and electrolyte imbalances, including fluid overload.

Hemodialysis, peritoneal dialysis, and exchange transfusions may be used in treatment, depending on the substance ingested. These modalities are reserved for children who are acutely ill from the toxic substance with neurologic and respiratory involvement. All of them are associated with special risks and, therefore, are used only in extremely ill children in acute care situations.

Immediate Nursing Care

The nursing care of the child who has been poisoned includes helping to identify the substance, breaking the child's contact with the substance through its elimination from the child's system or through interference with its absorption, and providing supportive care until the child's condition is stabilized. In the case of ingestion of a mildly toxic substance, these three phases may be short-lived. However, the phases of nursing care may be prolonged if the child has ingested an unidentified substance or if multiple body systems are extensively involved.

The nurse's assessment of the child must be very thorough. It is absolutely crucial in the case of ingestion of an unidentified substance. The condition of the child's skin and mucous membranes should be noted. Burns of the lips, tongue, or teeth would indicate ingestion of a corrosive substance. Excess salivation and difficulty swallowing may also indicate that this type of substance is involved.

The nurse should direct particular attention to the child's clothing. The odor of the clothing may indicate that gasoline or a petroleum product was involved. This odor may also be noticeable on the child's breath and mouth if it was ingested.

Careful and frequent assessment of vital signs is essential. Changes, such as the onset of hyperventilation and cyanosis, indicate a change in the status of the child. The possibility of such children becoming comatose or needing supportive measures, such as oxygen or intubation, should be anticipated.

Seizures and hematemesis are two signs that indicate involvement of the neurologic system and gastrointestinal tract, respectively. They should be anticipated as potential problems, particularly if the substance remains unidentified.

Laboratory tests are used to identify the substance. Blood, urine, and vomitus can be screened. Groups of drugs, as well as lead, aspirin, and some other preparations, can be identified by such screening tests. Other substances that can be ingested may not be detected through the screening tests that are available at individual hospitals.

Radiography may be used to confirm the presence of certain substances. Those that are radiopaque include chloral hydrate, heavy metals, iron, phenothiazines, and enteric-coated tablets. This group of substances may be remembered easily by using the mnemonic CHIPE. Chipe

Supportive Nursing Care

Supportive care for a child who has ingested a toxic substance is most consistently provided in an intensive care or acute care setting. The child's condition is monitored closely to detect even slight changes in functioning. Additional therapeutic measures are rapidly instituted if indicated by a change in the child's status.

Vital Signs. Frequent monitoring of vital signs is a mainstay of nursing care. This is accomplished with the aid of an apnea monitor, as well as a cardiac monitor. Temperature and blood pressure monitoring is also continued by the nurse.

Neurologic Assessment. An assessment of the neurologic status of the child is done along with the vital signs as a routine part of the care. The child's orientation to time and place, as well as recall of information, is documented. This information must be adapted to the child's developmental level to be accurate. The child's level of consciousness is also ascertained at this time. If the child is lethargic rather than alert, it is important for the nurse to describe the specific stimuli to which the child does respond.

Evaluation of the child's motor ability is one aspect of the neurologic assessment. Areas of weakness or actual paralysis, as well as hyperactivity, are noted. The child's pupils are assessed for equality and responsiveness to light. At the same time, the presence or absence of nystagmus should be noted and recorded. Other reflex activites, such as the gag and cough reflexes, should also be assessed by the nurse.

All children with altered neurologic status have impaired respiratory ventilation and should be placed on a regular routine of respiratory care. This should include turning, coughing, and deep breathing exercises on a regular basis, usually every two hours. In alert children, the deep breathing may be facilitated by bubble-blowing or a similar activity that provides diversion.

Working With Parents

At the time of poisoning, the nurse should calm the parents while obtaining the necessary information. The seriousness of the situation is a reality that must be accepted by the parents. This does not preclude honest concern on the part of the nurse.

In the initial interview with the parents, the nurse should avoid questions that convey judgmental attitudes. Questions that begin with "why did you . . . ?" or "how could you . . . ?" only add fuel to the parents' feelings of guilt and anxiety regarding the situation. Questions of this type also reduce the parents' inclinations to communicate openly with health personnel. A supportive, nonjudgmental attitude elicits the most accurate information regarding the incident. Allowing the parents to verbalize their anxiety helps them to reduce their stress level and to provide support for their child.

Parents should be informed that the care received in the emergency room may not be sufficient for all children. If signs of toxicity are present upon admission or if the substance was highly toxic, the child is admitted for continued care and close observation. The ability of the parents to cope with the child's potential hospitalization is enhanced if this possibility is identified early in the course of contact with the parents.

Parental teaching is also a nursing priority. If the accident occurred because the parents failed to recognize the child's developmental level, this information is reviewed with them. If the home environment is determined to be unsafe, information regarding home safety should be given to the parents and reviewed with them, Figure 16-4. The role of parental stress in such accidents should be emphasized in the teaching. Parents should be aware that once the child has been involved in an accidental poisoning, the possibility of recurrence is much greater.

If a child who is older than five years of age is involved in a poisoning incident, it may be a deliberate attempt at suicide or a cry for help. In these cases, the family should be referred to the psychiatric division of the hospital or to a local mental health agency for evaluation.

SAFETY CHECKLIST FOR PARENTS

Household Products

1. Are all soaps, detergents, and cleaners kept on high shelves, not under the sink?
2. Are drain cleaners and furniture polishes out of reach?
3. Are beauty supplies kept off windowsills and ledges?
4. Are all perfumes and cosmetics out of reach?
5. Are food and household products stored separately?
6. Are disinfectants and deodorizers on a high shelf?
7. Are all substances stored in their original container, rather than in containers that formerly were used for foodstuffs (such as pop bottles or milk cartons)?
8. Are weed killers, insecticides, and fertilizers stored in the garage kept out of reach?
9. Are gasoline and antifreeze stored in proper containers with appropriate caps?
10. Are instructions carefully read and followed when using bug sprays, insecticides, and other toxic products?
11. Are containers from bleach and drain cleaners rinsed out before they are discarded in the trash?

Medications

12. Are medicines kept off counters, windowsills, and bedside tables, and out of purses?
13. Are medicines properly and safely locked in a cupboard?
14. Have old, unused, or out-of-date medicines been discarded properly?
15. Are safety caps reapplied properly to medicine bottles?
16. Are medication labels legible, and are instructions read carefully before use to ensure proper administration?

General Information

17. Does everyone in the home who is old enough know how to contact the poison control center?
18. Is your child supervised more carefully when routines are disrupted?
19. Is Ipecac Syrup available for use in your home if you are so instructed?

FIG. 16-4 The safety checklist is a good teaching tool for parents.

LEAD POISONING

Lead poisoning, or plumbism as it is sometimes called, is distinctly different from other ingestive poisonings in that it is a gradual process rather than an acute one. Affected children are usually four years of age or younger, have a history of ingesting foreign substances (pica), and reside in or near structures built prior to 1940. Homes of that era were constructed with building materials that contained large amounts of lead, such as paint, plaster, and putty.

Children may also be exposed to lead as an inhalant. Lead is found in the environment as an industrial pollutant, as a residue in dust and dirt from auto emissions, and in the smoke from the burning of colored newsprint. Lead joints are used in some plumbing systems, increasing lead levels in the water supply. In the past, lead solder was used to seal commercially canned evaporated milk. Lead can also be leached from improperly fired and glazed ceramic products by pouring orange juice into them. All of these lead forms are potentially hazardous.

Toddlers are at risk for lead poisoning because of the nature of their explorations. Once they begin to ingest lead-containing paint chips, they frequently return to the same site. They often continue to ingest these chips secretly, even after being restricted from the site. The pleasant, slightly sweet taste of the lead chips attracts them repeatedly.

TABLE 16-6 Effects of Lead on Brain Tissues (Lead Encephalopathy)

EARLY EFFECTS
Persistent vomiting
Irritability
Clumsiness
Ataxia
Decline in learned developmental skills
LATER EFFECTS
Stupor
Coma
Convulsions
Death
RESIDUAL DAMAGE AFTER TREATMENT
Mental retardation
Learning disabilities
Convulsive seizures
Visual defects (optic atrophy)
Attention deficit disorders
Hyperactivity
Cerebral palsy

The highest rate of lead absorption occurs in very young children, as evidenced by the amounts accumulated in their soft tissues. Signs of toxicity are evident at far lower lead levels in this age-group than in older children. The circulating lead binds with erythrocytes, shortening the life span, reducing the amount of hemoglobin, and causing hypochromic, microcytic anemia. The initial symptoms of lead poisoning resemble those of anemia. Later, the cumulative effect is evident in the soft tissues of the brain and kidney, Table 16-6.

Diagnostic Evaluation

Samples of the patient's blood are drawn to determine lead levels, as well as the degree of anemia present. A twenty-four-hour urine is collected to screen for the presence of lead, as well as to determine the effects of the lead on the kidney. The urine specimen is collected only after two doses of calcium disodium edetate (EDTA) are administered intramuscularly twelve hours apart.

Radiographs are obtained to confirm the presence or absence of lead chips in the gastrointestinal tract. In addition, the long bones are examined for the presence of "lead lines." These are areas of increased density near the epiphyseal plates.

Treatment

Children with blood levels of lead ranging from 40 to 80 micrograms are followed in a clinic specializing in this problem. Contact with the lead is broken and the child is watched carefully. For children with levels exceeding 80 micrograms, chelation therapy is instituted. An initial dose of dimercaprol (BAL) is given. After the initial dose, a combination of BAL and EDTA is given every four hours for five days. Some form of procaine is usually given along with the deep intramuscular injections to relieve the discomfort for the child.

Parent Teaching

Parents should know what environmental clues to look for in lead poisoning. One of the most obvious is the presence of holes in the plaster, flaking paint both inside and outside the home, and the teeth marks of the child on painted surfaces. Signs manifested by the child may include loss of appetite, fatigue, headaches, stomachaches, constipation, and vomiting.

Parents can prevent lead poisoning by carefully removing all flaking and blistered paint. They should choose paint appropriately so that only indoor paint is used inside the home. The child should be encouraged to chew or suck on appropriate toys instead of painted surfaces. The assistance of the physician or clinic is essential if any question remains about the child's exposure to lead.

HEAD INJURIES

The activities of the toddler may result in a head injury. A fall from a high chair, a tumble down the stairs, or involvement in an auto accident are all potentially serious accidents.

Classification

Head injuries may be classified as open or closed lesions. Closed head injuries are identified as minor, moderate, or severe, depending on the level of consciousness of the child, Table 16-7.

Open lesions include scalp lacerations, compound fractures, and any other open destruction of the head from trauma. Open lesions generally prompt parents to seek medical assistance more quickly than do closed injuries.

Medical Treatment

Treatment of head injuries in the emergency room setting starts with a careful assessment of the child's status. Airway, breathing, and circulation are the first priorities of care. Careful assessment and monitoring of vital signs

TABLE 16-7 Classification of Closed Head Injuries

MINOR INJURIES	**Cerebral Concussion**
	Transient and reversible damage to nerve cells and fibers
	Momentary to brief loss of consciousness
	Rapid return to a normal level of alertness (amnesia for incident)
	No demonstrable abnormal neurologic signs
MODERATE INJURIES	**Cerebral Contusion**
	Damage to larger areas with small petechial hemorrhages and edema at the site of injury and directly opposite it
	Longer period of unconsciousness
	Demonstrated abnormal neurologic signs (focal disturbances)
	Lack of nerve function in bruised portion (temporal lobe)
SEVERE INJURIES	**Brain Stem Contusion**
	Damage to upper brain stem causing compression of the reticular activating system, which controls the level of consciousness, and the corticospinal tracts, causing motor abnormalities of the face and extremities
	Immediate onset of coma; improvement is very gradual
	Demonstrated abnormal neurologic signs, initially on the same side as the injury (for example, pupillary dilatation secondary to compression of the third cranial nerve)
	Cerebral Lacerations
	Damage involves tears and severe bleeding into and around the tear
	Associated with penetrating injuries and depressed skull fracture
	Deteriorating level of consciousness and subsequent coma which is severe and prolonged
	Demonstrated abnormal neurologic signs
	Permanent scarring of the injured area with some degree of disability

provide the baseline for evaluating changes in the child's status. An assessment of the child's neurologic status is performed as part of the vital signs routine. This should include an evaluation of the child's level of consciousness, orientation, and motor and reflex functioning.

Intravenous fluid therapy may be started, but fluids are run at a minimal rate to keep the vein open, with the maximal volume being about one-half the normal calculation according to body weight. Output is monitored closely. A Foley catheter may be inserted into the bladder to obtain a more accurate measurement of the output.

The child is examined carefully for any other potential injuries. X-ray studies are used to locate any fracture sites in the head or elsewhere in the body. A lumbar puncture is performed to determine the nature of the spinal fluid, as well as to detect changes in pressure. An electroencephalogram may be obtained to detect abnormalities as well as to establish a baseline measurement for future comparison. A computerized axial tomographic scan (CAT scan) may be done to determine the type of brain tissue damage.

Nursing Care

The nursing care given the child who has sustained a head injury is directed at early recognition of problems, with resultant treatment to prevent further complications.

Vital Signs. The aim of vital sign monitoring is the rapid detection of Cushing's triad of increased intracranial pressure, arterial hypertension, and bradycardia. Shifts in vital signs may be very slight or may occur gradually. However, when monitored over a period of time, vital signs are reliable indicators of a worsening neurologic status. Initially, neurologic assessment is performed every fifteen minutes.

As the intracranial pressure rises, other changes and signs indicating cerebral herniation are also noted. The third cranial nerve or oculomotor nerve and the cerebral peduncle are compressed. This is evidenced by unequal pupillary responses. To detect this response, the pupils are observed in a darkened room. A light from a penlight flashlight is shone into the child's eyes and the speed and type of pupil response is noted. A small, narrow beam of light yields the most accurate assessment. Pupillary changes are usually accompanied by changes in the level of consciousness. Abnormal responses should be recorded and reported. Absence of pupillary response in both pupils indicates brain damage that may not be reversible.

Abnormal Drainage. While assessing the vital signs, the nurse should note any drainage around the nose or the ears. Rhinorrhea or otorrhea may be seen with basilar skull fractures. The drainage is serous or serosanguinous. To determine if this drainage is actually leakage of spinal fluid, a Dextrostix may be used to determine the presence of glucose. Glucose is present in spinal fluid but is not present in normal nasal drainage.

Headaches. Headaches often accompany these signs, although children seldom complain about them. Rather, they are usually identified by the behavioral changes and the irritability observed in the child. An infant or young child with a headache may assume certain positions, refusing to move or to change position voluntarily. Careful use of the ordered medications and gentle cuddling or rocking may relieve some of the discomfort.

Vomiting. Vomiting may also accompany head trauma. The kind, frequency, and amount of emesis should be recorded carefully. A nasogastric tube connected to low suction may be inserted during the child's evaluation in the emergency room. Additionally, the child's oral intake may be restricted. If a nasogastric tube is inserted, the infant or child must be prevented from removing it. It may be helpful to keep it out of his or her sight as much as possible in order to reduce the chances for accidental removal.

Motor Control. Observations of motor control in children with head injuries should be closely related to their developmental age. The ability to move and use arms and legs should be comparable on both sides of the body. Offering a toy from either side is an easy way to assess the use of both upper extremities. Older children may be asked to raise their legs in order to touch the nurse's hand with their toes. Younger children may neither understand nor follow these directions. To assess the lower extremities, each leg is raised off the bed and allowed to drop again. Muscular weakness or paralysis is indicated if the child allows the leg to fall straight to the bed surface without any slowing or voluntary change in position.

Positioning. On admission to the unit, children with head injuries are restricted to bedrest. A side-lying position allows for mucous drainage and prevents aspiration in children who are prone to vomiting. This position is maintained with a pillow or blanket roll placed against the back. Care must be taken to turn and reposition these patients every two hours if they are unable to do so themselves.

Seizures. Because these children may develop seizures, it is wise to protect them from accidental injury caused by the side rails of the bed. This may be accomplished for small infants or children by placing bumper pads around the crib. For older children, a blanket roll or bath blankets may be taped to the inside of the siderails to provide cushioning.

Hygiene. Meticulous hygiene practices help prevent skin breakdown in children with head trauma. This is particularly true in children with bowel and bladder dysfunction secondary to a head injury. The use of mild soap and water to cleanse the perineal area after wetting and soiling is as important for older children as it is for infants. In older children, the use of a diaper should be avoided if at all possible. The implication of regressing to a baby stage again is distressing to these children even if soiling does occur. The judicious use of fruit juices and stool softeners may be effective for bowel evacuation if the child is allowed to drink liquids.

Mouth care is also an important part of hygienic care for all age-groups. If brushing the teeth is not possible, the use of lemon and glycerin swabs may be temporarily substituted. These swabs are more palatable to the child if they are chilled in the refrigerator. As oral hygiene is performed, the presence or absence of reflex activities, such as the gag, cough, and swallowing reflexes, may be determined. In infants, the rooting and sucking reflexes may be assessed as well.

Discharge. Many children with a history of head injury are observed for a brief period in the hospital and then sent home. These are children who have no neurologic signs that indicate increased intracranial pressure or

INSTRUCTIONS TO PARENTS ABOUT HEAD INJURIES

Your child has been thoroughly examined and it is considered safe to allow him to return home. Please observe him carefully during the next 48 hours and telephone your physician if any of the following signs develop:

1. *Excessive drowsiness.* Your child may be exhausted by what has happened since the injury. You should be able to arouse him by the method you normally use to get him up after a deep sleep. If you cannot do so, notify your physician.
2. *Persistent vomiting.* Your child may vomit once or twice following a head injury. If vomiting occurs more often than that, notify your physician.
3. *Use of arms or legs.* Your child should be able to use his arms and legs as well as he could before his head injury, including walking. If you observe unsteadiness or difficulty, notify your physician.
4. *Speech.* If your child's speech is slurred or he is unable to talk as he normally does, notify your physician.
5. *Vision.* If your child complains of seeing double, or if his eyes do not work together, or if one pupil is larger than the other, notify your physician.
6. *Headaches.* Your child may have a headache that can be relieved with aspirin. If aspirin is not effective in relieving it, or if the headache increases in severity, notify your physician.
7. *Seizures.* If a seizure occurs, turn the child on his side and protect him from injury. Stay with him until the seizure is over, and then notify your physician.

It is advisable to look for these danger signs every three hours, both during the day and during the night following the injury.

FIG. 16-5 Instruction sheet for parents of children with head injuries

altered neurologic function. Upon discharge, written instructions are given to the parent or other reliable person regarding observation of the child, Figure 16-5. The parents should be taught how to check the pulse and respiration rate and what signs indicate a need to return to the emergency care center.

DROWNING

Drowning can occur with children of any age; however, the factors associated with the incident and the outcomes vary. Some factors involved in the incident include the temperature of the water, the person's ability to swim, the state of health of the individual, and the ingestion of alcohol or drugs.

Regardless of whether the drowning occurs in the ocean's salt water or a lake's fresh water, the sequence of stages is from hypoxia, to hypercarbia, to acidosis which results in cardiopulmonary arrest. In those children who experience a near drowning because of the prompt intervention of a knowledgeable individual, the hazard is the formation of pulmonary edema. As a result of saltwater immersion, the edema is caused by the aspiration of a hypertonic solution. In freshwater drowning, it is caused by the washout of pulmonary surfactant.

Treatment

The treatment of the drowning victim is immediate cardiopulmonary resuscitation to reestablish oxygenation. This is begun immediately even in the water if at all possible, and continued. Attempts to drain the water out of the child are usually ineffectual and waste valuable minutes in which cardiopulmonary resuscitation should have been started. This is done even when the child has been submerged for a considerable length of time. Children have survived lengthy submersion in cold water because of the efforts of rescuers.

When ventilating an infant, both the nose and mouth are covered by the mouth of the individual performing the CPR. One small breath (sufficient to puff out the cheeks) is given after each five compressions. The infant's head should be tilted backward only slightly for this, as an exaggerated position will obstruct the airway. It is also important to have the infant's head level with or slightly lower than the trunk to improve cerebral perfusion.

Chest compression for the infant is done using the tips of the index and middle fingers at a rate of 80 to 100 compressions per minute. The sternum should be depressed no greater than 1/2 to 3/4 inch as lacerations to the liver are a real danger. For an older child, the heel of one hand may be used to depress the sternum 3/4 to 1 1/2 inches.

Once the child is in a care area, oxygen is usually delivered by means of positive-end-expiratory pressure (PEEP). This method provides the greatest improvement in oxygenation as more alveoli remain open rather than collapsing on expiration. This is usually administered by endotracheal tube and can be intermittent, mandatory, or controlled if the child will not initiate it spontaneously.

Intravenous fluids are also used with this child to combat the metabolic acidosis which has occurred. Blood gases are drawn and, on the basis of these, intravenous fluids including sodium bicarbonate are used.

Nursing Care

Participation in cardiopulmonary resuscitation and the treatment that follows is the nurse's role. This may take place in the emergency room or in the intensive care area. The nurse along with the respiratory therapist may be monitoring PEEP and the Swan-Ganz catheter for pulmonary circulation.

Maintaining the intravenous fluids and identifying subtle changes in status are important aspects of care. Documenting intake and output is always important with intravenous fluids, but is especially crucial with this child as decreases may signify a decrease in the cardiac output.

Support of the family is also extremely important. They need to know that the person caring for their child is knowledgeable and caring. Provisions should be made for their comfort during the many hours of waiting. Knowledge of where to find things, such as a lounge, snack bar, restrooms and telephone, is important to the family and takes but a few minutes in the orientation process. Families also need to know when and how often they may be with the child, if they may not stay continuously.

Prevention

The anticipation of a potential accident can do a great deal to eliminate the accident. New parents should be taught by the nurse to anticipate hazards that can occur at various stages in the child's development. For the infant and toddler it is important to provide continuous supervision. Potential hazards such as swimming pools should be fenced and locked. A child in a wading pool or bathtub requires continuous supervision. Teaching the child to swim and also to respect water are important measures.

Any child participating in water sports such as boating without the ability to swim should wear an approved lifejacket. The lifejacket should be an appropriate size for the child and should be put on when the child is on dry land prior to walking out on the dock. Children often fall off narrow docks into the water before ever having boarded the boat.

School-aged and adolescent children should be instructed to swim only in guarded areas when the lifeguard is on duty. They should also be taught to "buddy up" in pairs so that each child is watchful of the other and will go for help if anything happens. This age-group also needs to wear lifejackets when participating in boating and waterskiing even if they are good swimmers.

SUMMARY

Accidents of any type are traumatic for both parents and children. They necessitate rapid decision making about the child's care and often generate a feeling of loss of control once emergency treatment has started. Accidents also generate a strong sense of guilt, justified or unjustified, on the part of both parents and children. Nursing responsibilities are precise and demanding in the acute care setting. Changes in the child's condition may be subtle. However, these changes must be recognized and correctly identified.

Accidents involving burns and head injuries often require long-term hospitalization for the child. Such lengthy hospital stays are of concern to the nursing staff in terms of the child's developmental levels and concept of body image. Much time is spent promoting the child's image and reinforcing previously learned skills, as well as maintaining current skills.

Working with the parents requires a great deal of patience and empathy. Parents are not always receptive to safety education, and often it must be reinforced repeatedly. The nurse's supportive interaction with the parents has a direct bearing on the outcome of the child's care.

SUGGESTED ACTIVITIES

- Visit the nearest Poison Control Center. Observe how information is received and how calls are monitored. Find out what follow-up care is given to individuals who call in but who do not come in for treatment.
- Care for a child admitted to the hospital as a result of an accident. Review the circumstances of the accident. What could have been done to prevent it? What teaching should be done to prevent a recurrence of the same situation? Share the preventive safety measures and the teaching information with your student group.

DISCUSSION TOPICS

1. Ask a nurse from your local health department to talk to your class about referrals of and follow-up for children with suspected lead poisoning. Share with your class the information on lead poisoning that is available from public health agencies.
2. Arrange for a member of the nursing staff of an area burn unit to meet with your class and share the routines of the unit. In particular, discuss the supportive care of the parents and child during the resuscitative period.

REVIEW

A. Matching. Match the method of assessment in Column I with the parameter being assessed in Column II.

Column I	Column II
1. Use of a narrow-beamed light in a darkened room	a. Motor control in upper extremities
2. Offering a brightly colored toy just out of the child's reach	b. Pupillary response
3. Use of a Dextrostix to determine whether glucose is present	c. Spinal fluid in drainage

Match the nursing measure in Column I with the purpose in Column II.

Column I	Column II
4. Monitoring urinary output on an hourly basis	a. To reduce heat loss and energy expenditure
5. Placement of child in reverse isolation	b. To prevent paralytic ileus
6. Maintenance of room temperature between 80°F and 85°F.	c. To determine effectiveness of fluid administration
7. Limiting intake to intravenous fluids	d. To prevent infection

B. Multiple choice. Select the one best answer.

Situation: Harry is a nine-year-old boy who was admitted to the pediatrics unit after falling out of a tree. He was unconscious initially and now is responding slightly.

1. It is desirable that Harry's level of consciousness be checked immediately upon hospital admission in order to
   a. determine whether he can withstand a surgical procedure.
   b. provide a baseline to which later assessments of consciousness level can be compared.
   c. familiarize him with a procedure that will be performed repeatedly.
   d. enable the physician and nurse to observe his responses to routine tests simultaneously.

2. Which of the following characteristics of Harry's pupils should be noted and reported?
   1. Size
   2. Equality or inequality
   3. Response to light
   4. Speed of light response
   5. Color of eyes

   a. 2, 3, 4 and 5 c. 1, 2, 3 and 5
   b. 1, 3, 4 and 5 d. 1, 2, 3 and 4

3. Changes in Harry's pupillary size are regulated by which cranial nerve?
   a. Second c. Fourth
   b. Third d. Fifth

Situation: Sally, age eighteen months, swallowed some powder from a bottle of drain cleaner. The cleaner's active ingredient was lye.

4. The first thing Sally's mother should do is
   a. induce vomiting to prevent absorption of the toxic substances.
   b. dilute the lye with water and/or vinegar (acid) solution.
   c. give the antidote which is listed in the encyclopedia.
   d. take Sally to the nearest hospital emergency room.

5. Which of the following questions should the nurse in the emergency room ask Mrs. Watts?
   1. "Describe exactly what happened to Sally."
   2. "Explain why you left Sally alone in the kitchen when you went to answer the knock at the front door."
   3. "Do you know how much of the substance Sally ingested?"
   4. "Do you know that poisoning is the leading cause of death among children?"
   5. "Did you by any chance bring the container of the substance with you?"

   a. 1, 2, 3 and 5 c. 2, 3 and 4
   b. 1, 3 and 5 d. 1, 2 and 4

Situation: Jeff Jones, a two-year-old boy, was admitted to the hospital with a diagnosis of chronic lead poisoning. His mother stated that he had eaten paint from his crib rail over a period of weeks.

6. Jeff should be observed carefully by the nurse for
   a. convulsions.
   b. hemorrhage from the rectum.
   c. edema of the extremities.
   d. respiratory difficulty.

C. Short answer. Briefly respond to the following statements.

1. List four signs of inadequate fluid intake or dehydration in a child with burns.
2. Name three signs of metabolic acidosis in children with burns.

BIBLIOGRAPHY

Bailey, Judith. "Head Trauma." *RN,* Vol. 42 (May, 1979), pp. 44–51.

Bennett, Robert M. "Drowning and Near Drowning: Etiology and Pathophysiology." *American Journal of Nursing,* Vol. 76 (June 1976), pp. 919–921.

Campbell, Laura. "Special Behavioral Problems of the Burned Child." *American Journal of Nursing,* Vol. 76 (February, 1979), pp. 220–224.

Davis, Rene Clark. "Prevention of Childhood Accidents Through Safety Education." *Issues in Comprehensive Pediatric Nursing,* Vol. 2 (March–April, 1977), pp. 57–71.

Emig, Elaine, and James R. Lloyd. "How to Get Burned Children Home Sooner." *RN,* Vol. 77 (July, 1977), pp. 37–39.

Frye, Susan, and Julie Lander. "The Initial Management of the Acutely Burned Child." *Issues in Comprehensive Pediatric Nursing,* Vol. 1 (July–August, 1976), pp. 39–59.

Greensher, Joseph, M.D., and Howard C. Mafenson, M.D. "Emergency Room Care of the Poisoned Child." *Issues in Comprehensive Pediatric Nursing,* Vol. 4 (June, 1980), pp. 1–21.

Jacoby, Florence Greenhouse. "Individualized Burn Wound Dressings." *Nursing 77,* Vol. 7 (June, 1977), pp. 62–63.

Jones, Claudella A., and Irving Feller. "Burns – Avoiding and Coping With Complications." *Nursing 77,* Vol. 7 (November, 1977), pp. 72–81.

Jones, Claudella A., and Irving Feller. "Burns – The Home Stretch . . . Rehabilitation." *Nursing 77,* Vol. 7 (December, 1977), pp. 54–57.

Jones, Claudella A., and Irving Feller. "Burns – What To Do During the First Crucial Hours." *Nursing 77,* Vol. 7 (March, 1977), pp. 22–31.

Kinzie, Vickie, and Carol Lau. "What To Do For the Severely Burned." *RN,* Vol. 43 (April, 1980), pp. 46–51.

Kunsmon, Judith. "Nursing Care After Primary Excision." *RN,* Vol. 37 (August, 1974), pp. 23–25.

Langner, Barbara, and Mary Anne Modrcin-McCarthy. "Lead Poisoning: An Ongoing Pediatric Nursing Concern." *Issues in Comprehensive Pediatric Nursing,* Vol. 4 (June, 1980), pp. 23–35.

Lybarger, Patricia. "Accidental Poisoning in Childhood: An Ongoing Problem." *Issues in Comprehensive Pediatric Nursing,* Vol. 2 (March–April, 1977), pp. 30–39.

Ninman, Carolyn, and Pricilla Shoemaker. "Human Amniotic Membranes for Burns." *American Journal of Nursing,* Vol. 75 (September, 1975), pp. 1468–1469.

Proctor, Audrey. "Pediatric Arrest – Scaling Down CPR." *RN,* Vol. 42 (September, 1979), pp. 58–64.

Sheeky, Elizabeth. "Primary Excision: Innovation in Pediatric Burn Care." *RN,* Vol. 37 (August, 1974), pp. 21–25.

Stanley, Linda. "The Near Drowning Victim: CPR Is Not Enough." *RN,* Vol. 41 (June 1979), pp. 41–44.

Talabere, Laurel, and Patricia Philips. "A Tool for Assessing Families of Burned Children." *American Journal of Nursing,* Vol. 76 (February, 1976), pp. 225–227.

Wagner, Mary M. "Emergency Care of the Burned Patient." *American Journal of Nursing,* Vol. 77 (November, 1977), pp. 1788–1791.

Chapter 17

The Abused Child

OBJECTIVES

Upon completion of this chapter, the student will be able to

- describe the types of child abuse that occur and the proper method of reporting.
- identify some of the approaches a nurse might use with the parents of an abused child.
- discuss the various forms of nursing intervention that can be used to deal with a child's inappropriate behavior.

The abused child is not isolated to a particular environment, culture, or socioeconomic class. The signs of abuse listed here are not all-inclusive. The signs and behaviors are clues which raise a suspicion. This suspicion of abuse, upon investigation by the proper authorities, may or may not be confirmed. It is the responsibility of the nurse to report abuse with or without the permission of other professionals.

TYPES OF ABUSE

Child abuse is defined as any nonaccidental injury to a child caused by the caregiver. It can be classified in a variety of ways. Abuse involves the commission of an act. Abuse is subdivided further into physical, emotional, and sexual abuse. Neglect can be either physical or emotional. Neglect is an act of omission.

Physical abuse involves the use of one or more inappropriate methods of disciplining a child. The extreme of physical abuse is usually called battering, which designates severe and repetitive injuries to the child's central nervous system, internal organs, or long bones. Sexual abuse ranges from subjecting the child to sexual exposure to actual rape. Emotional abuse involves an inappropriate debasement of the child's feelings.

Whether or not it is combined with child abuse, a child may suffer from neglect. Physical neglect is defined as a failure of the parent or caregiver to provide adequate food, clothing, shelter, medical care, education, or proper supervision. Emotional neglect involves a failure to nurture the child's sense of self. A child suffering from neglect may also be subjected to willful injuries or abuse, or the neglect may be a separate entity.

SYMPTOMS

Physical Abuse

Injuries from physical abuse vary greatly from one child to another, Figure 17-1. A burn is one of the injuries that may be intentional. It may either be a form of discipline that was used or the result of a parent's rage. Cigarette burns are often inflicted to the child's fingertips and occasionally, to the child's scalp or other body regions. Hot liquids may be poured on a child who inadvertently but frequently spills things at mealtimes. The

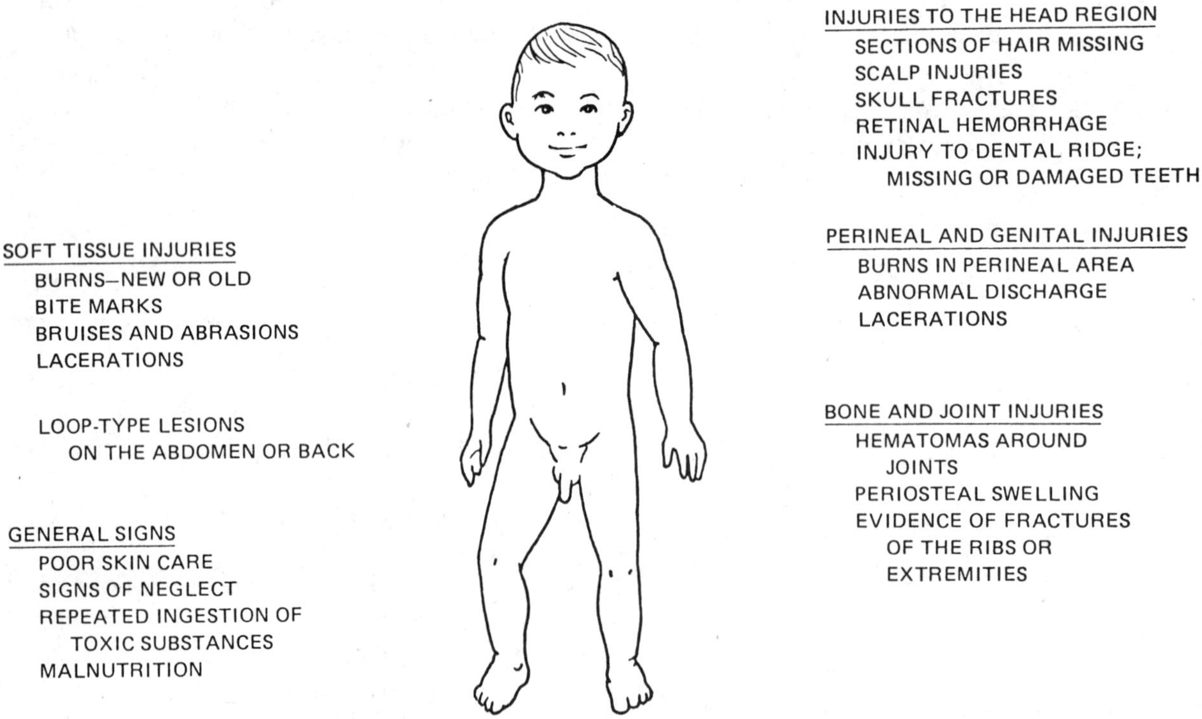

FIG. 17-1 Assessment for abuse

child who wets himself when toilet training is supposedly accomplished may be placed in an extremely hot tub of water "to teach him a lesson." Rope burns on body parts indicate binding or gagging of the child.

Beatings may be evident from the presence of abrasions, lacerations, or swelling of any part of the body. Soft tissue injuries are often more obvious when two extremities are compared for size. The instrument used in the beating, such as a hanger, a belt, or a strap, may actually be identifiable from the marks that are visible on the skin surface. The cluster of lesions to form regular patterns is significant.

Wringer injuries are those caused by the forceful twisting and compression of a child's limb, Figure 17-2. Damage in these instances involves the soft tissues. This type of injury may also be combined with rotation injuries that injure the bones as well. Epiphyseal separation usually occurs along with subperiosteal hemorrhage. X-ray studies may reveal that the child has multiple fractures of this type that are in various stages of healing. Fractures and dislocations in a child under two years of age that are inconsistent with the history are always suspect.

Head injuries are the most frequent cause of death in abused children. If the child survives the injury, he or she may still be left with severe brain damage. Skull fractures may result from the use of a blunt instrument or from the child being dropped or hit on the head, Figure 17-3. Children sustaining head injuries should also be examined for additional damage, especially to the mouth. Many small infants and toddlers sustain injuries to the

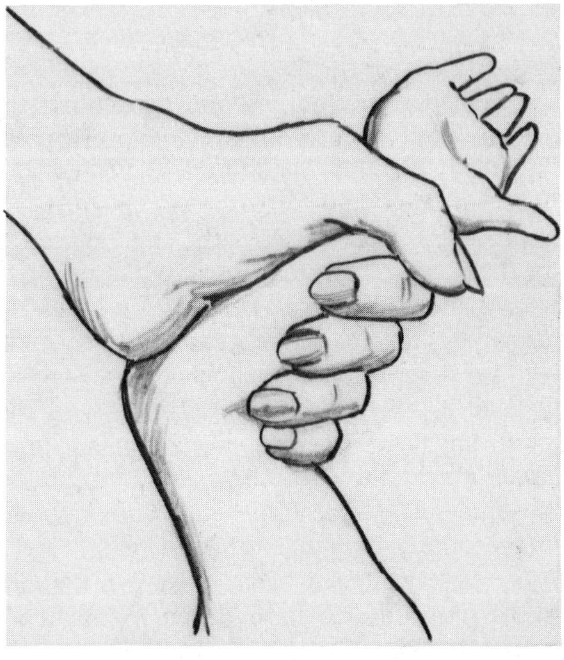

FIG. 17-2 Wringer injuries to the extremities result from jerking or twisting arms or legs.

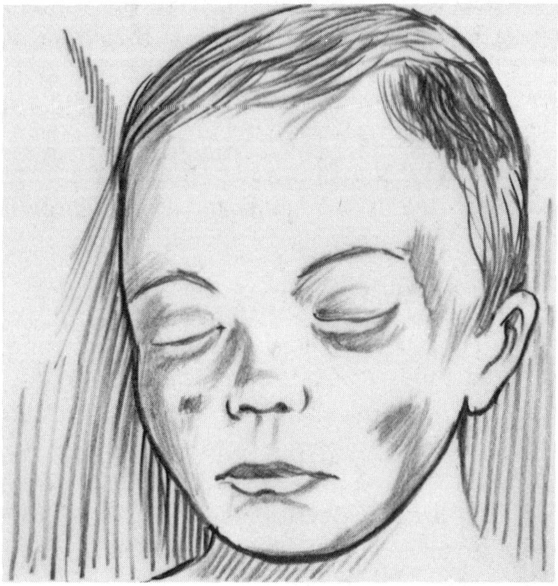

FIG. 17-3 Skull fracture with periorbital hematomas

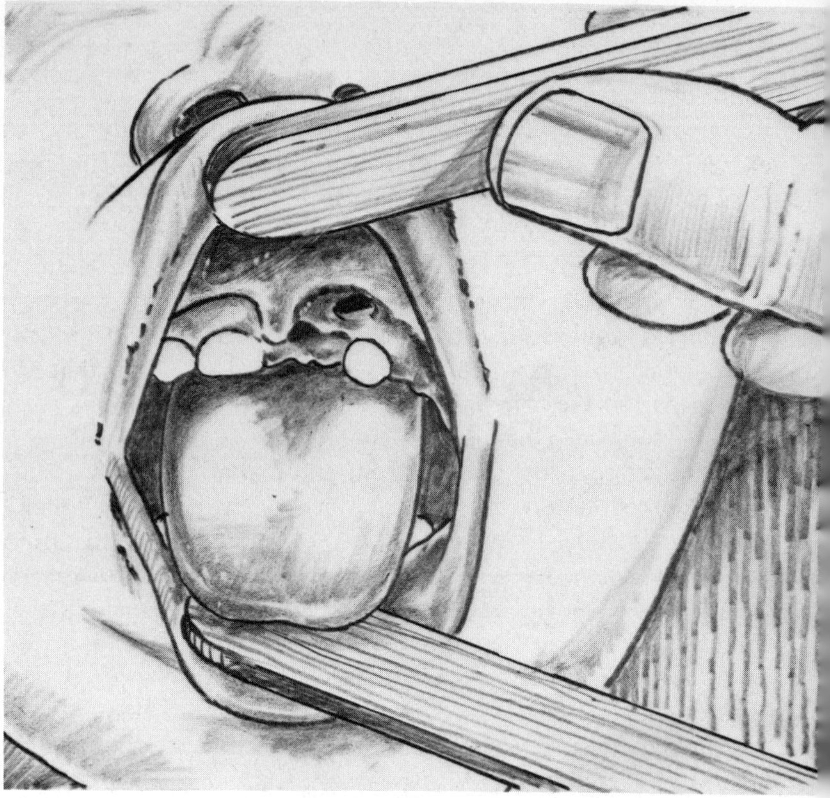

FIG. 17-4 The mouth and dental ridge should be inspected for injuries. Frequently, missing teeth, lacerations of the frenulum, and soft tissue injuries are evident.

tongue, teeth, or frenulum from the forceful insertion of a bottle or spoon into their mouths, Figure 17-4.

A large number of children are not identified because their injuries are less severe. They do not fit the preconceived notions that are well documented by the media and so are ignored.

Behavioral Observations of the Child

The nurse should also note the behavior of injured children. Do they appear to be unduly fearful of adults, especially their parents? Do they cling inappropriately to the parent? Are they unusually passive or withdrawn for their age and level of development? Does the child appear to be malnourished or poorly cared for? Does the child appear to be very protective of the parents, or does he or she try to meet their needs? Does the child respond inappropriately to painful procedures? Is the child overly compliant? Is the child unduly frightened by routine procedures that have been explained and repeated previously? Does the child appear to be thriving in the protected area of the hospital?

Children who have been abused often feel that they "deserved the punishment" in some way. A description of the incident may be verbalized with the child identifying why the punishment was given. This child may demonstrate uncertainty in dealing with adults in the hospital setting because they do not respond in the same fashion that he has learned. Provocative or very clinging behavior may be demonstrated toward all adults in the environment because of this uncertainty. His learned behaviors in the home setting do not elicit the same response from adults in the hospital setting.

Behavioral Observations of the Caregiver

Observation of the behavior of the parents may also be revealing. Are they unusually mistrustful of the members of the health care team? Do they appear to discourage social contact with anyone? Do they provide conflicting information about the child's injuries or reason for admission? Do they appear to be detached from the child, with little or no concern for the child's problems or discomfort? Do they voice frequent complaints about trivial or unrelated problems that are totally divorced from the child's current injury?

When talking with the parents, the nurse should also note their expressed beliefs about children. Do they feel that one should not "give in" to babies when they cry? Do they believe that a child must be shown "who is boss"? Do they believe that a child should obey the parents without question, or that they should not be allowed to "get away with anything"? Do they believe in the philosophy "if you spare the rod, you spoil the child"? Do the parents recount the harsh disciplinary measures used on them, and do they view such measures as appropriate for their own children?

SEXUAL ABUSE

Sexual abuse is often difficult to identify as the phyisical signs may not be readily visible. There is a reluctance to tell about it on the part of the victim. Incest is always a well-guarded family secret.

Physical indications of sexual abuse include bruises of or bleeding from external genitalia, vagina, or anal area; edema and erythema noted of the cervix, vulva, or perineum; pain or itching in the genital area; torn, stained, or bloody underclothing; presence of semen; and positive tests for the sexually transmitted diseases.

Behavioral indicators exhibited by the child include difficulty in walking or sitting, reluctance to participate in physical or recreational activities, poor relationships with children of a similar age, regressive behavior even to appearing retarded, delinquency, truancy, running away from home, and extreme interest in own sexual organs and those of other children or the parent. In older children indicators include seductive behavior, promiscuity, prostitution, and confiding history of sexual abuse to a friend, teacher, or the authorities.

Many of these children have common elements in their environment that can be noted. These factors include overcrowding in the home, prolonged absence of one parent, alcoholism, social and/or geographical isolation of the family, a pattern of incest in the family, and an abusive parent who demonstrates overprotectiveness, jealousy, and distrust of the child.

In taking the history it is important to obtain as much of it as possible from the child. The child's comments should be quoted directly to indicate the child's level of understanding of what has happened. When the child uses terms such as "dinkie," "privates," etc., he should be requested to point to the part and this information is also documented on the chart. Statements made by the parents are also included.

Many hospital emergency rooms and pediatric units have a special kit for documentation of sexual abuse. This includes an examination form and the equipment needed for the collection, labeling, and preservation of evidence. The nurse or a designated hospital employee is required to keep all evidence, including specimens in their personal possession until the law enforcement officer arrives. At that time it must be given directly to that person. Color photographs of the traumatized areas as well as radiological examinations, if medically indicated, may be done without parental consent. If the parent or guardian of the child is not present, the social worker is usually the person responsible for notifying them, telling them that an examination for suspected sexual abuse was performed.

NEGLECT

Neglect usually occurs over a longer period of time and consists of inadequate or dangerous child-rearing practices. There may not be specific, visible signs of the problem as in the other forms of abuse.

The physical indications of neglect include abandonment; lack of adequate supervision; lack of adequate clothing for the climate; lack of good hygiene; lack of adequate nutrition; lack of safe, warm, and sanitary shelter; lack of necessary medical or dental care; and failure to comply with necessary medical treatment for the child. An example of the latter would be the parent who fails to administer appropriate anticonvulsant medications to a child with recurrent generalized seizures. These indicators must be considered within the context of the cultural values, the parental capacity and the economic status in the home.

One or more behavioral indicators might include failure to thrive (in infants); poor learning; poor school attendance; falling asleep in school; chronic hunger or fatigue; begging or collecting leftovers or stealing other children's lunches; coming to school very early and staying inappropriately late; dull, apathetic appearance; engaging in vandalism; and engaging in sexual misconduct.

EMOTIONAL ABUSE

Emotional abuse is by far the most difficult to identify. The abuse or maltreatment may range from isolated situations to a lifelong pattern of destructive parenting. This child does not suffer the physical injury so often thought of as child abuse but incurs a mental injury that is cumulative.

The behavioral signs that give evidence of this type of abuse include hyperactivity or withdrawal, fire-setting, truancy or disciplinary problems, stuttering, enuresis, autism or failure to thrive, delinquency, psychosomatic complaints, aggressiveness, and suicide attempts.

Some environmental factors which may be related to emotional abuse are substance abuse, including both drugs and alcohol; disruption of the family unit, including frequent marriages, broken homes, continuous friction; inadequate parenting, including withholding love, inappropriate discipline, conflicting home values, discriminatory treatment of children, and immaturity of the parents. The child does not have the degree of self-esteem to withstand the stresses in these families and thus ultimately becomes the victim. The cumulative effects of this type of damage persist far beyond the limits of childhood years.

CHARACTERISTICS OF CHILD ABUSERS

The backgrounds of parents or individuals involved in child abuse share some similarities. They may have been unwanted as infants or young children. They may not have developed a sense of trust, a problem that will persist throughout their entire life. At a young age, they may have learned to "parent" their own parents in order to avoid being battered.

Most potential abusers learn to be self-reliant at a young age. This, in turn, tends to isolate them. This physical and social isolation interferes with their establishment of trusting relationships with others and so the isolative behavior persists. Having a poor sense of self-esteem, they usually select a mate who is of the same type. When both parents are unable to trust and support each other, the cycle is perpetuated. The child from such a union might be a wanted child, but it may be wanted for the wrong reasons. The parents may want the child so that the child can love them, rather than the other way around. This role reversal is very common in abuse situations.

This pattern is not limited to any one socioeconomic group. In fact, it pervades all levels of society. Child abusers from low socioeconomic levels may, however, be more visible than others because welfare and other social services mandate child abuse reporting. Individuals with higher incomes may seek the assistance of a private physician, and the cases may not be reported as accurately or as consistently.

Some other characteristics are also common to child abusers. Many lack control of their impulses. Others are action-oriented. The concept of "do it now" is foremost, and they would not necessarily anticipate the consequences or the harshness of the punishment of the child. Abusive parents are usually compulsive and rigid in their expectations regarding the child's performance or behavior. These expectations are unrealistic in terms of the child's developmental level.

Often, the object of the abuse indirectly contributes to the problem. Initially, parent-infant bonding may be weak or nonexistent. A premature infant who is initially somewhat isolated from the mother may be viewed as sickly, difficult to care for, and developmentally slow. Even full-term infants may be viewed as problems, particularly if they nurse poorly, cry more than they sleep, and are generally fussy. These children are incapable at this point of returning or bestowing the love that this immature parent is seeking. Any child who is viewed by the parent as being different, difficult to handle, or just plain "bad" has the potential for being abused. The combination of the parents' negative upbringing, their child's unique character and needs, and other social or economic pressures may ultimately result in a case of child abuse, Figure 17-5. In many families, the combination of drugs or alcohol, job instability or economic pressure, and isolation with no one to turn to for help or advice, contributes to the abuse situation.

ATTITUDES OF THE NURSE TOWARD ABUSE

In the hospital situation, the nursing care plan and the actual delivery of care have a two-pronged focus: the care of the child and the care of the parents. The care of the child should be marked by a positive attitude toward treatment of the child's injuries, an emphasis on decreasing the stress of hospitalization, a positive approach toward returning the child to a state of wellness, and an identification of ongoing needs that may be continued after the period of hospitalization.

The nurse's attitude toward the care of the child is most important. When initially confronted with the visible evidence of child abuse, the nurse's inclination or reaction may be an open display of anger and hostility toward anyone who might have been involved. The attitude of the nurse must, in fact, be just the opposite. In light of the devastating emotional impact of child abuse on everyone involved, nurses must first evaluate their

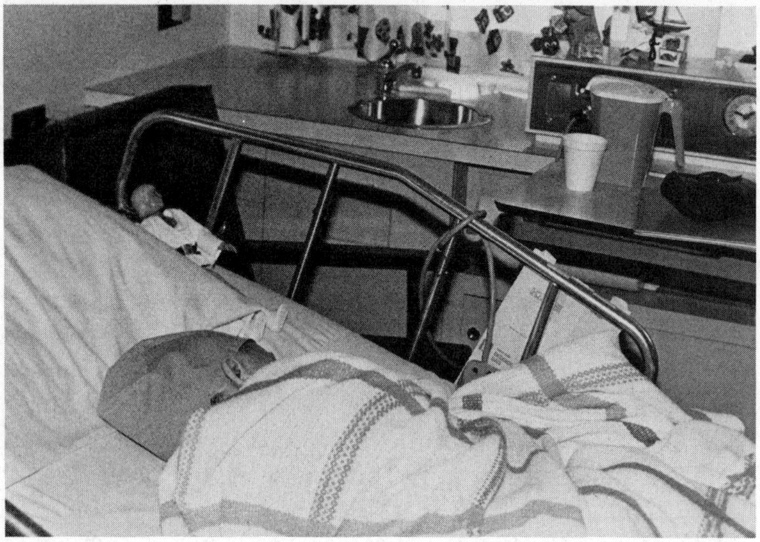

FIG. 17-5 This patient underwent a craniotomy following a skull fracture. The child refuses to interact with either adults or children.

emotional responses, objectively looking at their own attitudes and feelings and considering their validity, as well as their potential effect on the delivery of health care. They may then recognize that since a primary obligation in the care of any child is to preserve the family unit, if possible, punishment of the family or any of the individuals within it is counterproductive within the context of health care. A nonjudgmental attitude, therefore, must be fostered.

Anger and hostility toward the parents are not the only problems that may arise in abuse situations. These feelings are usually accompanied by a desire to compensate for the abuse by giving the child an extraordinary amount of attention. This overcompensation results in a failure of the nursing staff to set limits for the child. Ultimately, the child may be rejected by the nursing staff when he or she does not respond appropriately as the nurses expect.

This set of attitudes is sometimes referred to collectively as the rescue fantasy phenomenon. It has been described in many individuals working with families involved with child abuse. The health care worker's strong need to help people is in direct conflict with the incident of child abuse. The health care worker may begin to meet his or her own need to help without realistically considering the needs of the parents and the abused child. This rescue fantasy does not happen in all cases, but it should be recognized as an inappropriate, negative, and ineffectual way of dealing with the issue of child abuse.

Intervention with the Child

During the period of hospitalization, the abused child responds with behavioral patterns that have been learned elsewhere. The child may use very provocative behavior to gain almost continuous attention from staff members. This provocative behavior may become so irritating to staff members that they may wish to punish the child. It is not an isolated incident, but a repetitive pattern of response for the child. Such behavior may also be used in interaction with other children, often prompting those children to hit or hurt the abused child. If the behavior is ignored, the child usually tries harder to elicit a response from accessible adults.

The nurse should respond to the abused child with much warmth and affection, but limits must also be set. The child should know what behavior is acceptable and appropriate and what is not acceptable and for what reason. Throwing toys, for example, is inappropriate when they are directed at other children. A game that involves throwing a ball or a bean bag at a target uses the same energy and skills, but is a more appropriate outlet.

Nursing intervention should be planned and consistent. For this reason, the number of staff members caring for the abused child should be limited. These children may already demonstrate uncertainty in their interactions with adults other than their parents. Limiting the number of individuals who care for them promotes effective limit-setting and helps teach these children how to respond and behave appropriately.

Nursing intervention should also include ample opportunity for both the expression of feelings and the mastery of new behavior through play. Play should be both a positive and a pleasurable experience for the child. Depending on the child's age, an opportunity to play with other children should be provided, as should an opportunity to continue schooling if it is available. These opportunities may provoke intense negative feelings on the part of the child. During these times, the child should be removed from the group situation. It may only be necessary to draw the child aside to reassure him or her, or the child may have to be totally removed from the situation. Over a period of time, the nurses assigned to this child may be able to anticipate those situations that cause problems, intervening before the child acts inappropriately.

Decreasing the stress of the child's hospitalization is an ongoing process that begins with orientation to the unit and continues throughout the time of hospitalization, although with decreasing intensity. Both child and parents should be welcomed to the unit and oriented as any other family would be. Information may need to be repeated several times. The anxiety of the parents limits the amount of information that can be absorbed, and the age of the child may preclude his or her ability to absorb much more than the basics. A written booklet or form directed to the parents helps to reinforce this information and provides a ready reference for the parents.

Explanations should also accompany all procedures that are carried out on the child. The information should be appropriate to the child's age and developmental level. For abused children, unfamiliar procedures may be extremely frightening and overwhelming, particularly because they are performed by adults — the same age-group that inflicted the trauma. The nurse should allow ample time for an explanation, and should remain with the child during the procedure for reassurance, providing distraction or pleasant activities immediately afterward. Allowing abused children to participate in the procedure in some way may reduce their feelings of being victimized and may enhance their willingness to cooperate, particularly in such activities as whirlpool treatments for burns and dressing changes.

In planning the child's ongoing care following discharge from the hospital, it is important for the nurse to know whether the child will be returned home, or whether he or she will be placed in a foster home temporarily. The caregiver should be instructed in the physical care of the child, including bathing, feeding, dressing changes, and medications. This individual also should be prepared for the potentially regressive behavior of the child. They should know that this behavior is common with all hositalized children, and may involve disturbances of sleeping, eating, and behavioral patterns. The child, too, should be well prepared for discharge by the support team. This is particularly important when the child will be placed in a foster home. The child will have multiple fears and concerns regarding the temporary placement. The child should be helped to view the foster parent as a caring, supportive person, and should understand that this placement is not another punishment. This transition may be accomplished more easily if the foster parent visits the child in the hospital, or if a hospital staff member or social worker who has established good rapport with the child accompanies the child to the foster home initially.

WORKING WITH THE PARENTS

The nursing objectives for working with the parents include strengthening the parent-child relationship, providing a role model for alternative means of handling the child's behavior, and enhancing the identified parental strengths. These objectives overlap quite a bit and, as with the child, it is important that the contacts with the parents be both planned and purposeful. These contacts should be the responsibility of one or two staff members who have established a positive relationship with the parents and the child. Strengthening and supporting the positive aspects of the parent-child relationship requires careful, ongoing observation by the nurse. Initially, the parents may be angry, defensive, or mistrustful of staff members. It is the nurse's responsibility to provide the framework for developing a trusting relationship. This may be made more difficult by the large number of people with whom the family may have had contact. In many states, the disposition of child abuse cases requires that the parents have contact with many different individuals from the Children's Services division of the court, the police department, Social Services, and the hospital. Initially some parents avoid visiting the child because of guilt. The consistent, nonjudgmental support of one or two staff members usually helps the parents overcome this.

Parents should be made to feel comfortable on the unit and should have their questions answered. Time should be provided for them to obtain information regarding the child. It is important for the nurse to provide the parents with the same opportunity to care for their child as would be provided any other parent. This gives the nurse an additional opportunity to observe the parent-child interaction and to assist with the child's care.

Parents are seldom told what they do well. All too frequently, though, they are told what they are doing wrong. The nurse can strengthen the positive parenting practices observed, reinforcing them for the parent.

Parents must also be taught the behavior that is appropriate for the child's developmental age. It is included in the nurse's conversation just as it would be with any parent. The amount of teaching done in this fashion depends on the receptiveness of the parent. All such information should be presented in a nonjudgmental way, being careful not to imply that the parents' method of handling the child is incorrect or wrong. It should simply be presented by the nurse as another possible approach to the child.

In working with the parents, the nurse should keep in mind that this family needs help and that the abuse situation should not be dismissed lightly as a one-time occurrence. Over a period of time, the nurse may become aware of the various problems and needs that exist in the family and may tend to become sympathetic, rather than empathetic. It must be remembered that the parents or caregivers are not "bad," but that they need help. The nurse must be actively involved in seeing that they receive the necessary help.

As the time for the child's discharge approaches, the family may exhibit signs of increased stress and anxiety. Hospital discharge may mean the child's placement in a foster home rather than back in the parents' home. This plan may reinforce the parents' feelings of guilt and inadequacy. The nurse should allow the parents to express their feelings about what is happening. The child may demonstrate apprehension and fears of abandonment when placed in a foster home rather than returning with the parents.

THE HOSPITAL RECORD

The documentation of the individual incident of abuse usually initiates the hospital record. Included in this should be a factual description of the evidence of either abuse or neglect. The general appearance and emotional state of the child are included in this documentation. The parent-child interaction should also be recorded. Any explanations of the injury by either the parent or the child should be quoted if possible.

Specific documentation and descriptive charting avoids the subjective feelings of the staff member and is more acceptable in legal proceedings that may ensue. The child with failure to thrive should not be described as "small for age." A more appropriate method would be to list the height and weight, mark it on the grid of the growth chart, and include in the charting: "the child's weight and height are in the fifth percentile on the growth chart." Instead of saying the parent was angry with the child, describe the behavior or statement of the parent: "Parent sitting in child's room with back to child. Parent stated, 'you always cause me trouble!' as nurse entered room." Responses of the child to the care of the staff as well as participation by the parent should also be noted.

LEGAL ASPECTS

The legal aspects of child abuse relate directly to the Child Abuse Law which has been enacted by each state. The law establishes the criteria for child abuse and neglect and describes what constitutes violations under that state law. In most states, an abused child is one who is a victim of sexual activity; one who is endangered by cruel, excessive, or prolonged corporal punishment or discipline that creates a substantial risk of serious physical harm; or one who exhibits evidence of an injury or death, not considered accidental, that is inconsistent with the history. The Child Abuse Law applies to individuals younger than eighteen years of age, as well as to those who are younger than twenty-one years of age and are mentally or physically handicapped.

The obligation for reporting suspected cases of child abuse lies with individuals who are considered to be professionals, as well as those individuals employed in or by agencies that care for children. This includes physicians, nurses, clergy, employees of day care centers, among others. The report of suspected child abuse must be made to the Children's Services section of the County Welfare Department or to the local police department. A telephoned report may be made, but it should be followed by a written report. Within the hospital situation, nurses should follow the administrative policy established for reporting child abuse.

The report should include the name and address of the child and the names and address(es) of the parents or the person who has legal custody of the child. The child's age and the nature of the injuries or physical neglect should be included in the report. It is also helpful to note any evidence of previous injury or neglect. Any information regarding the cause of the abuse, or information that might be helpful in establishing the cause, should also be included. This report only indicates the possibility of abuse or a suspicion. The legally empowered agency then investigates to confirm or deny this suspicion.

These reports are considered to be confidential. The person reporting the abuse is immune from any civil or criminal liability for making the report. The law usually requires the agency to investigate every report in conjunction with the local law enforcement agency within twenty-four hours.

At the hearing, the person who filed the report may be called to testify. Precise and objective documentation is critical. The nurse in the hospital situation should remember that all nursing observations are extremely important, as is careful charting. The hospital record may be subpoenaed by the court and the information it contains may be decisive in determining the disposition of the case and the fate of the child.

Failure to Report Abuse

Occasionally, health care workers may not report child abuse, or may delay making the report. Usually, these individuals are those who are working in the community with families. Reasons for the delay may include a fear of being physically harmed by angry parents, difficulty in separating personal from professional responsibilities, a need to be liked by the client, denial of responsibility, or dissatisfaction with the disposition of previous court cases. These are all reasons for, but not excuses for, failing to meet one's professional responsibilities in an appropriate fashion.

Any individual who fails to report child abuse is subject to both a fine and a possible jail sentence. This is the prescribed penalty for a fourth-degree misdemeanor.

Because of a report of child abuse or of care administered during a child's hospitalization, the nurse may be called to court to testify. This may be either in juvenile or civil court. The only facts addressed are those that were directly observed. A nurse working in the area of child abuse may be called as an expert witness because of the knowledge and expertise acquired in this area.

Prior to the court appearance the nurse should review the medical record to refresh the memory of the incident. Notes should be made on pertinent information which can be taken to the hearing.

The questions directed to the nurse should be answered as carefully and specifically as possible. Professional terminology should be avoided if possible or, if used, clarified when giving answers.

Maintaining a calm manner is important even when cross-examined. Any display of anger or strong emotions tends to discredit whatever testimony that was given.

SUPPORT GROUPS

Parents Anonymous

One group that provides services to parents who have abused, or who fear they might abuse, their children is Parents Anonymous. This organization is structured into small, self-help groups. The chairman of the group is an individual who currently has or has had a child abuse problem. Each group has a professional sponsor who participates in the meetings and is available to the members when needed.

The philosophy of the organization is the belief that all humans can change and grow. Group members learn to support each other, to help other members recognize positive parenting practices in their lives, and to provide alternative families and support systems for the members. These groups do not, however, take the place of individual or family counseling from a professional person.

SCAN

SCAN, Inc. or Supportive Child-Adult Network is a multidisciplinary treatment team working with child abuse. It is located at the Children's Hospital of Philadelphia.

It provides for decision making, information sharing, and support by a team of professionals from more than one discipline. The advantage to the family is that there is a choice of workers; this enhances the establishment of a therapeutic relationship.

SUMMARY

In cases of child abuse, the nurse should not only know how to provide good nursing care to the child, but also how to deal effectively with the parents. This requires the use of appropriate techniques for intervention, as well as modeling alternative behaviors for the parent.

Nurses should be aware of their own feelings and attitudes toward the child and family so that they can deal effectively with them and approach the family in a nonjudgmental fashion. Along with this awareness of attitudes, nurses must be able to identify the socioeconomic conditions that may have precipitated the child abuse incident.

SUGGESTED ACTIVITIES

- Invite an individual from the Children's Services division of the county welfare agency or a protective services agency to speak to the class about working with families involved with child abuse.
- Attend a group meeting of Parents Anonymous in your area. Share with your class the goals of the group and the method by which an abusive or potentially abusive parent might join.
- Together with your class, stage a role-playing session that involves the interaction of a nurse, an abused child, and an abusive parent. Identify the attitudes that are displayed and determine their effect on the delivery of health care.

DISCUSSION TOPICS

1. Share with your class two or three cases of child abuse reported in the local newspaper. Discuss your feelings about what happened to the child.
2. Discuss appropriate methods of discipline that might be used for a toddler, a preschooler, and a school-aged child.

3. Determine the method used for reporting child abuse in your city. Describe the reporting procedure of the health agency to which you are assigned.
4. Discuss the various types of provocative behavior that may be displayed by a hospitalized abused child. Describe an appropriate nursing response for each type of behavior identified.

REVIEW

A. Matching. Match the description of abuse in Column I with the type of abuse in Column II.

Column I	Column II
1. Malnourished and poorly cared for	a. Physical abuse
2. Positive smear and culture for gonorrhea	b. Neglect
3. Burns on buttocks from hot water	c. Sexual abuse

B. Multiple choice. Select the one best answer.

Situation: George is a four-year-old victim of abuse who is admitted to your unit with a fracture and multiple skin abrasions. His language is verbally abusive to the staff as he demands constant attention.

1. The nurse's approach to George and his abusive parent should include
   a. open anger and hostility toward anyone involved in the abuse.
   b. rigid control of parent-child interactions on the unit.
   c. an implication that George could be removed from the home.
   d. nonjudgmental support of both parent and child.
2. The nursing care of George should include
   a. a demonstration of warmth and support, as well as setting of limits.
   b. allowing George free rein in his activities on the unit.
   c. giving George constant attention.
   d. ignoring George's verbal abuse toward the staff.
3. In the hospital setting, child abuse cases are reported to the
   a. medical staff.
   b. social service department.
   c. nursing director.
   d. hospital administrator.
4. Professional individuals are responsible for reporting child abuse in the community as well. It is reported to the
   a. city's Board of Health.
   b. Crippled Children's Association.
   c. Children's Services division of the welfare department.
   d. Children's Bureau of the Department of Health, Education, and Welfare.

C. Short answer. Briefly respond to the following statements.

1. List five signs of child abuse that would be evident on physical assessment.
2. List three of the inappropriate beliefs that abusive parents may have about their children.

BIBLIOGRAPHY

Besharov, D. "Building a Community Response to Child Abuse and Maltreatment." *Children Today,* Vol. 4 (September–October, 1975), pp. 2–4.

Broadhurst, Diane D. "Update: What Schools Are Doing About Child Abuse and Neglect." *Children Today,* Vol. 7 (January–February, 1978), pp. 22–24.

Copans, Stuart, et al. "The Stresses of Treating Child Abuse." *Children Today,* Vol. 8 (January–February, 1979), pp. 22–27.

Duryea, Perry, et al. "Child Maltreatment: A New Approach in Educational Programs." *Children Today,* Vol. 7 (September–October, 1978), pp. 13–16.

Flanzraich, Mark, and Irene Dunsavage. "Role Reversal in Abused/Neglected Families: Implications for Child Welfare Workers." *Children Today,* Vol. 6 (November–December, 1977), pp. 13–15.

Josten, L. "The Treatment of an Abused Family." *Maternal-Child Nursing Journal,* Vol. 4 (Spring, 1975), pp. 23–24.

Leaman, Karen. "Recognizing and Helping the Abused Child." *Nursing 79,* Vol. 9 (February, 1979), pp. 64–67.

Leistyna, Joseph A. "Advocacy for the Abused Rural Child." *Children Today,* Vol. 7 (May–June, 1978), pp. 26–27.

Ludwig, Stephen. "A Multidisciplinary Approach to Child Abuse." *Nursing Clinics of North America,* Vol. 16 (March, 1981), pp. 161–165.

Neill, Kathleen, and Carole Kauffman. "Care of the Hospitalized Abused Child and His Family: Nursing Implications." *Maternal-Child Nursing Journal,* Vol. 1 (March–April, 1976), pp. 117–123.

Olson, R. "Index of Suspicion: Screening for Child Abusers." *American Journal of Nursing,* Vol. 76 (January, 1976), pp. 108–110.

Scharer, Kathleen M. "Rescue Fantasies: Professional Impediments in Working with Abused Families." *American Journal of Nursing,* Vol. 78 (September, 1978), pp. 1483–1484.

Whiting, Leila. "Defining Emotional Neglect." *Children Today,* Vol. 5 (January–February, 1976), pp. 2–5.

Chapter 18

Health Care Problems

OBJECTIVES

Upon completion of this chapter, the student will be able to

- describe the proper assessment for each of the diseases discussed.
- identify nursing measures that are appropriate to the care of children with these illnesses.
- describe the dietary modifications that are instituted in children with respiratory problems and celiac disease.

The major focus of this chapter is respiratory disease because of its high incidence in toddlers. Long-term problems, such as cystic fibrosis and celiac disease, are also included. The malignant diseases that affect this age-group include Wilm's tumor and neuroblastoma. Diseases involving the special senses may not be recognized in this age-group until the child's communication abilities and mobility develop further.

ACUTE RESPIRATORY INFECTIONS

Respiratory infections are common occurrences in young children. The symptoms are often relatively mild and, if no complications arise, the child may be treated successfully at home after being examined at a clinic or in a physician's office. Because of the continuous nature of the mucous membranes throughout the system, the infectious process is not isolated to a single area of the respiratory tract. The term upper respiratory tract infection refers to those that involve the nose and pharynx, such as nasopharyngitis or the common cold. Lower respiratory tract infections affect the epiglottis, larynx, trachea, bronchi, and lungs.

Organisms that cause respiratory problems in children may be either viral or bacterial. Respiratory infections caused by viruses generally have a gradual onset, whereas those caused by bacteria arise more suddenly. The bacteria that are of greatest concern are the streptococcal organisms that are so abundant in the winter and early spring. Group A beta-hemolytic streptococcus is the organism that is responsible for rheumatic fever and nephritis. For this reason, throat cultures should be done in all children with pharyngitis in order to identify the organism and to eradicate the streptococcus before damage is done.

Nasopharyngitis

This infection, which is relatively common in young children, is caused by viruses to which the child has little resistance. Upon initial viral invasion, an inflammatory response occurs in the upper respiratory tract, causing copious amounts of clear drainage. When there is an invasion of bacteria, often the normal flora of the respiratory tract such as streptococcus, staphylococcus, or pneumococcus, the drainage becomes purulent.

The typical symptoms of nasopharyngitis in the child include an elevation of temperature to between 101°F and 102°F, anorexia, malaise, and cough. Young children may also develop vomiting and diarrhea. On physical examination, the child's throat is red and infected, the cervical lymph nodes are swollen, the nasal passages are congested, and the nose is completely obstructed, causing mouth breathing, Figure 18-1.

The treatment of the child is symptomatic. Antipyretics, decongestants, and antibiotics are commonly used. Without treatment, the infection can extend throughout the respiratory tract, requiring hospitalization of the child for care and treatment.

Croup or Acute Spasmodic Laryngitis

Inflammation of the larynx, causing a partial or complete respiratory obstruction, is

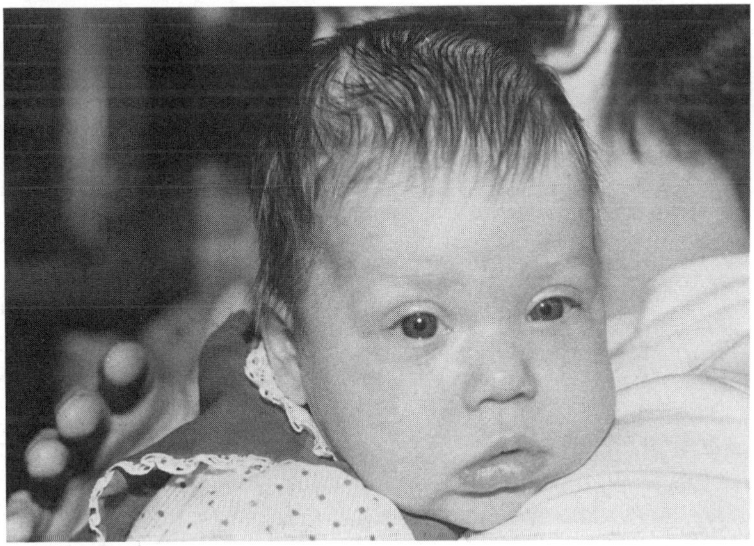

FIG. 18-1 Nasopharyngitis in this child is manifested by watery eyes and mouth breathing.

the most serious problem in croup. Croup is marked by a sudden onset of dyspnea, usually at night, and a barking cough. Onset often follows a mild upper respiratory infection or an episode of chilling. Stress and the child's response to it may also play a part.

The appearance of children with croup suggests suffocation. They are usually orthopneic, refusing to lie back because of the respiratory distress. Their voices are hoarse. Inspiratory stridor is audible, and a frequent, harsh, and barking cough is evident. On examination, other signs of respiratory distress, such as nasal flaring, retractions, cyanosis, and altered vital signs, are noted. The retractions are evident in the supraclavicular, substernal, and intercostal areas. Cyanosis is obvious in the nail beds, while observation of the mouth area reveals circumoral pallor. The child's temperature is elevated to about 101° F and the pulse and respiratory rates are also elevated.

The treatment involves reducing the laryngeal spasm with high humidity. Steam rooms, mist tents, ultrasonic nebulizers, and vaporizers can all be used to relieve the spasm and to liquefy the secretions, Figure 18-2. Cool mist is preferred. Emetics, such as Ipecac Syrup, may be used to reduce the laryngeal spasm and to cause the child to expel large amounts of the tenacious mucous secretions by vomiting. In the hospital setting, periodic treatments with intermittent positive pressure breathing and two percent racemic epinephrine may be instituted to alleviate the respiratory distress. Tracheotomy may be performed in some situations, but is less common because of the availability of other methods of treating the child's distress.

Acute Laryngotracheobronchitis

LTB

Laryngotracheobronchitis, which is often confused with croup, is an infection that in-

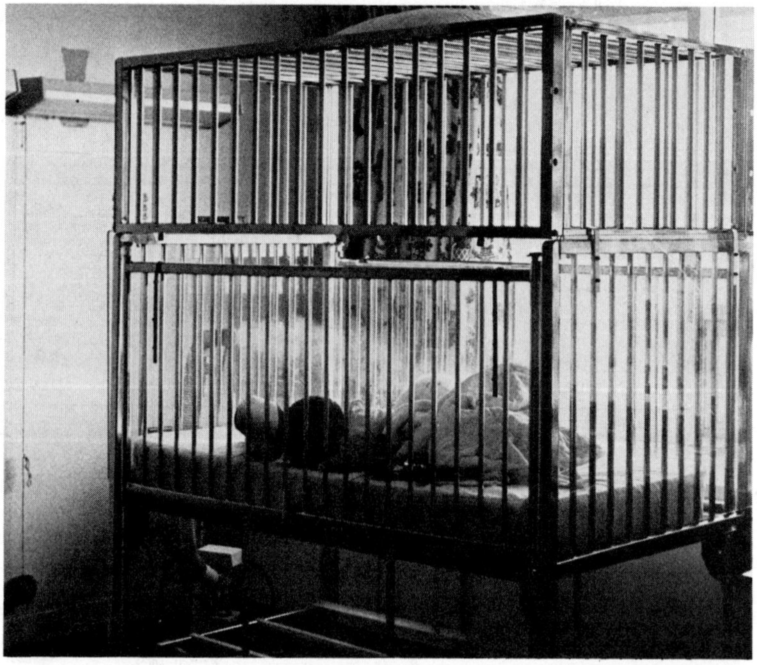

FIG. 18-2 This croupette is constructed of Plexiglas panels that line the outside of the crib. An ultrasonic nebulizer attached to one panel provides humidity.

volves the larynx, trachea, and bronchi. Affected children are prostrate with an acute infectious illness that is usually caused by *Hemophilus influenzae* or a hemolytic streptococcus. Staphylococcus or pneumococcus may also be the causative organisms.

This infection may or may not be preceded by an upper respiratory illness. Affected children are acutely ill with a temperature as high as 105°F, severe dyspnea, and minimal coughing. On assessment, an inspiratory wheeze or stridor may be audible which usually indicates obstruction of the larynx. As the infection extends to the bronchi and bronchioles, the wheezing becomes expiratory as well. On auscultation, breath sounds may be diminished or absent, indicating a large area involved with thick exudate, as well as the reason for the severe dyspnea. Nasal flaring, retractions, and hoarseness or aphonia may be present.

Antibiotic therapy is administered on the basis of culture and sensitivity studies. High humidity is necessary to loosen the secretions and oxygen is required to improve the respiratory exchange. Children with laryngotracheobronchitis may require digitalization because of cardiac failure. Until the child's status improves, fluids are administered intravenously to maintain adequate hydration and to facilitate administration of antibiotics, Figure 18-3. Tracheostomy or intubation may be necessary to maintain a patent airway.

Epiglottitis

Toddlers or preschoolers who are brought to the emergency room with a history of sudden onset of stridor accompanied by a high fever, drooling, and prostration show the classic signs of epiglottitis. This is an acute pediatric emergency.

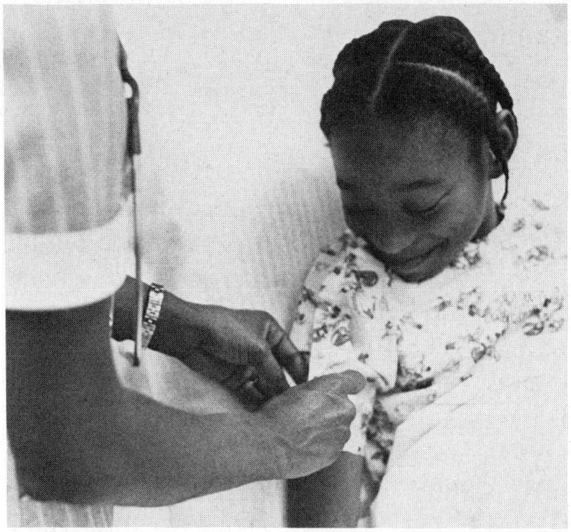

FIG. 18-3 Discontinuation of an intravenous line often brings relief and pleasure to the patient, as is obvious from this young girl's facial expression.

Because of the speed with which respiratory obstruction can occur in these children, the nurse should recognize this emergency problem promptly. Affected children should remain in an upright position, preferably on the parent's lap. Respiratory rate and quality are observed without handling the child. **Caution: No procedure that would cause the child to cry or to become upset in any way, including monitoring of vital signs, is initiated.** This also includes any examinations of the pharynx. (In many areas, this is referred to as a "no touch protocol.") Any incident that causes tears, or any change in the child's position that allows recumbency, will alter the position of the inflamed and edematous epiglottis and may cause obstruction of the airway.

The child is taken to a minor surgery room where, after induction of light anesthesia, the epiglottis is examined. If indicated, the child is intubated or a tracheostomy is performed. The child is then transferred to an intensive care setting.

Pneumonia

Pneumonia in toddlers is usually caused by pneumococcal or staphylococcal organisms. The disease is most prevalent in late winter and early spring. The child with pneumonia is acutely ill, with a rapid temperature elevation to 104°F or 105°F, dyspnea, and a nonproductive cough. The areas of involvement in the lungs may be identified by auscultation. The presence of rales should be noted along with gas exchange and any areas of consolidation.

X-ray studies are obtained to confirm lung involvement. Culture and sensitivity studies of the nose and throat, as well as of the sputum samples, help to identify the invading organism so that appropriate antimicrobial therapy may be started. A complete blood count usually reveals an extreme elevation of the white blood cell count (up to 35,000 or 40,000 per cubic millimeter).

Treatment involves appropriate antibiotic therapy, oxygen with humidity, and antipyretics. Analgesics may be effective in children with pleuritic pain. Hydration may be maintained orally, or intravenously if the child cannot consume an adequate amount. Complications, such as paralytic ileus and tension pneumothorax, can develop in these children. The nurse should be alert to this possibility.

Nursing Care of Children With Respiratory Infections

The care of children with respiratory infections depends on the severity of the illness. Many such children are cared for in the home if a responsible person is present to institute appropriate measures with the physician's supervision. Any child with signs of respiratory distress, however, is admitted to the hospital. The nursing care of children with respiratory infections has four main goals:

- to maintain an adequate air exchange
- to promote adequate hydration
- to control the body temperature
- to provide comfort

Maintenance of Adequate Air Exchange. Maintaining an adequate air exchange in children with respiratory infections often involves the use of a croupette, oxygen tent, or an ultrasonic nebulizer. Any one of these devices provides the child with a cool environment that is high in humidity.

It is essential that the nurse make careful and frequent assessments of the child's respiratory status. Frequent monitoring of vital signs and pertinent, close observation will prevent severe respiratory distress. The child who is increasingly restless may not be cyanotic, yet may require intubation or a tracheostomy. Cyanosis is a late sign of decreasing oxygen levels and rising carbon dioxide levels.

The symptoms of the child are very important in assessing the respiratory status. Cough, stridor, dyspnea, restlessness, and pallor all indicate decreasing levels of oxygen. A rising respiratory rate is evidence of the child's need for oxygen. The late signs of air hunger, cyanosis, and exhaustion provide stark evidence of the rising levels of carbon dioxide. At this point, the pulse rate begins to rise, the child develops respiratory acidosis, and respiratory arrest and death may ensue. Particularly in cases of croup and epiglottitis, the child's condition may deteriorate rapidly to a state of respiratory acidosis.

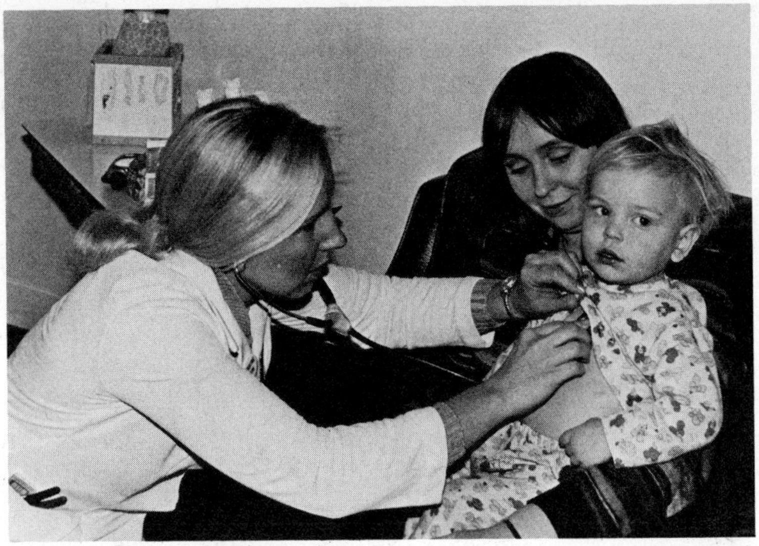

FIG. 18-4 Assessment of breath sounds is an important aspect of care for the pediatric respiratory patient.

When assessing the child for respiratory distress, the nurse should direct attention to three specific areas: the nares, the chest wall, and the abdomen, Figure 18-4. With normal respirations, there is no visible flaring of the nares, the respirations are quiet, the movements of the upper chest and abdomen are synchronized, and there is no evidence of any retraction. In children with moderate respiratory disorders, the nares flare slightly, the upper chest lags on inspiration, xiphoid retractions in the lower chest are evident, and an expiratory grunt is audible with a stethoscope. In cases of severe respiratory distress, the child's nares flare markedly, seesaw movements of the chest and abdomen are apparent, marked retractions are noted in the xiphoid, supraclavicular, and intercostal areas, and an expiratory grunt is audible.

Positioning of the child to promote adequate air exchange varies with the child's age. Young infants should be positioned on their sides with their heads slightly elevated by adjusting the frame of the bed. This allows for adequate expansion of the lungs and minimal compression from abdominal contents. This side-lying position also promotes drainage of secretions from the nose and mouth. This is extremely important in this age-group as the high humidity liquefies secretions that the infant is unable to handle. Older children usually find a semi-Fowler's position to be comfortable. They should be supported in this position and proper body alignment maintained. It is important to ensure that this position is changed often in order to facilitate proper lung expansion.

Postural drainage may be used both in the home and in the hospital as an aid in the removal of secretions. In the hospital setting, it is usually the responsibility of the respiratory therapy department. If it is to be carried out in the home setting, someone in the home must be taught the correct procedure. The nurse involved in the care of pediatric patients should know how to carry out this procedure, as well as how to answer questions regarding it, Figures 18-5 through 18-8.

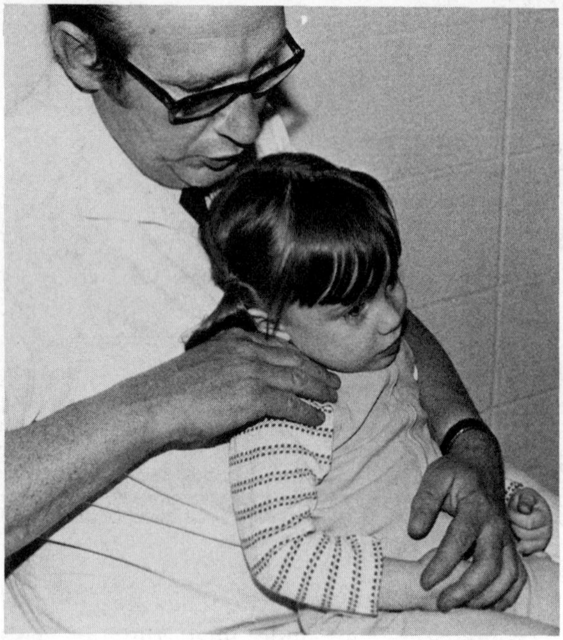

FIG. 18-5 This child is leaning approximately 30° backward while in a sitting position. This promotes drainage of the anterior apical segment of the right lung.

Conservation of energy also has an effect on maintaining adequate air exchange. Children with respiratory problems should not be allowed to exert themselves in any way. They should be handled as little as possible. In the acute phase, the number of procedures performed should be kept to a minimum. These children are often given small amounts of sedatives, such as phenobarbital, to promote rest. Narcotics are contraindicated because of respiratory depression. If these children are sleeping, they are not awakened for routine checks. The parents or some other significant person should be present continuously, if at all possible, to reduce the possibility of crying, as well as to allay the child's fears. During this early period, intravenous fluid therapy may also obviate awakening the child.

Hydration. The second goal involves promoting adequate levels of hydration. Because of illness and discomfort, children with respiratory

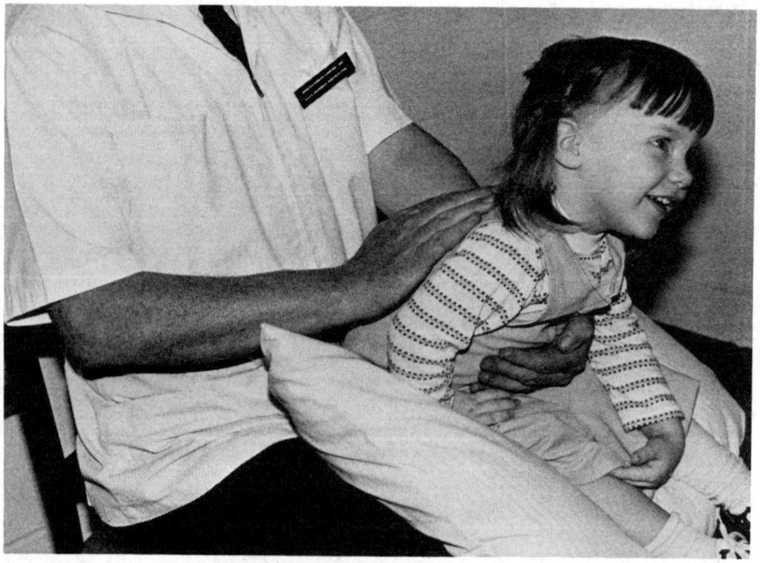

FIG. 18-6 Drainage of the posterior apical segment is promoted.

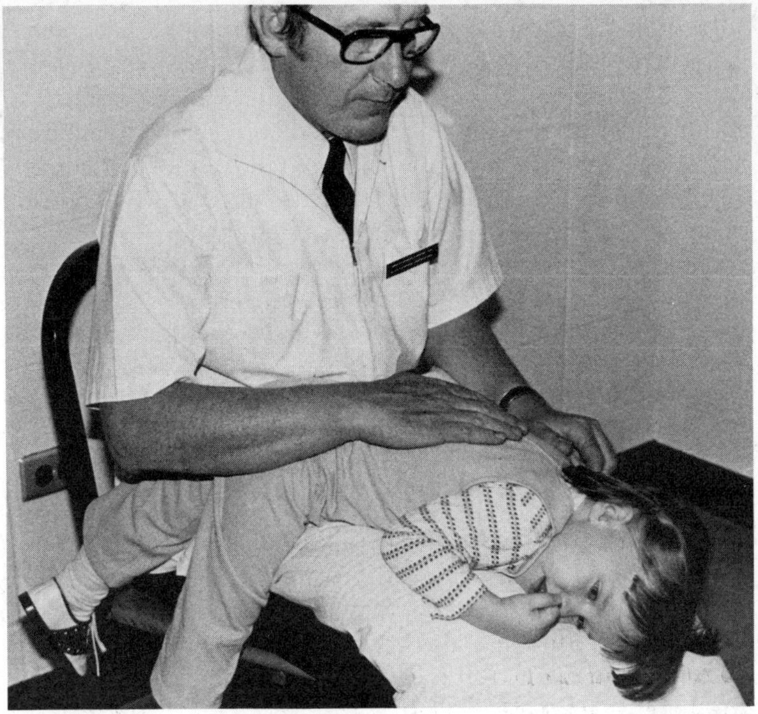

FIG. 18-7 Drainage of the right middle lobe of the lung is accomplished with the head tilted 30° downward. The pillow allays the child's fear of falling.

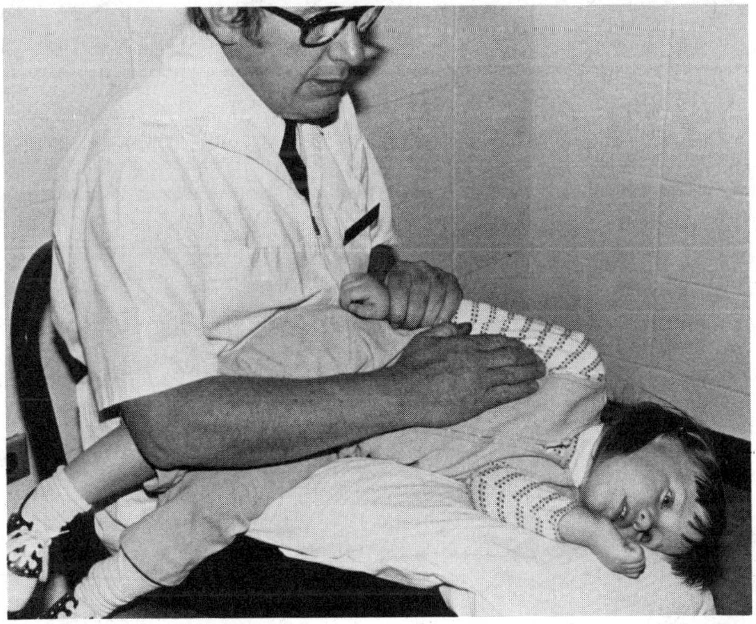

FIG. 18-8 This position allows drainage of the dorsal segment of the lower lung lobes.

infections often refuse any oral fluids or may only take sips of the liquids offered. The rate of fluid loss secondary to the child's rapid respirations, increased metabolic rate, and copious secretions far outweigh the intake. For this reason, fluids are usually administered intravenously at first in any child who is sick enough to require hospitalization for the respiratory illness. The volume of fluids administered over a twenty-four-hour period is usually one and a half times the normal maintenance volume. As the child's condition improves, this volume is reduced and the child is encouraged to take more fluids orally.

Initially, the liquids offered should be clear, such as strained fruit juices, carbonated beverages, or flavored gelatin water. They should be encouraged but not forced. Popsicles made of fruit juice may also be used to increase the child's intake. As the child improves and the appetite increases, milk shakes and eggnogs may be added to the diet if full liquids are permitted. These liquids are avoided initially because of the increased production of mucus that often occurs with the consumption of milk products.

Maintenance of an accurate intake and output record is essential in evaluating the adequacy of the liquids ingested. Parents are usually more than willing to help keep track of the child's intake, as well as the volume voided.

Because of the illness, the child's appetite is often depressed. This brief period of anorexia is seldom long enough to cause serious problems with the child's nutritional status. However, if the child had severe nutritional problems prior to the illness, other forms of nutritional therapy may be necessary to return the child to an optimal nutritional state. In this situation, predigested protein supplements may be used.

Temperature Control. The third goal of nursing care of the child with respiratory illness is control of the body temperature. Fever is a component of all of the respiratory conditions discussed. The severity of the temperature elevation varies with the problem. However, with any respiratory disease, the child's temperature can change rapidly. The nurse should be prepared for possible febrile convulsions in any child with a high temperature, and should take measures to reduce the child's fever. The child should wear light clothing and be covered lightly with a sheet rather than with blankets. The room environment should not be overly warm. Ventilation should be adequate, but drafts should not be allowed to blow across the child.

Antipyretics may be administered to the child as often as every four hours. It is important to teach parents how to administer an accurate dose of either the tablets or liquid suspension. If the tablet form is issued, parents should know how to dissolve or crush the tablet for young children in order to prevent aspiration. Older children may either chew the tablet or swallow it. At least one-half glass of water should be taken with the tablet to ensure adequate dissolving.

Cooling sponges may also be used to reduce the child's temperature. The nurse should use tepid water to sponge the child's body, making sure that the child is protected from too rapid chilling and drafts. Sponging should be discontinued if the child begins to shiver. Parents should be taught how to do this at home.

Comfort. The fourth goal of care for children with respiratory infections is the provision of comfort. The two most common areas of discomfort for this child are the nose and the throat. The nasal obstruction is most distressing to young children as it interferes with drinking from a bottle or a cup. Nose drops are often administered to alleviate this. For instillation of the drops, the child should be positioned horizontally with the shoulders elevated on a blanket roll to allow the head to fall back. This position is maintained for a minute or two after the drops have been administered. When using nasal sprays, the child should be in an upright position. Otherwise, the child receives a much larger dose of spray than intended. If possible, nasal sprays should be administered fifteen to twenty minutes prior to feeding times for the greatest benefit.

Throat discomfort is often relieved by the same medication given to control the fever. Other measures that provide relief include gargling (if the child is old enough), drinking cool liquids, and using topical sprays for the throat. Throat sprays may provide some relief but they also may interfere with the child's eating as they may also numb the tongue.

ASTHMA

Asthma is one of the most common pulmonary diseases caused by an allergic response. It is included in the group of allergies that account for one-third of the chronic conditions seen in children and adolescents. Mortality is low, but the morbidity of the disease is quite high, involving between two and three million children according to the U.S. Department of Health and Human Services.

The term allergy relates to the ability of an antigen to stimulate production of an antibody. Such antibodies are from the IgE class of immunoglobulins. These immunoglobulins attach themselves to the cell surface of both basophil and mast cells. When antigens interact with these antibodies, several types of chemical mediators are released. The most familiar of these mediators is a substance called histamine. Through some mechanism in certain individuals, the production of IgE is not maintained at normal levels but is synthesized at abnormally high levels. The sudden release of even small amounts of histamine as a response to an antigen stimulates an allergic response in the individual.

Allergic diseases are commonly thought to be inherited, although the exact mode of transmission is unclear. The form the allergic response takes in various family members may be different but the process is the same. Sensitive individuals react to a protein or a polysaccharide molecule. Antigens may be derived from varied extrinsic sources, including animal dander, pollen, parasites, food, mold, and insects. When both parents have allergic responses, their child has a seventy-five percent chance of becoming allergic. If only one parent is allergic, the possibility decreases to about sixty percent for each child.

Assessment

History. An accurate and detailed history should be included in the nursing assessment of the asthmatic child. This helps to identify the potential allergens and other stresses that may add to the child's problem. The nurse should first investigate the family history. What allergies do other family members have? Is anyone in the family sensitive to particular foods or medications? Does anyone have a history of hay fever, hives, or eczema?

The parents or child may be aware of particular situations or circumstances that contribute to the allergic symptoms. Does the problem occur in a particular season? House dust and molds or spores may create problems during the winter, whereas pollens and grasses may precipitate asthmatic attacks in the spring and summer. Does the attack follow exposure to aerosol sprays that might be used to propel paint, deodorizers, or perfumes? Do the symptoms occur following an infection? Do certain medications, such as aspirin or antibiotics, cause the symptoms or make them worse?

The nurse should encourage the parent to describe the child's past and present history in detail, beginning with the infancy period. Were there any medical problems associated with the mother's labor and delivery? Was the child breast-fed or bottle-fed? What type of formula was used if the child was bottle-fed? Were there any episodes of allergic problems as an infant, such as diarrhea from milk intolerance, eczema, or colic?

Determining the onset of the allergic symptoms is the nurse's next responsibility. The parents should be asked to describe the onset of the symptoms as completely as possible. This information should include the symptoms first noted by the parents, the time of day, and the environment the child was in at the time. The nurse should review the common allergic symptoms in the various systems and ask the parents specifically about the presence or absence of these. Have the parents noted excess tearing or itching of the eyes? Does the child sneeze or have coldlike symptoms that affect the nose? Does the child cough frequently, wheeze, or have difficulty breathing? Do skin irritations or hives occur frequently?

Attention should also be directed toward the child's environment. The location of the house in relation to industries or undeveloped areas, the presence or absence of pets, and the type of furnishings in the child's room are all important considerations.

For the child who has been treated in the past for the problem, the nurse should determine what actually was done for the child. What was included in the treatment? Was the child given prescription medications? Were they effective? Was skin testing done? Was the child given a course of desensitization therapy? Was an elimination diet prescribed? If so, what was the child permitted to have?

Physical Examination. In observing the child, the nurse should look for signs that indicate the presence of allergy in children. The "allergic salute," or the pushing of the palm of the hand upward on the tip of the nose to open the air passages, is frequently observed, Figure 18-9. In the same child, the nose may show a crease from the frequent "saluting." Dark circles around the eyes and frequent throat clearing are other signs of allergy. Paroxysms of sneezing, usually upon awakening, may also be noted. Inspection of the mucous membranes of the nose will reveal them to be pale and swollen. The skin should be inspected for a maculopapullar, erythematous, or pruritic rash. The most common sites are behind the knees and at the bend of the elbows. In the case of food allergies, the tip or the edge of the tongue often has shiny bald patches that are surrounded by an elevated "pearl" border. This is properly termed geographic tongue. Open-mouthed breathing and a V-shaped palate may also be seen in these children.

Laboratory Studies. Initially, the laboratory studies include a complete blood count. The total and differential white blood count is of significance because of its correlation with in-

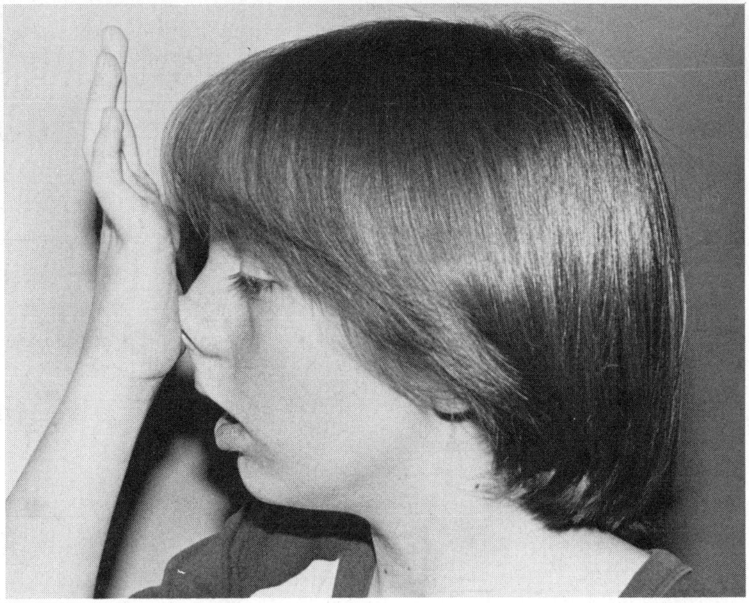

FIG. 18-9 The "allergic salute" is commonly used by allergic children to temporarily reduce the upper airway obstruction.

fection, as well as with signs of allergic response. In children with a history of inhalant allergies, a nasal smear is done to check for eosinophils. An allergic response is documented in the presence of greater than ten percent eosinophils.

Sinus and chest radiographs, as well as pulmonary function studies may also be performed depending on the type of allergy.

Skin Testing. Skin testing is a diagnostic tool used to confirm the allergens that have been identified through the patient's history. It is also used to determine appropriate concentrations for the course of immunotherapy to be used.

The cutaneous method of skin testing (the scratch or prick method) is done on the child's back. It involves the scratching of a small area of the epidermis with a needle or lancet and the subsequent application of an allergen extract to each scratch site. The sites are arranged in rows with a small space between rows so that the allergens can be identified. The prick method involves the application of a drop of the extract to the skin and subsequent pricking of the skin surface.

Erythema and wheal formation indicate a positive reaction. Positive reactions occur within ten to thirty minutes. The severity of the reaction does not necessarily correlate with the severity of the child's symptoms. When a significant skin reaction occurs, the extract is wiped off and an anti-inflammatory ointment is applied. Positive reactions may persist for up to twelve hours. In a few children, a delayed reaction may occur one to two days later. This should immediately be reported to the physician.

Intracutaneous or intradermal testing are also done. They involve the use of the volar surface of the child's arms. An allergen extract, in a strength of 1:1000, is administered in a dose of 0.02 milliliter. **Caution: During any skin test, the child should never be left unattended**

because of the potential risk of systemic reactions. If systemic reactions occur with the intracutaneous testing, a tourniquet is applied to the arm and aqueous epinephrine in a strength of 1:1000 is administered.

The nurse should clarify any medication orders prior to the skin testingprocedure. Some physicians and clinics prefer that antihistamines be withheld for three to five days prior to the testing. This restriction does not apply to bronchodilators that are used to treat asthmatic children. These medications are usually administered routinely until the day of the test. They are then withheld until the skin testing is completed.

One additional test may be ordered for the child. This is the radioallergosorbent test (RAST). It measures the quantity of IgE present in blood serum. It can also determine the quantity of antibodies produced in response to a specific allergen. The disadvantage of the test is its high cost (about $5.00 per test for each allergen). Its advantage is that it may be used in an acutely ill child in whom skin testing would be hazardous.

Treatment

Once the allergens have been identified, the treatment plan can be instituted. It includes food diaries and elimination diets, immunotherapy to produce hyposensitization, and environmental control. Each of these methods requires the full cooperation of the parent, as well as of the child. Hospitalization is necessary for acute attacks.

Food Diary. A record of everything that is eaten and what happens afterward should be kept for the child with identified food allergies. A repetitious pattern may emerge, identifying specific substances that cause problems. Ingestants that may cause problems include cow's milk, wheat, chocolate, eggs, seafoods, and drugs, such as aspirin and antibiotics.

Elimination Diet. The elimination diet is one in which all known offenders are removed for a period of two weeks. After that time, the foods are again introduced, one at a time, usually at four-day intervals. Any worsening of the child's symptoms would indicate that the substance is a possible allergen. The same items are retested to confirm that they provoke the allergic response in the child.

Immunotherapy. Immunotherapy is used to reduce the child's sensitivity to an allergen if it cannot be eliminated or controlled in the environment. It is a long slow process of injecting small quantities of allergens in increasing strength until the patient develops a tolerance for the substance.

The substance for the serial injections is prepared specifically for each child and is kept refrigerated. A tuberculin syringe is used. The upper arm is the preferred site of injection. Air is not added to the vial to prevent oxidation of the substance. The initial dose is usually 0.05 milliliter of a 1:100,000 strength solution and the amount is increased by 0.05 milliliter each week. If a local reaction larger than a nickel occurs, the dose is maintained at the same level the following week.

The child is observed closely for any signs of a systemic reaction, such as itching of the head, palms, or soles of the feet; sneezing; laryngeal edema; or shock. If such a reaction occurs, a tourniquet is placed above the injection site. Epinephrine in a strength of 1:1000 and a dose of 0.01 milliliter per kilogram of weight is given. One-half the dose is given into the same arm as the injection site. The remainder is given into the opposite arm to counteract the systemic reaction. It is for precisely this reason that these injections are administered in settings where emergency equipment and a physician are available.

Environmental Control. The concept of environmental control is very broad in children. It includes desensitizing the child's room and the home as much as possible. It also includes protecting the child from exposure to infections, as these often precipitate allergic responses in many children.

When discussing environmental controls with the parents, the subject should be presented in as positive a manner as possible. These are steps the parent can take to reduce the child's exposure to allergens. They do not mean that the child will never become ill, as some parents might believe.

In considering the child's room, special attention is given to anything that catches and holds dust. This includes items like upholstered furniture, shag rugs, feather pillows, and stuffed animals. Wall hangings or ornaments are also eliminated. All furnishings should be either wood or metal. The clothing in the closet should be in current use with nothing stored. The mattress and box springs should be covered with an allergy-proof covering. All blankets and bedding should be washable synthetics or cotton blends. All washable items should be laundered every few weeks to eliminate dust collection.

Initially, the room is cleaned from top to bottom, with particular attention directed toward moldings, lights, shelves, and closets. The outlets for the heating system in the room should be sealed. With forced air heat, it may be preferable to cover the vent with a filter that is changed every one to two weeks. The room is damp-dusted on a daily basis.

Live pets, with the exception of those from the reptile and fish families, are unacceptable to these children because of their sensitivity to animal dander. Asthmatic children should also avoid exposure to other children's pets if at all possible.

Medication. A number of medications may be used in children with asthma. These include epinephrine hydrochloride for the acute wheezing attack, theophylline preparations, cromolyn sodium for prophylactic use, and corticosteroids. The use of these drugs must be considered individually in light of the child's increased susceptibility to infection, the level of growth and development, and the necessity for careful monitoring to avoid toxic reactions.

During an acute wheezing attack, the drug of choice is epinephrine hydrochloride (1:1000) in a dose of 0.01 cubic centimeter per kilogram injected subcutaneously. Administration of this drug according to the physician's order can usually be repeated twice at twenty-minute intervals after the initial dose.

Theophylline and ephedrine preparations are usually given to the child at the onset of a respiratory infection because these so often lead to acute asthmatic attacks. Effective therapeutic doses of theophylline may be very close to the toxic level. For this reason, blood levels must be checked. The child's metabolic requirements change with maturation and the theophylline dose is usually decreased at about nine years of age. Toxic reactions to this drug include nausea, vomiting, diarrhea, headache, and, possibly, seizures. Aminophyllin is often administered intravenously in acute attacks.

Caution: Cromolyn sodium is never administered to patients in the midst of an acute

attack of asthma with sneezing. It has no intrinsic anti-inflammatory or bronchodilating effect. It prevents exercise-induced bronchospasm, however, as it inhibits the release of histamine. The dosage is one 20-milligram capsule used with a special inhaler two to three times a day to control the symptoms. The nurse must emphasize to the child's parents the necessity of continuing this drug to prevent acute episodes. The parents also need to know that the drug is not effective if the capsule is swallowed, as it will not dissolve.

Corticosteroids may also be used selectively in some patients. They are for short-term use during an acute attack. Prednisone may be used in a dose of 2 milligrams per kilogram per day, given in three divided doses. Any long-term use of the drug requires a slow, tapered withdrawal to avoid adrenal problems. A short course over a period of two to three days does not require this tapering. Its undesirable systemic side effects account for the cautious dispensation of the drug. Aerosol inhalations of steroids carry less risks of side effects. Live vaccines are not administered to the child during this course of therapy. Barbiturates also are not given during this time as they diminish the full effect of the steroid.

Behavioral Considerations

Several behavioral considerations must be dealt with in children having a long-term chronic problem such as asthma. During this entire process of identifying specific allergies and developing a treatment plan, the child should be included and information shared at the child's level. Emphasis should be placed on positive measures that can be taken to reduce the incidence and severity of the attacks.

The identified restrictions, whether a particular food, a type of pet, or a certain activity, should be minimal. Children should know about these if they are old enough to understand, but the restrictions should neither rule their lives nor alter their self-concepts.

In sharing information about immunotherapy, children should know that it is an injectable medication. It is also important that they know that each injection teaches their bodies how to act when the allergen is present. The use of puppets, with Mr. Allergen as the bad guy, is often an acceptable and effective means for conveying the message about immunotherapy.

Older children should be encouraged to maintain contact with their peer group and to socialize as before. The need for identification with the group is especially strong. Alternatives may have to be considered when a child cannot participate in an activity. Again, emphasis should be placed on what can be done, rather than what cannot be done. The nurse may facilitate acceptance of such limitations by exploring the child's interests and encouraging those activities that are within the child's physical abilities.

Support Groups

Agencies that provide information regarding allergies include the American Lung Association, the Allergy Foundation of America, and the National Institutes of Allergy and Infectious Diseases (part of the National Institute of Health). There are regional or local chapters of the American Lung Association. The Asthmatic Children's Foundation, headquartered in Ossining, New York, has nineteen residential-treatment facilities in the United States and Canada, for children with severe, long-term disease.

CYSTIC FIBROSIS

Cystic fibrosis is a disease of the exocrine glands which is inherited through an autosomal trait. Both parents must be carriers for the disease to be transmitted. The disease varies in severity among those affected, with minimal involvement in some children and severe involvement from the time of birth in others.

Symptoms

The basic defect in cystic fibrosis is obstruction of the exocrine gland ducts. The major areas of involvement in the gastrointestinal tract are the salivary glands, pancreas, biliary system, and small intestine. The damage to the pulmonary system occurs in the bronchi, bronchioles, paranasal sinuses, and the entire mucociliary transport system. The problem involves abnormal mucus, bronchospasm, edema, and inflammation in the airway structures. The combination leads to stagnant, viscid mucus which obstructs the airway and provides a perfect media for infection. Treatment is aimed at interrupting this cycle to prevent the tissue damage that will otherwise occur.

The earliest signs of the disease are present in neonates and represent involvement of the gastrointestinal tract. Meconium ileus occurs in five to ten percent of the infants with cystic fibrosis. It is suspected early in the postdelivery period because of the failure of the infant to pass a meconium stool. Other signs in the infant include abdominal distention and vomiting. It is surgically correctable.

Later in the infancy period, the child may show signs of failure to thrive or a malabsorption syndrome. These children have ravenous appetites, but appear to be pale and undernourished and have protuberant abdomens. Obstruction of the pancreas eliminates the necessary digestive enzymes. Less than sixty percent of the ingested food is used. On inspection, the child's stools are large, bulky, foul-smelling and often have obvious fat globules on the surface. Steatorrhea occurs as a result of the lack of protease, amylase, and lipase. These children do not have the loose, watery stools that are characteristic of various forms of diarrhea. Other gastrointestinal symptoms include hypoproteinemia with edema and rectal prolapse.

The pulmonary manifestations of the disease begin with obstruction of the bronchi and bronchioles. This process causes areas of atelectasis, uneven ventilation, and impairment of the mucociliary transport mechanism. As this process recurs and tissue damage increases, trapping of air and overinflation of the lungs occur. These signs are evident in certain physical changes in the child's appearance, such as an increase in the anterior-posterior diameter of the chest, a flattening of the diaphragm on radiographic examination, and a hyperresonance on percussion of the chest wall. Ultimately, the child develops the barrel-chested appearance that is typical of individuals with chronic obstructive lung disease.

Signs of respiratory involvement in young infants include the presence of a dry, hacking cough. This changes to a chronic, more frequent, productive cough in older children. An increased respiratory rate, poor exercise tolerance, anorexia, and wheezing, which is common with infection, may also be noted. Infants with repeated respiratory infections should be evaluated for cystic fibrosis.

Diagnostic Tests

The diagnosis of cystic fibrosis is based on the abnormal salt loss demonstrated by a quantitative method of the sweat test. The method of choice is the Gibson-Cooke method whereby a small area of the skin surface is stimulated with pilocarpine and the sweat is collected. The exact quantities of sodium and chloride are then determined through iontophoresis. This particular method has been in use since 1959. (The previously used palm print test was a screening test that did not identify quantities of sodium and chloride.) Sodium levels greater than 70 milliequivalents per liter and chloride levels greater than 60 milliequivalents per liter are considered to be diagnostic. The normal level for both substances is less than 40 milliequivalents per liter. Any child whose test results are between the normal and diagnostic levels should be retested.

Other diagnostic tests include stool analysis to detect the presence of pancreatic enzymes and the amount of fat. Chest X-rays and pulmonary function studies are done to determine the extent of pulmonary involvement. The diagnosis is then made on the basis of the family history, abnormal laboratory findings, and the chronic pulmonary and gastrointestinal pathologic processes.

Medical Treatment

Once the diagnosis of cystic fibrosis has been made, the parents and child should become involved in a comprehensive program of care and education designed to help them deal with their lifelong problem. An individualized program is set up for each child. The program takes into account the manifestations of the disease in the child and the educational needs of the parents and child. Initially, this is accomplished in a hospital setting as a follow-up to the diagnostic evaluation.

Children with pulmonary involvement are started on a program of postural drainage and exercise, treatment with medication, and mist tent therapy. Postural drainage and percussion are used prophylactically, as well as therapeutically, to remove the thick, viscid mucus. This regimen is carried out two to four times a day, depending on the program, Figures 18-10 and 18-11. Most of the routines include the use of mist and a bronchodilator approximately one-half hour before postural drainage to improve its effectiveness.

Medications included in the treatment of the pulmonary manifestations of cystic fibrosis include the previously mentioned bronchodilators. These are usually administered through nebulization. Antibiotics are used to treat infections. They are seldom used on a continuous basis. In some children, they, too, are administered in an aerosol form. Expectorants may be given to these children, but higher-than-normal dosages may be required. Antihistamines or steroids are used in children with additional allergy-type problems.

Aerosol or mist tent therapy for these children aids in liquefying secretions. Ultrasonic nebulizers are most effective in reducing the size of the droplet particles so that they can enter the alveoli rather than just saturate the bronchi. In the past, all of these children slept and napped in mist tents. Although this method is still used, the implementation of the mist treatments have changed somewhat. Oxygen is used along with mist, for acute care in the hospital setting.

Treatment of the gastrointestinal problems involves dietary control, as well as some supplementation. The diet is high in carbohydrates as these are best tolerated, high in protein to supply growth needs, and restricted in fats. Pancreatic enzymes, such as pancrelipase (Cotazym and Pancrease) or pancreatin (Viokase), are given with each meal. Both powder and capsule forms for older children are available. Supplementation of fat-soluble

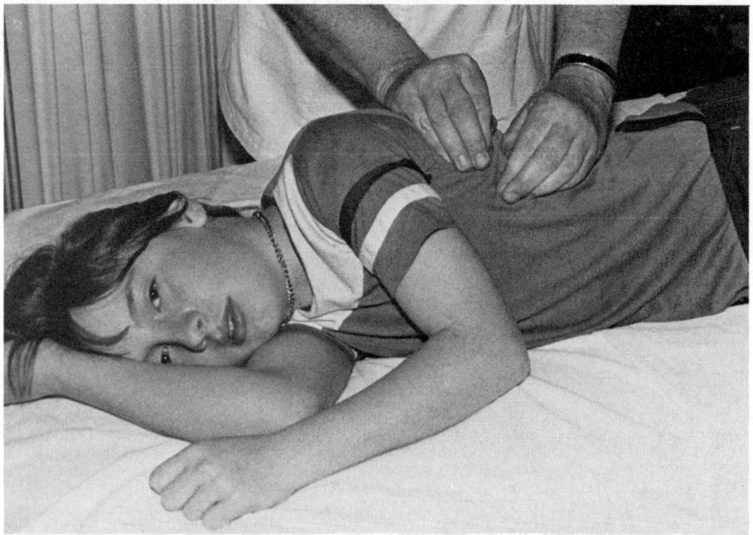

FIG. 18-10 The parents can be taught the appropriate positions for postural drainage to be carried out at home. Here, the position for the left middle lobe is modified slightly.

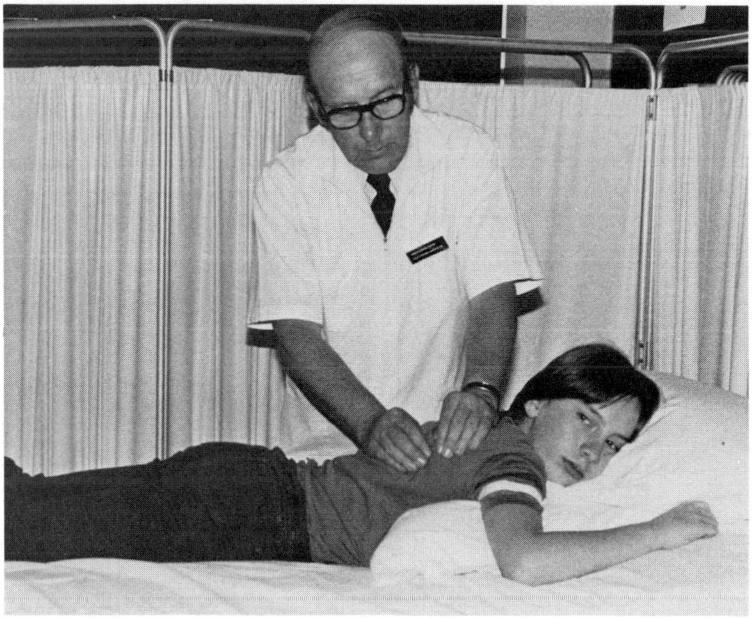

FIG. 18-11 The posterior segment of the right upper lobe is drained while the patient is positioned on pillows.

vitamins A, D, E, and K is also necessary. These are given in a water-miscible form. During hot weather, additional supplementation of salt is necessary. If the child is still being fed formula, one without butterfat such as Progestimil or Portagen is preferred as it is more easily digested.

Nursing Care

During the initial phase, the care of the child with cystic fibrosis differs somewhat from the follow-up care that is given on a routine basis. At the outset, the nurse is usually part of a multidisciplinary team that is involved in the care and education of the parents and child. During that initial period, the parents are trying to cope with all the details of the involved treatment of the child while they are absorbing the full implications of the diagnosis itself. The implications of a genetically transmitted disease are far more complex than those of an isolated acute illness.

The nurse should encourage an open discussion of the parents' feelings about the disease. What comes forth from the discussion most often is a feeling of guilt for having "given" their child something they never intended. Parents and relatives should know that the disease is not inherited from one side of the family or the other, but that both parents transmitted the trait. This trait cannot be detected until a child is recognized as having the disease. Genetic counseling is essential for these parents.

Some parents experience a sense of relief when the diagnosis is confirmed. Often, they have suspected something was wrong for some time. This is particularly true of parents with other children who have developed a basic knowledge of normal development and behavior.

Parent groups may be helpful in providing support for the parents by allowing them exposure to a wide range of feelings and concerns identified by parents whose children have the same disease.

As these children grow, the nurse should encourage them to assume more responsibility for their care. The frequency of their hospitalization, the restrictions on some of their activities, and the daily regimen of medications may lead to strained relationships with their peers and siblings. They should be encouraged to find and develop areas of skills that are compatible with their condition and in which they can excel.

Some long-term concerns for this child involve procreation. Sterility in both the male and female can occur as a result of obstruction rather than hormonal factors. Young people should know that this does not affect masculinity or femininity. Pregnancy, however, with its normal stresses on pulmonary function, may be a real problem for a young woman with cystic fibrosis.

Support Groups

Agencies that provide education, research, and support for families affected by cystic fibrosis are the local chapters of the National Cystic Fibrosis Foundation. Assistance with job training skills for adolescents or young adults may also be obtained through the Bureau of Vocational Rehabilitation.

CELIAC DISEASE

Celiac disease is often called gluten-sensitive enteropathy, which describes exactly what the disease involves. Affected children show signs of malnutrition and deficiency diseases.

Other signs include stunted growth, wasted extremities, distended abdomen, irritability, and behavioral changes.

On assessment, the nurse will note poor skin turgor, a large amount of gas in the distended abdomen and watery, foul-smelling stools. Stooling occurs frequently. The child is pale in appearance and quite irritable. Bruising of the skin from a vitamin K deficit may be evident. Hypoproteinemia also occurs in these children.

Treatment

The treatment for children with celiac disease is primarily dietary. The gluten portion or protein fraction, gliadin, of wheat, rye, barley, and oats is eliminated from the diet. The child is permitted proteins, a small amount of fat, and carbohydrates containing monosaccharides or disaccharides. Polysaccharides or starches are forbidden. Initially, because of poor weight gain and protein deficiency, this child is given 6 to 8 grams of protein per kilogram of body weight. Other supplements include water-soluble vitamins A, D, E, and K.

Implementation of the diet does not bring about an immediate cure of the symptoms. Improvement is a gradual process that will be evident in two to six weeks. The first signs in order of appearance are improved appetite, a decrease in stools to near normal, and a gradual weight gain.

Nursing Care

The difficulties encountered by parents in caring for an irritable, fussy baby, are immediately apparent to the nurse. Babies with celiac disease are seldom satisfied by the food that is offered. Whatever is ingested causes abdominal discomfort and frequent stools. Initially, during the period of hospitalization, food may be withheld. This further increases the child's irritability. When foods are reintroduced, they are usually not what the child is accustomed to eating.

The nutritionist is the one who teaches the parents about the dietary restrictions for this disease. However, the nurse should also know what is restricted and what is allowed in order to reinforce this information for the parents. Parents must be taught to read ingredient labels very carefully, as many items may contain small amounts of wheat flour. Rice and rice flour, although more costly than other flours, are permitted for the child. Treats, such as cookies, that are commonly given to children must be avoided unless they are made specially with rice flour.

If there are other children in the family, difficulties may arise with the accessibility of restricted foods. Some families affected by celiac disease find it easier to restrict the whole family to breads, desserts, and other preparations made with rice flour than to constantly single out the child whose intake must be restricted.

Liberalization of the diet usually is effected during the late school-age period or during adolescence. Previously restricted foods are gradually reintroduced into the diet with sufficient time in between to determine the child's tolerance. If this liberalization is done too early or too rapidly, the disease may occur again, even in adulthood.

URINARY TRACT INFECTIONS

UTI

Urinary tract infections can occur at any time in the child's life cycle. However, they are most common in the late toddler and early preschool period in female children. This does not mean that male children do not have these infections, but the ratio of female to male children with urinary tract infections is approximately 30 to 1. The major structural difference that may explain the higher incidence in girls is the length of the female urethra, which is less than 2 centimeters long.

Other problems that ultimately lead to urinary tract infections in children include anatomic abnormalities. Obstructive lesions may occur at the ureteropelvic or the ureterovesical junction. The presence of vesicoureteral reflux forces bacteria-laden urine back to the kidney, with potential scarring and increased damage.

Symptoms

Children with urinary tract infections may have very vague symptoms. The typical symptoms of dysuria, frequency, and urgency may not be present, or may be caused by perineal irritation rather than a urinary tract infection. Common symptoms in a young child include fever, hematuria, and enuresis. Vomiting and abdominal or flank pain may also occur. The urine may be described by the parents as very concentrated, musty, and odorous.

Diagnostic Tests

The method of urine collection for urine culture and sensitivity testing is of the utmost importance in the positive identification of an infection. In young children, a clean, voided urine specimen is obtained by cleansing the perineal area carefully and then applying a sterile urine collection bag. In older children who are toilet trained, a midstream specimen is preferred. The perineal area is cleansed with soap or benzalkonium chloride (Zephiran) and then rinsed thoroughly with sterile water. The child is then asked to void. The initial portion of the voided urine is discarded. The urine for the specimen is then obtained from the midstream of the voiding. It is important to attempt this procedure when the child has not voided for approximately one hour or the bladder may not be sufficiently full to obtain a specimen.

In some situations, catheterization may be required to obtain urine for culture. A sterile technique and the smallest possible catheter are used to minimize trauma to the urethra. Again, the initial portion of the specimen is discarded and the middle portion of the specimen is sent for culture and sensitivity. It is important to remember that any form of instrumentation, such as catheterization, can predispose a child to subsequent urinary tract infection, even when one did not already exist.

Characteristic findings in the urine of a child with a urinary tract infection include a high bacteria count and the presence of abnormal elements. The bacteria count is considered diagnostic of a urinary tract infection when it contains more than 100,000 bacteria per milliliter. This count may not be valid if the specimen was allowed to remain unrefrigerated for a long period, enabling the bacteria to multiply. Red blood cells may be present in the urine as well as casts which indicate an infectious process within the kidney itself. In most of the children, there is a decreased ability of the kidney to concentrate urine.

Other diagnostic tests may include an intravenous pyelogram (IVP) to detect structural abnormalities as well as functional problems. A voiding cystourethrogram (VCUG) may be performed to detect evidence of reflux. Surgical correction such as a urethral reimplantation or a ureteroneocystostomy may be required for obstructive anomalies.

Treatment

Treatment involves the use of an antibiotic to which the infecting organisms are sensitive. Oral forms of sulfisoxazole, ampicillin, nitrofurantoin, and amoxicillin are commonly used. Treatment is continued for ten to fourteen days. A repeat urine culture is done after two to three days of treatment to determine the effectiveness of the antibiotic. These cultures are then repeated one week and six weeks after the antibiotic therapy is discontinued. Follow-up cultures may then be done at three-month intervals for the next year or, in some children, even longer.

Nursing Care

Nursing care of the child with a urinary tract infection includes both the care given during the acute phase and the preventive health teaching thereafter. During the acute phase, it is important for parents and children to understand the need for careful specimen collection, as well as the rationale for any diagnostic tests. Parental participation in care is helpful to children, particularly since they usually have just completed or are completing toilet training.

The recording of intake and output is essential in this situation. Enlisting the help of the child and parents in this recording ensures its accuracy. A visual record, such as a star for every glass of liquid consumed, offers encouragement to the child to drink an adequate amount as well as to record it accurately.

Preventive teaching primarily involves good hygiene. Careful cleansing of the perineum from front to back in girls is a must after toileting. Use of bubble baths and perfumed soaps in the tub should be discouraged. Underwear should be of the absorbent cotton variety rather than nylon or other material that allows moisture to accumulate and provide a better growing media for organisms. Daily changes of underclothing are also necessary. Encouraging the child to void every two hours rather than waiting for longer periods prevents accumulation of large amounts of bacteria-laden urine in the bladder. Adequate fluid intake is also important. Such preventive measures will not eliminate infections that are caused by anatomic obstructions to flow. However, they will help maintain the body's natural defenses against infection.

NEUROBLASTOMA

Neuroblastoma is a tumor that arises from the adrenal medulla or from the chain of sympathetic ganglia. It may be intrathoracic, cervical, or pelvic. It is one of the few tumors which may be present at birth. About twenty-five percent of these tumors are discovered before the child reaches one year of age. The remainder are usually identified before the age of five years.

Initially, the tumor is encapsulated. However, neuroblastoma spreads rapidly and usually metastasizes before the primary tumor has been recognized. Metastasis is to the liver, bones, and lymph nodes, as well as to the adjacent tissues and the viscera.

Symptoms

Children with neuroblastoma are acutely ill. Their temperature is elevated, hypertension is present, and hepatomegaly is also evident.

They may complain of bone and joint pain. Many of these children have exophthalmos and severe ecchymosis in the periorbital area. Lymphadenopathy is present in the cervical and axillary areas. The child looks pale, feels ill, and has usually lost weight prior to admission. The abdominal mass in these children is irregular in shape and extends across the midline.

Diagnostic Tests

Diagnostic evaluation includes a complete blood count including platelets, a bone marrow aspiration, a radiographic survey of the long bones, and a twenty-four-hour urine screen for catecholamines (VMA). This neoplasm frequently metastasizes to the bone and its marrow. The catecholamine levels are elevated.

Treatment

Treatment involves surgery, irradiation, and chemotherapy. During surgery, all or part of the neoplastic mass is removed. The operation is followed by irradiation and the use of chemotherapy. The drugs of choice for chemotherapy include vincristine, cyclophosphamide, dactinomycin, and dacarbazine. In some children, spontaneous remissions have been documented.

Nursing Care

Nursing care for this child involves preparing the child and the parents for the diagnostic tests that will establish the diagnosis, as well as the treatment regimen that will be instituted if the diagnosis is confirmed. The feelings of the parents at this time, which may include grief, anger, and despair, should be recognized and accepted.

Physically, the child requires comfort measures to reduce pain, careful monitoring of the elevated blood pressure, and maintenance of an adequate fluid and food intake. Careful handling and positioning of the extremities in a neutral position, as well as the use of analgesics, are important. Parents should be taught how to lift and move these children, as well as how to position them to reduce pain. Parents should know the chemotherapeutic agents that will be used, as well as their side effects. Parents need a great deal of support and encouragement from the nursing staff when caring for their child, as they must deal with their own feelings about this potentially fatal illness, at the same time they are providing support for their child.

NEPHROBLASTOMA

Nephroblastoma, or Wilm's tumor as it is more commonly called, arises in the kidney as an encapsulated mass of abnormal epithelial tissue. Its growth may begin in utero or after the birth of the baby. It is one of the most common neoplasms present in early life. Two-thirds of the cases occur before the age of three years.

The tumor may expand, causing the connective tissue capsule to rupture. However, the mass is not palpable beyond the midline of the abdomen. The lungs are the most common sites of metastasis, which occurs via the renal vein or the lymphatic system. For this reason, palpation of the abdomen is avoided in this child once the tumor is identified.

Symptoms

The child who is admitted with a diagnosis of Wilm's tumor seldom appears to be ill. The symptoms are usually related to pressure of the expanding tumor mass, and may include anorexia and constipation. Medical attention may be sought as a result of the parents' observation that the child's abdomen is increasing in size or that his or her clothes no longer fit. On palpation of the abdomen, the physician notes a smooth, encapsulated mass on one side of the abdomen.

Diagnostic Tests

The diagnostic evaluation for nephroblastoma includes an IVP, a twenty-four-hour urine collection for catecholamine screening (VMA), a bone marrow aspiration, and a long bone survey. The IVP shows the distortion of the renal pelvis and caliceal system. The bone marrow aspiration and bone survey, as well as the urine screen, are done to rule out the presence of neuroblastoma.

Other tests which would aid in the diagnosis include a complete blood count, blood serum electrolytes, and kidney and liver function studies.

Treatment

The treatment of this condition involves surgery, irradiation, and chemotherapy. A radical nephrectomy, with removal of the ureter to the bladder and the perirenal fat, is performed. The renal vein is ligated carefully before the tumor mass is handled. The chemotherapy of choice is dactinomycin or vincristine. Some surgeons administer one-fifth of the total dose during surgery and the remaining four-fifths at scheduled intervals postoperatively.

Irradiation is used to eliminate any sites of metastasis. The side effects of this are numerous as irradiation of the growth centers of bones causes growth suppression. Bone marrow depression can also occur. The child's gonads are shielded during the radiation therapy to prevent sterilization.

In this particular condition, the younger the child, the better the survival rate. This is because the tumor appears to be more susceptible to the chemotherapy, and less time has elapsed to permit metastasis. Two-year survival after treatment is considered to be curative for this disease.

Nursing Care

The preoperative nursing care given the child is the same as for any other child with two exceptions. First, palpation of the abdomen is avoided because of the possible seeding of the tumor cells. The second exception involves the recognition of the malignant nature of the tumor itself.

In working with parents postoperatively, the nurse should be prepared for the intense feelings generated by the diagnosis. These are often further intensified by the child's response to the radiation and the chemotherapy. Even when prepared for the side effects, parents are often upset by the child's lethargy, nausea, alopecia, and weakness. The parents need consistent support and frequent reminders that the treatment is necessary in order to eliminate any residual cells and to prevent recurrence or metastasis.

DISORDERS OF THE SPECIAL SENSES

Problems with sight or hearing are causes for concern in children because of the limitation of sensory input that accompanies distortions of vision or sound. Children learn through their experiences in the environment. To limit the sensory input is to limit or impede the learning that takes place.

Otitis Media

Otitis media is an infection that affects the middle ear. It occurs most commonly in young children because of the short, wide, and straight nature of their eustachian tubes. It usually occurs as a sequela of an upper respiratory infection.

Symptoms. At first, the inflammation causes obstruction of the eustachian tube. This is followed by the formation of a serous exudate in the middle ear and infection. A high fever (about 104°F) and pain are the characteristic symptoms. Older children may complain of a sharp pain in the ear. In younger children, pain may be demonstrated by their irritability and restlessness. Young children may or may not pull at their ears or rub their heads as they lack the ability to discriminate pain loci.

Assessment. Otoscopic examination of the ear reveals slight bulging of the eardrum, disappearance of the landmarks, and distortion or absence of the light reflex. Drainage is present only if the tympanic membrane was ruptured. If it is present, a culture should be done.

Treatment. Treatment involves warm applications to the ear, administration of antibiotics, and sometimes, the use of nasal sprays or decongestants. Analgesics and antipyretics may also be used. Decongestants may help to shrink the mucous membrane and allow for drainage through the eustachian tube.

Nursing Care. Nursing care for this child involves reducing the child's temperature and providing comfort measures until the antibiotic takes effect and the pressure on the middle ear is reduced. The child with recurrent infections of the middle ear should be referred to a specialist for evaluation.

Chronic Infections. With chronic infections or the development of a serous exudate in the middle ear, the child's hearing may become impaired.

A myringotomy and insertion of ventilating tubes are used to correct chronic accumulations of fluid in the middle ear. For children with possible hearing impairments, a number of other diagnostic tests may be done. Audiometry, using pure tone air conductive stimulation, can be done. Tympanometry may be performed to identify the limited mobility of the tympanic membrane. It is a more sensitive indicator of slight changes in hearing acuity and can also be used to evaluate the effectiveness of the ventilating tubes.

Visual Disorders

In children, visual impairment may result from congenital problems, such as cataracts or amblyopia; the retinopathic effects of other diseases, such as sickle cell or diabetes; maternal infections, such as rubella; prematurity; retrolental fibroplasia; and iritis secondary to juvenile rheumatoid arthritis. Visual problems are not always easily detected in children, especially in younger ones.

At the time of birth, the eyes are immature as a result of their short diameters and small size. For the infant, clear vision is only achieved at very close range. As the infant grows, the eye increases in size and the skills needed for normal vision improve. Normal accommodation and refraction are present in the beginning school years between the ages of five and six years. This does not mean, however, that the child's visual acuity should not be tested earlier. The child should have good coordination of eye movements at the end of the first year of life.

It is important to identify visual disorders in children as early as possible to prevent sensory deprivation and the resultant loss of abilities already achieved. Two factors have a key role in the adaptations made by the child with visual loss. One of these factors is the rate of progression of the disease. The child whose problem is relatively stable or changes very gradually has time to make adjustments and to adapt to the changing visual acuity. In contrast, the child who sustains a rapid loss of vision, such as from a traumatic injury, does not have the opportunity to use this coping ability. The second factor is the age at which the visual loss occurs. In very young children significant visual impairment may go undetected until the problem is quite severe. For the purposes of education, such children are often placed in classes for the visually impaired. They are considered to have a congenital disorder simply because it occurred prior to school entry.

For those children with decreased acuity of vision rather than complete loss of vision, a number of visual aids may be helpful. Increased magnification is important, particularly for the skills of reading, writing, and mathematics that are learned in the early years. Good lighting enhances the benefits of magnification for the child. Other optical aids, such as a video magnifier, large-type materials, and writing guides assist the children in learning and using their abilities to the fullest.

In the hospital setting, it is important for the nurse to include questions regarding vision when performing assessments. These problems must be detected early and assistance offered to the child. In children with a known visual impairment, the nurse should identify any adaptations of the environment that are required to allow the child to function at a maximal level. Careful orientation of the child to the surroundings is critical. Maintaining consistency in the environment is also important. Parents provide much support for the child, but may not be present at all times. In their absence, the nurse should know how to adapt the care to meet the child's special needs.

Other sensory stimulation should be provided in the hospital setting. The nurse may read to these children as well as play tapes and records for them. The talking books program is available for individuals with visual loss through most libraries. Tape recorders, record players, and radios provide auditory stimulation. In conversations with the family, it is important to talk with these children, rather than talking about them in their presence. They should be allowed to touch and feel objects in order to facilitate their orientation.

Agencies that can be of assistance to the family include the regional offices of the American Foundation for the Blind, as well as Centers for the Visually Impaired.

SUMMARY

A wide variety of conditions affect toddlers. The acute forms of respiratory distress caused by partial obstruction are some of the most serious. Careful assessment is the key to survival in many of these situations. Children with allergies or asthmatic problems have both acute and chronic respiratory problems. These conditions require ongoing identification, hyposensitization and treatment.

Initially, children with cystic fibrosis and celiac disease are much alike in that failure-to-thrive symptoms are the first signs of both disorders. Once the diseases are identified, however, the treatment is divergent.

Neuroblastoma and Wilm's tumor are both malignant neoplasms that affect children. Surgical excision, radiation therapy, and chemotherapy comprise the treatment regimen for both of them. Survival rates are best in younger children.

Impairment of the special senses is another major problem that can occur in young children. Not only is the sense that is lost of concern, but also the learning or perception that does not take place because of the impairment.

SUGGESTED ACTIVITIES

- Together with your classmates, devise an in-service program on respiratory therapy for hospital nurses. Explain and demonstrate proper postural drainage techniques, as well as the correct operation of respiratory therapy devices. Provide a review of the medications commonly used in respiratory conditions, including their dosages, routes of administration, rationale for use, interventions that enhance their effectiveness, and possible side effects.

- Visit a health care center or hospital that specializes in pediatric eye care. Observe the methods of assessment used, the family teaching that is done, and the special adaptations in care that are made. Share your observations with the class.

DISCUSSION TOPIC

Research several of the special agencies that assist families of children with the diseases discussed in this chapter. What services do they provide? What are their identified goals? How can families initiate contact with them? Are there any qualifications that must be met before assistance is given? Report your findings to the class.

REVIEW

A. Matching. Match the disease in Column I with the treatment or diagnostic test in Column II.

Column I	Column II
1. Celiac disease	a. Sweat test
2. Serous otitis media	b. Actinomycin D
3. Laryngotracheobronchitis	c. Gluten-free diet
4. Cystic fibrosis	d. Myringotomy with ventilating tubes
5. Wilm's tumor	e. Tracheostomy

B. Multiple choice. Select the one best answer.

1. Jeff is a two-year-old boy who was admitted for possible cystic fibrosis. The nurse may expect the physician to do which of the following groups of tests?
   a. Chest radiographs, blood urea nitrogen, and pulmonary function tests
   b. Pulmonary function tests and a barium enema
   c. Examination of the urine and sputum
   d. Examination of the stools for fat and enzymes

2. Which of the following best describes the stool of a child with cystic fibrosis?
   a. Consists largely of undigested food
   b. Foul, bulky, and greasy, containing unabsorbed fat
   c. Green, watery, and odorous
   d. Hard, dry, and offensively odorous

3. Marie is a 1 1/2-year-old girl with a nephroblastoma. Her preoperative nursing care should include
   1. postural drainage, clapping, and vibrating to reduce secretions.
   2. an avoidance of any manipulation of the abdominal wall.
   3. normal care related to her developmental age.
   4. an explanation of the protein and sodium restrictions in her diet to her parents.
      a. 1 only
      b. 2 and 3
      c. 1 and 3
      d. 4 only

4. The most effective treatment for Marie's condition includes
   1. radiation therapy
   2. Actinomycin D
   3. surgical removal
   4. Amphotericin B
   5. renal dialysis
      a. 1 and 5
      b. 2, 3, and 4
      c. 1, 2, and 3
      d. 4 and 5

5. Jackie was admitted with the diagnosis of croup. A bath blanket has been placed in his croupette tent to absorb the moisture. His clothing should be changed
   a. once a day with his bath.
   b. every four hours.
   c. whenever his clothing becomes damp.
   d. just before his mother comes to visit him.

6. Which of the following nursing observations would indicate severe respiratory distress?
   a. Synchronized respirations, absence of retractions
   b. Absence of nasal flaring, expiratory grunt
   c. Absence of xiphoid retraction, occasional nasal flaring
   d. Seesaw respirations, xiphoid retraction

C. Short answer. Briefly respond to the following statements.

1. List three means of effecting environmental control of particles for a child with asthma.

2. List three aspects of teaching involved in the education of a mother of a two-year-old girl with a urinary tract infection.

BIBLIOGRAPHY

Bridgewater, Sharon C., et al. "Allergies in Children: Recognition." *American Journal of Nursing,* Vol. 78 (April, 1978), pp. 614–616.

Bridgewater, Sharon C., and Ruth R. Voignier. "Allergies in Children: Teaching." *American Journal of Nursing,* Vol. 78 (April, 1978), pp. 620–621.

Brown, Marie S., and Carol Grunfeld. "Otitis Media." *Issues in Comprehensive Pediatric Nursing,* Vol. 3 (August, 1978), pp. 35–53.

Dudding, Burton A. "Problems Related to the Common Cold." *Issues in Comprehensive Pediatric Nursing,* Vol. 3 (August, 1978), pp. 1–11.

Fries, Peter C. "Nursing Skills in the Outpatient Management of Childhood Inhalant Allergy." *Issues in Comprehensive Pediatric Nursing,* Vol. 3 (August, 1978), pp. 24–34.

Gold, Warren M. "Asthma." *Basics of RD.* Evansville, IN: American Lung Association, 1976, pp. 1–6.

Huber, Helen L. "Draining the Fluid Ear with Myringotomy and Tube Insertion." *Nursing 78,* Vol. 8 (July, 1978), pp. 28–31.

Krause, Marie V., and L. Kathleen Mahan. *Food, Nutrition and Diet Therapy.* Philadelphia: W. B. Saunders Company, 1979.

Mikkelson, Cynthia, et al. "Cystic Fibrosis: A Family Challenge." *Children Today,* Vol. 7 (July–August, 1978), pp. 22–26.

Organ, Alan E. "Lower Respiratory Tract Infection in Childhood." *Issues in Comprehensive Pediatric Nursing,* Vol. 3 (August, 1978), pp. 12–23.

Pinney, Margo Ann. "Review of Cystic Fibrosis." *Issues in Comprehensive Pediatric Nursing,* Vol. 3 (August, 1978), pp. 54–65.

Richerson, Hal B., and Sheldon C. Siegel. *Asthma: Which Drug When?* Evansville, IN: Mead Johnson, 1975.

Rosen, Ellen, and Monnette Viau. "Pediatric Allergy Nursing Assessment and History Guide." *Pediatric Nursing,* Vol. 2 (March–April, 1977), pp. 37–38.

Stapleton, F. Bruder, and Michael A. Linshaw. "Urinary Tract Infections in Children: Diagnosis and Management." *Issues in Comprehensive Pediatric Nursing,* Vol. 2 (March–April, 1978), pp. 1–10.

Stern, Elizabeth J. "Helping the Person With Low Vision." *American Journal of Nursing,* Vol. 80 (October, 1980), pp. 1788–1790.

Voignier, Ruth C., and Sharon C. Bridgewater. "Allergies in Children, Testing and Treating." *American Journal of Nursing,* Vol. 78 (April, 1978), pp. 617–619.

Wieczorek, Rita R., and Bernice Horner-Rosner. "The Asthmatic Child: Preventing and Controlling Attacks." *American Journal of Nursing,* Vol. 79 (February, 1979), pp. 258–262.

Wilson, Theresa. "Judy R.: A Child With Wilm's Tumor." *RN,* Vol. 41 (April, 1978), pp. 67–73.

Section VI

The Preschooler

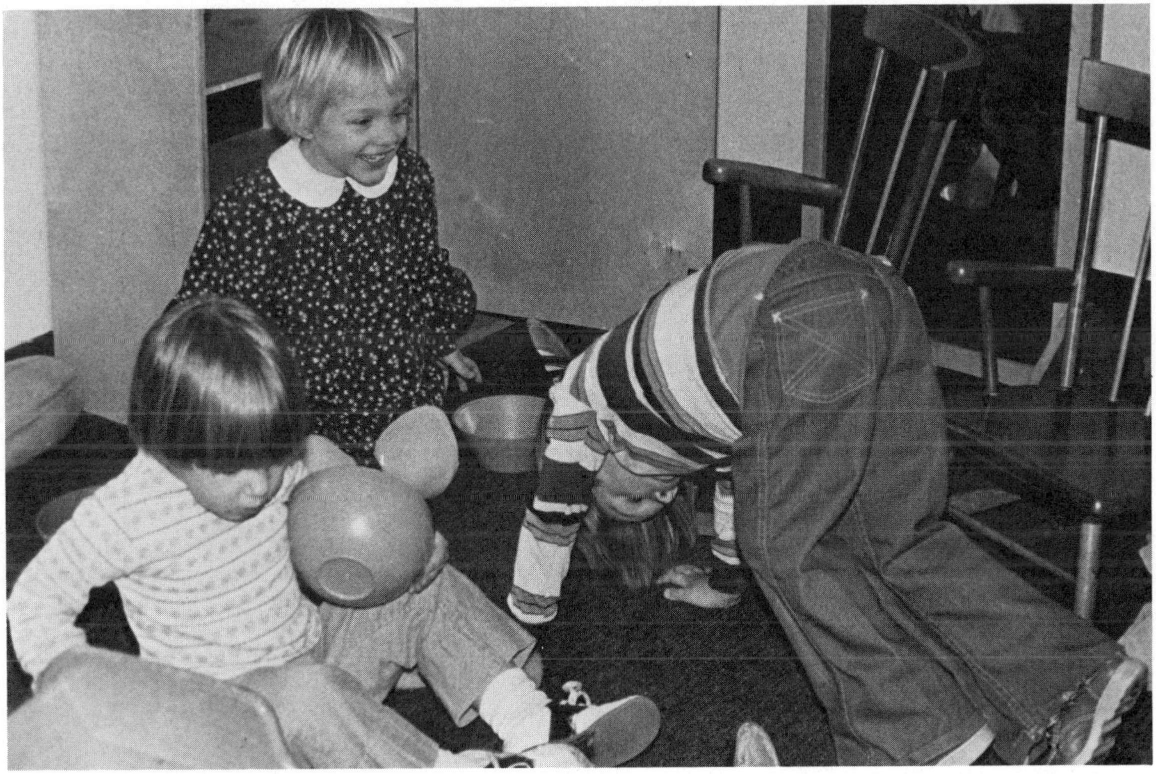

Chapter 19

Growth and Development

3-5 yrs.

OBJECTIVES

Upon completion of this chapter, the student will be able to

- contrast the physical development of a three-year-old child with that of a five-year-old child.
- describe conflicts that might be encountered in the hospitalization of a preschooler.
- list specific toys or activities that would be suitable for a preschooler admitted for diagnostic tests.
- identify the child who might require further testing because the achievement level is not consistent with the chronologic age.

The preschool period is characterized by relatively slow physical growth but enormous changes in other areas. This is particularly true of the child's acquisition of knowledge and perception of the world. This is a period of transition from the autonomy of the toddler to the industriousness of the school-aged child. It is a time of motor skill development, a rapid increase in vocabulary, and imaginary friends and playmates. Erikson describes this period as one of initiative, and it is this initiative which pervades all aspects of the child's life.

DEVELOPMENTAL TASKS

Erikson's Stage of Initiative

Learning takes place in the preschool child primarily through a process of reinforcement or conditioning. The environment and the culture exert an unusually strong influence on children and their actions. Erikson identifies this stage as one of initiative versus a sense of guilt.

All of the child's energies are directed toward actual and imaginary problems with which he or she is confronted. The exploration is focused on both people and things in the child's immediate environment. If the exploration cannot actually be attempted, such as driving a car, it is done through the imagination. The preschooler's delight is obvious as the child sits in a cardboard box, manipulating an unseen steering wheel and making the sounds of a horn or conversing with invisible passengers. The little girl dressed up in adult clothes and making mud pies is exploring a world that she is not yet able to enter but can explore through imagination.

The environment that best meets the child's needs in developing a sense of initiative is one that is stimulating and free for exploration. This does not mean to imply the child has no limits. Adult supervision is required but it must be more subtle, allowing the child freedom and encouragement. Protection from injury or hazards in the environment is important, as is the protection of the child from his or her own aggressive impulses.

The alternative to developing a sense of initiative is the development of a sense of guilt. The child whose explorations are suppressed, whose activities are limited, and whose environment is dull and repetitious begins to feel defeated and angry. The absence of positive recognition for achievements eventually stifles the sense of initiative. The child becomes timid and afraid to attempt new activities. These behavioral patterns may persist even into adulthood.

The sense of guilt is sometimes reinforced verbally by the adult who recognizes the child's accomplishment by saying, "That's good, but why didn't . . ." The adult who adds to the child's drawing, fixes the alphabet letters, and "improves" on the sand castle conveys the same negative message to the child.

Piaget's Preoperational Stage of Cognitive Development

The preschool child is in the preoperational stage of development which extends from ages two to seven years. The two phases within this stage include the preconceptual phase from two to four years and the intuitive phase from four to seven years.

During this period the child increases the ability to use symbols, and is able to distinguish between the symbol itself and the event or action it conveys. The sand pail and shovel may convey a trip to the beach for a young child whereas the older child recognizes multiple uses for the same items. The bib that is first identified with eating later is recognized as an item to keep the clothing clean.

The preschooler does not have the ability to reason except in a primitive fashion. This ability encompasses a global concept of ideas which can be used to explain any other element within that global collection. The child in the hospital for elective surgery may then explain his presence as "I'm here because I didn't wear my coat outside like Mommy said." Both inductive and deductive reasoning seen in the adult are not present at this age. This child demonstrates transductive reasoning which is from particular to particular. It permits the identification of relationships that do not exist and further enhances the distortion of reality that is unique to the preschooler.

The egocentricity of the toddler continues in this period and the child sees everything in his own world as either happening to him or caused by him. The world is then shaped to the preschooler's needs rather than the needs shaped to the world. This egocentricity interferes with the child's ability to criticize himself. It also interferes with his ability to recognize another's point of view.

In specific situations the child lacks the ability to focus on some aspects as being more important than others. The term "field dependency" is used for this phenomenon. In the child's life, objects, people and routines all have equal value. It is for this reason that routines are consistently maintained to provide sameness and security for the child.

To cope with his environment the child may use animistic thought. In this process the familiar inanimate objects are endowed with human or animal qualities. The stuffed rabbit that speaks or cries and the doll that becomes a real baby are common examples. The child may also assume animal characteristics to master or control a stressful situation. The roaring lion can then accept the dressing change in the hospital setting.

As the child moves into the intuitive phase, the thought processes are marked by centration, a lack of reversibility, and a static quality. The centration allows the child to focus on one aspect of a situation and ignore all other aspects. The lack of reversibility is demonstrated by using various sized containers with the same amount of water in them. Even pouring the same amount into each, in front of the child, does little to convince him that they are all equal amounts. The recognition of static quality occurs when the child focuses on the state of an object rather than its transformation of size or shape.

PHYSICAL GROWTH AND DEVELOPMENT

Three Years of Age

The preschool child grows slowly, gaining 4 to 4 1/2 pounds per year, and 2 1/2 to 3 1/2 inches in height per year. The three-year-old boy ranges in height from 35 inches to 40 1/2 inches, with the average being about 37 1/2 inches. Girls of the same age are slightly shorter,

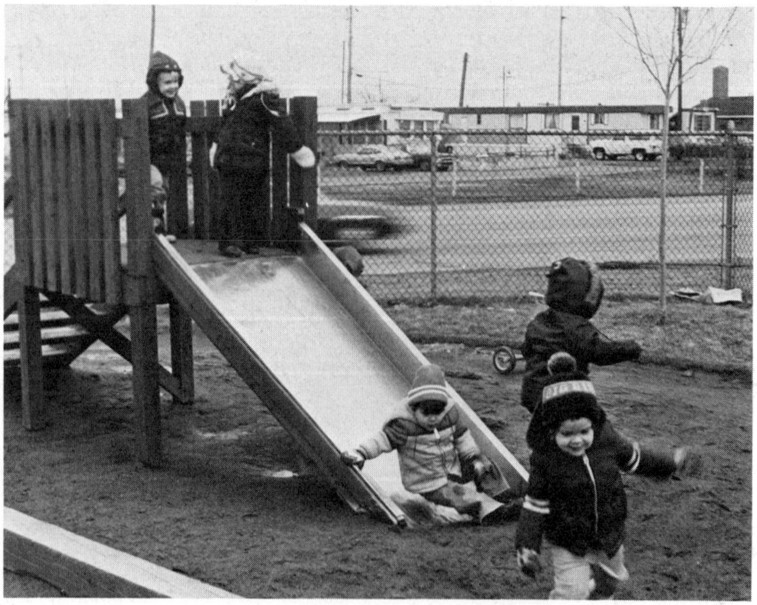

FIG. 19-1 Three-year-old children come in a variety of shapes and sizes, as evidenced by this playground group.

with a normal range of 34 3/4 to 39 1/2 inches and an average height of 37 inches, Figure 19-1.

The weight of a three-year-old boy ranges from 26 1/2 to 39 1/2 pounds, with the average being 32 1/4 pounds. On an average, a girl of the same age weighs 31 pounds. The normal weight range for girls in this age-group is 25 1/2 to 38 pounds.

Height and weight changes during this period are accompanied by distinct changes in body configuration. The lordosis and the protuberant abdomen that are characteristic in the toddler disappear dramatically in the preschool period, as does the toddling gait.

If one were to watch this child for a period of time, many other changes would be evident. For instance, three-year-old children can ascend steps using alternate feet. They can also stand for a short period on one foot and continue to maintain balance. They also can assist with dressing themselves, including unbuttoning their clothing and putting on their shoes without tying their laces, Figure 19-2. Washing hands, feeding oneself, and brushing teeth demonstrate fine motor development. A beginning ability to write in scribbles, as well as to copy geometric figures and draw pictures, provides evidence of fine motor skill development.

Typically, three-year-old children are more organized in abilities, better coordinated, and show less frustration and aggression than do toddlers. They try very hard to do what is expected. They need assistance in learning to take turns and share in group play, as previously, they have primarily been involved in parallel play, Figure 19-3. The appetite of the three-year-old child lags during this period, and

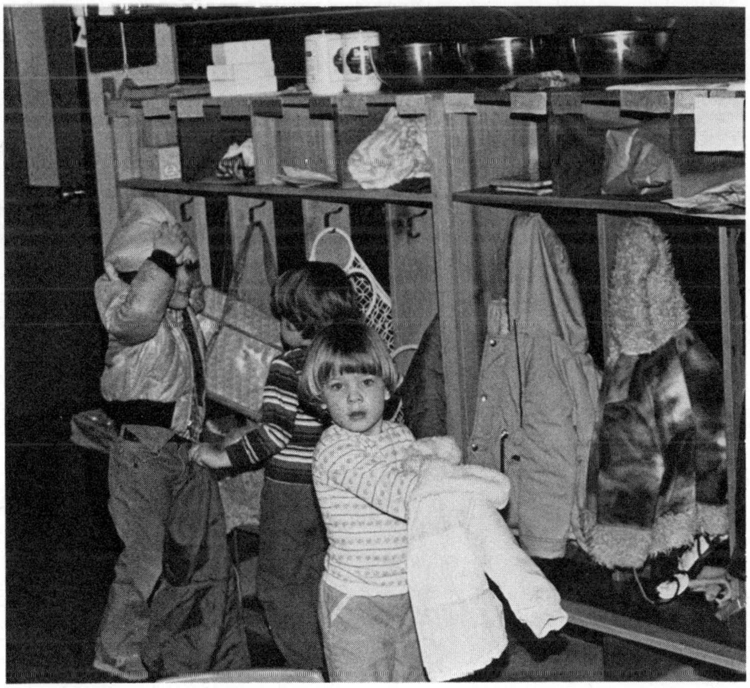

FIG. 19-2 Clothes that are stored within reach encourage the child to develop the ability to dress and undress.

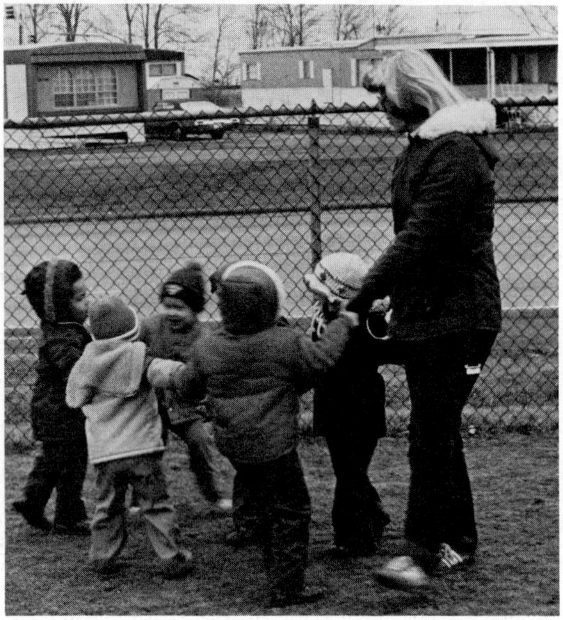

FIG. 19-3 Group play for a three-year-old child can be as simple as a circle game.

encouragement to eat appropriate foods may be needed. If allowed to select foods from a balanced diet, in a week's time, the child would consume an appropriate amount of nutrients.

Four Years of Age

Four-year-old boys range in height from 37 3/4 inches to 43 1/2 inches. Average height is 40 1/2 inches. Girls of the same age are 37 1/2 to 42 3/4 inches in height, with an average height of 40 inches. The weight of a four-year-old boy ranges from 30 to 44 3/4 pounds, with 36 3/4 being average. The weight of girls this age ranges from 29 to 44 pounds with the average being 35 1/2 pounds.

Four-year-old children can be characterized by one word – doing. This child has a high level of energy and a great deal of motivation. As a result, many projects are started and seldom finished. It may be difficult to differen-

FIG. 19-4 String art painting is an excellent choice of activity for a four- or five-year-old child either in nursery school or in the hospital. (Courtesy of the Department of Health and Human Services)

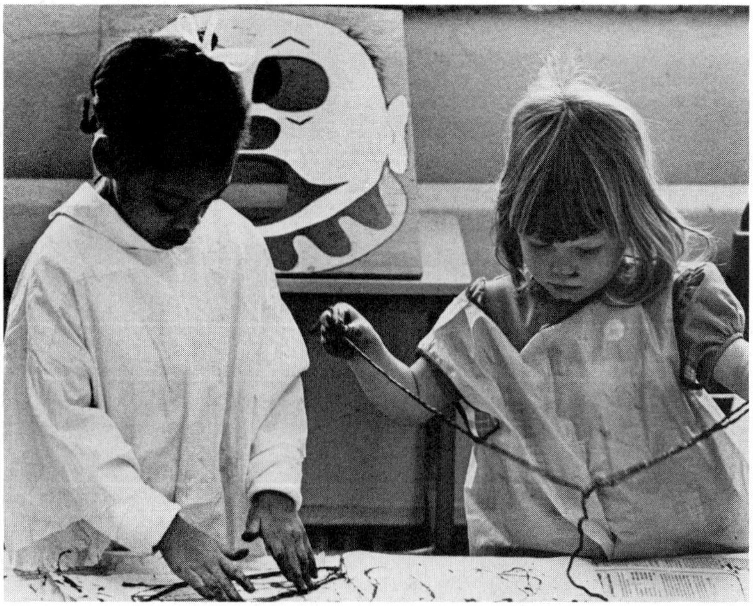

tiate between craftmanship and destructiveness. The child has a longer attention span and the ability to concentrate. Because of this, the child plays quietly for longer periods than before, Figure 19-4.

Behavior of the child may seem to deteriorate during this period. It usually relates to the child's observant, questioning manner. Through this testing, the child spots inconsistencies and may reject rules or guidelines set down by parents or others in authority.

The ability to run easily, climb on a jungle gym, hop on one leg, and skip (even clumsily) are all examples of the gross motor development of this age. The fine motor skills are demonstrated by the ability to dress and undress oneself, including buttons and laces. The ability to tie laces is not yet present. Being able to draw a three-part man in crude form is part of the child's artistic ability along with other drawings that are recognizable to an adult. The ability to use scissors and manipulate play materials also give evidence of fine motor skills.

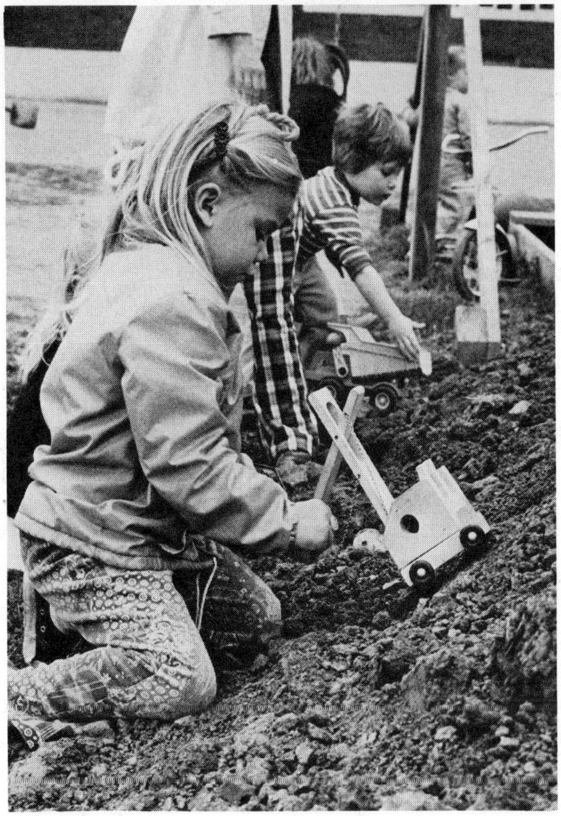

FIG. 19-5 Learning by doing is as much play as education. (Courtesy of the Department of Health and Human Services)

Five Years of Age

Five-year-old boys range in height from 40 1/2 inches to 46 inches, with an average height of 43 1/4 inches. The average height of girls of the same age is about 42 3/4 inches, with a range of 39 3/4 to 45 1/2 inches. Weight for boys ranges from 33 3/4 to 51 pounds with 41 1/4 pounds being the average. For girls, the average weight at this age is 39 pounds, with the range being 32 to 49 3/4 pounds.

Five-year-old children are distinctly different from three- and four-year-old children in the abilities they display as well as in their sense of newfound independence. These children demonstrate both a willingness and an ability to help others and to learn through "doing" types of activities, Figure 19-5. In this period, formal schooling is initiated, Figure 19-6. Their ability to cooperate, their lengthened attention span, their love of routines, and their interest in learning serve to make this a positive experience for most children. These children continue to be highly imaginative. Although they attempt to answer questions accurately, their answers may reflect their wishful thinking. Fellow students may become aware of this tendency as they listen to elaborate stories about the care and feeding

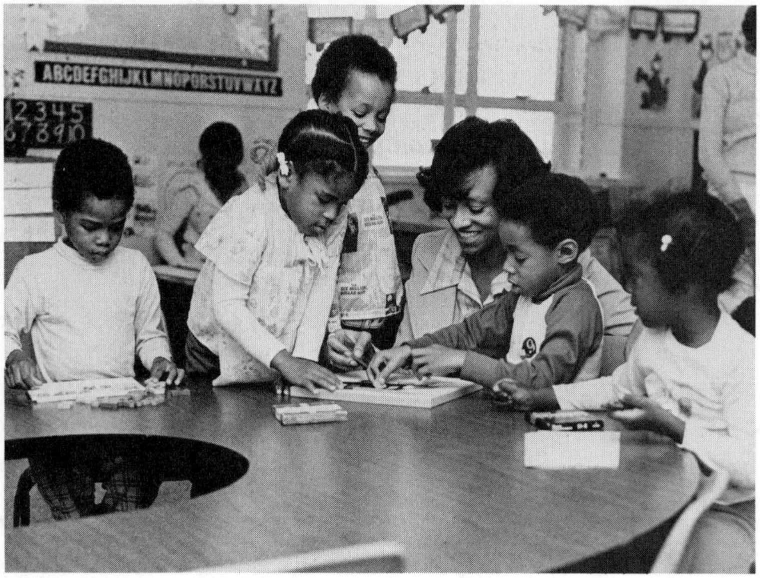

FIG. 19-6 Kindergarten means the beginning of formal schooling for the child. (Courtesy of the Department of Health and Human Services)

of a beautiful horse named Brandy, only to find that it is fiction, not fact.

Evidence of the skills in gross motor ability include backward heel-to-toe walking, hopping well, running with speed and agility, jumping rope, and roller skating. The ability to dress without assistance and tie shoelaces is typical of the fine motor ability of this child. Crude printing of some letters, numbers, or one's own name demonstrates further skill in this area. Drawings depict lifelike representations.

EMOTIONAL AND SOCIAL DEVELOPMENT

Speech Development

Speech development is very complex and unfolds rapidly. Preschool children increase their vocabulary from 900 to 2100 or more words, with an understanding of up to 20,000 words. Speech is used in a variety of ways, including exploring the environment, controlling others, and, when angry or frustrated, as a substitute for former crying behavior.

Sex Role Identification

During this period, children learn sex differences as a part of their acquired knowledge of body image. They examine themselves and others and make comparisons as a part of the learning process. One preschooler made this fact vividly clear at the supper table when she announced "I know the difference between boys and girls." Her parents, recognizing her preschool experiences, encouraged her to elaborate. "Boys stand up and girls sit down when they go potty," was her reply.

Establishment of a gender role begins about eighteen months and is usually well established by three years of age. Identification occurs when the child imitates and later acquires attributes of a particular individual. The process of identification is enhanced when the individual is nurturing, when there is a physical or psychologic similarity, and when the individual has a desirable position or quality. This may or may not be a parent. It can also be a sibling or other individual.

During this time, preschoolers are increasingly aware of stereotyped sex roles, and of advantages and disadvantages of their own particular role. The degree of role-typing is dependent on the family group and on exposures to others with diverse or more flexible roles. In this context and others, the child is quite sensitive to social messages that depict adult expectations of the ideal child. Peer acceptance beginning at this age and extending into later childhood is to a large degree dependent upon conformity to the sex role behaviors considered appropriate.

During this period, the beginning questions about "where babies come from" usually occur. The manner in which the parent responds to the questions will lay the groundwork for the child's attitudes in this area. A parent who is flustered by the questions, who responds with anxiety, and who overwhelms the child with detailed information creates as many problems as the parent who gets upset and changes the subject. Both imply that the subject is "off limits" or "taboo" in some way.

Clarifying the child's request for information by asking what he thinks aids the parent. It also focuses on what the child actually is interested in finding out. Short, simple explanations that answer only the question asked are most appropriate. The impending arrival of a sibling often initiates the need for information and reassurance that they were and are wanted. Both language and information must always be adapted to the child's level of understanding.

Fears of the Preschooler

With their increased knowledge, these children are very vulnerable to fear. Some of their fears reflect those of their parents or other siblings, such as thunder and lightning, pain, hospitals, and dogs. However, preschoolers usually develop fears of their own that reflect certain situations or conditions. Fears of desertion or abandonment by their parents may be very strong. Likewise, fear of the dark and of being alone are prevalent. Their fears may also be related to their culture, as reflected in the threats of a monster or "bogeyman" that may be used to control the child's behavior. Most preschool children are apprehensive about verbalizing their fears. They continue to believe in the magical power of words, believing that "if I say it, it may come true."

These fears are often reflected vividly in the nightmares of the child. The adult can assist the child in coping with nightmares by recognizing when they occur and talking about them when the child has calmed down. Initially, the child needs to feel the strength and protection of the parent or the caregiver. This should be provided until the child has regained composure. Offering opportunities for children to act out their fears in a play situation also helps them to deal with the fears. In all situations, the nurse and the parents should provide comfort and a great deal of support.

Play Activities

Appropriate play materials for the younger preschooler include large riding toys, such as fire engines, police cars, tricycles, wagons, and rocking horses, Figure 19-7. Their interest in rhythms may be enhanced by the use of drums, tambourines, sturdy music boxes, and

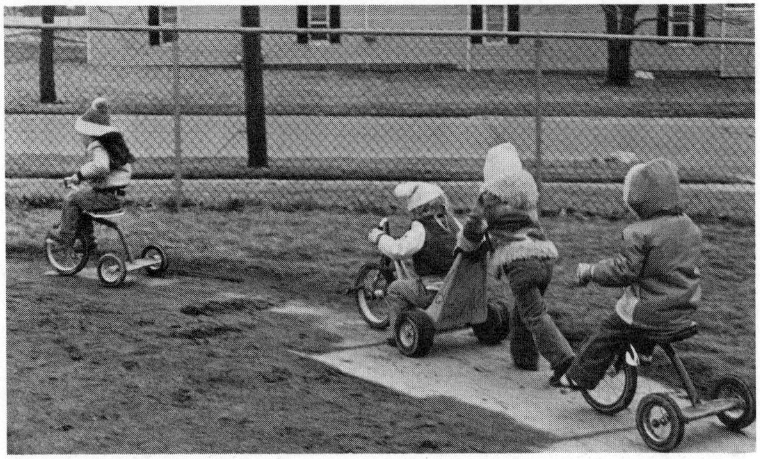

FIG. 19-7 Preschoolers enjoy riding toys outdoors.

phonographs and records. For adult imitative play, the child might enjoy a child's tool box with safe tools, dolls and cribs, a table and chairs, and dishes, Figure 19-8. Fine motor skills may be enhanced with the use of clay, finger paints, flannel or chalkboards, age-appropriate puzzles, and simple board games that do not require reading.

Additional toys for older children in this preschool period include more complex puzzles, the use of small building blocks or construction-type kits, and small boat, truck, or car sets. In order to help the children act out their fantasies, clothing and equipment identifying a variety of adult occupations can be provided. Dollhouses, as well as play schools

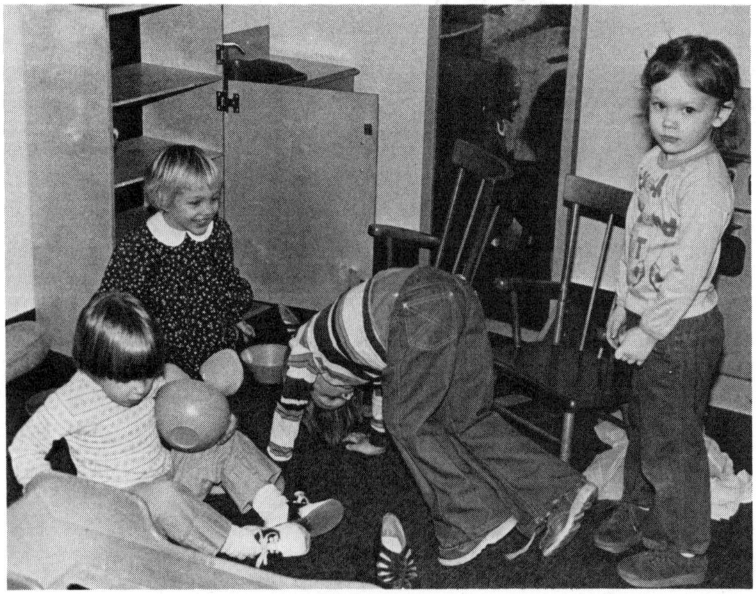

FIG. 19-8 This day-care center's make-believe kitchen area is in use, but activities are disrupted by an impromptu somersault.

and hospitals with play people, may be used for both entertainment and play therapy for children of both sexes. It is important to avoid any sex role stereotyping with these activities. Play materials should promote creativity and use of the imagination as well as symbolism.

Developmental Lags

A number of characteristics may signal a lag in development or some type of disability. The nurse should be aware of them so that appropriate testing may be done and referrals made. Some of the identifiable lags seen in the preschool years include the following:

- an inability to follow simple directions
- an inability to focus visually on pictures of familiar objects
- avoidance of interactions with others in a group
- use of repetitive motions or gestures with excitement
- an inability to tolerate any change in routines
- an inability to complete toilet training

A number of disturbances in speech may be revealed during this period. The child with limited or absent speech, or those whose speech is only partially understandable, should be identified. Because the family adapts to the child's speech pattern they may be unaware of its inappropriateness. This is particularly true of articulation problems that involve distortions of sounds or substitutions of consonants. This child may also continue to use jargon and babbling that are normally present in the toddler period but are inappropriate at this age. Family members should be reminded to avoid baby talk and to speak clearly and distinctly to the child. The child copies adult speech patterns and needs appropriate role models.

THE NURSE'S APPROACH TO THE CHILD

The nurse's approach to the preschool child should reflect a knowledge of the child's level of growth and development, as well as recognition of the child as a unique individual. If there is ample time to develop rapport slowly, the child should be approached with a suitable toy, book, or game. The nurse can sit down or kneel so that eye contact with the child is maintained. Initially, a more distant approach may be more acceptable. The nurse can first talk with the parent in the child's presence. When the child demonstrates an interest in participating in the exchange, the nurse should then speak to him or her quietly, avoiding condescending or teasing remarks.

Any procedure that may evoke fear or extreme stress should be avoided, if possible, until the child has developed trust or confidence in the ability of the nurse, as well as of the parents, to provide support. Simple, direct explanations should be used in these situations. Shaming the child, or using demeaning comments, force, or scare tactics only adds to the child's fear and may actually terrorize the child. Regressive behavior while in the hospital is a normal occurrence in children this age, and should be accepted as such.

SUMMARY

The preschool child is not a small adult. He or she is an entirely unique individual with a multitude of abilities and some limitations. The nurse should be aware of each child's functional abilities in order to assess needs and to adapt care accordingly. The nursing care of these children involves assessing their physical status, determining which developmental tasks have been achieved, recognizing their fears, and approaching them in a supportive manner. Only in this way can the nurse help the child face a health care problem positively.

SUGGESTED ACTIVITIES

- Visit a preschool group in a local nursery or day-care center. Compare the physical development and motor activities of the various age-groups.
- Observe one three-year-old, one four-year-old, and one five-year-old child whom you know. Compare the development of each child with the established norms.
- Visit the playroom setting in your assigned hospital. Identify ten different toys that are suitable for use by a preschool child. Interview the play therapist or child-life worker regarding other suitable toys for this age-group.
- Interview four hospitalized preschool children. After establishing rapport with each of the children, ask them to play a game with you by finishing the following statements: "I don't like ..." "When my mommy and daddy leave ..." "Scary things are ..." "I'm afraid when ..." "When it's dark .... " Share their responses with your student group.

DISCUSSION TOPICS

1. Identify the various ways in which sex stereotypes may be reinforced by parents or other individuals with whom the preschooler comes in contact. Discuss what types of play activities and materials may be encouraged to counter this stereotyping.
2. Perform a Denver Developmental Screening Test on a preschool child. Have your class discuss the performance of the various children. Identify those factors which may have enhanced or hindered the child's performance.

REVIEW

A. Matching. Match the activity in Column I with the age at which it normally occurs in Column II.

Column I	Column II
1. Balancing on one foot	a. Three years
2. Starting many projects that are seldom finished	b. Four years
3. Ascending steps using alternate feet	c. Five years
4. Fabricating imaginative stories	
5. Buttoning and unbuttoning clothing	
6. Helping others and learning from doing	

B. Multiple choice. Select the one best response.

1. The average weight gain for a preschooler per year is
   a. 10 to 15 pounds.
   b. 8 to 10 pounds.
   c. 4 to 5 pounds.
   d. 1 to 2 pounds.
2. Erikson described the preschool period as a stage of
   a. independence versus dependence.
   b. initiative versus guilt.
   c. autonomy versus inferiority.
   d. trust versus mistrust.
3. Appropriate play materials for a preschool child who is confined to bed include
   a. a tricycle, puzzles, and dolls.
   b. a wagon, tool box, and "dress-up" clothes.
   c. puzzles, simple board games, and modeling clay.
   d. mobiles, finger paints, and large construction toys.

C. Short answer. Briefly respond to the following statements.

1. Identify four characteristics of developmental lag in preschoolers.
2. List three strategies that may be used in the nurse's approach to a preschool child.

BIBLIOGRAPHY

Adair, M. "Speech and Language Development in Preschool Children." *Nursing Care,* Vol. 10 (August, 1977), pp. 22–23.

Belsky, J., et al. "What Does Research Teach Us About Day Care? A Follow Up Report." *Children Today,* Vol. 8 (July–August, 1979), pp. 21–26.

Chinn, Peggy, and Cynthia J. Leitch. *Child Health Maintenance: A Guide for Clinical Assessment.* St. Louis: C. V. Mosby Company, 1974.

Fleming, R. A. "Developing a Child's Self-Esteem." *Pediatric Nursing,* Vol. 5 (July–August, 1979), pp. 58–60.

Gelhard, Hil. "Drawing and Development." *Pediatric Nursing,* Vol. 4 (November–December, 1978), pp. 23–25.

Johnson, Thomas R., et al. *Children are Different: Developmental Physiology.* Columbus: Ross Laboratories, 1978.

Newman, Barbara M., and Philip R. Newman. *Infancy and Childhood.* New York: John Wiley and Sons, 1978.

Petrillo, Madeline, and Sirgay Sanger. *Emotional Care of Hospitalized Children.* Philadelphia: J. B. Lippincott Company, 1979.

Vaughan, Victor C., et al. *Nelson's Textbook of Pediatrics.* Philadelphia: W. B. Saunders Company, 1979.

Chapter 20

Health Care Problems

OBJECTIVES

Upon completion of this chapter, the student will be able to

- differentiate between the type of nursing care required by a child with idiopathic thrombocytopenic purpura and that required by a child with leukemia or hemophilia.
- identify the specific types of medications and treatments used for the two most common types of acute leukemia.
- describe the nursing care of a child with nephrosis, including the appropriate diet and medications.
- describe the method of transmission of sickle cell disease, the diagnostic tests used to detect it, and its implications.
- describe the inheritance pattern of Duchenne's muscular dystrophy as well as the signs and symptoms.

The health problems discussed in this chapter are typical conditions that may affect preschool children. This does not in any way imply that the conditions may not be observed in younger or older children, or that the infections of the respiratory tract or other conditions discussed earlier cannot occur in the preschool child. When any condition occurs in a child, it is the responsibility of the nurse to adapt the care as well as the assessment to the growth and development level of that individual child.

IDIOPATHIC THROMBOCYTOPENIC PURPURA

Idiopathic thrombocytopenic purpura causes a severe disruption in platelet production as well as a premature destruction of red blood cells. The acute form of idiopathic thrombocytopenic purpura is seen in children of ages two to six years.

Those children who are at high risk for developing this condition are those with bone marrow infiltration from leukemia, those with aplastic anemia, and those on myelosuppressive drugs, such as 6-mercaptopurine and methotrexate. Additionally, thiazide diuretics act

TABLE 20-1 Possible Causes of Idiopathic Thrombocytopenic Purpura

Sensitization through bacterial or viral infections such as rubella, rubeola, mumps, chickenpox, or respiratory infections
Bone marrow infiltration secondary to diseases such as leukemia
Sensitization from multiple blood transfusions which cause increased destruction of antibody-coated platelets
Chemicals or drugs that may alter bone marrow activity, such as antineoplastics like methotrexate

directly on platelet production and may also cause the primary form of thrombocytopenic purpura, Table 20-1.

Symptoms

The disease has an abrupt onset following a viral infection. The child has symptoms of bleeding, including petechial or pinpoint hemorrhages in the skin, ecchymoses or larger areas of hemorrhage or bruising, and obvious bleeding from the gums, gastrointestinal tract, and the urinary tract. The pathophysiology involved includes a low platelet count, a short platelet lifespan, abundant megakaryocytes in the bonc, and a possible immune response.

The bleeding may be either spontaneous or traumatic. Spontaneous bleeding is confined to the microcirculation and to involvement of the mucous membranes. It is seen as petechiae and ecchymoses. Traumatic bleeding is the result of injury to arterioles and small arteries, and is usually marked by the development of hemarthrosis.

Diagnostic Tests

The diagnostic tests that may be performed to confirm or rule out this disease include a blood smear, a bone marrow study, and determinations of platelet count, prothrombin time, clot retraction, and capillary fragility. The normal platelet count ranges from 200,000 to 400,000 platelets. Thrombocytopenia occurs with a platelet count of less than 100,000. Any count that is less than 50,000 is associated with distinct hemorrhagic phenomena. A platelet count that is less than 10,000 is considered life-threatening and may indicate the need for immediate platelet transfusion.

Platelet production within the bone marrow is the result of the giant multinucleated cells called megakaryocytes, which are the precursors of thrombocytes. Their maturation takes four to five days. Each megakaryocyte releases 2000 to 7700 platelets. Their life span is about eight to twelve days. In the case of an antigen-antibody reaction, the platelets become coated with antibodies and are then sequestered by the spleen and destroyed.

Nursing Considerations

The major care problem in this condition is hemorrhage and its assessment. The child should be observed closely for hematuria, tarry stools, nosebleeds, and gingival bleeding. The skin should be observed closely each day and assessed for tenderness of ecchymotic areas and the distribution of petechiae. One method of detecting changes involves the marking of a body figure chart, such as that shown in Figure 20-1 at the time of admission and every twenty-four hours thereafter. Increases in tenderness of the ecchymotic areas and a changing distribution of petechiae indicate increased bleeding.

Bleeding into an organ or a joint may be identified by limitation of movement, pain or weakness of the part, and, in the case of thoracic cavity involvement, shortness of breath or dyspnea. The bleeding may extend to involve the nervous system as well. If it does, weakness or numbness of an area or body part may be noted. Patients with continued bleeding in an area or body part in the nervous system may develop increased intracranial pressure. Persistent bleeding may also cause shock, which is commonly heralded by restlessness, agitation, decreasing blood pressure, and lowered skin temperature.

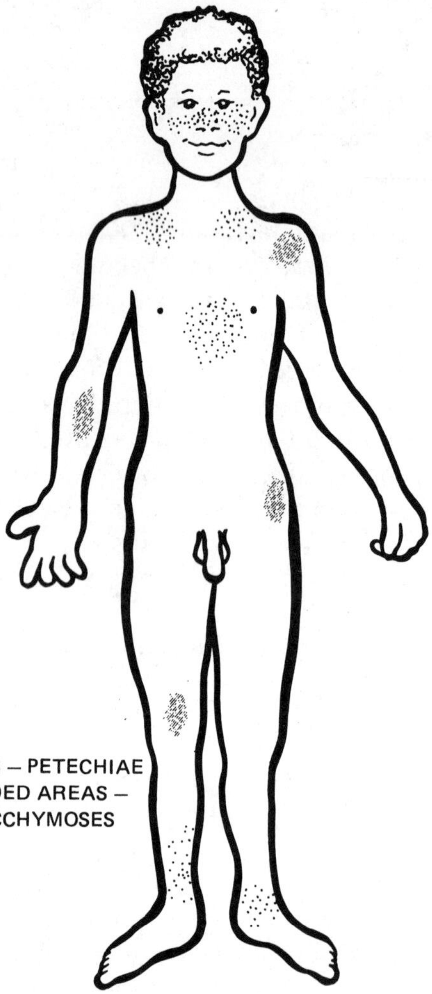

FIG. 20-1 Areas of ecchymoses and petechiae may be marked on a body figure chart, both front and back views. Any change in the distribution of these areas signifies increased bleeding.

Nursing intervention for the child should have as its primary aim the avoidance of any exertion. This necessitates complete bedrest, avoidance of coughing or straining during defecation, and the implementation of relaxation techniques. Stress from the external environment should be controlled or eliminated as much as possible.

Medical Treatment

During the acute phase of this disease, medical treatment may include platelet transfusions for the control of hemorrhage. However, these transfusions may be rendered ineffective by antibodies in the child that cause rapid destruction of the newly transfused platelets. For this reason, treatment with steroids, usually a form of prednisone, is the most common initial intervention used to control bleeding. The usual dose is 0.5 to 2.0 milligrams per kilogram of body weight per day. The main goal of therapy is to prolong the life span of the antibody-coated platelets in order to prevent them from being sequestered in the spleen and destroyed.

If this treatment is not effective, a splenectomy may be performed to stop the early destruction of platelets. After surgery, treatment will include transfusions, if necessary; the use of steroids to increase the platelet count; and careful observation for signs of hemorrhage because of the child's increased bleeding tendencies. The steroids are withdrawn after several weeks. The platelet count will return to normal as their production is taken over by the liver, lymph nodes, and bone marrow. Occasionally, splenectomy may not be effective, and the child may continue to have bleeding problems. In this situation, the child receives a course of immunosuppressive therapy.

SICKLE CELL ANEMIA

Sickle cell disease is a chronic, hereditary, hemolytic anemia that predominately affects the Black community. The disease is a syndrome of several problems that are directly related to a chemical defect in the hemoglobin caused by a mutant autosomal gene. This defect allows a residue of valine, one of the essential amino acids, to be substituted for glutamic acid. This minor molecular substitution which occurs in a specific position on a polypeptide chain, causes serious consequences. Deoxygenation results in surface changes that allow the sickle hemoglobin molecules to elongate and distort the shape of the cell. Distortion does not allow the cells to move freely through the blood vessels. Instead, they cling and obstruct the vessels, causing further deoxygenation, increased clumping of cells, and pain.

Children who receive the hereditary trait from both of their parents are considered to be homozygous and will invariably have some form of the disease, Figure 20-2. Children receiving the trait from only one parent are heterozygous, and will inherit the trait, rather than the disease. Their blood contains twenty-five to forty-five percent hemoglobin S which does not sickle under normal conditons. Individuals who inherit the trait only are generally asymptomatic, although some may develop idiopathic hematuria without any other symptoms. During the latter part of the first year when the transition is made from fetal hemoglobin (Hgb F) to the adult form (Hgb A), the child with the disease will have eighty to one hundred percent sickle hemoglobin (Hgb S) mixed in with the Hgb A.

Symptoms

Children who inherit the disease have a variety of symptoms depending on the stage of the disease. Newborn infants are asymptomatic at first since they are in a transition period and still have a high percentage of fetal hemoglobin present. Near the end of the first year, when Hgb S accounts for the majority of hemoglobin, the symptoms of pallor, lymphadenopathy, hepatomegaly, splenomegaly, and jaundice become evident.

Diagnostic Tests

Diagnosis of sickle cell anemia can only be confirmed after obtaining a careful history, assessing the child's physical status, and performing several laboratory tests. The diagnostic tests that are most commonly used to detect sickle cell disease are the oxygen reduction test, the solubility test, and hemoglobin electrophoresis. The Sickledex test, a solubility test, is one example of a mass screening test. It is often used because it yields rapid results in approximately five minutes and because its cost is reasonable. It is not accurate in children younger than six months of age or in those with severe anemia. Hemoglobin electrophoresis, the most

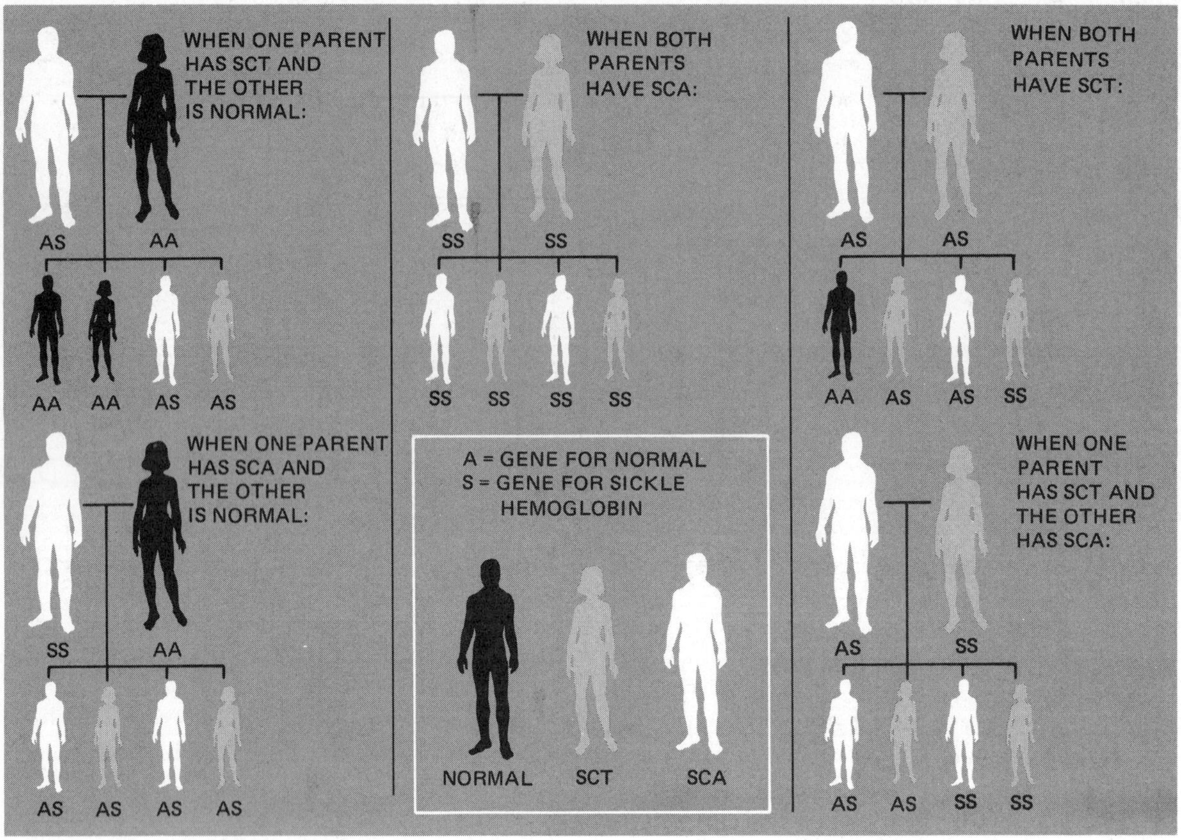

FIG. 20-2 Inheritance patterns for sickle cell anemia and sickle cell trait

accurate test, is used to determine the percentages of normal and abnormal hemoglobins present. This test usually reveals ninety percent Hgb S, two to ten percent Hgb F, a small percentage of Hgb A_2, and no Hgb A. The oxygen reduction test or sickle cell prep does not differentiate between the trait and the disease.

When a routine blood count is performed, these children are found to have hemoglobin concentrations of 6 to 8 grams, and their hematocrit is between twenty and thirty. The peripheral blood smear reveals sickled cells. Additionally, abnormal liver function, hyperbilirubinemia, and hyperplasia of the bone marrow are evident.

Sickle Cell Crisis

In children with sickle cell disease, the breakdown of red blood cells and the resulting anemia and jaundice are continuing problems. These problems are often complicated by viral or bacterial infections, severe chilling, dehydration, or emotional upsets. Any one of these can trigger one of several types of crises.

The four major types of crises are hemolytic, aplastic, thrombotic (or occlusive), and sequestration. In the hemolytic crisis, the child's body begins to destroy red blood cells at a more rapid rate than normal. This type of crisis results in a worsening of the ever-present anemia and jaundice, and is the least common of the four types. Aplastic crises occur when the bone marrow stops production of red blood cells and the anemia becomes increasingly severe. Thrombotic crises, the most common type, are caused by the occlusion of the blood vessels with sickle cells. This, in turn, causes deoxygenation and resultant tissue destruction, swelling, and areas of infarct. Thrombotic crises cause a great deal of pain for the patient. Sequestration crises are critical and require blood transfusions. They occur when the blood pools in the child's liver and spleen, causing a precipitous drop in blood pressure and circulatory collapse. Sequestration crises occur most commonly in toddlers and preschoolers, and may cause death. The common symptoms of a sickle cell crisis include abdominal pain, arthralgia, and unexplained swelling of the hands and feet.

Medical Treatment

Medical treatment is directed toward control of the crises that occur and prevention of sickling when possible. The treatment is primarily supportive and includes prevention of tissue hypoxia through adequate rest and reduced oxygen consumption. Adequate hydration of the patient by oral and parenteral means is also important as hemoconcentration results in increased blood viscosity, and hence, a greater potential for thrombotic crisis. Electrolyte replacement therapy is also essential, Figure 20-3. Metabolic acidosis is the end result of tissue hypoxia and will cause increased sickling. Transfusions are not used on a routine basis for every patient because of the additional risks of hepatitis, blood incompatibilities, and hemosiderosis, which is the accumulation of iron stored in the liver after breakdown of large numbers of red blood cells. Analgesics may be prescribed for the joint and abdominal pains that accompany the crises.

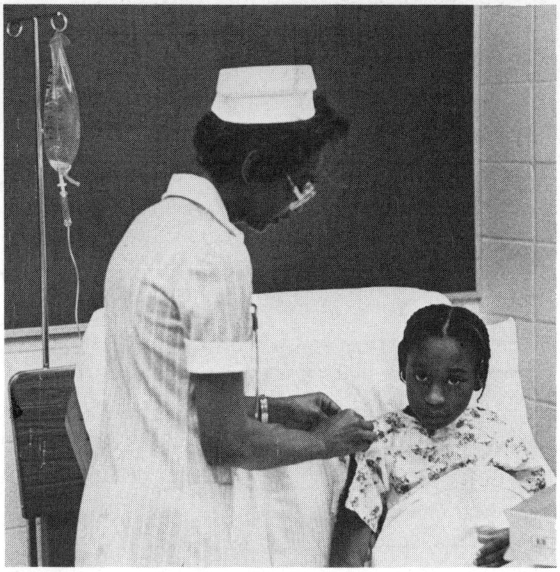

FIG. 20-3 Intravenous fluids are used in patients with sickle cell anemia to reduce blood viscosity, correct acidosis, and replace electrolytes.

Nursing Care

Nursing care of the child with sickle cell anemia involves helping to implement the prescribed treatment program, educating the parents about the disease, and assisting the parents and child in coping with a long-term disease process.

Implementing the Treatment Regimen. One of the primary aims of nursing care in these children is the prevention of sickling. Maintaining the child on bedrest initially is extremely important. The child should be observed carefully for any signs of overexertion or emotional stress. Oxygen may be administered, but it is of limited value at the tissue level. It is usually administered on a short-term basis to children who have problems with cardiac failure. Careful monitoring for infection is necessary. Infection and fever increase sickling.

Maintaining the fluid and electrolyte balance also prevents sickling. The nurse should calculate an adequate fluid intake for the child and provide this amount as a minimal daily intake. Oral fluids that are acceptable to the child should be offered in small amounts on an hourly basis during the waking hours to maintain hydration. Intake and output must be recorded carefully. Intravenous fluids must be monitored throughout. The child should be observed for signs of electrolyte imbalance as well as of metabolic acidosis.

Assessment of pain should be an ongoing process, and the child should be medicated accordingly. Very young children may be more difficult to assess, but will usually demonstrate any distress through their behavior. Careful positioning as well as the use of both diversional therapy and distraction may provide additional relief.

Parent Education. The education of the parents should be a multidisciplinary effort. The nurse may be involved in clarifying information previously received, or in reinforcing information presented by others.

Genetic counseling should be a distinct part of this process. The parents should be told of the risks for this child, as well as for any subsequent children. Nurses should be prepared to cope with the parents' feelings of grief and depression, particularly at the time of initial diagnosis. Parents often derive support from the nurse's calm presence and understanding attitude during their frequent contacts. Continuous coordinated care provides the most effective support for parent and child.

Nurses should help the parents plan the home care of the child as well. In particular, they should stress those aspects of care that prevent sickling, such as avoidance of chilling and infections, adequate rest, avoidance of overly strenuous activities, and adequate consumption of liquids. The parents should also know the symptoms that indicate a crisis and the need for immediate treatment. Education of parent and child should stress the positive aspects of what can be done. Maintaining the child's participation in school and appropriate activities is necessary.

The prognosis for the child is dependent on the severity of the disease and the frequency and type of the crises. A child younger than five years of age is at the greatest risk. The risk then decreases somewhat as the child grows older and reaches adulthood. Severe anemia and infections are the primary causes of death.

CHILDHOOD LEUKEMIA

The leukemias seen in childhood are differentiated according to the cytologic type. The most common type is acute lymphocytic, or ALL. It is potentially the most responsive to current treatment methods. The myelocytic type, also called granulocytic, is the least responsive to treatment. Presently, it is associated with the poorest survival rate. Together, they comprise ninety percent of the cases seen. A monocytic form of the disease exists, but it is very rare.

Symptoms

The leukemic child usually has symptoms of fever, malaise, anorexia, lethargy, pallor, and abdominal and bone pain. In addition, these children may have petechiae and ecchymotic areas visible, and hepatosplenomegaly may be evident on palpation. Four major manifestations of the disease are usually seen, including anemia, hemorrhage, infection, and leukemic infiltration of organs.

Anemia. The anemia may be the result of several influences on the child. It may be caused by blood loss over a period of time. It may also be caused by crythropoietic failure, or a failure to develop sufficient numbers of red blood cells as a result of bone marrow suppression.

Hemorrhage. Hemorrhage may manifest itself in a variety of ways. Initially, the child may appear to have more bruises than usual, particularly on the extremities. The parents may attribute this to trauma, however slight. Bleeding from the nose, mouth, or gums may also occur. The petechiae may appear to be a rash to the untrained eye rather than evidence of bleeding. All of these bleeding disturbances are the direct result of platelet reduction secondary to leukemic invasion of the bone marrow.

Infection. Infection is also related to bone marrow suppression. Because of the disease, the number of granulocytes is decreased, which affects their ability to fight infection effectively. Additionally, the child may be at risk of superinfection as a result of antibiotic suppression of normal flora, particularly in the gastrointestinal tract.

Leukemic Infiltration. Leukemic infiltration of various organs not only causes the enlargement of certain organs, such as the liver and spleen, but also causes bone and joint pain. Leukemic cells invade the central nervous system, resulting in headaches, nausea, visual changes, and seizures.

Medical Treatment

The goal of all therapy for leukemia is to induce remission. Chemotherapy, as well as a small amount of radiation therapy, is used for this purpose. The chemotherapy is given orally and intravenously. Because leukemic cells invade the central nervous system, some of the chemotherapy is given intrathecally as, otherwise, it would not cross the blood-brain barrier in a sufficient concentration to destroy the leukemic cells. For the same reason, radiation of the cranium is used as a prophylactic measure.

During the child's initial hospitalization, treatment includes the correction of any major hematologic deficiencies, such as anemia; the control of metabolic derangements, such as hyperuricemia; the elimination of existing infections; and the reduction and control of the proliferating leukemic cells through induction chemotherapy. The initial remission induction takes approximately four to six weeks to achieve. During this time prophylactic therapy to the central nervous system is also administered. Radiation therapy to the cranium, as well as the intrathecal administration of drugs, such as methotrexate, is included in this phase of therapy. Maintenance chemotherapy is part of the discharge routine, and includes oral medications that are given to maintain the remission. During the first two years, the child will be rehospitalized every three months for reinduction chemotherapy, which includes oral, as well as intravenous medications. In some areas, this is done on an outpatient basis in a clinic setting. This is usually more acceptable to the child and less disruptive to the entire family than inpatient treatment. After the child has been in remission for two years, reinduction chemotherapy is administered every six months.

The drugs that are commonly used to treat children with leukemia are listed in Table 20-2. These drugs must be given in sufficient amounts to eradicate the leukemic cells and to allow the bone marrow to resume its normal functioning.

TABLE 20-2 Drugs Commonly Used for Chemotherapy in Patients with Leukemia

Antimetabolites
Cytarabine (Cytosar-U, Cytosine arabinoside)
6-Mercaptopurine (6-MP, Purinethol)
Methotrexate (Amethopterin)
Thioguanine (TG)
5-Azacytidine (5-Aza-C)
Alkylating Agents
Cyclophosphamide (Cytoxan, Endoxan)
Chlorambucil (Leukeran)
Mechlorethamine (nitrogen mustard, Mustargen)
Mitotic Inhibitors
Vincristine sulfate (Oncovin)
Vinblastine sulfate (Velban)
Antibiotics
Dactinomycin (Actinomycin-D Osmegen)
Doxorubicin (Adriamycin, Doxyrubicin)
Daunorubicin (Daunomycin, Rubidomycin)
Bleomycin (Blenoxane)
Enzymes
L-asparaginase (EC-2)
Hormones
Cortisone
Hydrocortisone
Prednisone
Adrenocorticortropic hormone (ACTH)

General Side Effects

The side effects of chemotherapy are numerous and can cause some of the same problems as the leukemic infiltration itself. The most common side effects are nausea, vomiting, diarrhea, alopecia, and bone marrow depression.

Nausea and vomiting which may occur one-half to five hours after the injection of a particular medication, may be controlled in some children by an alteration in the time at which the medication is given. In the case of an intravenous preparation, scheduling the treatment for late afternoon or early evening allows the child to partake of some food during the day without feeling nauseous. Use of antiemetics prior to the infusion may also be beneficial. Providing frequent small meals that are easily digested may also help.

Diarrhea is a concern because of the fluid and electrolytes that are lost. It is also of concern because leukemic children are predisposed to skin breakdown. The perineal and anal areas must, therefore, be cleansed carefully. Sitz baths may also help. As rectal ulceration and rectal prolapse can also occur, the nurse should avoid taking rectal temperatures and administering suppositories. Those children receiving Vincristine or vinblastine may develop constipation from an adynamic ileus.

Bone marrow depression is a major problem. In some children, as much as ninety percent of the bone marrow may be replaced by leukemic infiltration. The onset of chemotherapy also causes bone marrow depression because of the toxic nature of the drugs. The child must be observed carefully for signs of increased bleeding. The period of greatest risk is during the initiation of chemotherapy.

Protection of the child from any source of infection in the environment is also a nursing consideration. Because of the child's decreased resistance to infection, the normal flora within the body may act as pathogens. Good skin care is mandatory. Puncture sites, whether for an intravenous line, a bone marrow aspiration, or blood analysis are common sources of infection. Dressings should be removed and the underlying areas checked carefully on a daily basis. Swelling or red streaks on the arm denoting phlebitis may be the first indication of infection. A slight cough is also cause for concern, as the child may easily develop fungal respiratory infections which are difficult to treat.

Alopecia is a side effect of several of the drugs. The child and the parents may be able to cope with this better if they are made aware of its likelihood before the treatment. In this way, they may select an acceptable wig for the child before a significant amount of hair is lost. Another method that is used by some physicians to control alopecia is a scalp tourniquet. A rubber tubing tourniquet is applied circumferentially at the hairline just prior to the intravenous infusion. It is maintained during the infusion until approximately five minutes after completion of the infusion. The purpose of it is to occlude the arterial blood flow to the scalp, thereby preventing the drug from destroying the hair follicles. A showerlike cap containing crushed ice is also used to reduce blood flow in the same manner.

Buccal ulceration may also be caused by some of these medications. The mouth is a good indicator of the condition of the gastrointestinal tract. The child's mouth should be inspected daily with a flashlight for any signs of redness, white patches, or areas of ulceration. Frequent mouth care and the use of mouthwash and irrigations should be initiated at the onset of chemotherapy. If areas of irritation develop, effective debridement may be accomplished by the use of oxygen-releasing preparations that cleanse the mouth. The use of half-strength hydrogen peroxide is usually acceptable. Some form of antifungal preparation, such as nystatin (Mycostatin), may have to be included in the regimen. Cleansing must be thorough but gentle. Toothettes, rather than a soft toothbrush, may be used in order to cause less gum irritation. A device such as a Waterpik may also be used for cleansing. In very young children, bottles and pacifiers must be sterilized in order to prevent the introduction of harmful organisms into the mouth.

Specific Side Effects of Chemotherapeutic Agents

Some side effects are specific to individual drugs. Cytoxan, for instance, may cause hemorrhagic cystitis. In this instance, fluid intake should be increased and voiding should be encouraged every two hours, even during the night. Parents should be told to report any symptoms of burning or pain on urination, as well as any color change in the urine that would indicate bleeding.

Methotrexate and thioguanine may cause dermatitis and photosensitivity. Children receiving these drugs should not be exposed to the sun without adequate protective clothing. Topical sunscreen agents are also helpful.

Vincristine and vinblastine may cause neurotoxicity, which is first evidenced by a weakened hand grasp, foot drop, numbness, ataxia, or depression.

Adriamycin in large doses causes cardiac arrhythmias, which show up in electrocardiographic changes, and may cause heart failure. This drug also turns the child's urine red for ten to twelve days after administration. This should not be mistaken for hemorrhagic cystitis.

The child receiving both 6-mercaptopurine and allopurinol (Zyloprim) may have additional problems because they are both xanthine analogues. Zyloprim may delay the metabolism of 6-mercaptopurine, thus increasing the potency of the drug when it is metabolized.

Lethal Complications

Two potentially fatal complications of treatment are infection and hemorrhage. The period of greatest risk for the leukemic child is during the initial remission induction chemotherapy when bone marrow depression is greatest, both from the disease and from the treatment. Infections are treated immediately with massive intravenous doses of broad spectrum antibiotics. Hemorrhages may be treated with the infusion of several units of packed red blood cells or platelet transfusions. Four to six units of platelets may be transfused for several days if the platelet count is 10,000 per millimeter or less.

Bone Marrow Transplants

The myelocytic or myeloblastic type of leukemia is responsive to a different type of treatment. In this child, bone marrow transplants may be used. Some of the disadvantages of this method include the difficulty of finding a compatible donor, prevention of infection in the child during the time that the child's bone marrow is nonfunctioning, and prevention of rejection of the foreign protein. The treatment does offer some hope to individuals despite the difficulties.

Nursing Intervention

Initially the care of the child is related to the establishment of a definite diagnosis. This would include careful observation and documentation of any signs of the disease, protection from infection, maintenance of the nutritional status including hydration, and emotional support for the parent and the child.

Observations. The hemorrhagic potential in leukemia dictates frequent and careful observations of the child. The skin should be checked in the normal process of care for signs of pallor, petechiae, and ecchymoses. The inside of the mouth should be inspected for bleeding as well as any potential for infection. The characteristics of urine and stools should be noted and documented for changes that would indicate the onset of additional bleeding. Special attention should be paid to complaints of pain, such as headaches, which could indicate involvement of the central nervous system. Parents' observations should not be discounted as parents are much more attuned to the early behavioral changes that indicate potential problems.

Infection. The selection of the child's room aids in infection control as does the limitation of contacts. A private room would be advantageous but this may not be possible. The child can share the room with another child with no obvious signs of infection. Visitors and staff members with respiratory infections or any other signs of illness should be kept away from this child.

Careful attention should be paid to the blood work. The granulocyte count is especially important to prevention of infection. A count that is below one thousand per cubic millimeter is a life-threatening emergency.

Strict adherence to careful handwashing and the principles of medical asepsis is a must with this child. The frequency of diagnostic tests that require skin punctures alters the integrity and provides a site for the entrance of organisms.

Nutritional status. Many of these children are admitted with weight loss, fatigue, and muscle wasting that indicate a poor nutritional status. This can occur even with an adequate intake in a child. The rapidly proliferating leukemic cells make inordinate demands on the metabolism.

The child should be provided with small, frequent feedings along with supplements. All of these feedings should be of good quality proteins as well as high in calories. The child's likes and dislikes must be considered. The provision of a normal mealtime routine is helpful. The assistance of a parent or other caregiver in providing dietary information about the child as well as helping with meals and snacks is advantageous.

Maintaining an adequate fluid intake in the child is also necessary. The intake and output should be monitored carefully. An adequate intake not only prevents dehydration but also promotes adequate renal function and the elimination of bacteria-laden urine. The adequate output also aids in excretion of uric acid.

Emotional support. Throughout the period of diagnosis and initiation of therapy both parent and child need a great deal of support. The use of primary care facilitates the open exchange of feelings and a continuity of information. The nurse must convey an acceptance of the very real fears and anger that are a part of this process.

Information that is provided to the parents about the diagnostic procedures should be accurate and supportive. If the parents are to participate in the care, they need to know what is to be done and how they can help. Initially, they may be hesitant for fear of hurting the child. Information that is conveyed to the child should be adapted to the developmental age of the child.

Play therapy is a very effective means of allowing the child free expression regarding the hospitalization and the diagnostic procedures. Both the staff and the child-life worker or the play therapist may use this means for the child to express anger. Parents often need help to see that this expression is both normal and healthy for the child. Adjusting to changes in body image can also be accepted more readily through play therapy.

Support for parents may come from a number of sources. Individual nursing staff members may provide some of this. Referral to the social service department of the hospital may aid in financial problems and provide counseling of a limited or an ongoing nature. Some agencies provide group counseling sessions for families and address such issues as home care, helping the siblings cope, and dealing with ongoing stress. Many families have identified the staffs of the Ronald McDonald

Houses as being especially supportive. (These houses are located near major medical centers and provide low-cost housing in a homelike atmosphere for the families of children hospitalized with acute or life-threatening problems.)

Home Care. At some point the child will return home and the major portion of the care will be thrust upon the parents or caregivers. They need to be prepared for this role. They should know the care, the medications, and the signs of infection or complications that indicate the need for medical assistance.

If the child is of school age, parents or caregivers need to know when the child may return to the classroom. They should be prepared to help the child deal with attitudes of classmates about the disease as well as the child's altered body image. Normalization of activities is often difficult as the child and parents have daily reminders of the illness in the oral medications that are taken on an ongoing basis.

DUCHENNE'S MUSCULAR DYSTROPHY

Duchenne's muscular dystrophy is characterized as a progressive, symmetric, muscular weakness. It is seen most commonly in boys and is inherited as a sex-linked trait. The disease is usually diagnosed between infancy and the early school years. In most children it is identified prior to the age of six years. A rare form of the disease affects females. This form is carried as an autosomal dominant trait, Figure 20-4.

Symptoms and Diagnosis

Weakness of the skeletal muscles occurs as normal tissue is replaced with ineffective

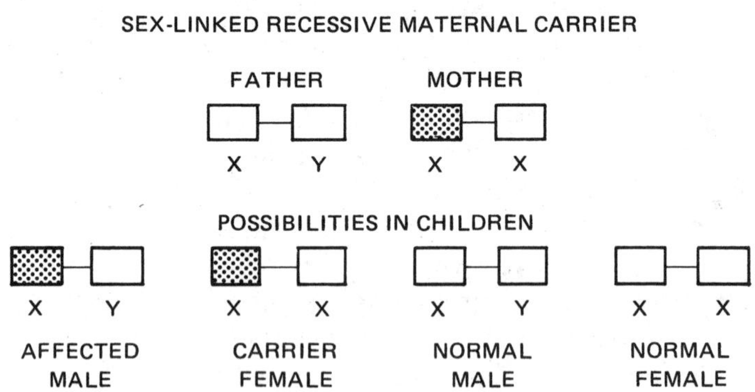

FIG. 20-4 Inheritance pattern of Duchenne's muscular dystrophy

50% change that any girl will be a carrier
50% chance that any boy will be affected
(The Y chromosome directs testicular development. It does not block the action of the paired defective recessive gene.)
50% chance that either the male or the female will be normal

fibrotic tissue. The child may exhibit weakness and fatigue prior to diagnosis. Early in the disease, the child may appear to be gaining weight or improving in muscular size. This apparent increase in muscle mass is actually pseudohypertrophy which becomes evident as the muscle undergoes fibrotic changes. Frequently, the calf muscles of the leg are the first site of this hypertrophy. Other symptoms that may cause the parent to seek medical assistance include a loss of coordination, an inability to climb stairs, frequent falling, and an inability to participate in previously mastered activities or games.

The diagnosis is made on the basis of three tests. A blood test is used to determine the elevation of an enzyme, cephalophosphokinase (CPK), which is secreted by the skeletal muscles. This elevation may be detected as part of a routine screening exam very early in the disease, even before symptoms are noted. The second test is electromyography, which differentiates between nerve conduction damage and muscle damage. The third test is a muscle biopsy to determine the amount of muscle replaced with fibrotic tissue. This test is also repeated at periodic intervals to determine the progression of the disease.

Nursing Care

The nursing care of children with Duchenne's muscular dystrophy and their parents initially involves being supportive during the stressful period of diagnosis. The parents may use a wide variety of defense mechanisms in dealing with this period of testing and determination of the diagnosis.

Once the diagnosis is made, the parents require continued support because of the implications of a genetic disease. Their other children may be affected by the disease, although they may be undiagnosed as yet, either as victims or as carriers. Their plans for future children may be altered by the implications of this disease. During this period of major stress, they are also expected to be supportive to the child undergoing the testing. Genetic counseling is essential for these families in order to provide accurate information so that they are able to sort out their feelings and make logical decisions.

For the child with Duchenne's muscular dystrophy, the goal of treatment is to maintain the highest functional level possible. The treatment is supportive and palliative, but not curative. Braces, splints, and crutches are used to maintain mobility. Eventually, the child will be limited to a wheelchair for ambulation. Physical therapy is usd to maintain full range of joint motion and to prevent the development of contractures.

The major focus of the care of these children is the prevention of infection. Their forced immobility predisposes them to bladder infections and other genitourinary problems. A high fluid intake and the use of acid ash juices, such as cranberry juice, may help prevent some of the problems. Voiding every two to three hours also prevents statis of large amounts of bacteria-laden urine in the bladder. The respiratory system is also compromised by the condition. Poor gas exchange leaves the child prone to infections. Deep breathing, coughing, postural drainage, and reduced exposure to infections are helpful. The prognosis of the disease is poor; the child does not survive to adulthood.

NEPHROSIS

The condition referred to as nephrosis is frequently called idiopathic nephrotic syndrome, or childhood nephrosis. The terms are used interchangeably, but all identify a noninflammatory disease of the renal tubules and the characteristic picture of a severely edematous child with multiple problems. The condition is most commonly seen in male children during the toddler or preschool period. However, it can occur in older children, as well as in adults.

Pathophysiology

The exact cause of the disease is unknown. It is thought by some to be a type of autoimmune response and by others to be the result of a toxic state. The result is a defect in the permeability of the glomerular membrane which allows large quantities of protein to be excreted.

The proteinuria is usually in excess of 0.1 gram per kilogram of body weight per day. This tremendous outpouring of protein exceeds the rate of synthesis of albumin in the liver. The child will also have hypoalbuminemia. The loss of protein also occurs in the gastrointestinal tract with symptoms of a malabsorption syndrome. During this period, there is an increased rate of protein catabolism or breakdown as the body attempts to maintain some degree of stability.

As the albumin leaves the circulatory pathways, the level of the blood lipids rises. This accounts for the hyperlipidemia or very high blood cholesterol levels seen in these children.

The massive shift of proteins and lipids causes significant changes in the osmotic pressures within the circulatory system. The intravascular pressures decrease as the protein is lost. The fluid held in the capillaries crosses into the extracellular spaces and the child appears severely edematous. Theoretically, this edema is a protective mechanism, whereby enough pressure is exerted around the capillaries to prevent a massive circulatory collapse.

Treatment

The treatment for nephrosis is aimed at producing diuresis. The most common method of treating the child involves the use of corticosteroids, particularly prednisone. It is administered daily in dosages based on 60 milligrams per square meter of body surface. Prednisone, rather than another corticosteroid, is used because it is well tolerated and has less of a tendency to cause increased salt retention and potassium loss. In addition to the prednisone, a potassium-sparing diuretic is administered. These medications are administered daily for about four weeks and then discontinued abruptly.

The diuresis begins about one to two weeks into the treatment. It is characterized by a gradual increase in urine output, a loss of weight, and changes in the pH of the urine from acid to alkaline. The steroid treatment is continued until the child has near normal levels of serum albumin and the proteinuria has resolved or been greatly reduced.

After diuresis has been achieved the corticosteroids are administered on a decreased dosage and alternate day schedule for between eight and twelve months. This minimizes the undesirable side effects of corticosteriods and avoids suppression of the child's own adrenal function.

An antihypertensive medication may also be used if the child's blood pressure is elevated. Antibiotics are not used routinely as a prophylactic measure.

Nursing Care

Edema. One of the major nursing care problems identified for children with nephrosis relates to the child's severe edema, Table 20-3. Meticulous skin care is a necessity. The skin should be observed carefully for any signs of irritation or breakdown. It should be cleansed frequently with a mild soap and patted dry. Opposing skin surfaces are kept separated using cotton or lamb's wool in order to prevent the skin from rubbing together and breaking down. Powder is used sparingly to prevent friction between surfaces. Overuse of powder can cause irritation.

Special attention must be directed to the severe edema in the scrotum and thigh areas. A T-binder or a scrotal support is used even in very young children. The binder is removed and the skin checked carefully for any signs of irritation. The frequent checking of the area around the genitalia may be very upsetting to the preschooler, who already is concerned with his penis. **Caution: Injections are avoided in children with nephrosis.** The tissues are so edematous that they do not absorb the drug. Therefore, as diuresis occurs, the rate of drug absorption accelerates causing a massive overdose.

Periorbital edema, which is particularly upsetting to both the young child and the parents, is minimized by proper positioning of the patient. Encouraging the child to sleep with the head of the bed elevated in a semi-Fowler's position helps to reduce the periorbital edema.

Large amounts of fluid in the abdomen, or ascites, is also controlled with positioning. The semi-Fowler's position aids in reducing the pressure on the diaphragm. In addition,

TABLE 20-3 Nursing Care Problems in Children with Nephrosis

Edema
Meticulous skin care
Maintenance of bedrest
Positioning of patient with the head slightly elevated (semi-Fowler's position)
Provision to T-binder or scrotal support, if needed
Avoidance of injectable medications
Administration of diuretic as ordered
Observation for malabsorption syndrome (indicating edema of the gastrointestinal tract)
Decreased Resistance to Infection
Elimination of undue exposure to others with infection
Observation for signs of infection in any body system
Observation for areas of skin breakdown
Administration of antibiotics as ordered
Anorexia
Provision of small, frequent meals
Determination of child's dietary preferences
Selection of high protein snacks
Assistance with feeding
Provision of brief rest periods before meals
Maintain sodium restriction

pillows and bath blankets are used for positioning the child in order to prevent irritation from opposing skin surfaces. Abdominal paracentesis may be used to reduce the ascites.

Dietary Control. The severe protein depletion associated with nephrosis results in a major nutritional loss for affected children. Ideally, a high-protein diet should be consumed. Realistically, children rarely will eat any diet that is vastly different from what they are used to having. On this basis of acceptance, the child is offered a diet containing 2 to 3 grams of good-quality protein per kilogram of body weight. The food is offered in several small meals rather than in large quantities all at once. The combination of ascites and fatigue makes it difficult for the child to eat adequately. In children with excess potassium losses, the diet is also supplemented with oranges or bananas, which contain larger amounts of potassium. One-half of a small banana equals 4.8 milliequivalents of potassium; one-half cup of orange juice contains 5.1 milliequivalents.

Because of fluid retention, sodium is restricted to 1 gram daily. Any restriction that is more stringent is usually poorly tolerated by the child. The child should consume at least a portion of every meal so that the restriction does not exceed this level. Fluids may not be restricted for the child. However, the nurse must be careful to offer fluids that are not high in sodium content. In those children who have fluid restrictions, the intake is calculated on the basis of the previous day's output plus insensible losses.

Infection. Protection from infections is also important. Children with nephrosis are highly susceptible to infection. For this reason, it is imperative that contact with large groups of people be avoided. In the hospital, the child should be protected from other patients with infections. Upon discharge, the school-aged child may or may not be permitted to return to school. If unable to return to school at this time, the child may be tutored to remain current with classwork.

In those children who do not respond to corticosteroids, other agents such as immunosuppressive or antineoplastic drugs, such as Cytoxan, may be used. These drugs are usually reserved for those children who suffer two relapses in the first year after the onset of treatment. Such children are usually near adulthood and have hematuria, hypertension, and a history of lengthy bouts of acute disease lasting six months or more.

Parental Support. Throughout the entire disease process, the nurse must work positively with the parents. Initially, they should be provided with an explanation of the diagnosis and should be helped to adjust to the child's long-term problem. During the child's hospitalization, the nurse should reinforce positive parenting skills, as well as support the parents. It is important that the nurse make a special effort to prepare the parents for the home care of the child. The dietitian may also assist the parents by reinforcing the dietary information that was shared and by adapting this information to the family's eating patterns.

Play Activities. Play activities in both the home and the hospital should be used to help children with nephrosis adjust to their appearance and health problems. Initially, these children may have realistic concerns regarding their body image. The negative aspects of their appearance may inadvertently be reinforced by the comments of the staff or other children.

The nurse should try to emphasize the positive aspects of the child's appearance and personality. The nurse should also acknowledge any improvements in the child's condition.

HEMOPHILIA

Hemophilia is a term that designates a group of diseases. It is actually a syndrome that is the result of several distinct inherited congenital defects in clotting. In each form of the disease the defect involves the factors that are necessary for a normal clotting mechanism. The defect interferes with thromboplastic activity and results in inadequate clot formation.

Classification

The classic type of hemophilia is referred to as hemophilia A, or Factor VIII deficiency, and involves a deficiency of antihemophilic globulin (AHG). This is a sex-linked recessive disease that transmits the disease to males and renders females asymptomatic carriers. Each pregnancy in an affected woman is associated with a fifty percent chance of producing a male who has the disease. The disease is rare in families but can occur with a carrier mother and a father with the disease.

Hemophilia B is a deficiency of the plasma thromboplastin component (PTC), or Factor IX. It is also called Christmas disease. The mode of transmission of the disease is the same as for Factor VIII deficiency, and the clinical symptoms that are manifested are the same.

The third type, hemophilia C, involves a deficiency of Factor XI, or plasma thromboplastin antecedent (PTA). This type of hemophilia is unique in that it appears as an autosomal dominant trait and, as such, can occur in both males and females. The bleeding tendencies in children affected by this form is also unique. Bleeding occurs only as a direct result of trauma. This is in contrast to the spontaneous type of bleeding that occurs with the other hemophilias. Moreover, the bleeding, when it occurs, is less severe.

Symptoms

The major symptom exhibited by children with hemophilia is prolonged bleeding caused by an extremely delayed clotting time. The bleeding, which may be either internal or external, can occur anywhere in the body. Hemorrhage within the nervous system or the joints is the most serious type. Hemarthrosis is most common in the early school years. Bleeding may also occur in the skin, the urinary tract, and in any part of the mucous membranes lining the gastrointestinal tract.

The bleeding may result from minor injury and may not always be recognized by the parent initially. It can also occur spontaneously, as in type A and B hemophilias. The massive bleeding that occurs in some children may be fatal. The severity of the disease depends on the percent of the clotting factor involved. The mild forms have twenty-five to fifty percent of the clotting factor, while the most severe have less than one percent.

Treatment

Bleeding from small wounds may cause major problems for hemophiliac children. In the case of a wound, the parents should know what to do immediately. Small cuts or injuries should be packed with a fibrin foam, such as Oxycel or Gelfoam, and have pressure applied. The child should be taken to a medical facility if the bleeding persists. Nosebleeds, or epistaxis, are usually controlled in the same fashion with the addition of gentle pressure. These children do not bleed faster than a normal child, but bleed for a longer period of time.

Joint hemorrhages are of greater concern than wounds elsewhere in the body. The joint should be immobilized until the bleeding subsides. This is accomplished through the use of a posterior splint, ice packs, and elevation of the part. These measures should be applied by the parents prior to transport of the child to the hospital. The blood in the joint capsule causes severe pain for which narcotics may initially be administered. When the bleeding subsides, gentle passive range of motion is initiated to help maintain full joint mobility. Replacement therapy with the missing clotting factor is necessary to prevent a recurrence of the bleeding. Joint impairment can occur in these children as a result of the multiple injuries to the same joint and the gradual development of joint contractures.

Special Considerations

Surgical procedures require extreme caution in these children. A procedure as simple as a tooth extraction may require admission to the hospital. The administration of transfusions of fresh, whole blood or the missing clotting factor is required. Whole blood administered as an emergency measure or as a preoperative or postoperative measure, can cause a volume overload before therapeutic effectiveness is achieved. For this reason, it is preferable to administer fresh frozen plasma or a form of dried and reconstituted plasma that contains the necessary clotting factor. Cryoprecipitate is used for the patient with mild hemophilia involving a Factor VIII deficiency. Concentrates, such as Profilate and Factorate, are used in children with the severe bleeding problems. Initially, it is important to determine whether the child is receiving any antiplatelet medications, such as aspirin or aspirin-containing products, or any nonsteroidal anti-inflammatory drugs.

Nursing Care

The nursing care of hemophiliac patients involves protection of the child and control of the environment. The disease may be recognized at the time of birth or shortly thereafter, but early detection is uncommon. In these situations, the baby should be observed closely. A circumcision should not be performed in affected infants. The infant's crib should be padded and all sharp toys avoided. As the infant becomes more mobile, it is important to protect the head from injury by the use of a football-type helmet and to protect the knees with knee pads.

Arrangement of the child's surroundings is also important in avoiding injuries. Toys are selected both at home and in the hospital with the child's unique safety needs in mind. The use of a mesh playpen to restrict the child's movements is acceptable when adequate supervision is not possible. When the child is allowed out of this environment to explore, the constant and alert attention of either the parent or the nurse is required.

Hemophiliac children receive frequent transfusions of blood and blood products. Because of this, many of these children carry the hepatitis virus. The nurse should take special precautions in handling needles and syringes after infusions.

Parent Teaching

The parents of hemophiliac children should be taught not only information about the disease itself and home care, but also about alternative ways to handle their child. To grab hemophiliac children by the arm or to swat them lightly on the seat can be life-threatening. On the other hand, if discipline is totally lacking these children may learn very early that they can do anything they wish as no one is likely to intervene because of their disease. This manipulative behavior may become a lifelong characteristic if not altered early.

Along with discussing growth and development with the parents, therefore, the nurse should discuss as well as demonstrate alternative methods of disciplining the child. Emphasis should be on positive reinforcement of desired behavior. This role modeling can reinforce effective parenting skills. The more effectively this is done, the less inclined the preschooler will be to threaten "if you don't give me that toy, I will poke this straw in my mouth and bleed to death." These negative behaviors should be ignored completely until the child realizes they do not work. Consistency is the key to reinforcement.

Parents, as well as the child, should be helped to accept the limitations of the condition and to be realistic about the child's accomplishments. The child should be encouraged to pursue appropriate activities in school and elsewhere. The debating team and chess team, for example, are realistic pursuits, but the basketball team is not. Frequent absences from school may require the use of a tutor to keep the child at the appropriate grade level.

The parents should also be informed of the services of the National Hemophilia Foundation. This agency can provide them with up-to-date information about the disease and current research. Financial help, provision of medical supplies, counseling, patient advocacy, and group meetings are offered through the state and local chapters.

SUMMARY

The child with idiopathic thrombocytopenic purpura has a potentially life-threatening illness. The assessment for the areas of bleeding and the protection of the child during the acute phase are priorities for nursing care in this condition.

Sickle cell disease has a slower more insidious onset in children and the extent of the problem may not be recognized initially. In addition to the effects of chronic illness, the nurse must be acutely aware of the genetic implications of this disease and its impact on the family unit.

Children with leukemia presently have an optimistic prognosis because of the multiple types of chemotherapy that are available and the aggressive approach to treatment. A major nursing responsibility in this disease is a knowledge of the side effects of the drugs that may be administered to the child.

Duchenne's muscular dystrophy is another hereditary disease whose transmission is sex-linked. The child appears to be quite normal for the first few years of life until the disease insidiously appears. The goal of all care and treatment is to maintain the child in a mobile state as long as possible.

Recurrences of acute nephrosis are not uncommon in some children. The nurse's attention must be directed toward the relief of symptoms related to the disease, such as severe edema. The nurse must also be knowledgeable about the prescribed diet and the medications for the child.

Hemophilia is an inherited disease characterized by the absence of a specific clotting factor. The severity of the disease is reflected in the percent of the clotting factor available in the plasma. The problem is lifelong. Care involves control of the environment to prevent problems and prompt treatment of emergency situations.

SUGGESTED ACTIVITIES

- Care for a child with one of the diseases discussed in this chapter. Share with your group the symptoms you observed and the treatment program that was instituted as well as any specific information about diet or medications. Also discuss the child's perception of the reason for hospitalization.
- Talk with three or four Black Americans in your community. Find out what they know about sickle cell disease and how they feel about sickle cell screening tests. What do they see as the advantages or disadvantages of mandatory testing?
- Plan a twenty-four-hour balanced menu for a five-year-old child with nephrosis. Remember to include snacks between meals and at bedtime.

DISCUSSION TOPICS

1. Discuss with your group the impact of the knowledge of a hereditary disease on a preadolescent child or an adolescent. How would the parents respond to this child's concerns?
2. What agencies are available in your community to assist children with the diseases mentioned in this chapter? What type of assistance would be provided for the family?

REVIEW

A. Matching. Match the name of the disease in Column II with its description in Column I.

Column I	Column II
1. Inherited congenital defect of blood coagulation	a. Idiopathic thrombocytopenic purpura
2. Noninflammatory disease of the renal tubules	b. Sickle cell anemia
3. Self-limiting disease affecting platelet production	c. Leukemia
4. Disease characterized by proliferation of immature leukocytes	d. Duchenne's muscular dystrophy
5. Inherited disease characterized by progressive, symmetrical muscle weakness	e. Nephrosis
6. Inherited disease characterized by defective hemoglobin	f. Hemophilia

B. Multiple choice. Select the one best answer.

Situation: Larry is a four-year-old boy with acute lymphocytic leukemia. He is currently hospitalized and is being treated with methotrexate and prednisone. Larry has large areas of ecchymosis over portions of his skin.

1. A decrease in which one of the following types of blood cells causes severe ecchymosis?
   a. Erythrocytes
   b. Neutrophils
   c. Platelets
   d. Lymphocytes
2. Which of these breakfast menus would be most suitable for Larry, considering that he has buccal ulcerations?
   a. Apple juice, a fried egg, and shredded wheat
   b. Stewed prunes, rye toast, and bacon
   c. Orange juice, cream cheese, and whole wheat toast
   d. Applesauce, cream of wheat, and a soft-boiled egg

Situation: Christopher is a three-year-old boy with nephrosis who is currently hospitalized. He is anorexic and must be encouraged to eat.

3. What type of diet would you expect the doctor to order for Christopher?
   a. A normal diet with increased protein and moderately restricted salt
   b. A low-protein diet with no restriction of salt intake
   c. A normal diet with slightly reduced carbohydrate content
   d. An elimination diet similar to that used for allergic patients

4. Because of Christopher's edema, you are very careful about maintaining an accurate intake and output record as well as a daily weight record. In addition, his daily skin care includes
   1. frequent bathing of the genitalia and application of cornstarch.
   2. support of the scrotum with a soft dressing and T-binder.
   3. separation of opposing skin surfaces with cotton material.
   4. gentle massage of pressure points with lanolin-containing lotion.
   5. avoidance of intramuscular injections in the buttocks.
      a. 1 and 2
      b. 3, 4, and 5
      c. 1 and 5
      d. 1, 2, 3, 4 and 5

5. Characteristic signs and symptoms of idiopathic thrombocytopenic purpura include
   a. an abrupt onset of the disease following a viral infection, petechiae, ecchymoses and gingival bleeding.
   b. a gradual onset of the disease with no history of infection, abdominal pain, or vomiting.
   c. ecchymosis, gingival bleeding, diarrhea, dehydration, and a rapid onset of the disease.
   d. fever, malaise, petechiae, epistaxis, and a gradual onset of the disease.

6. Symptoms that would indicate increased bleeding in a patient with idiopathic thrombocytopenic purpura would include
   a. decreased coloration of ecchymotic areas, vomiting, and diarrhea.
   b. a sudden drop in blood pressure, diaphoresis, and tachycardia.
   c. a changing distribution of petechia and increased tenderness of ecchymotic areas.
   d. an increased pulse rate and signs of shock.

7. Symptoms that herald a sickle cell crisis include
   1. loss of appetite.
   2. pain in the arms and legs.
   3. swelling of the joints.
   4. diarrhea.
      a. 1 and 4
      b. 1, 2, and 3
      c. 2 and 3
      d. 1, 2, 3 and 4

8. The diagnostic tests used to determine the presence of HbS include
   1. oxygen reduction blood tests.
   2. SGOT and SGPT enzyme tests.
   3. Sickledex test.
   4. hemoglobin electrophoresis.
   5. skeletal surveys.
      a. 2 and 4
      b. 1, 3, and 4
      c. 1 only
      d. 1, 2, 3, 4 and 5

C. Short answer. Briefly respond to the following statements.

1. Describe the difference between the inheritance of sickle cell trait and the inheritance of sickle cell disease.

2. Describe the nursing care of a child with Duchenne's muscular dystrophy.

3. List three measures that may be used to protect an infant with hemophilia.

BIBLIOGRAPHY

Bloomfield, Karen. "Johnny Is My Most Difficult and Dearest Patient." *Nursing 74,* Vol. 4 (October, 1974), pp. 68–70.

Doswell, Willa M. "Sickle Cell Anemia: You Can Do Something to Help." *Nursing 78,* Vol. 8 (April, 1978), pp. 65–70.

Foley, Genevieve, and Marie McCarthy. "The Child with Leukemia: The Disease and Its Treatment," and "In a Special Hematology Clinic." *American Journal of Nursing,* Vol. 76 (July, 1976), pp. 1105–1119.

Foster, Sue. "Sickle Cell Anemia – Closing the Gap Between Theory and Therapy. Part II." *American Journal of Nursing,* Vol. 71 (October, 1971), pp. 1952–1954.

Greene, Patricia. "The Child with Leukemia in the Classroom." *American Journal of Nursing,* Vol. 75 (January, 1975), pp. 86–87.

Greene, Patricia. "Teaching Aid for Children with Sickle Cell Disease." *American Journal of Nursing,* Vol. 77 (December, 1977), p. 1953.

Marlow, Dorothy R. *Textbook of Pediatric Nursing.* Philadelphia: W. B. Saunders Company, 1977.

Martinson, Ida M. "The Child with Leukemia – Parents Help Each Other." *American Journal of Nursing,* Vol. 76 (July, 1976), pp. 1120–1122.

McFarlane, Judith Medin. "The Child with Sickle Cell Anemia." *Nursing 75,* Vol. 5 (May, 1975), pp. 29–33.

McFarlane, Judith. "Sickle Cell Disorders." *American Journal of Nursing,* Vol. 77 (December, 1977), pp. 1948–1954.

Pochedly, Carl. "Sickle Cell Anemia – Recognition and Management, Part I." *American Journal of Nursing,* Vol. 71 (October, 1971), pp. 1948–1952.

Scipien, Gladys, M., et al. *Comprehensive Pediatric Nursing.* New York: McGraw-Hill Book Company, 1980.

Whaley, Lucille F., and Donna L. Wong. *Nursing Care of Infants and Children.* St. Louis: C. V. Mosby Company, 1979.

Wiley, Loy, ed. "Muscular Dystrophy: A Nursing Point of View." *Nursing 80,* Vol. 10 (January, 1980), pp. 44–49.

Chapter 21

Children With Special Needs

OBJECTIVES

Upon completion of this chapter, the student will be able to

- describe the adaptations in care that are necessary for a mentally retarded child based on the child's functional level.
- identify specific concerns and nursing approaches relating to the continuity of care for a chronically ill child.
- compare the child's response to terminal illness with his or her developmental age.
- describe ways in which the nurse may assist the parents in coping with the terminal illness of their child.

Children with special needs are those children who have overriding problems or conditions that directly influence the care that is given to them. Their growth and development and their adaptive behaviors are altered by their special problem. Considered in this area are those children with mental retardation, chronic illness, and those who are terminally ill.

MENTAL RETARDATION

The child with mental retardation is one who is below average in intellectual function and who exhibits delays in adaptive behavior. In the past, this child's problems, if not recognized at birth or with follow-up pediatric care, were usually identified during the school-age period. Presently, the majority of children with mental retardation are still identified between the ages of six and sixteen years. However, with the current increased emphasis on developmental assessment, these children should begin to be identified earlier and assisted to achieve more. Use of such tools as the Denver Developmental Screening Test enables the nurse to recognize intellectual and developmental delays earlier. The parents can then be taught how to work with the child to achieve an optimal functional level.

Causes of Retardation

Multiple factors have been identified which are associated with retardation. These include such prenatal infections as toxoplasmosis, chromosomal abnormalities such as Down's Syndrome, encephalopathy caused by infections or bilirubinemia, and cranial anomalies. During the delivery and immediately afterward such factors as anoxia, hypoglycemia, hemorrhage, and actual trauma can cause retardation. In the period of infancy and childhood, retardation can be the end result of cerebral infections, trauma, cerebrovascular accidents from congenital defects, lead poisoning, and postimmunization encephalopathy. For this latter group, if the problem occurs very early in infancy the damage will usually be much greater.

Other factors which are not as easily or clearly defined may interfere with a child's ability to develop intellectually. Nutrition cannot be overlooked as a contributing factor. The low-birth-weight infant born to a nutritionally deprived mother is already in a high risk category. The child who has been deprived economically, socially, and emotionally does not enter the learning situation with the same skills and tools as an advantaged child.

Chromosomal Abnormalities Associated with Retardation

The development of improved techniques for the study of the chromosomes has allowed for better recognition of those diseases resulting from chromosomal aberrations. The possibility of a mechanical error in the process of cell division is very great because of its complexity. The addition or loss of a chromosome or a portion of one occurs during the formation of the gamete or in the early stages immediately after fertilization. The three specific diseases associated with retardation which will be discussed here are Down's syndrome or Trisomy 21, Klinefelter's syndrome, and Turner's syndrome.

Down's Syndrome

Trisomy 21 or Down's syndrome is the most common of the chromosomal abnormalities occurring once in 770 births. The abnormal reproductive cell occurs when the pair of number 21 chromosomes fail to separate during normal division for egg or sperm cell production. The end result upon fertilization is a zygote with three chromosomes rather than two of number 21. There is a strong correlation of this occurrence with advanced maternal age. At age twenty the incidence is 1/2000. By age thirty the incidence is approximately 1/900. By age forty it has risen to 1/100. Some studies have also identified advanced paternal age as being a factor. Translocation of a chromosome or extra genetic material from the number 15 to the number 21 is less common but can produce the same clinical result with a higher incidence regardless of maternal age.

The child with Down's syndrome can be recognized by certain characteristic features. These include a flattened occiput; inner epicanthal folds; abnormally shaped, low-set ears; flattened nasal bridge; and protruding tongue. The hands are characteristically short and broad with incurving of the little finger, a single palmar or "simian" crease across the palm, and a single crease in the fifth finger indicating hypoplasia of the fifth phalanx. A gap exists between the first and second toes along with distinctive changes in the whorls on the ball of the foot. Hypotonia is distinctive in these children. Congenital heart disease is a common occurrence and is usually a septal defect. Other features include a high-arched palate; strabismus; a broad, short neck; small teeth; and a furrowed tongue. In those children who do not have brown eyes, there are characteristic light-colored specks on the iris called Brushfield spots. Intestinal atresia and imperforate anus also occur more commonly in these infants.

Klinefelter's Syndrome

This particular syndrome, although caused by a chromosomal aberration, is often called primary gonadal failure or hypogonadism. The syndrome is usually identified in adolescence when the young person seeks health care for delayed puberty or perhaps for infertility. The individual has a chromosomal complement of 47 XXY which is an additional X chromosome. There are variants of this syndrome with additional X chromosomes, the severity of the mental retardation being associated directly with the number of additional X chromosomes. It occurs in 1/500 live male births.

Characteristic features include a tall male with legs disproportionately long in relation to the trunk; sparse facial and pubic hair, often with a female distribution; and undeveloped testes, penis, and prostate with decreased or absent sperm production. Gynecomastia occurs in more than half of these males. Buccal smears are chromatin-positive and chromosomal analysis readily identifies the additional X chromosome.

Turner's Syndrome

Turner's syndrome is another syndrome of gonadal dysgenesis occurring less often than Klinefelter's syndrome. It occurs in 1/3000 live females. Chromosomal studies identify this individual as having a single X chromosome instead of the normal XX in females. The chromosome constitution is then 45X and is referred to as a monosomy. This condition, unlike Down's syndrome, has no relationship to maternal age. It also has distinctive characteristics which allow for its recognition at birth rather than at puberty.

Characteristic findings which would identify this child at birth include lymphedema of the hands and feet, and loose skin folds at the nape of the neck (webbed neck). Low birth weight and short stature are also evident at that time. During childhood, additional characteristics can be identified: micrognathia; low posterior hairline; low set, malformed ears; increased carrying angle at the elbow (cubitus valgus); broad chest with hypoplastic nipples; vision and hearing problems; hyperconvex fingernails; and mental retardation. Cardiovascular problems include hypertension as well as a high incidence of coarctation of the aorta. The failure of sexual development may be the problem which brings the child into the health care system, however, this is less common than in the past because of the better recognition of the syndrome.

Buccal smears usually indicate a sex-chromatin negative individual and confirm the diagnosis of Turner's syndrome. The gonadotropin plasma levels are elevated even in infancy. Urinary excretion of estrogens is low. Anabolic steroids such as synthetic androgenic hormones are used to enhance linear growth in either continuous or intermittent therapy over several years duration. Without this, most individuals do not achieve five feet in stature. At age fifteen oral estrogens are administered daily for a period of six months to initiate sexual maturation. Once menstruation begins the estrogens are given in a cyclic pattern thereafter. The moderate degree of learning disabilities or retardation is not affected by treatment of the infantile sexual development.

Developmental Classification

Severe Retardation. Children who are classified as severely retarded have an intelligence quotient (IQ) of twenty to thirty-five. These children require nursing care. They have severe sensorimotor handicaps. They may be unable to be toilet trained because of the immaturity of their nervous systems. As these children reach six to eighteen years of age, they are usually able to communicate simple wants, they may be able to walk, but they are totally incapable of self-care. One of the major problems in caring for these children is their total dependency, which may cause economic as well as emotional strain for the family. Their functional level is that of a toddler, and temper tantrums, negativism, and preoccupation with bodily functions are evident, Table 21-1.

The child with an IQ of less than nineteen is identified as profoundly retarded. This child may have been identified as needing custodial care because of the severity of the retardation. It is important to remember that these categorizations are limited to children with isolated retardation and not those with other handicapping conditions. The child with a severe sensory handicap, such as blindness or deafness, or a child with marked motor impairment, such as cerebral palsy, may initially test within these ranges because of the handicapping condition.

Moderate Retardation. Children who are classified as moderately retarded are semidependent and have an IQ of between thirty-six and fifty-one. These children can perform activities of daily living and self-care, as well as sim-

TABLE 21-1 Characteristics of Various Degrees of Mental Retardation

Severe Retardation	Moderate Retardation	Mild Retardation
IQ range of 20 to 35	IQ range of 36 to 51	IQ range of 51 to 68
Severe sensorimotor handicaps	Considered to be trainable in simple tasks	Considered to be educable in more complex tasks
Inability to carry out activities of daily living	Ability to carry out activities of daily living	May not be identified until school-aged
Minimal speech abilities (basic needs only)		Prone to conduct disorders
Total dependence on others	Ability to interact with others	Influenced strongly by peers
	Low tolerance for frustration	
	Benefits from occupational training in a sheltered workshop setting	
Highest functional level is that of a toddler	Highest functional level is that of a child in second grade	Highest level of functioning is that of a child in the sixth grade

ple tasks when supervised. They are considered trainable, and function at a second-grade level. When these children achieve their highest potential, they are able to get along with others and to conform to some social rules, and may be able to travel independently within a clearly defined setting. Some of the problems that are present in these children include a low tolerance for frustration, a need for immediate satisfaction, bed-wetting, masturbation, and destructive behavior. The destructive behavior may involve either persons or property, but it is seldom willful and usually is a result of the child's lack of judgment. Delinquent behavior may occur, but it is usually directed by others with a higher level of intelligence. Not all of these children mature sexually. Emotionally, they function at a below-average level and are generally not interested in a heterosexual relationship. They should be considered for occupational training for specific skills in a sheltered workshop-type situation.

Mild Retardation. Mild retardation is associated with an IQ of fifty-one to sixty-eight. Mildly retarded children exhibit a far greater level of functioning than those with more severe retardation. Their abilities are largely dependent on their home environment, their culture, and their personal motivation. Their maximal functioning is at the sixth-grade level. These children frequently develop conduct disorders, usually evidenced by failure in the classroom and poor emotional control. They develop strong ties to their peer group and may be participants in delinquent behavior. These children know right from wrong but may do wrong to gain acceptance by their peer group.

This child has more potential ability for independence than children in the previous classifications. The ability to care for himself, communicate needs, and perform more complex tasks permits a degree of independence not available to the others. The child realistically should attain the basic academic skills that permit functioning in the environment. Using public transportation with some limitations, making purchases and paying for them, and performing repetitive skills in a job situation are all appropriate long-term goals for this child. The degree to which the child achieves independence is a reflection of the home environment, the acceptance of the child, the learning opportunities available, and the onset of the appropriate intervention.

Hospitalization

When working with mentally retarded children in the hospital setting, it is imperative that the nurse determine their developmental age and capabilities. The parents should be asked specific questions regarding all of the activities and routines of the child's day. Application of this information serves a twofold purpose. First, maintenance of home routines reduces the anxiety the child experiences in the strange environment of the hospital. Second, once the child's current level of functioning has been determined, the nurse can then work to maintain those skills and abilities that have already been mastered. If the child is being followed routinely in a clinic setting, the nursing staff may also act as a liason between the hospital staff and the family. The nursing care plan must focus on both the current medical problem and the child's developmental status, Figure 21-1.

Working with the Family

After the initial meeting with and testing of the child, serial observations are made to

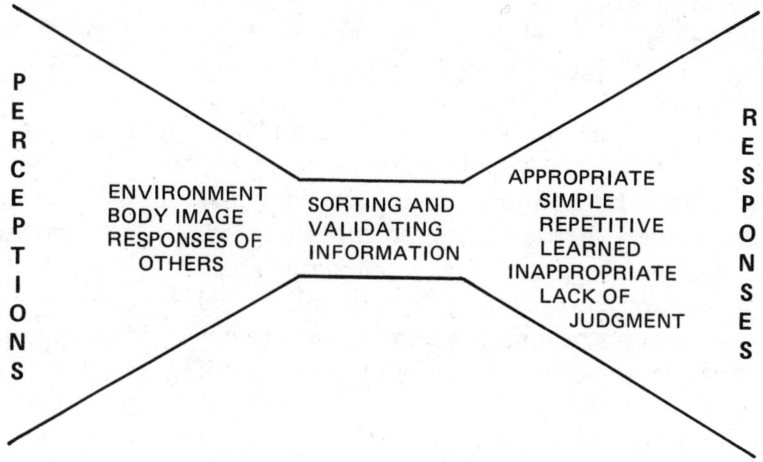

FIG. 21-1 Retarded children's responses are dependent upon the accuracy of their perceptions as well as their ability to process information.

validate the baseline assessment. At the time the actual diagnosis is confirmed, the parents will need a great deal of support. They generally go through a grieving process for the perfect child they might have had. During the stage of denial, they may refuse to recognize that a problem exists. Once they have completed the grief process, they can actively seek assistance and participate in the child's care.

If the diagnosis is confirmed in the hospital setting, the nurse is often the one to identify strengths and weaknesses in the child and to reassure the parents of the adequacy of their parenting skills. This is done in a variety of ways, depending on the time of the child's diagnosis. Early in the assessment period, the child should be observed within the home environment. Interactions with other family members can be observed along with assessing the child's current level of functioning.

Once the initial assessment has taken place, the health care team and the parents should discuss the results and plan for the child's future. This planning should include an identification of skills to be reinforced and behavioral patterns to be altered in some way. The parent is taught how to achieve these objectives in a step-by-step fashion. Realistic goals should be set based on the parents' motivation and the child's readiness.

If the period of assessment takes place in a hospital setting, the parent should be shown how to care for the child, and should be allowed to implement these techniques prior to discharge while supervision is available. The parent is taught to positively reinforce acceptable behaviors. In this situation, the nurse assumes a major role in working with the parents on various approaches to the child. For instance, a variety of methods may be developed for increasing the learning activities of the child, such as increasing environmental stimulation to enhance the child's achievement potential. The nurse or home tutor may also help the parent to establish multiple short-term goals for each desired activity in order to facilitate measuring the progress of the child. All tasks should proceed from simple to complex.

Progress should be recorded to reinforce the child's achievement.

One of the major difficulties faced by these parents is the lack of effective role models. They may have had other normal children with whom their parenting was effective, but they may be unsure of their ability to parent a retarded child who has difficulty with receiving and sorting out stimuli, and then reacting appropriately. Parent groups provide invaluable support to the parents of a newly diagnosed retarded child.

Other siblings should also be included in the discussions and sharing of information regarding the retarded child. In the past, other children were frequently excluded from these discussions for a number of reasons. The parents may not have known how to explain the problem or may have avoided it because of their own feelings. If excluded, some siblings may come to believe that they caused the child's condition, or they may become unduly upset because of the negative attitudes or ridicule of their peer group. Group discussions allow for a sharing of knowledge as well as a common sharing of feelings. They also promote the concept of personal involvement with the child.

This teaching, which should be geared to the developmental level of the siblings, is best accomplished in small group settings. Siblings should know that this child will learn but that the learning process will be slow; that the child will develop but at a different rate than normal children; and that their brother or sister is not entirely unique but is like many other such children. They can also be shown what can be done to help their retarded brother or sister learn new skills.

An assessment of the child's functional level should be done at periodic intervals by a multidisciplinary team. The child's learning activities initially are focused on activities of daily living, including self-feeding, dressing, and toileting once the child has sufficient motor ability to accomplish them. The ability to communicate is an ongoing learning activity. The use of play materials, selected appropriately, enhance functional abilities. The services of a child life worker or an occupational therapist are helpful. Consistent limit setting must be used throughout to aid the child in achieving the desired behavior.

As the child grows there should be opportunities to establish relationships with peers. In the past these children were often isolated in their own homes and when they were taken out the situations may have been traumatic. Participation in day care or school settings for the preschool and school-age child allows and encourages the establishment of a peer relationship in a nonthreatening environment.

Community Resources

The nurse should also notify the family of the available community resources. At the onset, the family may require counseling services provided through local mental health centers or other agencies. This counseling should include genetic counseling regarding the cause of the child's retardation and the possibility of its recurrence in future children. Later, parents may use the services of specialized nurseries and day-care centers. Some retarded children may also be enrolled in special classes offered in public or private schools. As the child grows and learns, sheltered workshops, group homes, and vocational training should be made available on the basis of the degree of retardation, Table 21-2.

TABLE 21-2 Community Resources for Mentally Retarded Children

FACILITY	SEVERE RETARDATION	MODERATE RETARDATION	MILD RETARDATION
Nurseries	Residential	Residential or day care	—
Preschool	Residential or private day care	Same as above	—
School	Same as above; also institutionalization	Special education, either public or private	Special education, either public or private
Occupational Programs	—	Sheltered workshops	Vocational training programs

Agencies which provide additional information about mental retardation include the National Association for Retarded Children and the Joseph P. Kennedy, Jr. Foundation, as well as mental health services groups throughout the country and state boards of health. An organization called Caring from Milton, Washington, DC 98354 is a support group for parents of children with Down's Syndrome.

CHRONIC ILLNESSES AND DISORDERS

Long-term problems may be evident from the time of an infant's birth. Children with congenital anomalies frequently require multiple surgical procedures. Other children during the course of a lifetime develop recurrent illnesses that present special problems. The potential achieved by the child will depend, in great measure, on the attitude and adjustment of the parents of that child.

The initial disappointment of some parents may be replaced by serious depression. If so, the parents may exhibit rather destructive attitudes toward the child and others. The stress of chronic illness is not merely emotional, however. Stress also becomes economic through the burden of prolonged or frequent hospitalization. It becomes physical through the ongoing, physically taxing process of caring for the child day after day, year after year. For all this effort, the parents receive little gratification from the child and often, little positive feedback from others, Figure 21-2.

Cultural influences also play a part in this stress. In the United States, a parent's status is not increased by the birth of a child as it is in some cultures where the child is a necessary contributor to the family. Society's focus on perfection and beauty further endangers the well-being of a family with a handicapped child.

Effects on the Child

Long-term health problems generally necessitate frequent hospitalizations. The effect on the child depends on the child's developmental age at the time of the separation from parents. Ideally, the parent of a very young child, such as a toddler or preschooler, will choose to room-in to provide support for the child. Even with this support, however, many

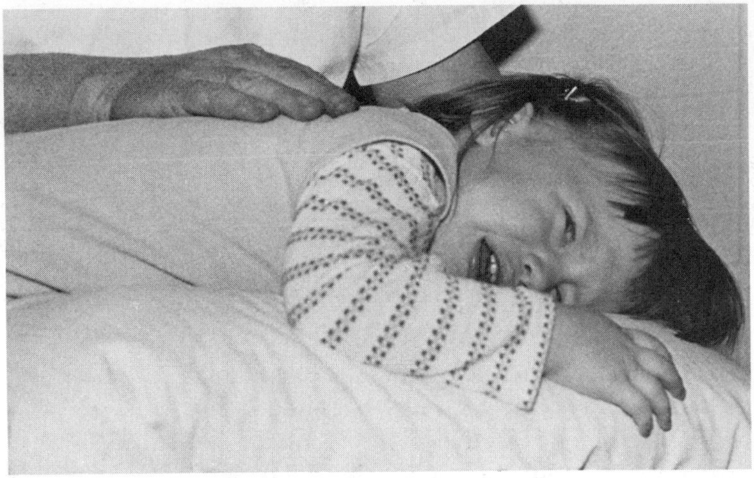

FIG. 21-2 The frustrations of frequent, daily postural drainage techniques can be overwhelming to the toddler with cystic fibrosis, as well as physically and emotionally taxing for the parents.

children experience depression after an illness. As the symptoms of an illness subside, the child very gradually returns to the previous level of functioning.

Between hospitalizations, the child and parents are continually reminded that the child is not totally well. The child may be maintained on a daily regimen of medications to maintain the state of well-being. There may be dietary restrictions or alterations. The child may not be able to engage in activities which were a source of enjoyment in the past. The parent or child may fear any activity which might precipitate a premature return to the hospital, Figure 21-3.

The adjustment of the family is enhanced when both the parent and the child are willing to discuss the difficulties openly. In the case of an infant or a very young child, the parents should be allowed the freedom to vent their feelings about the difficulties without fear of repercussions. However, if they are encouraged to share this type of information before they have developed a sense of trust in the nurse, the parent may not be able to work productively in the future with that same person.

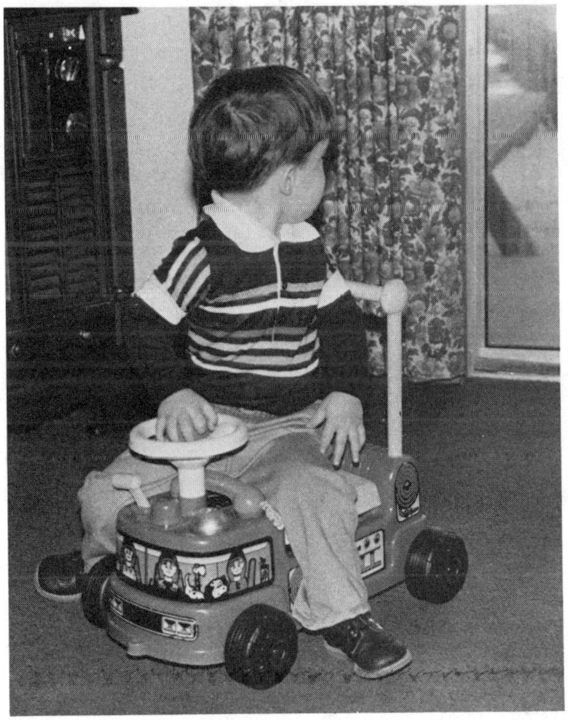

FIG. 21-3 Riding a truck may not be very appealing to a child who would much rather be outside playing with brothers and sisters.

Knowledge should be shared as early as possible with both parents and children. This allows children and parents time to adjust to the illness or disorder. Children may be helped to develop a sense of control over what is happening by being permitted to make some decisions, whether about times for rest periods, fluid restrictions, or planning the diet.

In some clinical settings, the chronically ill child's care is overseen by a single individual, usually a pediatric nurse practitioner. This nurse acts as a liaison between the schools, the community agencies other than the clinic, the hospital staff, and the family. The advantages of this arrangement are the continuity of information shared between agencies and the enhancement of long-term planning. The parents also view this arrangement very positively as a long-term relationship is established. The primary advantages of this system for the child are the resultant continuity of care and the awareness that one person knows their ability levels.

TERMINAL ILLNESSES

The child's response to a terminal illness is influenced by several factors. The primary influence is the child's developmental age. Other influences that must be considered are the reactions of those around the child and the disease process itself. The incidence of death from children's diseases has been altered dramatically in recent years. At one time, the diagnosis of leukemia meant only a few months to live. Currently, some young people with leukemia appear to be in a permanent state of remission. Early diagnoses and the more effective treatments have actually extended the process of dyng. This pattern continues to change with newer advances in medicine and treatment.

Developmental Responses to Dying

Newborn babies or infants have no concept of themselves as separate from their mother. They consider themselves an extension of the parents. Their response to dying is primarily physiologic. The touching and warmth of a mother figure may provide temporary comfort, but it cannot totally relieve the pain or discomfort.

The response of toddlers to dying is closely tied in with separation anxiety. These children are fearful of separation from the home and from parents. Strangers are usually associated with pain and punishment. The anger toddlers feel may be expressed in "bad thoughts" about anyone hurting them. All of the traumatic events that occur in the hospital situation, such as blood work, lumbar punctures, and medications, thus become punishment for the bad thoughts. Because these intrusive procedures invoke even more anger in the child, the intensity of the cycle increases progressively.

Preschool children may show very little overt response to their plight. This is denial in its purest form. The true feelings of the child may be reflected in the nightmares that reflect stress. These may be so severe and intense that they become night terrors. Because of the child's increased verbal skills and comprehension, the child may have accumulated a great deal of information about the terminal nature of the diagnosis through viewing television, overhearing conversations of parents and the staff, and accumulating clues from cultural experiences. Parental behaviors add to the insecurity. For example, the child may dream of a trip to Disneyland and may be told by the parents that this is an impossibility. Suddenly, he or she is released from the hospital and takes the trip that had been "impossible" a short time before. This child tolerates ambiguity but now recognizes the limits are changing from those previously set.

School-aged children who are aware of their diagnosis view the pronouncement by the doctor or authority figure as an absolute verdict from which there is no reprieve. Depending on the child's life experience, death may be viewed as a biologic process or as the result of violence. Exposure of the child to the death of a pet or other members of the family, such as aunts or grandparents, focuses the child's thinking on the reality and finality of death itself. Daydreams and fantasies about living forever and being lucky are quite common. The child's belief in luck is so strong that he may tell the nurse, "If I'm lucky, I might not get caught." This also reflects the concept of death as an intervention by a supernatural being, which is very common. School-aged children have developed some concept of what is socially acceptable to others. For this reason, they avoid openly discussing their condition and avoid discussing pain or showing open wounds unless they feel the individual is accepting of this behavior.

Adolescents with terminal illnesses have the greatest emotional investment. Any type of disfiguring surgery conflicts with the adolescent's body image of perfection. Moreover, the major source of support for this group is their peers. Unfortunately, the peers may also be unable to cope with the concept of dying and so may withdraw their support from their dying friend. The young person may regress, developing the need to be cared for like a baby. When parents and staff respond appropriately, the adolescent may respond with much bitterness. This reversal is emotionally difficult for the parents and the staff to deal with effectively.

Shared Responses of the Child

Children with terminal illnesses may be willing to share some of their feelings with trusted nurses. The feelings that are shared depend on many things that have happened over the course of their growing years. These children's life experiences, particularly their method of coping with separations (such as that of a parent), changing residence, and hospitalizations, influence their ability to share their feelings. The child's view of the current circumstances and his or her concern for obtaining more knowledge or honest answers may also prompt sharing.

Initially, these children recognize that they are sick but feel strongly that they will get better. As the number or length of the hospitalizations increase and they are less physically able to do things than before, these children view themselves as well, but abandon the expectations that their current level of functioning will improve. Eventually, they recognize that they will not get better, and many actually consider dying as an imminent possibility. In conversation with these children, there is a noticeable decline in discussions about long-range goals, their condition, their progress, and their future.

Responses of the Family

When the family is first confronted with the child's diagnosis and poor prognosis, they begin to go through the stages so clearly identified by Kübler-Ross as denial, anger, bargaining, depression, and acceptance. During the period of shock and denial, the family may seek other medical opinions in an attempt to disprove the original diagnosis or to be assured of a more favorable outcome for their child.

The family's anger may be directed at a variety of people. For instance, the child may bear the brunt of the parents' anger because they may feel that the child is the cause of their suffering. Other family members, as well as members of the health care team, may also be targets of the family's displaced anger. Nurses and other members of the health care team should recognize this anger as a necessary venting of strong feelings. During this period, the family is overwhelmed by a sense of helplessness and an inability to control their own destiny and that of the child.

The concept of bargaining is an attempt to postpone the inevitable death of the child by promising "good behavior" in return for an extension of the child's life. This period allows the parent to cope with the reality of the diagnosis while trying to delay the end result by the process of bargaining.

As the family moves into the stage of depression they begin to mourn for both past and future losses. A father might feel sad about the lack of time he spent with a school-age son and may regret that he will never see his son drive the family car or graduate from high school.

The acceptance of the family is a recognition that death is inevitable. Most recognize the preciousness of the remaining time and are content to sit and hold or rock the child in silence savoring the closeness. Most families prefer to do as much of the child's care as possible during this time.

Members of the family group identify closely with one another. Because of this feeling of personal vulnerability, the family may withdraw their support from a terminally ill child for a period of time or may avoid visiting the child in a hospital setting. Some members of the family may never have experienced death before, and may need to sort out their own feelings and adopt coping mechanisms before they can support their child.

During the period of time when the child is at home, away from the hospital environment, both parents and siblings need a great deal of support and guidance. Parents, for instance, may hesitate to discipline the child in any way. They may become overprotective to the point that they allow the child to be destructive and aggressive toward other children, as well as toward inanimate objects. This period away from the hospital is one of great tension because of the parents' fears of being unable to care for the child properly, as well as the threat of rehospitalization. Moreover, the parents may have great difficulty coping because of the unpredictability of the situation. Consistent support from nurses and other health professionals throughout the hospitalization should alleviate these problems somewhat.

Siblings in the home may resent the terminally ill child because he or she is accorded special privileges and attention. They may view their brother or sister as capitalizing on the illness. They may also feign illness themselves in an attempt to regain their parents' attention. Their resentment and anger may build to the point that they silently wish the child dead, or at least back in the hospital and out of the picture. When their wishes come true, these siblings feel intense guilt. The nurse should alert the parents to the problems of the siblings. Involving them in the care of their sick brother or sister and recognizing their feelings alleviates much of their anger.

Nursing Care of the Dying Child and the Family

Care of terminally ill children must be adapted to provide maximal comfort for them and emotional support for their families. The hospital room should provide privacy, but should not isolate the child and family from the staff on the unit. The parents must be supported in their efforts to care for their child. Some parents are fearful that they will inadvertently do something that will hasten the child's death. The presence of a nurse may allay these fears and enable them to feel comfortable providing care. The nurse should be available to help with the child's care, as well as to answer the parents' questions, Figure 21-4.

Home care or hospice care is generally more acceptable to the child than hospitalization, but neither may be feasible. Home care is not accepted by every family, and may be emotionally exhausting without adequate support from health care professionals. Hospices, although increasingly common, are not as available in this country as they are in England.

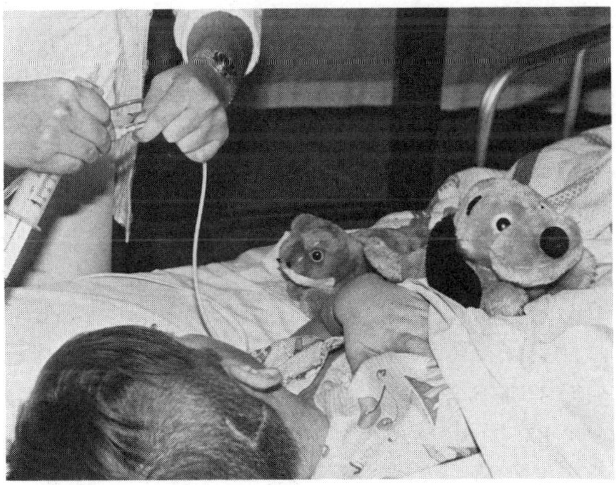

FIG. 21-4 The parents of this terminally ill child preferred that the nurse do the tube feedings for the child. The family assumed responsibility for the remainder of the child's care.

Behaviors Exhibited by the Dying Child

As death approaches, the child may demonstrate an increase in restlessness. This usually indicates the increased weakness of the child. Many of these children react to the slightest stress with angry outbursts or inappropriate behavior. Some of this behavior may be a response to pain, but much of it indicates the child's inability to control anxiety over his or her failing strength. The child should be reminded that the nurse, the parents, or all will be present at all times.

Some adolescents may continue to demonstrate resentment and anger over what is happening to them. Others may deny the serious nature of their illness in spite of failing strength. These defenses should not be challenged but should be accepted as that individual's coping mechanism.

Many of these children demonstrate an increase in their emotional bonds to their parents or caregivers. Their withdrawal or disinterest in other family members and visitors is obvious.

Difficulties in Providing Care

The nurse faces many problems when caring for terminally ill children. The first and foremost problem is recognition and integration of the nurse's own feelings about dying. Culturally, the nurse has been indoctrinated with such concepts as the old dying before the young, the focus of all health care being cure, and the dictum that a nurse should never get emotionally involved with the patient. Despite all of these cultural contradictions, the nurse must function as a caregiver. This is often accomplished by acting as if the child will recover.

Nurses use bargaining just as the parents may have done. "Please, Lord, not on my shift" is, in effect, an admission by the nurse that the child might die but it is also a wish for some "distancing" from the reality of death. Nurses may also try to control their feelings by increasing their efficiency or by controlling the care of the child. Whether or not they realize it the nurse is thereby usurping the role of the parent. This is particularly noticeable in intensive care areas where complex equipment or monitors are in use. In such environments, the parents feel inadequate and may hesitate to make known their preferences regarding the child's care. The child is thus caught in the middle of a power struggle of two authority figures, and no one, particularly the child, benefits.

When the nursing staff is able to accept the child's death as inevitable, they usually focus on relieving pain and keeping the child from feeling isolated. If the staff is unable to meet these two goals, feelings of failure, as well as of guilt and frustration may arise. If this occurs repeatedly, the nurse may avoid future emotional investment in other patients because of the personal pain that it brings.

Grief and Mourning

Grief and mourning for the child who has died is a process that is shared by the nursing staff as well as the family. In some families, the process may be initiated very early, close to the time of the initial diagnosis. In anticipation of the child's death, some parents may complete funeral arrangements, give away the child's belongings, and become emotionally distant, thereby isolating the child as he or she is dying.

Children who are involved in health crises several times in the course of their illness cause great stress for the family. The family begins to grieve for the child who is dying, and suddenly the child is better. Their emotions cannot be turned on and off rapidly enough to accommodate these changes. As a result, the parents may cease to show any happiness over the child's improvement, whereas the nursing staff will likely be elated because the child is meeting their needs of a "cure." These emotional extremes and the unpredictability of the situation prevent the family from planning for the future.

After the death of the child, well-meaning friends and relatives frequently make statements such as "he is better off now." The intent of the statement is to console the parent that the child is free of pain and possible suffering. However, it has the opposite effect, as parents cannot readily accept that their child, who was a part of them, is better off dead. Another statement that causes distress is "you can always have another baby." The well-meaning individual often forgets that each child is unique, and one can never replace the other.

The relationship between the parents may be very strained at this point. They may experience a sense of failure in their responsibilities as parents. The blame and guilt may become overwhelming, and divorce may be seen as the only alternative. All of these feelings may be shared openly with support groups that assist families in this time of crisis. Groups, such as the Candlelighters and Compassionate Friends, have local chapters all across the country that are prepared to provide this support. Religious beliefs and organizations may also provide comfort.

Ideally, support will have been provided by nurses and other professionals throughout the child's frequent hospitalization. Other families who have gone through this or who are currently involved in the same situation may provide additional support. Many families in this same situation avail themselves of temporary residences, such as the Ronald McDonald House, that are located near most pediatric medical centers. The residence staff provide empathy based on a realistic awareness of each family's needs.

SUMMARY

Children with special problems have unique nursing care needs. The nurse must carefully assess the developmental levels and recognize the long-term needs of these children. Parents and staff must work together to provide the best treatment for these children, emphasizing quality as well as continuity.

SUGGESTED ACTIVITIES

- Make arrangements to observe a special education class in your local public school. These are usually listed as Educable Mentally Retarded (EMR) classes. Determine the size of the class and the children's developmental characteristics. Describe the special problems or adaptions you observed.
- Visit a residential treatment center for multihandicapped children. Identify how continuity of care is maintained for these children, particularly if they must be hospitalized. Share your observations with the group.
- Invite a member of the nursing staff from a hospice to meet with your group to discuss their philosophy of care. How do they meet the needs of the terminally ill patient?
- Contact the local chapter of either Candlelighters or Compassionate Friends. Find out how they are able to assist the parents of terminally ill children, where they get referrals from and how the nurse can assist them in their work.

DISCUSSION TOPICS

1. Discuss with your classmates how you felt when you learned of the death of a friend or relative. Ask them about their feelings in the same situation. Identify the stages of grief.
2. Ask several parents of retarded children to visit your class and share information about their children. How can a nurse assist these parents to care for their children?

REVIEW

A. Matching. Match the characteristics of mental retardation in Column I with the level of retardation in Column II.

Column I	Column II
1. Considered trainable with an IQ of thirty-six to fifty-one	a. Child with mild retardation
2. Has problems with conduct disorders	b. Child with moderate retardation
3. Highest functional level is that of a toddler	c. Child with severe retardation
4. Usually not identified until school aged	
5. Inability to carry out activities of daily living	
6. Ability to function in a sheltered workshop setting	

B. Multiple choice. Select the one best answer.

1. Jimmy is a 2 1/2-year-old boy who is dying of a malignant tumor. You would expect his primary response to dying to be related to
   a. fear of injections and treatments.
   b. separation from home and parents.
   c. anger at his parents.
   d. limited life experiences.
2. The fears of a toddler regarding death are usually related to
   a. "bad things" caused by "bad thoughts."
   b. a concept of heaven or hell.
   c. anxiety about mutilation and annihilation.
   d. a concept of punishment and loss.

3. Methods the nurse can use to avoid isolating Jimmy include
   1. allowing unlimited visiting hours for parents.
   2. permitting sibling visitations, if possible.
   3. making staff members available to answer questions.
   4. ensuring that nursing care is administered only by the nursing staff.
   a. 1 and 4
   b. 1, 2, and 3
   c. 3 and 4
   d. 2 and 3

4. Kübler-Ross describes five stages of reaction to imminent death. The usual sequence of these stages is
   a. anger, bargaining, denial, acceptance, and depression.
   b. acceptance, denial, bargaining, anger, and depression.
   c. denial, anger, bargaining, depression, and acceptance.
   d. bargaining, denial, depression, anger, and acceptance.

5. Some of the problems encountered by Jimmy's parents in the home situation might include
   1. an inability to discipline the child.
   2. parental anger at the child.
   3. the child taking advantage of his "sick" role.
   4. sibling resentment of any special attention directed toward Jimmy.
   a. 1 and 3
   b. 2 and 4
   c. 1, 2, and 3
   d. 1, 2, 3 and 4

6. Jimmy dies while you are caring for him. Which of the following would be an acceptable means of conveying your concern to the family?
   a. "He is much better off where he is."
   b. Standing silently and holding the parent's hand.
   c. "Now things can get back to normal at home."
   d. "Would you be willing to sign the autopsy permit?"

C. Short answer. Briefly respond to the following statements.

1. List three stresses that occur with the family of a child who has a chronic disease.

2. List three ways in which a nurse might be supportive to a family of a child with retardation or chronic illness.

BIBLIOGRAPHY

Barnard, Kathryn E., and Marcene L. Powell. *Teaching the Mentally Retarded Child.* St. Louis: C. V. Mosby Company, 1972.

Begab, Michael J. *The Mentally Retarded Child.* Washington, D.C.: U.S. Department of Health, Education, and Welfare, 1967.

Bloch, Judith. "Impaired Children: Helping Families Through the Critical Period of First Identification." *Children Today,* Vol. 7 (November–December, 1978), pp. 2–6.

Brown, Marie Scott. "The Gordons Needed All the Help They Could Get." *Nursing 77,* Vol. 7 (October, 1977), pp. 40–43.

Bullington, Becky Page, et al. "Working with Families of Multihandicapped Children in a Residential Institution." *Children Today,* Vol. 5 (September–October, 1976), pp. 13–17+.

Easson, William M. *The Dying Child.* Springfield: Charles C. Thomas, 1970.

Golden, Deborah A., and Jessica G. Davis. "Counseling Parents After the Birth of an Infant with Down's Syndrome." *Children Today,* Vol. 3 (March–April, 1974), pp. 7–11+.

Goldson, Edward. "The Family Care Center." *Children Today,* Vol. 10 (July–August, 1981), pp. 15–20.

Grove, Sheryl. "I Am a Yellow Ship." *American Journal of Nursing,* Vol. 78 (March, 1978), p. 414.

Gurmand, Joyce. "We Knew Our Child Was Dying." *American Journal of Nursing,* Vol. 74 (February, 1974), pp. 248–249.

Gyuley, J. Eileen. *The Dying Child.* St. Louis: McGraw-Hill Book Company, 1978.

Hardgrove, Carl, and Louise Warrich. "How Shall We Tell the Children?" *American Journal of Nursing,* Vol. 74 (March, 1974), pp. 448–450.

Hobbs, Nicholas, et al. "Classifying Children." *Children Today,* Vol. 4 (July–August, 1975), pp. 21–25.

Horoshak, Irene. "Where Hope for Mental Retardees Grows Brighter." *RN,* Vol. 39 (June, 1976) pp. 39–43.

Kittleson, Judith A. "In Spite of Everything, Tommy Died in Peace." *RN,* Vol. 78 (February, 1978), pp. 97–102.

Klepser, Mary Jo. "How Long Does Grief Go On?" *American Journal of Nursing,* Vol. 78 (March, 1978), pp. 420–422.

Kovalesky, Andrea. "That Night in the Neonate Nursery." *American Journal of Nursing,* Vol. 78 (March, 1978), pp. 414–416.

Lacasse, C.M. "A Dying Adolescent." *American Journal of Nursing,* Vol. 75 (March, 1975), pp. 433–434.

Martinson, Ida M. "Home Care for the Dying Child." *American Journal of Nursing,* Vol. 77 (November, 1977), pp. 1815–1817.

Miller, Christina. "Working With Parents of High-Risk Infants." *American Journal of Nursing,* Vol. 78 (July, 1978), pp. 1228–1230.

Mills, Gretchen Curtis. "Books to Help Children Understand Death." *American Journal of Nursing,* Vol. 79 (February, 1979), pp. 291–295.

Murphy, Ann, et al. "Meeting with Brothers and Sisters of Children with Down's Syndrome." *Children Today,* Vol. 5 (March–April, 1976), pp. 20–23.

Riccardi, Vincent M. *The Genetic Approach to Human Disease.* New York: Oxford University Press, 1977.

Rodgers, Bechett M. "Comprehensive Care for the Child with a Chronic Disability." *American Journal of Nursing,* Vol. 79 (June, 1979), pp. 1106–1108.

Stutz, Sara. "When the Baby Isn't Normal." *RN,* Vol. 34 (November, 1971), pp. 40–43.

Suarez, Margarita, and Jeanne Q. Benalld. "Coping With Failure: The Case of Death in Childhood." *Issues in Comprehensive Pediatric Nursing,* Vol. 2 (September–October, 1977), pp. 3–15.

Vaughan, Victor C., et al. *Nelson's Textbook of Pediatrics.* Philadelphia: W. B. Saunders Company, 1979.

Section VII

The School-Aged Child

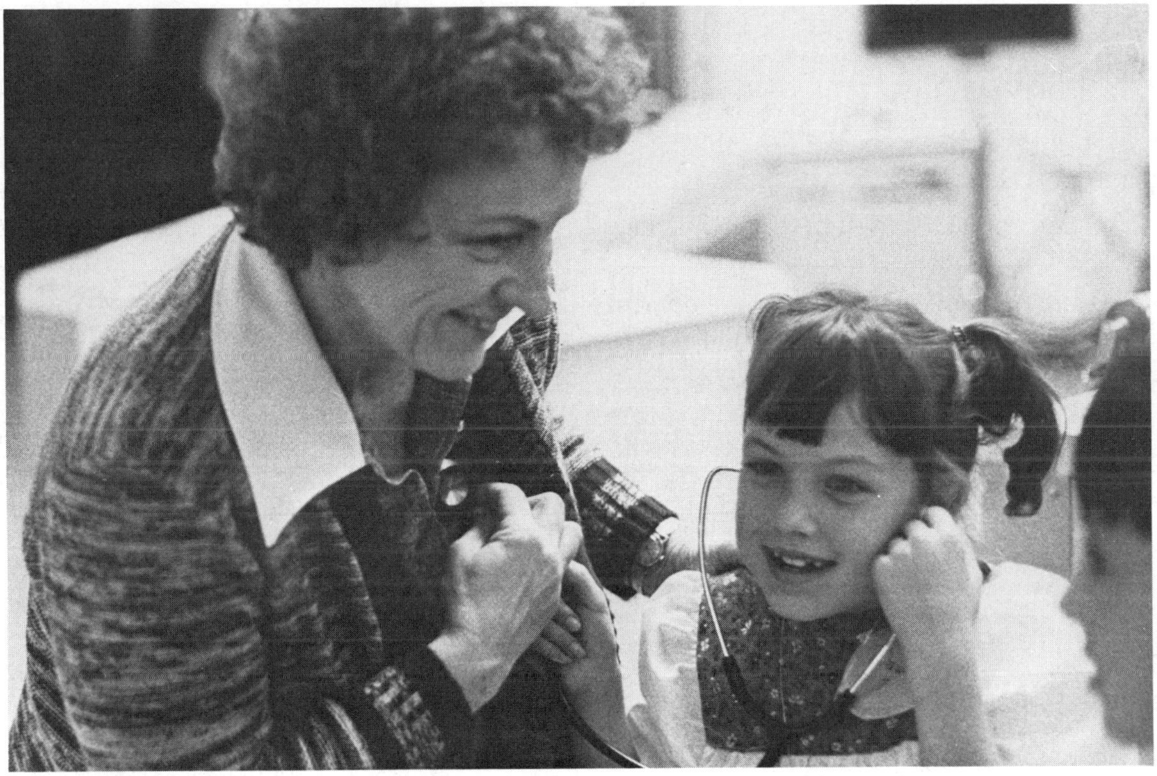

Chapter 22

Growth and Development

OBJECTIVES

Upon completion of this chapter, the student will be able to

- describe characteristics of the school-aged child's physical growth patterns.
- differentiate between the developmental tasks of the school-aged child cited by Erikson and those cited by Piaget.
- list some of the problems that affect this age-group.

The term school-age refers to the period in life that extends from the age of six years to the age of ten years. Some authors refer to school-age as the middle years of childhood, denoting the interim period between early childhood and preadolescence. Traditionally, school-age is marked by entrance into a formal process of education and ends with the onset of puberty. This period has also been described as the period of latency or sexual tranquility. The child is comfortable forming intimate relationships with a peer of the same sex. This period may be identified by specific dental changes, beginning with the shedding of the first deciduous tooth and ending with the final permanent teeth (other than the wisdom teeth).

DEVELOPMENTAL TASKS

The developmental tasks of school-aged children reflect the three main changes that occur in this period of their lives. The first change involves an increased relationship with their peer group and subsequent movement away from the family. The second is an improvement in the motor skills necessary for participation in games, work, and other activities. The third is a rapid change in their cognitive skills.

Peer Relationships. Within the context of their evolving relationship with their peer group, several specific tasks are accomplished. Learning to get along with others is very important in this child's development. It involves a certain amount of give and take, as well as adherence to the rules of the relationship. Skills related to cooperation and the social skills and habits that are developed during this time are carried throughout the lifetime of the individual. The degree of acceptance or approval received from the peer group depends on how well the child conforms to the standards of the group.

An assimilation of attitudes also accompanies this peer relationship. These attitudes are dictated by the culture. The child reinforces those values that are espoused regarding religion, politics, occupations, and the economy itself, Figure 22-1. These values are not automatic endowments from the time of the child's birth, but are learned values reinforced in many ways from infancy to adulthood by parents, peers, and significant others. The increased conscience formation is another aspect of this same developmental task.

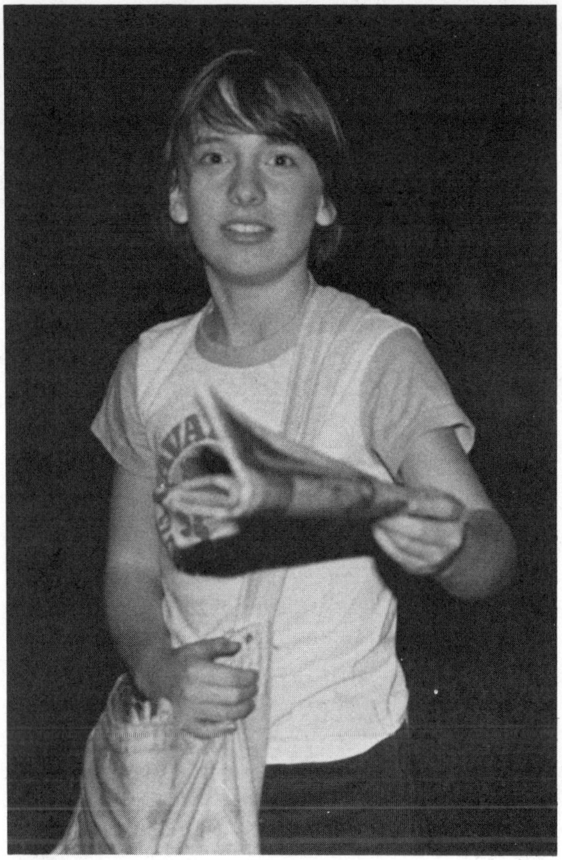

FIG. 22-1 Delivering newspapers brings both a sense of satisfaction and monetary reward for the school-aged child.

Motor Skills. The second major area of change is the development of motor skills to participate in work and games. The gradual changes that have occurred in growth contribute greatly to this child's ability to participate in games. The learning of rules is important and is typical of this child's development, but the ability to perform is even more important. The child's abilities and achievements are either reinforced by the peer group or altered to mesh with the group's standards. Children who lack the neuromuscular coordination to succeed in such activities become alienated unless they can interact with and become members of a group in which their particular skills are valued.

Cognitive Skills. The third area of development is in cognitive skills. In the school years, one of the major tasks of the child is to learn to read, write, and to calculate, Figure 22-2. These are the basic skills that allow these children to communicate and to function in society. Along with these skills, they must

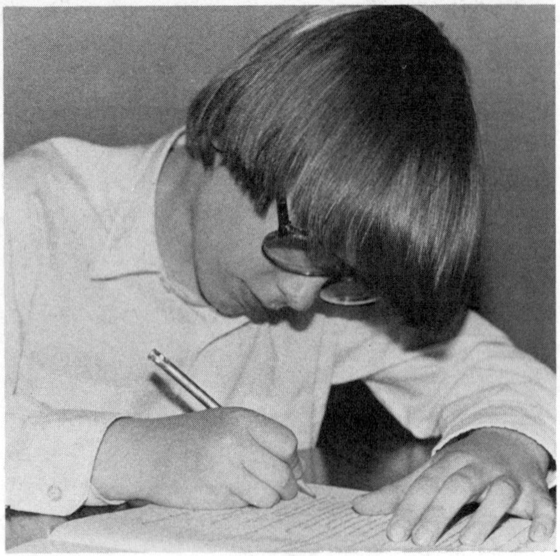

FIG. 22-2 The ability to write is a major accomplishment in terms of cognitive skill.

learn those concepts that are necessary for them to function on a daily basis in society. Giving, taking, and sharing responsibility are important components of these particular tasks.

One important aspect of cognitive development is skill in the use of the language. The use of humor or jokes is typical of this age-group. Initially, the jokes are long and rambling. As the child develops, they become more concise, with a distinct punch line or surprise ending. Perhaps the best example of this development of humor is the frequency with which the child relates riddles. The "stupid" jokes that are told are usually directed at adults, rather than at another child, and are used to relieve tension. The telling of "dirty" jokes about body parts and functions is another aspect of this development.

Gender Role. The learning of a masculine or feminine social role is continued through this period of the school years. By the end of the preschool period, gender identity has been established. The culture within which the child and family operate has clearly defined ideas relating to gender role and what is acceptable behavior for an individual. Children this age constantly evaluate and compare their role and behavior to the acceptable norms.

Erikson's Stage of Psychosocial Development

The period of the school years is described by Erikson as engendering a sense of industry versus a sense of inferiority. During this period, children use new-found skills to increase knowledge and to maintain control over their environment. They attempt to use the skills in many ways, bringing either satisfaction or dissatisfaction with their personal performance.

The attempts at mastery that produce a sense of industry pervade the child's contacts with peers, family, teachers, and the community at large. These children direct all their energies to a particular endeavor in order to succeed. The threat of personal failure is very real, and any hint of unsatisfactory work in school or on the playing field is usually met with increased vigor and motivation to improve and succeed with the next encounter.

Academic achievement is not the singular index of achievement for this particular stage. The child often succeeds in some academic areas, such as mathematics, but may be weak in language skills. Some children may develop a musical skill with a particular instrument in order to offset their minimal academic skills. Another child may score twenty-four goals in a year of soccer competition, yet never make a basket during basketball season. Success in one area usually compensates for a feeling of inferiority in another area, thereby allowing the child to maintain a sense of adequacy.

Piaget's Stage of Cognitive Development

The school years are described by Piaget as the third stage, or the stage of concrete operational thought. During this period children complete the transition from mere experience with physical reality to solving problems that have close ties to the physical sphere, Figure 22-3. They learn to classify objects, use symbols, apply rules, and understand the principles of cause and effect. The relationship between objects and ideas permits the child to compute mathematical problems, solve simple science experiments, and apply a system of classification to a group of objects.

During this period, children also learn the concept of conservation or permanence. If, for instance, they take a large ball of clay and roll it into a snakelike form, they know that the clay is the same substance and the same weight, but that the shape has changed because of their manipulation. Through this process of classification and ordering of elements, the child internalizes the concept of relations that are a necessary part of the final stage of cognitive development.

New-found thought processes also allow these children to consider the views of other individuals without necessarily altering their own views. The young boy learning the rules of baseball may have been batting a particular way for some time. When the coach, as well as his father, suggests that he position himself in a slightly different fashion, he may accept the suggestion without believing that it will help. The subsequent reinforcement of the change by a base hit or home run will alter his thinking process considerably. School-aged children typically use inductive reasoning. When this task is achieved, their mode of reasoning will change from inductive to deductive.

The thinking abilities of these children continue to be quite literal, especially during the early part of the school-age period. Problems related to imaginary situations are difficult for them to solve. This is also true for problems with several variables or with

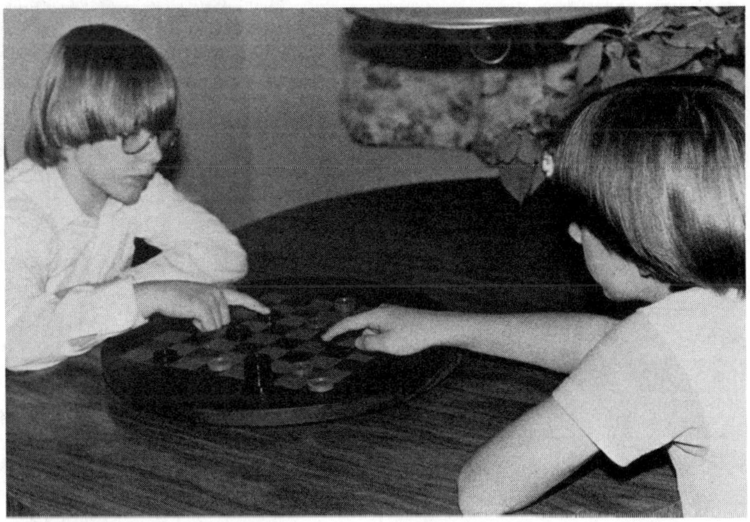

FIG. 22-3 Playing a competitive game, such as checkers, enhances the problem-solving aspect of cognitive development.

multiple correct solutions. The ability to be flexible and diverse in their thinking is limited. When they solve problems incorrectly, they also have difficulty using this information to identify a new solution to the problem.

PHYSICAL GROWTH

In the beginning of the school-age period, changes in stature, weight, and body contour occur. The soft contours that are so typical of the toddler and preschool period are lost at the beginning of the school years. The arms and legs become longer in proportion to the trunk. The facial contours are slimmer as well. All of these changes result in a "gawky" or "spindly" appearance of the child.

The average six-year-old girl is about 45 inches tall and weighs about 43 pounds. During each of the succeeding four years, the child will grow 2 to 3 inches per year and gain between 3 and 8 pounds per year. By age ten, a girl with a steady growth rate will be about 54 inches tall and will weigh 71 to 72 pounds. Six-year-old boys are usually half an inch taller than girls of the same age (45 1/2 inches tall) and several pounds heavier, weighing 45 1/2 pounds. The normal range of weight for six-year-old boys is from 37 1/2 to as much as 58 1/2 pounds. By age ten, the average boy's height has increased by 9 inches and his weight by 24 pounds, thus measuring 54 1/2 inches tall and weighing 69 1/2 pounds.

The growth pattern is slow and consistent, resulting in a gradual lengthening of the skeletal structure. This change in body proportion with its associated lower center of gravity is beneficial for the type of physical activities and skill development that occurs in this age-group. The ability to participate in such sports as bicycle riding, climbing, and skating is enhanced by this change in structure and motor skills, Figure 22-4.

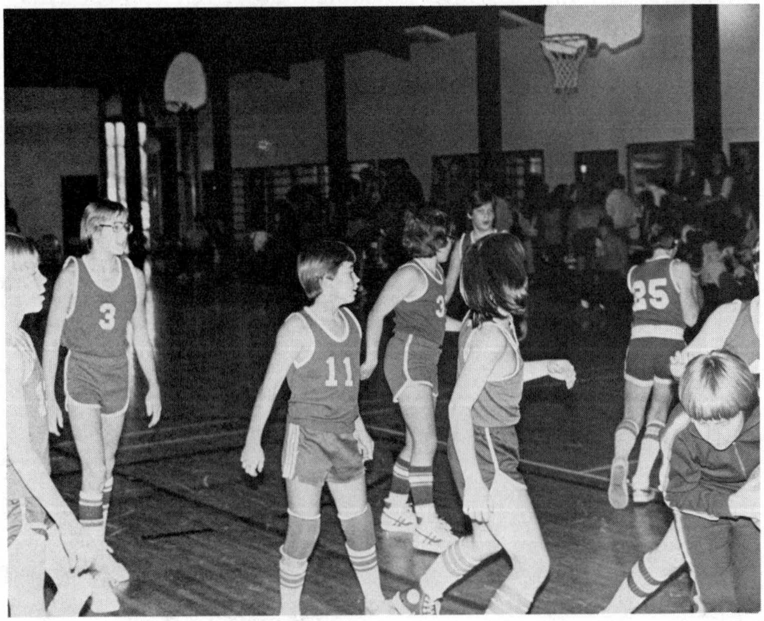

FIG. 22-4 Changes in body structures increase the ability to participate in sports such as basketball that require well-developed motor skills.

AGE CHARACTERISTICS

Children of each age included in this period have some unique characteristics that mark the child's development. Although one child may proceed rapidly through the tasks, another child may advance at a much slower rate. Development is individualized, depending on endowment, experiences, and the encouragement of others.

Six Years of Age

Six-year-old children are still very egocentric individuals. They have boundless enthusiasm and energy for initiating projects, but seldom finish them. They are the original "perpetual motion" machines — continually wriggling, climbing, and banging. Speed and motion are exciting extensions of their energy level. Girls are superior in movement accuracy, while boys are superior in forceful, less complex acts at this age.

Interpersonal relationships are also undergoing significant changes at this time. Six-year-old children gravitate toward others their age, moving away from their family sphere. Their attitude toward mother fluctuates widely. They are often frustrated with and resentful of the close supervision of either parent. They are also rigidly demanding, wanting things to go precisely according to their plans. This rigid attitude often leads to tears and temper tantrums from the frustration. The ability to adapt and compromise does not develop until later in this period.

In the school setting, these children can participate in games, but are not capable of handling competition. This is either because the necessary physical coordination is lacking or because they have a strong need to work cooperatively with others. Decision making is quite difficult at this age.

The incidence of infectious illness is increased in this age-group because of the increase in contact with other six-year-old children having a variety of organisms in their noses and throats. Somatic complaints may sometimes be used to avoid school. Playing "doctor" or "hospital" is quite common in this age-group. It answers some questions, but many more questions related to sex differences arise at this age. Body functions and "bathroom" activities are common subjects for jokes during this period.

Seven Years of Age

Seven-year-old children are much more intense individuals. They are more cooperative and have learned a measure of compromise in activities. Motor skills and coordination have increased. There is a seriousness about their responsibilities in school and at home. Their standards are often set rather high, which presents problems at times.

Friction with the family develops when seven year olds feel that they are not given sufficient choice in matters. They are usually negative toward the family while at home, but staunchly defend or boast of them in public. This is particularly true when older brothers and sisters who are openly admired for their skills and abilities are involved.

Privacy, personal belongings, and collections are all high priorities for seven-year-old children. Luck or magic are generally seen as important influences on events in their lives. Magic tricks are sheer delight for children of this age.

As with six-year-old children, these children continue to have fears about body injury or physical harm affecting them or their loved ones. Some of these fears may be triggered by the violence on television and in the movies to which the child is exposed. The child's environment also plays a part in this fear.

Increased maturation permits this age-group to perform jumping-jack exercises accurately, walk a narrow balance beam, balance on one foot with eyes closed, and hop and jump in small squares. Both sexes show these improvements in skill levels.

Eight Years of Age

Eight-year-old children are generally outgoing and enthusiastic, ready to tackle any project. Unfortunately, this quality may get them into trouble as they often take on projects or activities that are somewhat beyond their capabilities. By nature they are gregarious, preferring the company of their age-mates. A stable relationship with one or two valued friends usually forms at this age. Gangs and clubs take on added importance, Figure 22-5.

School is the focus of many of the activities of this age-group. The child strives to succeed in academic areas. The ability to make things and to perform with peers are important aspects of this child's life.

Eight-year-old children are usually willing to work at small jobs for pay. They place a great deal of value on monetary rewards. Many bargains and deals are made with both peers and parents. They may be quite fascinated by what money can buy at a garage sale or flea market. Involving them in the choice process enhances their decision-making skills.

Games participated in by both sexes are greatest at this age. The ability to throw a ball more than 40 feet is more easily accomplished by boys than girls.

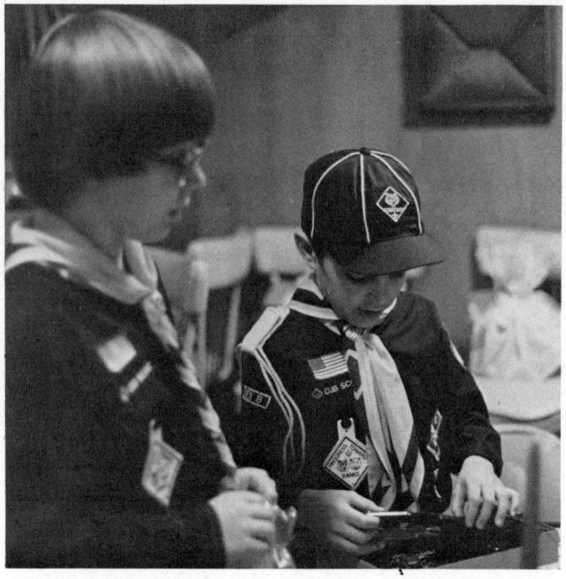

FIG. 22-5 Participation in group activities, such as scouting, is enjoyed by eight-year-old children. Note the differences in physical size.

Nine Years of Age

Children of this age-group have the ability and motivation to complete tasks that are initiated. They are self-motivated and are able to make decisions. The peer relationship continues to be very strong. Hero worship and prejudices are more evident at this age. They are aware of adult expectations regarding manners and conduct, but generally conform only in the presence of others.

Some negative attitudes are displayed toward parents at this age. The peer group is valued and family attitudes or values are de-emphasized. These children feel a strong sense of loyalty toward select friends.

Motor skills are much improved in children this age. They are able to participate in almost all competitive games. They work as hard at play as they do at actual work.

FIG. 22-6 Participation in organized outdoor sports shows the increased skill level of nine-year-old children.

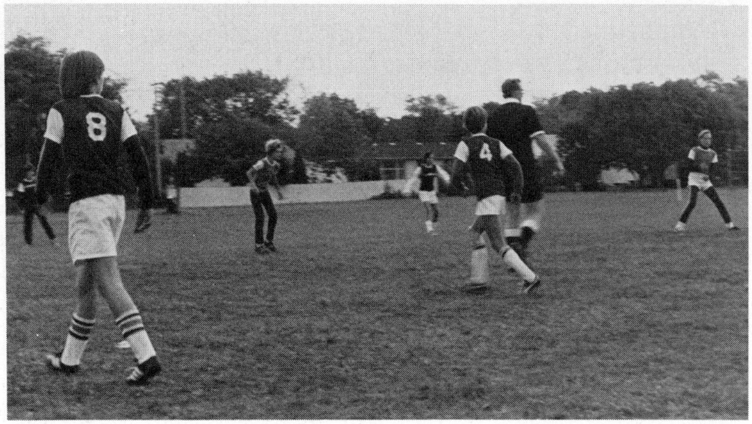

Their participation in outdoor sports underscores their improved skill level, Figure 22-6. Boys at this age begin to outdistance girls in the ability to jump, run, and throw in controlled situations.

Ten Years of Age

Ten-year-old children are rapidly approaching adolescence, and many of their behavioral patterns reflect this. At this point they are aware of many of their strengths and abilities. They know that they can do well in certain activities, whether they are academic or physical in nature. They continue to be highly competitive both inside and outside the classroom.

In the home setting, they tend to continue to be somewhat messy, leaving a trail of clothing, games, and other belongings in their wake. This messiness extends to personal care, and frequent reminders to bathe and brush their teeth may be needed. Some supervision may be appropriate in this area, as some young people may attempt to "dry clean," running the shower so their parents can hear it, but never actually showering.

Most of the child's time is spent in the school setting or with the peer group. In school, these children tend to budget their time better for activities and are more receptive to learning than before. Factual information is easily memorized. However, there is still a need for someone else to point out cause and effect relationships, as the ten-year-old child cannot do this in all areas. Gifted children may need additional support and guidance as a result of achievement levels that are in advance of the peer group.

At this age, group activities are high priorities. The child is often involved in structured groups and organizations, such as the Boy Scouts or Girl Scouts. The child may also be involved in other less formal groups, such as clubs formed by neighborhood children. These groups surface and disappear rather rapidly, and their membership shifts from time to time. All of these groups are formed with children of the same sex.

In terms of attitudes toward family, these children are both fiercely loyal and strongly attached to the family group. Their interaction is most positive with parents and least positive with younger siblings of the same developmental age. They often have a good relationship with very young children in the home, but compete strongly with those close to their own age.

NUTRITION

School-aged children normally consume about 2400 calories per day. Their protein requirements in relation to their total weight are decreasing to nearly adult levels. At this time, they need 1.2 grams of protein per kilogram of body weight. The parents should recognize the necessity of a balanced diet for these children.

Unfortunately, many of the calories consumed by school-aged children are in the form of junk food, and hence, are often "empty" calories. Two major factors influence this behavior. One is the sales pitch of the mass media and the other is the influence of the peer group and what they are allowed to eat. The child with spending money who stops at the bakery or candy store on the way home after school each day seldom is ready to eat a nutritious evening meal. The large amount of calories consumed in this way may lead to obesity in the child, as well as nutritional deficiencies.

Enlisting the child's interest in the quality of food substances may be helpful. They can then select foods and snacks that are most appropriate, such as nuts or peanut butter, fruits, and cheeses. This interest in food is encouraged in the school setting.

Nutritional assistance can be provided for those children who need it. The National School Lunch Program and the breakfast programs that are available in some areas provide free or reduced-cost meals to the child. The lunch program provides one-third of an adequate day's intake for the school-aged child.

LEARNING DISABILITIES

Children within a school setting may have a number of problems in their interactions with others, their ability to learn, and their motor skills. Because the child's future success in life is dependent on the knowledge and skills developed at this time, it is important to recognize problems in children and to determine the reason for their existence.

Five to twenty percent of all school-aged children have a form of learning disability. These are children who have impairments in perception, conceptualization, language, memory, control of attention, impulse, or motor function. The term *learning disabilities* emphasizes the potential positive implications of education and training of these children. It is preferred to the term minimal brain dysfunction. The term "attention deficit disorder" is also appropriate for learning disabilities.

Identification. The child with a learning disability must be identified, the problem delineated, and treatment approaches planned by a multidisciplinary team. In the school setting, this usually involves a parent-teacher conference during which the child's classroom behavior and areas of weakness are discussed. At this point, the decision may be made to have the child undergo a complete physical examination by a pediatrician. This should include a neurologic evaluation as well. An unidentified physical health problem may be the cause of the disability.

If this testing does not identify a clear-cut cause, the family or teacher may request that the school district evaluate the child's psychological status. This is done in an effort to determine both strengths and weaknesses and to find out what might be hampering the child's progress in the school setting.

Federal Legislation and Testing. In 1978, a federal law called the Education for All Handicapped Children Act was legislated. Responsibility was thereby given to public schools to seek out, identify, and evaluate those children needing special assistance. The law included a provision to keep both handicapped and nonhandicapped children in regular classrooms whenever possible. It specified composition of the team that would evaluate the child and make placement decisions. It clarified the needs of parental information, the confidentiality of the data, open access to records by the parent, and the opportunity for a formal appeal process on the basis of the educator's decision.

The nurse in the school setting is often involved as a member of the multidisciplinary team in the evaluation of a given child. The nurse may also be observing the child in the school setting prior to the evaluation. Assessment by the pediatric nurse frequently involves administration of the Denver Developmental Screening Test, if the child is younger than age six.

Other tests performed by the school psychologist might include the Bender-Gestalt Test, which identifies deficits in perceptual learning skills; The Wechsler Intelligence Scale for Children (WISC-R), which is composed of twelve subtests of both the verbal and the performance areas of the child's cognitive ability; achievement tests, such as the Wide Range Achievement Test (WRAT) and the Peabody Individual Achievement Test (PIAT); and the Vineland Social Maturity Scale, which is administered to the parent or guardian rather than the child. Additionally, specific areas of skill development may be pinpointed by such tests as the Key Math Diagnostic Arithmetic Test, the Woodcock Reading Mastery Tests, which includes one part on auditory perception; and the Frostig, which measures visual-motor perceptual skills.

Treatment Programs. Once the testing is completed, the combined observations, test results, and parental input allow the diagnostic team to identify what kind of help the child needs. A recommendation or diagnostic prescription is then made. The parents may request a formal hearing if they feel the results of the testing are inaccurate in some way.

The educational programs that are available for the child with learning disabilities range from supplemental tutoring for the child with a deficit in one specific area to learning disabilities classes for the child with more extensive needs. In addition, programs for slow learners and for retarded students are available in many school districts. Additional programs are also available for children with hearing impairment, visual impairment, or orthopedic handicaps.

The treatment of the individual child with learning disabilities is based on the results of the total evaluation. The treatment may be biochemical, nutritional, functional, or any combination of these, depending on the specific needs of the child. In the process of the testing, some children are identified as having endocrine imbalances, low blood sugar levels, or anemia. These conditions must be corrected initially.

Some children may be sensitive or allergic to specific foods or to food additives, and an elimination diet can be developed for them. This is the underlying principle of the Feingold Diet — all foods containing a natural salicylate radicle, or any artificial flavorings or additives are eliminated. Controlled studies have raised some questions regarding this diet's effectiveness.

In some situations, family counseling may be the preferred mode of treatment. In others, behavioral therapy is the treatment of choice. Medical treatment may include the use of stimulants, such as amphetamines or caffeine. These are used selectively to improve the child's functional level.

Children with functional problems may need help in one or more areas. In some children, the perceptual-motor area is impaired. In other children, auditory skills may be lacking. A specific developmental program is established for each child to enhance the skills that are already developed and to improve the ones that are impaired.

A number of agencies work specifically with children who have learning disabilities. One agency is the New York Institute for Child Development. Another group with local as well as national and state organizations is the Association for Children with Learning Disabilities (ACLD).

WORKING WITH SCHOOL-AGED CHILDREN AND THEIR FAMILIES

The pediatric nurse should be able to recognize the normal patterns of development in the school-aged child, as well as some of the individual variations that may occur. When working with families, it is important to identify the strengths of the child and to encourage both the child and the family to work toward an improvement of skills in the weaker areas.

In the hospital setting, the child's skills in some areas may not be clearly evident because of the nature of the illness. An attempt should be made to maintain those skills that have already been acquired. The child's ability to make decisions, even on a limited scale, should be respected. Individual achievements should be recognized and in older children a spirit of competition should be maintained. The skills learned in the academic setting should be maintained in the child who is hospitalized for a long-term illness. This may be accomplished by a visiting teacher, a special tutor, or a hospital-based teacher if available.

For hospitalized children with learning disabilities, it is important for the staff to learn what is being done for the child in the classroom. Limitation of environmental stimuli may help some of these children while in the hospital setting. Instructions to the child may have to be both verbal and written and presented in concrete terms. Some children may benefit from simplified directions and the consistency of care that is afforded by having the same staff members give the child care. If this child was on an elimination diet at the time of admission, it must be carefully maintained during hospitalization in order to reduce the possibility of any behavioral disorders occurring.

SUMMARY

School-aged children undergo a period marked by rapid increases in cognitive skills and abilities; new relationships with their peer group rather than their family as the pivotal focus; and a distinct increase in motor abilities. The majority of their time is spent in the school setting with their peer group and away from their family.

During this period, they have the opportunity to test the family's attitudes and values against the standards of their new group. They move into and out of informal groups rather easily at this age, depending on their ability to conform to the group's standards. Language skills and academic achievement are distinct components of the developmental tasks of this age-group.

Learning disabilities or an inability to function at adequate levels in the school setting may occur at this time. These disabilities may be the result of motor deficits, impairment of memory, or other perceptual-motor problems. Their cause must be explored and a specific treatment program developed to ensure that this child achieves his or her optimal potential.

SUGGESTED ACTIVITIES

- Investigate the method by which a tutor may be retained for a child involved in a long-term hospitalization. What criteria must be met? How are these activities funded?
- Ask a learning disabilities teacher to speak to your group. What types of programs are available in your local schools?
- Invite a teacher from a Talented and Gifted (TAG) Program to share information about their local program with your class.

DISCUSSION TOPICS

1. Discuss the activities and games that should be made available for a hospitalized school-aged child who is confined to bed. Devise a list of six acceptable, age-appropriate activities for this child.
2. Together with other members of your group, investigate the activities and functions of several organizations for school-aged children, such as the Boy Scouts, Girl Scouts, and Indian Guides. Share this information with the rest of your class. Note the appropriateness of the activities in terms of the child's developmental level.

REVIEW

A. Matching. Match the developmental task in Column I with the developmental theory in Column II.

Column I	Column II
1. Altering the shape of an item	a. Piaget's stage of concrete operational thought
2. Striving to get good grades in school	b. Erikson's sense of industry
3. Arranging and classifying a rock collection	
4. Identifying the permanence of matter	
5. Attempting to improve shooting ability in basketball	
6. Enjoying riddles	
7. Helping to deliver newspapers	

B. Multiple choice. Select the one best answer.

1. Jeff is a six-year-old boy of average height and weight. You would expect his height and weight to be approximately
   a. 33 inches and 33 pounds.
   b. 38 inches and 38 pounds.
   c. 45 inches and 45 pounds.
   d. 60 inches and 60 pounds.
2. In selecting appropriate games, you should encourage Jeff to
   a. participate in complex, skill-oriented games.
   b. develop individual skills rather than competitive ones.
   c. participate only in competitive games with all ages.
   d. play only board games to increase manipulative skills.
3. Jeff's questions related to sex differences are frequently answered by
   a. asking the teacher questions.
   b. reading about the differences in children's books.
   c. watching other children of both sexes.
   d. playing "hospital" or "doctor" with others.

4. Infectious illnesses are common in Jeff's age-group because of
   a. increased exposure to a variety of other children, and hence, to their organisms.
   b. decreased resistance to infection at this age.
   c. poor nutritional intake of vitamins and minerals.
   d. inadequate health care secondary to ignorance or poverty.
5. Bill is Jeff's ten-year-old brother. If he is of average height and weight, you would expect him to be
   a. 50 inches tall and weigh 51 1/2 pounds.
   b. 54 inches tall and weigh 69 pounds.
   c. 58 inches tall and weigh 61 pounds.
   d. 60 inches tall and weigh 54 pounds.
6. Because of his age, you would expect Bill's peer relationships to be
   a. strongly related to the activities of a group of the same sex.
   b. strongly related to a single person of the same sex.
   c. strongly related to a single person of the opposite sex.
   d. weakly related to the activities of a group of the same sex.

C. Short answer. Briefly respond to the following statements.

1. Name three of the impairments classified as learning disabilities.
2. List three nursing interventions that are appropriate for the care of a hospitalized child with learning disabilities.

BIBLIOGRAPHY

Binder, Florence Z., and Joan E. Butler. "Children With Learning Disabilities." *Issues in Comprehensive Pediatric Nursing,* Vol. 3 (September, 1978), pp. 1–14.

Bolden, Billie K., and Ada Shannon. "The Nurse Practitioner and the Child on the Feingold Diet." *American Journal of Nursing,* Vol. 75 (May, 1975), p. 801.

Cochran, Audrey. "Recognizing MBD in the Problem Child." *RN,* Vol. 35 (May, 1972), pp. 35–39.

DiPalma, Joseph. "Drugs for the Hyperactive Child." *RN,* Vol. 35 (May, 1972), pp. 61–69.

Elkind, David, and Irving B. Weiner. *Development of the Child.* New York: John Wiley and Sons, Inc., 1978.

Feingold, Ben F. "Hyperkinesis and Learning Disabilities Linked to Artificial Food Flavors and Colors." *American Journal of Nursing,* Vol. 75 (May, 1975), pp. 797–803.

Hymovich, Debra P., and Robert W. Chamberlin. *Child and Family Development: Implications for Primary Health Care.* New York: McGraw-Hill Book Company, 1980.

Johnson, Thomas R. (ed.), et al. *Children Are Different.* Columbus: Ross Laboratories, 1978.

Newman, Barbara M., and Philip R. Newman. *Infancy and Childhood: Development and Its Contexts.* New York: John Wiley and Sons, Inc., 1978.

Siemon, M. "Mental Health in School-Aged Children." *Maternal-Child Nursing,* Vol. 3 (July–August, 1978), pp. 211–217.

Chapter 23

Health Care Problems

OBJECTIVES

Upon completion of this chapter, the student will be able to

- describe the type of health care problems that occur in school-aged children.
- identify appropriate nursing interventions that can be used in the care of school-aged children with specific health problems.
- differentiate between the care given a child with an acute problem and one with a chronic problem.

The conditions included in this chapter are both acute and chronic diseases occurring in the school-aged child. Initially, all of these require hospitalization for diagnosis and establishment of a treatment plan. The child with diabetes, glomerulonephritis, rheumatoid arthritis, a brain tumor, or epilepsy will require ongoing supervision to control the problem as well as adjust the treatment and care. The children with Legg-Calvé-Perthes disease, cryptorchidism, rheumatic fever, and precocious puberty also require hospitalization initially but the course of the problem is more limited rather than permanently affecting the child's life-style.

JUVENILE RHEUMATOID ARTHRITIS

Juvenile rheumatoid arthritis is a chronic systemic disease with characteristic joint involvement. The presence of a persistent synovitis in one or more joints for a period of six weeks or longer is necessary to confirm the diagnosis. Pain or tenderness in a joint is not sufficient as a diagnostic sign. The joint must be involved with swelling or limitation of motion, heat and pain, or tenderness. In some children, a coexisting, recurrent, daily fever is noted. Low normal temperatures are common in the morning, with a subsequent rise to 102°F to 103°F in the late afternoon.

Other symptoms include the rheumatoid rash which characteristically accompanies the fever. It is an erythematous, maculopapular rash. The lesions vary in size and are found mainly on the chest, axillae, thighs, and upper arms. It is seldom present on the face or on the distal portions of the extremities. It is frequently pruritic.

Classification

Three types of juvenile rheumatoid arthritis have been identified. These include the systemic form, which is commonly called Still's disease, the pauciarticular form, and the polyarticular form. Each of these types has distinctly different characteristics and prognoses in children.

Systemic Form. The systemic type accounts for about twenty percent of all the cases. With this form, the child appears to be quite ill. Intermittent fever spikes occur and a rheumatoid rash is usually, although not always, present. At the onset of the disease, the child may not have any identifiable joint involvement. Joint involvement occurs within the first six months of the illness, however. Its incidence is equal in both boys and girls.

Pauciarticular Form. The pauciarticular type of juvenile rheumatoid arthritis refers to the child with involvement of one to four joints. About fifty percent of all patients with this disease belong to this group. They may have a low-grade fever, with or without a rash. The age ranges of children affected by this form of the disease include girls in the toddler and early preschool periods and boys who are early school-age.

Polyarticular Form. The polyarticular form of the disease, as its name suggests, affects multiple joints. This classification identifies those patients in whom five or more joints are involved. These children rarely have a rash unless fever is present. Some do have a low-grade fever. This form can affect girls or boys of any age.

Signs and Symptoms

The original joint changes associated with juvenile rheumatoid arthritis include inflammation which is localized in the joint capsule. This inflammation eventually spreads through the capsule to the surrounding cartilage. With progression of the disease, fibrotic changes and bony fusion occur, Figure 23-1. Involvement of the tendons and muscles in this process is common. Growth centers, which are adjacent to the affected joints, may either be suppressed or accelerated in the growth process.

Diagnosis

A number of laboratory studies are performed to differentiate juvenile rheumatoid arthritis from other similar diseases, such as rheumatic fever. In all affected children, the sedimentation rate is elevated. The hematocrit and the complete blood count reveal anemia and an increased leukocyte count. This is most common, with high elevations of the white blood cell count, in children with the systemic form of the disease.

The rheumatoid factor is identified in a small percentage of affected children. It is

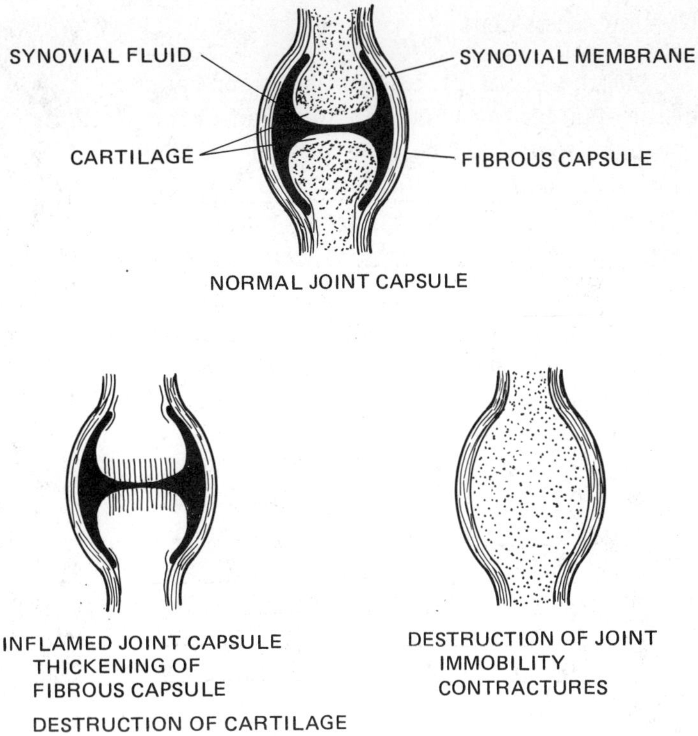

FIG. 23-1 Joint changes in juvenile rheumatoid arthritis

positive in girls with the polyarticular form, but negative in boys with the same form of the disease. It is negative in all other forms, regardless of sex of the child. Antinuclear antibodies are present in up to forty percent of patients with juvenile rheumatoid arthritis. They are usually found in male children with the pauciarticular form of the disease who are older than five years of age. These children commonly have eye involvement. Another diagnostic test may also be positive in this age-group. It is the HLA-B27 histocompatibility antigen test.

Radiographs of the involved joints are obtained. The first changes seen are soft tissue swellings. Erosive bone changes and narrowing of the joint spaces occur later in the disease process. These changes are most common in children with a positive rheumatoid factor. Electrocardiograms and echocardiography may also be performed. Some of the children have pericarditis. It is more prevalent in children with the systemic type of disease onset. An analysis of synovial fluid is important in children with involvement of only one joint. The aspirated fluid is analyzed, and usually demonstrates the inflammatory process characteristic of this disease.

Initial eye examinations are important for all of these children as are examinations at regular intervals. Uncontrolled eye involvement can cause cataracts, glaucoma, and eventual blindness. Eye involvement is most common in those children with the pauciarticular form of the disease.

Nursing Assessment

In the initial process of assessment and history-taking, the nurse should obtain information about any recent exposures of the child to infections, particularly streptococcal infections. The family is also questioned about trauma to the joints, as well as recent immunizations, such as rubella. It is also important to know whether there is a family history of arthritis — in parents, grandparents, or in siblings.

During the physical assessment, particular attention is paid to all areas of the musculoskeletal system. Range of motion and muscular strengths and weaknesses are also of special note. Joints that are hot, red, swollen, painful or tender are identified carefully. Joint deformities are also carefully documented. Any signs of lymphadenopathy should also be noted.

During the period of initial hospitalization following diagnosis, both short- and long-term goals for treatment are established. The long-range goal for the treatment of all affected children is to maintain as high a functional level as possible. They should be encouraged to become functioning members of society, even though they may have to undergo hospitalization and treatment periodically. For this reason, they are maintained in their home environment and kept in regular school classrooms, Figure 23-2.

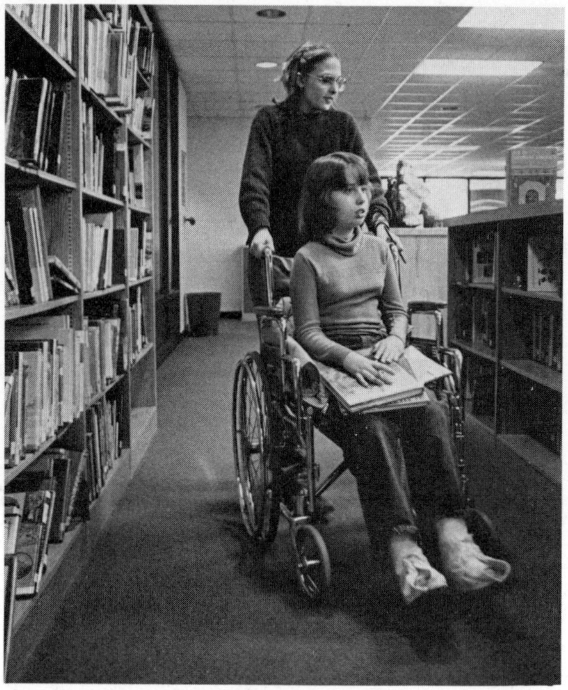

FIG. 23-2 With some assistance, participation in school is possible for this young girl with juvenile rheumatoid arthritis. (Courtesy of Larry Lambert)

Medical Treatment

The goal of medical treatment is to keep the child as free as possible from deformities and contractures. This is accomplished through a treatment plan that includes drug therapy, physical therapy, orthopedic corrections, and regular eye care. Good nutrition, adequate rest, and education of parents and child are also necessary parts of this program.

Drug therapy includes the use of pharmacologic agents to reduce joint pain and inflammatory response. Initially, the drug of choice is either aspirin or one of the nonsteroidal antiinflammatory drugs. Aspirin is administered in doses of 80 milligrams per kilogram per day in divided doses. The exact dosage is calculated according to body weight as well as the dosage necessary to maintain a blood salicylate level of 25 milligrams per 100 milliliters. The disadvantage of the aspirin is its toxic effect on the liver. For this reason, the child may be given other rapid-acting drugs, such as indomethacin (2 to 4 mg/kg/day), tolmetin

(20 mg/kg/day), naproxen (10 to 12 mg/kg/day), or sulindac (5 mg/kg/day). More than one drug may be tried before finding the one that is the most suitable drug for a particular child.

For children who have a poor response to the rapid-acting drugs, other, slower-acting drugs may be used. These include D-penicillamine, hydroxychloroquine, and gold salts. Many of these drugs, such as hydroxychloroquine, may be given on a regular basis for as long as two years. D-penicillamine is contraindicated for use in conjunction with gold therapy, and has many side effects. Gold therapy is parenteral only, and may be maintained for years.

Steroids are used to control the disease process in children who are acutely ill. They are used selectively to suppress the signs and symptoms of the disease, but they do not inhibit the joint destruction and so cannot be used on a long-term basis. Steroids also have multiple systemic side effects in both children and adults. One side effect that is of major concern in children is growth suppression or stunting, which can occur from long-term use. To minimize the side effects of corticosteroids, the selected drug is often given on an alternate day schedule.

In some children who are resistant to the usual forms of drug therapy, antineoplastic drugs may be administered for short periods of time. The most common drug used for this purpose is methotrexate. Others that may be administered include cyclophosphamide and nitrogen mustard.

Physical Therapy

Physical therapy for children with juvenile rheumatoid arthritis begins with a complete assessment. Incorporated in this assessment is an evaluation of joint range of motion. This assessment is necessary to obtain baseline information. An evaluation is also done of muscular strength around the involved joints, as well as the noninvolved extremities. Functional abilities are also determined at this time. They include the gait and the distance the child is able to ambulate. The ability to use stairs or transfer from a wheelchair or a bed is also assessed. Activities of daily living, such as dressing, feeding, and bathing are included in the evaluation.

Exercise Program. Once the baseline assessment has been completed and an exercise program has been structured for the individual child, the therapist carries out the program with the assistance of the nursing staff and parents. If the child is old enough, he or she becomes part of the treatment team and is involved in the education process as well. The exercise program progresses from passive motion, to active motion with assistance, to active motion. The exercises are designed for the involved joints, as well as the areas immediately above and below the joints. Parents are taught how to do the exercises, as well as how often they should be repeated and what constitutes a realistic schedule in terms of the child's daily activities.

Gradually, as these children grow, they assume full responsibility for the exercise program. The advantage of this approach is that it allows them to regain a degree of control over their lives and their health care. These children often resist the efforts of the parent to carry out the program, but will not object to doing the exercises themselves.

Splints and Assistive Devices. Maintaining joint alignment usually involves splinting. The parents and the child, if old enough, are taught the proper application of splints, associated skin care, the proper maintenance of the splint, and what exercises are to be done. In addition, they may be shown how to make simple adjustments in using the splint.

Children with juvenile rheumatoid arthritis may require assistive devices for ambulation, in the home and the school situation. Crutches and walkers may be used for this purpose. It is imperative that both the technique and the equipment allow the child independence as well as ease in carrying out daily activities. All age-appropriate activities are encouraged, including adapted forms of physical education in the school system.

Control of Stiffness. Reduction of pain and joint stiffness in the morning is accomplished with warm compresses or soaks and exercises. Many children have fewer problems with stiffness if they are kept warm during the night. This may be achieved by the use of extra coverings, blanket sleepers in young children and gloves or warm mittens for the hands. For acute episodes of stiffness or pain, a whirlpool or dry heat may be used. Paraffin baths can also be used, but they carry a risk of a burn if not used correctly.

Working with the Family

Communications between children with juvenile rheumatoid arthritis, their parents, and the members of the health team must be open and honest. Their discussions should encompass the physical status of the child, the treatment plan, and education regarding the disease process itself. Even the youngest child should be included in these office conversations in order to initiate the long-term trusting relationship that must develop. Information should be presented in terms that are understandable to both parents and child. Both should be encouraged to ask questions.

Attitudes within the home influence the child's abilities to function in all areas. The child cannot be protected from life itself. Except for the necessary adaptations or special arrangements, the parents should treat the child as if no problem existed. This may be particularly difficult for parents so health team members must reinforce this concept repeatedly. Consistency within the health care team should foster this ideal. Children should be helped to develop a positive attitude of "I can do it" with regard to decision making on appropriate levels, involvement in the treatment program, and relationships with others. Their level of self-confidence is a reflection of the attitudes of the adults involved in their care, whose opinions they value.

Special concerns of the child usually involve school and the problems of body image. In the school setting, the concern of others may be excessive, and the child may not be allowed to function at a normal level. This overprotective attitude is frequently related to the perception of a handicapped child as a novelty, which usually impedes the child's ability to function. The necessity of taking medication during school hours places undue emphasis on the concept of the child's illness rather than a state of wellness. Special arrangements may be made to allow the child to leave the classroom earlier to avoid the rush in the hallways, or to enter the cafeteria at a different time with another student along to help carry a tray. The use of crutches or a walker necessitates many small adaptations for any child, regardless of whether a leg is fractured or arthritic.

In older children, the problem of body image creates the most stress. They do not want to be considered sick, yet they realize that they do feel different. This is reinforced in many ways. Teenagers often need to test activities and then set their own limits. Long-standing attitudes of pity or overprotectiveness are evident in school-aged or teenaged children who use their illness to manipulate others. Much of this is a reflection of what these children hear about themselves from significant others in their lives. These are the same problems that can occur in any child with a long-term or chronic illness.

LEGG-CALVÉ-PERTHES DISEASE

Legg-Calvé-Perthes disease was first described around the turn of the century. It occurs most often in preschool or school-aged Caucasian boys. It rarely occurs in the Black community and seldom occurs in girls. The ratio of affected males to females is about four to one.

Pathophysiology

The exact cause of this disease is unknown, but the symptoms result from an occlusion of the blood supply to all or part of the proximal femoral epiphysis. Trauma is thought to play some part in this, although it is not always clearly identified. Boys in this age-group are quite active and may suffer mild injury without recognizing its potential severity.

The major pathologic finding is aseptic necrosis of the head of the femur. The femoral head may be only slightly misshapen or it may be very flattened, larger in size than normal, and abnormally broad and short at its neck. The term *coxa plana* is used to describe this type of manifestation. The course of the disease is studied by obtaining punch biopsies from the epiphysis at various stages during the disease.

The three stages of the disease, each of which last nine to twelve months, are aseptic necrosis, revascularization, and reossification.

Aseptic Necrosis. During the stage of aseptic necrosis, microscopically the bone shows extensive necrosis in the area of the femoral capital epiphysis. The cellular changes are consistent with bone death, with no attempt at repair. The epiphysis shows increased density, the joint space of the hip is widened, and the outline of the epiphyseal plate is irregular.

Revascularization. During the period of revascularization, or during the healing stage, the dense areas in the capital epiphysis begin to reabsorb. This allows new bone to replace the necrotic portion. The bone appears to be fragmented and mottled. The neck of the femur may continue to widen, and the epiphyseal plate becomes more irregular.

Reossification. The last stage is the period of reossification. Healing and replacement are completed in this phase. The contour of the femoral head that is established during this stage will persist throughout the individual's adult life. Ideally, normal bone and a normal femoral contour develop, and, at about the age of sixteen years, the epiphyseal plate closes. Without treatment, the head remains flattened and the joint grossly abnormal. The individual is then subjected to mechanical changes, and osteoarthritis occurs in early adult years.

Assessment

On assessment, several characteristic signs are identified. The child and parents usually seek help because of pain in the hip or in the knee. The referred pain in the knee results from mechanical alteration of the gait pattern on the affected side. Young children may ignore the pain at first. The parents may seek help for the child because of a detectable limp.

In comparison with the normal extremities of the child, the midthigh circumference of the affected leg differs. Limited abduction is noted in the affected limb, as well as impaired internal and external rotation and extension. All laboratory tests are within normal limits. Findings are confirmed by x-ray examination.

Treatment

All forms of treatment are aimed at prevention of deformity of the joint. The force of gravity in the process of weight-bearing can cause destruction of the femoral head. For this reason, the treatment specifically excludes any weight-bearing activities. In the past, these children were restricted to complete bedrest for up to two years. At the present time, a short period of bedrest is usually accompanied by light traction to eliminate weight-bearing. These children are then placed in weight-bearing braces or bilateral, long leg, abduction casts. The abduction casts have crossbars that maintain a forty-five degree angle and walking heels so that the child is ambulatory with crutches.

Nursing Care

Initially, the nursing care of this child involves implementation of the weight-bearing restriction and reinforcement of its importance for both parents and child. For children who are initially maintained on bedrest without traction this means avoidance of kneeling as well as standing. For those children in light traction (usually Buck's extension with a 4- to 6-pound weight), the nurse must maintain proper alignment of the child's body in a position of abduction. Nutrition and elimination are important considerations of care in addition to the routine care given an immobilized child.

As the child progresses, nonweight-bearing exercises may be added to the program. The use of a pool is particularly suited for this purpose. For those children whose legs are in casts, the nurse should teach cast care, impressing upon their parents the necessity of observing the cast closely for any signs of constriction secondary to the child's growth. The cast must also be checked for any softening. Most of these casts must be replaced every two months. The physical therapist teaches the child and parents the proper method of walking with crutches. The nurse should reinforce this teaching as much as possible.

SLIPPED FEMORAL CAPITAL EPIPHYSIS

The child with a slipped femoral capital epiphysis may present signs and symptoms that resemble those associated with Legg-Calvé-Perthes disease. Pain in the knee and a demonstrated limp is evident. This child may also become unusually tired after walking or standing for long periods of time.

This condition occurs in adolescents or preadolescents. Usually, it affects children who are very large, possibly overweight, or those who have recently undergone a rapid growth spurt. Characteristic age-range for this condition is ten to sixteen years.

X-ray findings demonstrate a displacement of the capital epiphysis, usually in a posterior and inferior position. The treatment involves surgical correction. Internal fixation is accomplished with the use of a nail or pins to maintain the position. This child spends only a short time on crutches — until the area heals — and then there is no restriction on weight-bearing.

BRAIN TUMORS

Brain tumors in children, as in adults, are localized space-occupying lesions. Their peak incidence is in male children between the ages of five and ten years. They are most commonly infratentorial, which means they occur below the structure known as the tentorium cerebri. The tentorium cerebri is a fold of the dura separating the cerebrum from the cerebellum. Approximately seventy-five percent of brain tumors in children originate in the brain tissue itself as gliomas.

Classification

Four common classifications of brain tumors exist: meningiomas, neuromas, gliomas, and metastatic lesions. Meningiomas are encapsulated tumors that do not invade the brain tissue itself. However, they cause problems with compression of brain tissue. Neuromas arise from the cranial nerves. The early symptoms relate directly to the functioning of specific nerves. Gliomas are infiltrating tumors that originate in brain tissue. The three most common gliomas are astrocytomas, medulloblastomas, and glioblastoma multiforme. Each of these types is further classified according to the predominant cell type in the lesion. Metastatic lesions are usually the result of a primary lesion in the lung.

Symptoms

The symptoms produced by a brain tumor are dependent on the location of the lesion and on the rate and pattern of its growth. Rapidly growing tumors produce early signs of increased intracranial pressure. Other early signs and symptoms may include weakness or paralysis of one side (hemiparesis), impaired sensation or numbness of one side (hemiparesthesia), reduction of the normal visual fields (hemianopsia), double vision (diplopia), altered gait patterns (ataxia), and alterations in mental status, such as lethargy, drowsiness, and behavioral changes.

Because of the common infratentorial location of these lesions, the majority of children have manifestations directly related to increased intracranial pressure. The most common signs of increased intracranial pressure include headaches, vomiting, ataxic gait or weakness, and alterations in vital signs. Other signs include cranial neuropathy, head tilting or posturing, cranial enlargement before eighteen months, papilledema, behavioral changes, and seizures.

Children usually do not complain of headaches. In very young children, crying, irritability, anorexia, and possibly, head-banging may indicate the child's discomfort. Typically, the headache is most severe in the morning and is aggravated by lowering the head or by straining in any way. The child shows a preference for remaining both still and quiet.

Vomiting is also most severe in the morning. It may become projectile later in the child's course. It occurs without nausea and most often with position changes from supine to upright positions.

The ataxic gait or weakness is often not recognized until detected on physical or neurologic examination. At the onset, the child simply appears to be clumsy and uncoordinated. Parents and teachers may not recognize the severity of the child's problem until increasing difficulty in moving and turning quickly and frequent falls are witnessed. Loss of fine motor skills is also evidence of ataxia.

The alterations in vital signs that are consistent with increased intracranial pressure include an increase in blood pressure, a decreased pulse and respiratory rate, and a widened pulse pressure (the difference between the systolic and diastolic reading of the blood pressure). The changes are directly related to the space-occupying lesion in the brain. As the lesion compresses tissue, it offers greater resistance to normal blood flow through the brain. The body attempts to compensate by raising the blood pressure, causing the tissues to become more edematous. The edema increases the resistance to blood flow and the cycle is perpetuated, Figure 23-3. This is less of a problem in young children, as the suture line and fontanelles expand to allow greater flexibility. In the older children, however, the skull resembles a closed container, allowing no room for expansion. Seizures and coma result as the pressure increases to a point at which the brain herniates through the foramen magnum and death ensues.

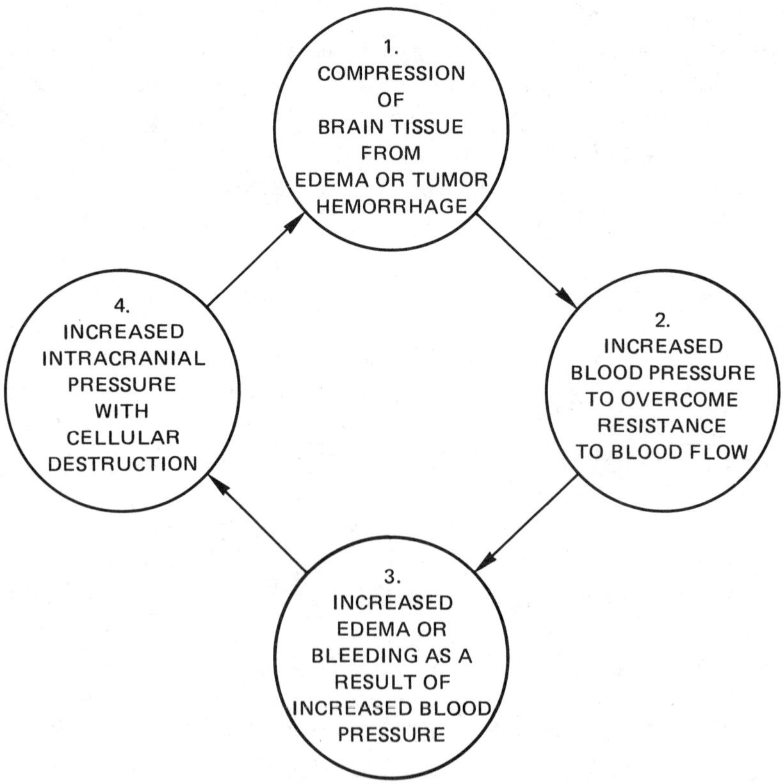

FIG. 23-3 The cycle of increased intracranial pressure. The cycle continues unless appropriate intervention is instituted.

Assessment and Treatment

The diagnostic evaluation of a child with a suspected brain tumor includes a complete neurologic examination. Additionally, a noninvasive procedure called a CAT scan (computerized axial tomography) may be performed. It provides information about the tumor, such as its size, its exact location, and its type (solid or cystic). The advantage of this procedure is that few reactions to the injected dye occur. The child is often sedated to prevent any movement during the examination. Diagnostic tests such as ventriculography or angiography, may also be used, but are associated with greater risk.

The treatment of choice for any of these tumors is dependent on the rate of tumor growth, the degree of malignancy, and the involvement of other structures. However, surgery is often performed.

Nursing Care

Initially, the nursing care of children with suspected brain tumors involves assisting with the preoperative observations and diagnostic preparations that will confirm or exclude the diagnosis. During this process, parents and children should be given the utmost in support because of the critical nature of the diagnosis.

Once surgery is scheduled, the preparation and support of the child and parents must be continued. Children, depending on their age, have varying perceptions of their brain and what it actually does. The nurse's explanation of its function should be geared to their developmental level. They should also be told that the removal of all or part of the tumor may not resolve all of the symptoms. Also, they should know that some of their skills and motor abilities may be lost temporarily, but that the doctors, nurses, and therapists will be working with them and their parents to help them regain these skills.

Immediate preparation for the surgery involves shaving of the child's head. This may be done the night before or the morning of the surgery. Both parents and children should be adequately prepared for this procedure as it is quite upsetting. The child's hair should be saved in an envelope or plastic bag and given to the parents. Children are usually less upset after the shaving if they are encouraged to wear some type of head covering. A surgeon's cap is a very acceptable head covering for some children.

Postoperatively, the child will be in the intensive care unit. Careful observation of vital signs and periodic neurologic checks are continued in this setting. Neurologic assessment includes the child's level of consciousness, pupillary responses, and response to stimuli. Seizure precautions should also continue during this postoperative period. Dressings are observed for any signs of drainage.

The child is positioned carefully to protect the operative site. In the case of an infratentorial lesion, the child's dressing will extend down the neck and over part of the upper back. The child is kept lying flat and is not permitted to flex the neck. Alternate positioning on either side is usually effected. Children who undergo removal of a supratentorial lesion will have a dressing that encircles their head, without extension onto the neck or back. Their head should be elevated approximately thirty degrees at all times to reduce edema.

Intravenous fluids are also administered to these children. Fluid calculations must be very specific and accurate. They are calculated at 2/3 to 3/4 of the maintenance rate.

As cerebral edema is present postoperatively, overhydration will cause additional problems. Before the child begins taking oral fluids, he or she should be assessed for a gag reflex. Fluids are not offered until this reflex has returned. Output is monitored carefully with the aid of a Foley catheter. If cerebral edema increases, rapid administration of hypertonic solutions or osmotic diuretics is often initiated to reduce the edema.

Hyperthermia is frequently seen after this type of surgery because of the disturbance of the heat-regulating center. The use of a hypothermia blanket is effective, as is the administration of antipyretics, either orally or in suppository form.

Rehabilitation and discharge planning time varies, depending on the patient's response to the surgery and recuperative abilities. Physical and occupational therapy are frequently used to retrain muscles, regain muscle tone, and maintain functional abilities. During this recovery period, the child and the parents should be helped to recognize small achievements and gains, as well as major ones. Because malignant tumors may not be curable, some of these children may be terminally ill.

JUVENILE DIABETES MELLITUS

The onset of juvenile diabetes can occur at any point throughout childhood. It is most common, however, in the school-age or adolescent periods. Characteristically, juvenile diabetes involves insulin dependency or Type I diabetes.

Symptoms

The classic symptoms associated with diabetes — polyuria, polydipsia, and polyphagia — do occur in children. However, they are not usually recognized as signs of diabetes initially. Other signs that are commonly seen when the child is admitted to the hospital relate to the fluid and electrolyte problems that occur with ketoacidosis. These signs include fatigue, muscle weakness, and malaise. They are related to losses of sodium and potassium, and to the depletion of calories. Vomiting may also occur, causing increased losses of chlorides and electrolytes. The child may be comatose on admission to the emergency room.

Cell starvation occurs in diabetic children, and continues for a period of time after the regulation of insulin and the diet has begun. One primary sign of this is the child's weight loss prior to the diagnosis, despite a ravenous appetite. Most affected children experience a five to ten percent loss of weight during the two weeks prior to actual diagnosis.

Other signs that occur during the two to four weeks preceding the actual diagnosis are abdominal pain, which simulates appendicitis, and blurred vision. The abdominal pain is caused by increased fat content in the intestinal blood vessels. The blurred vision is caused by the altered shape of the lens. This change in shape occurs as a result of high levels of blood glucose which cause a change in the osmotic pressure.

Diagnosis is made on the basis of the history and fasting plasma glucose levels above 140 mg per deciliter. A five-hour glucose tolerance test may also be done.

Acceptance of the Diagnosis

When the diagnosis of diabetes is first made, parents and children are usually overwhelmed. The term itself may bring to mind diabetic individuals they know (usually adults, not children) whose disease-related problems are multiple. While trying to learn about the disease, they may waver between feelings of denial, guilt, frustration, and depression. It is important for the nursing staff to recognize these feelings, acknowledge them openly, and encourage the parents and child to express them. Only then can they be channeled into a more constructive direction.

The attitudes of diabetic children are a reflection of their developmental level. They also reflect, to a great extent, the parental anxiety that has been either expressed or identified nonverbally. Preadolescents and adolescents often have the greatest difficulty adjusting because of their intense involvement with their peer group and their need for peer acceptance. If this interaction with peers can be nurtured in the hospital setting, their return to both home and school settings may be facilitated.

Lack of acceptance of the disease by parents and children promotes an ongoing state of emotional turmoil and crisis for the family. Some families never achieve a realistic acceptance of the disease and its limitations. As a result, the family may be rigid and compulsive about control. Children from these families are likely to return to the hospital frequently because the family lacks the ability or the motivation to adjust the diet appropriately to compensate for increased exercise or illness.

Dietary Control

The diet of the juvenile diabetic patient may be controlled in a number of different ways. The aim of all of the diets is to minimize the use of concentrated sweets. The most commonly used diet is that devised by the American Dietetic Association. It uses an exchange list for planning meals. Another diet that might be used is the liberal diet, which uses the basic four food groups and restricts the child's milk to a maximum of one quart per day. Another diet involves a total calorie restriction for meals and snacks. Still other diets involve the calculation of total available glucose or the control of carbohydrate intake each day.

Regardless of the dietary pattern that is used, parents and children must know what foods are permitted and what foods are restricted. They also should know what substitutions may be made in the diet and how to allow for these substitutions. Any of the diets that are based on an exchange system must specify not only the exchange sizes, but also the sizes of the portions allowed. Each of these diets provides a plan for meals plus additional snacks for the child, particularly at bedtime.

The appetite of the child should also be respected. If the child complains of hunger, additional acceptable foods should be allowed. This hunger may signify the particular growth needs of the child at that point. Adjustments are made on an ongoing basis for both growth and increases in activity.

Many of the diets have a meal pattern that supplies 2/7 of the total intake at breakfast, 2/7 at lunch, and 2/7 at dinner. The remaining 1/7 is supplied in the evening snack. It is important that some portion of this snack be protein as, otherwise, the child may become hypoglycemic in the early hours of the morning. This condition is often identified by the parents of young children when the child is found in the crib convulsing from hypoglycemia.

Adjustments are made in the diet of school-aged children. The standard school lunch menu may be inadequate for this child. Adaptations may have to be made. The child can carry a lunch from home or can supplement the school lunch menu. A type A school lunch contains 2 ounces of a complete protein, such as meat, but the other carbohydrates may be incompatible with the dietary pattern. An additional consideration is the time of the lunch period. This child should eat regular meals at the same time each day. The lunch period in school should be after 11:00 AM and before 12:30 PM. In some schools, an adjustment in the schedule must be made.

Insulin Regulation

Because the child is usually admitted to the hospital in a state of ketoacidosis, the insulin dose that is initially administered is higher than the maintenance level will eventually be. An initial dosage of regular insulin is approximately 2 units per kilogram of body weight. As the child is brought under control and food is better utilized, insulin requirements will decrease. The child is usually placed on a long-acting insulin for home use.

This period of decreased need for insulin is referred to as a remission or "honeymoon" period. It generally occurs one to three months after the initial diagnosis. It is not a permanent reduction in insulin need, and its duration varies from child to child. It is important to explain this phenomenon to the child and the family as it usually occurs outside the controlled environment of the hospital. The family should anticipate the possibility of a hypoglycemic reaction and should also realize that this episode will not eliminate the ongoing need for insulin. Eventually, the insulin dosage will stabilize. Some juvenile diabetic patients are quite brittle or difficult to control, and stabilization does not occur until growth is completed in adulthood.

Insulin Administration

The technique of administering insulin is taught to the parents, as well as the child, if the child is school-aged or older. Generally, one or two staff members work with the family to teach them the technique, eventually supervising the actual administration of the insulin. It is important to limit the number of individuals presenting information to the family in order to decrease the confusion that results from slight variations in instruction and in technique.

The nurse should know exactly what equipment the child will be using in the home situation. If a glass syringe is to be used, it should be sterilized by boiling every two weeks. In the interim, it is stored in a glass jar of alcohol, Figure 23-4. If plastic disposable syringes are to be used, the family should know how to handle them and should dispose of them properly. They are not reusable.

Site rotation is an extremely important concept for diabetic children, Figure 23-5. The use of the abdominal site should be introduced very early. It is a routine site for injection and should not be reserved for when there are problems with the standard arm and leg sites. Injection sites are considered to be one-inch square, and the same site is used no more than once every fourteen days. If lipoatrophy occurs, the site is not used. This condition can be avoided by using pure beef or pure pork insulin.

School-aged children who are encouraged and taught to administer their own insulin treatments generally have a sense of control of their health care and their bodies. They are less likely to feel victimized by adults. This, in turn, reduces their inclination to use their condition to manipulate others for their

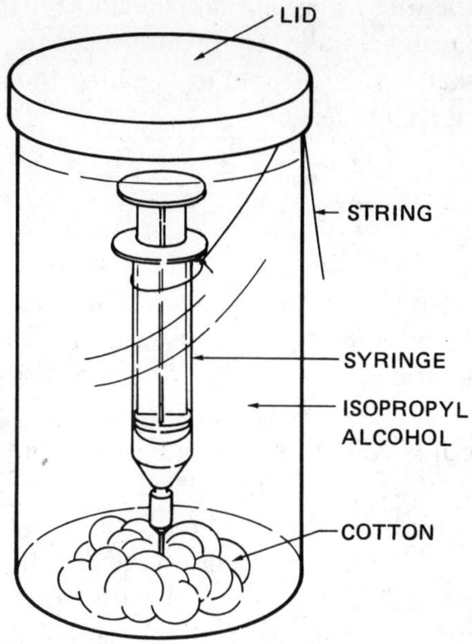

FIG. 23-4 Proper storage method for reusable glass syringes

The syringe is stored in a glass jar that has a lid and that is tall enough to hold it.

The jar is filled with isopropyl alcohol.

Several cotton balls may be placed in the bottom of the jar to protect the needle.

A string may be attached to the barrel of the syringe to facilitate its removal from the jar.

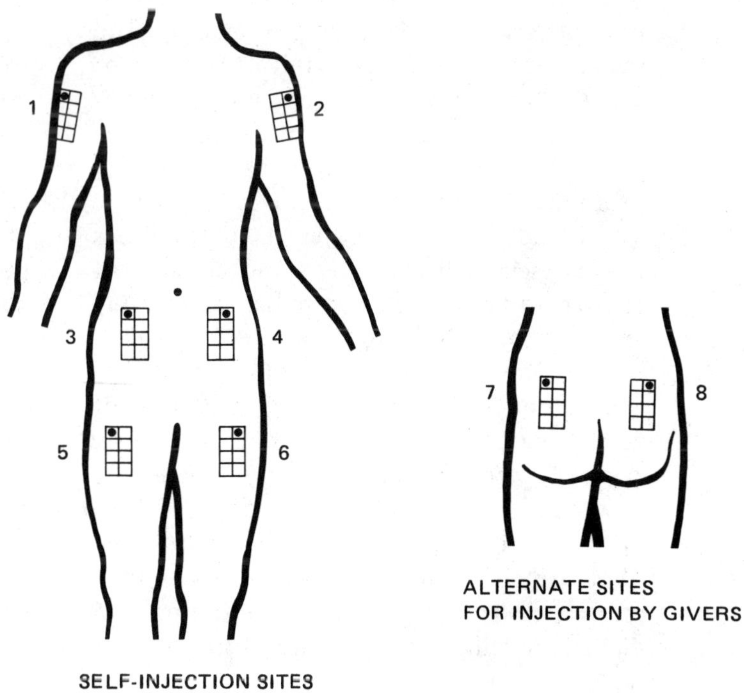

FIG. 23-5 Rotation of injection sites

own gain. Many young people do extremely well when they are individually taught to administer insulin to themselves and then are asked to participate in teaching their parents the technique.

Urine Testing

Urine tests for glucose and ketones are performed in the hospital as well as at home. For teaching to be consistent, the same testing method should be used in both settings. For accuracy, the technique should involve a double-voided specimen. The child is first asked to empty the bladder. One-half hour later a urine specimen is obtained for the test.

The use of Clinitest tablets for glucose testing is preferable. The two-drop method is a reliable indicator of the percentage of glucose spilled. The two-drop method measures up to five percent spillage. The advantage of this type of test is that its timing is not critical to the accuracy of the results. It is also important that the family use the proper color chart.

Acetest tablets are used to detect the presence of ketones. A color chart is used to read these results as well.

The disadvantage of these testing methods for the school-aged child is the amount of equipment needed to perform the tests if they are to be continued throughout the school day.

Another method of testing for glucose and ketones is the tape method. A number of tape preparations are available for this purpose. The influence of accurate timing on the results should be stressed to the child. Usually, these methods are most acceptable to adolescents. They are also easy to use when traveling or camping or while in the school setting. All diabetic children should know how to use both methods.

Insulin Reactions

Both hypoglycemic and hyperglycemic reactions can occur with diabetes, Table 23-1. All who are involved with diabetic children should be aware of the signs of these reactions and the proper treatment for them. Hypoglycemic reactions pose the greatest problems. The child may inadvertently increase the level of activity, burning more calories than usual and resulting in a hypoglycemic reaction.

Both children and parents should know what to do in the event of a reaction. Ten grams of glucose may be provided rapidly by the administration of 4 ounces of orange juice, one-half tube of instant glucose paste, two Lifesavers®, or two square sugar cubes. Any one of these can easily be made available in the school situation with written directions from the parent for their use.

In the school setting, the child should be treated for a reaction but should not be sent home. Sending the child home each time a reaction occurs further reinforces the concept of the child as sickly. It also provides a ready excuse for some children to leave school at a moment's notice. The parents should be notified of the insulin reaction by the school nurse.

In addition to having some form of glucose readily available in school, diabetic children should carry some glucose source with them, along with their diabetic identification card, bracelet, or tag. Sugar cubes or glucose paste are preferred to a candy bar as the child with a candy bar in his or her pocket may have difficulty resisting the temptation to eat it when a nondiabetic friend also consumes one. The child is much less likely to eat sugar cubes or glucose paste in this situation.

TABLE 23-1 Insulin Reactions and Diabetic Coma

INSULIN REACTION	DIABETIC COMA
Causes Omission of a meal Vomiting a meal after taking insulin Too much exertion or exercise Error in insulin dose Symptoms* Nervousness Weakness Hunger Sweating Cold and clammy skin Double vision Numbness of tongue or lips Confusion Appropriate Intervention Take some form of sugar immediately: orange juice, 4 oz hard candy (2 pieces), warm tea or coffee, with 1 Tbsp of honey or 2 cubes of sugar Characteristics of Urine Negative for sugar and acetone	Causes Insufficient insulin Dietary indiscretion Infection Symptoms* Thirst, no appetite Flushed face, dry skin Drowsiness Nausea or vomiting Blurred vision Frequent urination Fruity odor on breath Appropriate Intervention Test urine for sugar and acetone Call a doctor immediately; get proper insulin instructions Rest in bed Look for evidence of infection Characteristics of Urine Positive for sugar and acetone

*The symptoms of an insulin reaction occur rapidly, whereas the onset of the symptoms of a diabetic coma is more gradual.

Both parents and children should be able to anticipate the potential for a reaction in some situations. An increase in activity signals the need for an increase in the diet. This is particularly true in children who are involved in a sports program with intermittent increases in their activity level. These children should increase their intake by one bread exchange for each increase of thirty minutes in the activity level.

Rapid identification of an approximate blood sugar level may be obtained through the use of a new test tape method. Both Dextrostix and Chemstix provide approximate blood sugar level determinations when a drop of blood obtained from a finger stick is applied to the tape. This is especially helpful in the control of a brittle diabetic patient. Glucometers are also available for exact blood glucose measurements in the home. These require only a finger stick for blood.

The Somogyi Effect

Rebound hyperglycemia, or the Somogyi effect, can occur in diabetic children, as well as diabetic adults. It involves the increased production of glucose by the liver and a peripheral resistance to insulin. It can be caused by any one of the following three mechanisms: (1) growth hormone may depress glucose uptake at the cellular level; (2) cortisol may depress glucose transport into the cells or decrease cellular utilization; or (3) epinephrine may increase the breakdown of glycogen.

This type of rebound hyperglycemia is identified by its characteristic signs. Within an interval of three or four hours, the child's urine tests may change rapidly from negative to strongly positive. The blood glucose levels may fluctuate greatly, with no relationship to food ingestion. The early morning signs of headache and hypothermia, as well as nocturnal sweating generally herald the elevated levels of glucose and ketone that day.

Rebound hyperglycemia is treated by a gradual reduction in the amount of insulin administered. The reduction is no greater than two or three units at one time. During this treatment period, the nursing staff should review with the family the importance of regularly spaced, balanced meals; general compliance with the dietary pattern; replacement of uneaten foods; and careful documentation of all signs of a reaction.

Care During Illness

Both parents and children are taught how to cope with diabetes in the presence of minor illness. The dose of insulin is never altered unless the doctor specifically orders a change. Parents and children are taught that self-treatment is for one-day illnesses only. If, because of the illness, the child is having difficulty consuming the regular diet, fruit juices, crackers, and other foods that are better tolerated may be substituted on a temporary basis.

Urine glucose levels are monitored carefully throughout this period. Increases or decreases in food intake are based on these determinations. If the child cannot tolerate any food or fluids, the physician should be notified.

Long-Range Goals

The long-range goals for a diabetic child include normal growth and development, both physically and psychosocially; a sense of well-being reflecting adequate control of the diabetes; good nutrition; and an appropriate degree of independence.

The long-range goals cannot be accomplished without a concerted effort by members of the health care team and the family. The family should be optimistic about the child's future as well as flexible about the changes that must be made.

The achievement of these goals depends on the age of the child at the time of the diagnosis. Very young children are often more compliant with the necessary routines of care than are adolescents. The impact of the diagnosis itself may be initially greater for adolescents as they seek perfection in themselves and in others.

These same goals are achieved and reevaluated over a period of years. Progress is not measured in weeks or months of care. For some families, this period is marked by frequent hospitalizations. For others, the hospitalizations may be sporadic. For all of them, it is a time to relearn and redefine the goals.

RHEUMATIC FEVER

Rheumatic fever is a disease that affects many systems. It is triggered by a streptococcal infection in the upper respiratory tract. Acute attacks are initiated by group A beta-hemolytic streptococci. The disease is considered to be a hypersensitivity reaction or autoimmune response to that particular organism.

Rheumatic fever generally occurs in children five to fifteen years of age. The first attack usually occurs during the beginning school years, or around the age of six years. The condition is most prevalent in the winter months and in early spring, which coincides with the peak incidence of the streptococcal organisms in the general population. This pattern is also consistent with the close contact that accompanies cooler weather patterns.

Symptoms

The symptoms of rheumatic fever are grouped into major and minor categories. The diagnosis is usually based on the observation of two major manifestations or one major and two minor symptoms. These are the Jones criteria established by the American Heart Association. The knees, ankles, wrists, and elbows are involved more often than are the other joints, and the pain is aggravated by movement, massage, or any form of pressure.

Major Symptoms. Polyarthritis, carditis, subcutaneous nodules, chorea, and erythema marginatum are all classified as major signs of the disease.

Polyarthritis in this disease is usually migratory in nature and affects the large joints. The joint will be swollen, hot, red, and painful for one to two days during the acute phase. As this joint improves, another one will manifest the same symptoms.

Either pericarditis or endocarditis may be present. Inflammation secondary to the disease causes lesions within the heart, called Aschoff bodies, which produce damage in the connective tissue layers of the heart. As the endocarditis subsides, certain areas in the heart remain scarred, such as the aortic and mitral valves. Because of the scarring, the valve structure may be fused or may close incompletely. The symptoms of carditis include tachycardia, which is consistently disproportionate to the child's age, activity, and degree of temperature elevation. Cardiomegaly is often evident on the chest radiography. A change in heart sounds also occurs, such as a pericardial friction rub, muffling of the heart sounds from pericardial effusion, or an accentuated third heart sound, called a prediastolic gallop. When an electrocardiogram is done, a change in the conductivity of the heart such as an increased P-R interval is evident.

Subcutaneous nodules are less than 1 centimeter in size and cluster in small groups over the bony prominences. They are usually evident on the extensor surfaces of the joints, such as the elbow. The lesions are hard, painless nodules that eventually subside without treatment when the febrile course of the disease is completed. Microscopically, they resemble Aschoff bodies, although they do not cause any permanent damage.

Sydenham's chorea, more commonly called St. Vitus' dance, is an example of central nervous system involvement by this disease. It is usually seen after the febrile course of the disease. Chorea denotes involuntary, purposeless movements, such as facial grimaces, aimless movements of the extremities, and speech disturbances. It develops gradually, and any attempts to suppress the movement or getting the child to be still only exaggerates it. In the school situation, it may be recognized by a loss of fine motor skills that had previously been accomplished, or by difficulty in counting or pursuing any activity rapidly. Emotional lability is also characteristic of this problem.

Erythema marginatum is a distinctive skin rash. It consists of a macular rash with a clear center and a wavy, well-marked border. The snakelike or wavy pattern occurs only on covered or protected parts of the body, such as the trunk. There is no pruritis with this rash.

Minor Symptoms. The minor manifestions of rheumatic fever are general and may occur in combination with other symptoms. They are not diagnostic by themselves, but they often support a past history of the disease.

The minor symptoms of the disease include fever, which is present in the afternoons without visible inflammation, epistaxis, pallor, and malaise.

Diagnosis

The laboratory test that confirms the precipitating streptococcal infection is the antistreptolysis-O (ASO) titer. This blood test measures the antibodies formed in the blood against an extracellular product secreted by the organism. Normal values range from 0 to 120. Any value exceeding 166 Todd units is considered to be diagnostic. The child with rheumatic fever will have values considerably higher than this even if no previous streptococcal sore throat or other infection is cited. The titer begins rising about a week after the infection and continues to rise to a maximal level after four to six weeks.

Other laboratory tests that may be done include a sedimentation rate and a C-reactive protein test. Chest x-ray studies are performed to detect cardiac enlargement. Electrocardiograms are done in any child with evidence of carditis. Echocardiograms may be done to determine the area of valvular damage.

Medical Treatment

The medical treatment of rheumatic fever involves the eradication of any residual infection, the protection of the child from the recurrence of infection, the reduction or elimination of any permanent damage from carditis, and palliative treatment for other manifestations. These objectives are accomplished through the use of antibiotics, both for treatment and prophylaxis; bedrest, cardiotonics for carditis, and salicylates for the inflammatory joint involvement.

The antibiotic of choice is penicillin, usually procaine penicillin G, administered intramuscularly in a dose of 600,000 units daily for ten days. For long-term therapy and as a follow-up medication, 1.2 million units of Bicillin may be given once a month. In those children who are sensitive to penicillin, erythromycin agents may be substituted. The usual oral dose is 1 gram daily for ten days.

Implementation of bedrest for carditis varies from a strict enforcement to a modified form, depending on the physician as well as the cooperation of the child. The activity restriction is maintained until all signs of acute illness have subsided, as evidenced by the absence of C-reactive protein and a falling sedimentation rate. Digoxin may be administered in children with signs of congestive heart failure. A dosage of 0.06 milligram per kilogram of body weight is used as the initial digitalizing dose.

Salicylates are used to control the inflammatory process in the joints. They also exert an analgesic and antipyretic effect which is helpful. Dosage is regulated through blood level determinations. The daily dose is 60 milligrams per pound with a maximal dose of 10 grams or a blood level range of between 25 and 35 milligrams per 100 milliliters. Corticosteroids may also be used to control the acute manifestations of the disease. They are particularly helpful in congestive heart failure. Prednisone is usually given in a dosage of 50 to 75 milligrams per day.

Nursing Care

Implementation of bedrest is the most difficult of all the aspects of this child's care. Once the acute manifestations of rheumatic fever have subsided, the child may not understand the rationale for the activity limitation. In the hospital setting, the nurse should first clarify the restrictions with the physician. Is self-feeding allowed? Is the child permitted the use of a bedside commode? This type of clarification promotes consistency in implementation by all members of the staff.

Both the child and the parents should be given an explanation of the reasons for the restrictions of activity. The explanation should be appropriate for the child's developmental level. As the child improves, the restrictions will become more difficult to accept unless the parents and child understand the amount of time it takes for the heart to heal. They should be told that the slightest increase in activity increases the workload of the heart. Nurses may demonstrate this concept by allowing them to listen to the difference in their heart rate while standing quietly and then after thirty seconds of running in place.

The child's schedule is planned to provide periods of complete rest throughout the day. For maximal benefit, these rest periods should remain uninterrupted. It is the nurse's responsibility to plan the rest periods and to see that they are not interrupted by other members of the health care team. These periods of additional rest are identified for parents as a part of the home care program for children with carditis.

Home Care

Home care activities must be clearly defined for the parents and child. Together with the family, the nurse can help structure a schedule that incorporates the appropriate restrictions, yet conforms to the usual activities within the home. Because of the increased susceptibility to infection, the child's need for a separate room or bed should be identified. Dressing, bathing, meals, rest periods, and medication administration should all be included in this schedule. For children with carditis, the limitation of activity may extend for a period of up to three months.

Equipment for home care may be rented, borrowed, or adapted. For instance, a small tray table or an improvised sturdy cardboard box can be used as an overbed table for meals. An elevated backrest can be provided by using a wooden chair tipped upside down and padded with pillows. A large cardboard box can also be cut and taped at a 45-degree angle to provide the same support. A wagon can provide the same mobility as a wheelchair, provided it is large enough for the child.

Diversional activities during this period are extremely important. Books, crayons, a radio, and other sources of diversion should be easily accessible at the child's bedside. Board games and siblings in the home can also be an appropriate combination for diversion. These approaches may not be suitable if the child's fine motor skills are impaired by chorea. In these cases, the presence of a single goldfish in a bowl may provide an excellent source of diversion for some children. For others, growing plants or watching outside activity from a window relieves some of the boredom associated with bedrest.

Joint pain is an ongoing problem and a source of discomfort in some children. The parents should be taught how to position the child to provide maximal comfort and to maintain proper body alignment. Bed cradles may be used or adapted to keep heavy bedding away from sore joints. The parent should realize that minimal handling of the child, as well as the use of aspirin, may help. Use of heat or cold and massage of the joint seem to cause increased discomfort for the child and are thus avoided.

Nutrition

Nutrition is also an important aspect of care. Children with rheumatic fever have poor appetites and are too tired to feed themselves. Initially, they are offered small, frequent feedings. They should be fed if they are unable or not permitted to feed themselves. Many children will allow others to feed them if they are permitted to feed some food, such as a piece of bread, to themselves. They should not be forced to eat, but should be encouraged through food selection.

The dependency aspects of being fed are very upsetting to some children. The rationale for this should be stressed to both the parents and the child. Adaptations, such as allowing the child to consume all liquids, including soups, through a straw, may make it more acceptable. The parents should be aware that feeding times may signal a battle if the child is allowed to control them.

Long-term Care and Prevention

The long-term care of children with rheumatic fever involves either the intramuscular administration of prophylactic doses of penicillin on a monthly basis or the oral administration of it on a daily basis. The injectable form of the drug is often preferred as the child's compliance with the medication regimen is thus ensured. This prophylactic therapy may be lifelong, or it may be discontinued at some point during adulthood. The rationale for discontinuing the medication is that adults are much less susceptible than are children to the streptococcal organism. The antibiotics must be resumed, however, prior to any dental work or any intrusive procedures involving the genitourinary or gastrointestinal tracts.

Parental education is the most important aspect of prevention of rheumatic fever. Streptococcal infections, manifested by lymphadenopathy, temperature elevations, sore throat, and pain on swallowing, are cause for seeking medical assistance. A throat culture should be obtained to identify the infective organism. The prescribed antibiotic should be taken for the recommended ten to fourteen days without interruption. A follow-up throat culture may then be done to determine the effectiveness of the treatment.

A public service program called SOS, which stands for Stamp Out Strep, operates in some areas. It is usually located in schools. Any individual with any sign of a sore throat can come in to have a culture done. The culture is then sent to a state laboratory and the results are reported to both the family physician and the parents. The advantage of this type of program is that the individual is more likely to seek assistance early.

GLOMERULONEPHRITIS

Acute glomerulonephritis is the most common form of nephritis seen in children. It follows an infectious process and is related to antigen-antibody reaction. The organism most commonly implicated is the streptococcal organism, although its involvement may be declining with the increased emphasis on the treatment of streptococcal infections.

Symptoms and Incidence

Symptoms include hematuria, edema, oliguria, and hypertension. Children may also have an elevated temperature, headache, malaise, loss of appetite, and sometimes, vomiting. These latter signs are less specific as they could relate to many of the childhood diseases.

Glomerulonephritis most often affects children in the late preschool or early school-age group. More boys than girls are affected. The signs of kidney disease may be so slight that the disease may go unrecognized for a considerable period of time. Signs of fever and gastrointestinal upset may not be attributed to kidney disease until irreversible damage has been done.

Diagnosis

Urinalysis is an important diagnostic tool in these children. The amount of urine is significantly altered in this condition so the child will be anuric. Microscopic examination reveals hematuria even if gross observation does not. High specific gravity and the presence of casts of red cells in the urine are common. Protein levels are not elevated in all patients.

Blood studies reveal an elevation of non-protein nitrogen (NPN) and blood urea nitrogen (BUN). Along with these tests that distinctly identify impaired kidney function, other test results, such as an elevated sedimentation rate or elevated antistreptolysis titer may also help to confirm the diagnosis.

Nursing Care

The major focus of this child's care is to reduce potentially life-threatening hypertension and to maintain the function of the kidneys. Protection of the child from infection is also important.

The hypertension may be reduced through the use of antihypertensive agents. An attempt is made to reduce the diastolic pressure to less than 100 mm of Hg. Fluid and sodium intake is also reduced for this purpose.

Maintaining kidney function begins with a careful recording of intake and output. Fluids should be accurately measured, not just estimated. The parents' cooperation may be enlisted in keeping track of what the child has consumed. Daily weights are also important in this endeavor and should be checked at the same time each day.

Dietary controls may also help to maintain kidney function. In all children who exhibit signs of renal failure, protein and potassium intake should be restricted. The child and the parents should be told the purpose of the dietary restrictions, as well as what foods are permitted on the diet. In this way, the parents will not inadvertently provide something for the child which is not in keeping with the dietary restrictions.

Complete bedrest also helps to maintain renal function. It is important that the child understand the purpose of the bedrest as he or she may not feel particularly ill.

Frequent changes of position are also a necessary part of care. Oxygen therapy is used for the child with cardiac involvement.

Prevention of infection is accomplished through the use of antibiotics, an adequate diet, and bedrest. In addition, exposure of the child to anyone with a respiratory infection should be limited.

Many of these children recover completely without demonstrable damage. Other children who may have a less severe form of the disease may suffer from chronic kidney failure and may ultimately require dialysis or a kidney transplant.

PRECOCIOUS PUBERTY

Precocious puberty refers to the early or premature development of the structures associated with sexual development that normally begin changing in early adolescence. In girls, the changes may include breast enlargement, menarche, and the presence of pubic and axillary hair. In boys, an enlargement of the penis and scrotum, a change in the hair distribution over the genitalia and face, and voice changes may be evident.

Characteristics

The condition is more common in girls than in boys, and in a large percentage of these children no identifiable cause is found. Precocious puberty exists when the changes occur prior to the age of eight or nine years. The rate of change, however, is variable. Some children manifest these changes within the first year of life, with other changes progressing at a slower rate. Other children may begin later and progress at an extremely rapid rate.

Sexual development is not the only area of change. These children are advanced in height and weight, as well as in osseous (bone) maturation. The major concern with osseous maturation is that it leads to early epiphyseal closure. If this continues, the child may not attain a normal height. Both dental age and the child's mental age are consistent with the child's actual chronologic age.

Diagnosis

Diagnostic tests are used to confirm the changes and also to rule out the presence of any type of tumor. Urine is collected in twenty-four-hour specimens to assess gonadotropin excretion. Levels of plasma testosterone and plasma estradiol are also evaluated and are usually consistent with the identified pubertal level. Both cerebral and adrenocortical tumors can cause this problem.

Nursing Care

Once the possibilities of a tumor have been ruled out, nursing care is based on psychologic support of the parents and the child. The parents should know what changes have taken place and which changes will continue. A great deal of support is needed initially, and this support should be maintained as long as necessary. The parents should be reminded that by the age of ten or eleven years, the child's own peer group will be undergoing the same changes.

During the period of hospitalization, the nurse should be supportive of the child relating to him or her according to chronologic development rather than in keeping with the advanced physical development. A child of six or seven years of age who looks quite mature may inadvertently be treated as an adolescent by members of the nursing staff. The child's physical size often causes others to have greater expectations for the child's ability and accomplishments than would normally be expected.

In some cases, small doses of progesterone may be administered to inhibit gonadotropin production. This has a twofold effect. It slows the rate of sexual development and it also slows the rate of osseous maturation. Epiphyseal closure does not occur as soon and the child's ultimate stature is improved. Without treatment, many of these children would not attain an adult height of five feet at maturity.

CRYPTORCHIDISM

The term cryptorchidism refers to undescended testicles. In the male, the testes begin their descent into the scrotum about the eighth month of intrauterine life. In the majority of full-term male infants, they are present in the scrotum at the time of birth. In one-third of premature infants, they are undescended at the time of birth. This is because the delivery occurs at about the time of normal descent. In some infants, the testes retract into the inguinal canal when an attempt is made to palpate them.

Treatment

Initially, the child is treated conservatively with gonadotropin if the testes do not descend by the age of five years. Dosages of up to 5000 units of gonadotropin are administered three times a day. This regimen is continued for six to eight weeks. If this treatment is not successful, surgical correction is undertaken. The surgery is called an orchiopexy and involves anchoring of the testicle in the scrotum. The repair should take place prior to the onset of puberty as the body temperature may severely damage the sperm-producing capabilities of the testicle. The temperature within the body cavity may destroy cells for sperm production. The normal temperature of the scrotum is several degrees less. The increased potential for testicular cancer is another reason for the corrective surgery.

Nursing Care

Preoperatively, the child should be offered a precise explanation of what will be done during surgery. Surgery frequently is scheduled during the late preschool period. The child already has fears and fantasies about his genitalia. Explanations that are appropriate to the child's developmental level and recognition of the child's fears often allay much of the child's anxiety. The parents should also be given a factual explanation using appropriate terminology. Parents may not be able to discuss this condition openly with the child, so the nurse should initiate the discussion with both parents and child present.

Postoperatively, the child returns to the unit with a traction suture attached to the inner aspect of the thigh. This tension or traction suture is a rubber band that is sutured to the testicle. The rubber band is then stretched, and taped or sutured to the inner aspect of the thigh. This should not be removed or disturbed in any way. It is also important to maintain the child in a horizontal position in bed. This serves to maintain the appropriate tension on the suture. Elevating the child's head to a semi-Fowler's position reduces the traction and thus is not done unless the physician orders it.

In addition to positioning, the nurse is usually responsible for applying ice to the scrotum to reduce pain and edema and for the routine postoperative monitoring of vital signs. The area should be kept free of infection, so it is imperative to prevent fecal contamination. During the cleansing after a stool, or during routine assessment of the operative site, the child should be encouraged to look at the operative site so as to allay any residual fears of genital mutilation.

CONVULSIVE DISORDERS

Convulsive disorders are classified in a number of different ways. If classified by

TABLE 23-2 Seizure Classification Comparison Chart

Old Terminology	International Classification
	I. PARTIAL SEIZURES (seizures beginning locally)
	A. with elementary symptomatology (consciousness usually unimpaired)
	1. with motor symptoms
Focal motor, Jacksonian seizures	2. with special sensory or somato-sensory symptoms
	3. with autonomic symptoms
	4. compound forms
	B. with complex symptomatology (consciousness usually impaired)
	1. with impaired consciousness only
	2. with cognitive symptomatology
Temporal lobe or psychomotor seizures	3. with affective symptomatology
	4. with psychosensory symptomatology
	5. with psychomotor symptomatology (automatisms)
	6. compound forms
	C. partial seizures secondarily generalized
	II. GENERALIZED SEIZURES (bilaterally symmetrical without local onset)
Petit Mal	1. Absence (pronounced ab-sons')
Grand Mal	2. Tonic-clonic
Limited Grand Mal	3. Tonic
	4. Clonic
	5. Myoclonic (bilateral massive)
	6. Atonic
Minor Motor	7. Akinetic
	8. Infantile spasms
	III. UNILATERAL SEIZURES
	IV. UNCLASSIFIED SEIZURES

cause, they may be divided into acute or nonrecurrent seizures and chronic or recurrent seizures. Acute seizures include those caused by poisoning, metabolic disturbances, intracranial hemorrhage, central nervous system infections, and febrile conditions. The chronic type of seizures include those caused by epilepsy, either idiopathic or organic, and by epilepsy-stimulating states, such as hypoglycemia and migraine, as well as others.

Another classification system that is used categorizes seizure disorders according to the types of seizures that occur. Five major seizure groups have been identified: (1) grand mal, or generalized seizures; (2) petit mal seizures; (3) minor motor attacks; (4) psychomotor episodes; and (5) focal seizures. There is now an internationally accepted classification of seizures.

Grand Mal Seizures

The grand mal seizures are the most easily recognized. Generally, this type of seizure is associated with an aura, loss of consciousness, tonic and clonic phases, and a distinct postseizure state. The aura consists of a sensory phenomenon unique to each individual that precedes the loss of consciousness. It may be an odor, a taste, a visual phenomena (such as flashing lights), or a buzzing sound in the ears. A cry or strange laughter may also be elicited. There is some question as to whether children experience an aura. It may be that the child is simply unable to describe the aura or to relate it to the impending seizure.

During the alternating tonic and clonic phases, the tongue may be bitten as the teeth clamp down. Periods of apnea and irregular respirations, as well as cyanosis, occur. During this phase, frothy saliva may be evident on the lips. Incontinence also occurs at this time.

In the period after the seizure, the nurse should document the activities of the patient. There may be transient confusion, complaints of a headache, or recognition of the need for a period of sleep. Changes in the speech pattern should be noted, as well as any unusual behavior. Any weakness or inability to move the extremeties should also be assessed.

Febrile convulsions often occur as grand mal seizures in the preschool age-group. They are usually the result of an infectious process and a lowered seizure threshold. The child may have an isolated seizure or several that are related to an excessively high temperature. Measures should be instituted to maintain the child's temperature below the level at which the seizure usually occurs. These seizures are not the same as those that occur in children with epilepsy, and are usually outgrown by the age of five or six years.

Other Types of Seizures

The minor motor seizures are of four types: akinetic, myoclonic, atonic, and infantile spasm. Akinetic seizures are sudden, atonic episodes that occur with falling. Myoclonic seizures involve involuntary muscle contractions of the trunk and limbs. Both of these seizures are very brief in duration and may occur several times per day in the child. These children do not lose consciousness during the brief period of seizure activity. The atonic and infantile spasms may indicate brain damage. Any of these may be additionally associated with mental retardation.

Petit mal or absence seizures are the most common type seen in children. They consist of brief episodes of altered consciousness. The child may appear to be staring or to be distracted for up to thirty seconds. Because there is no obvious motor involvement, the child may have many of these seizures per day and the parent or the professional may only identify a few of them. In school-aged children, these recurrent seizures are often mistaken for inattention. These children may be reprimanded or punished for an event over which they have little control.

Psychomotor seizures occasionally occur in children. They involve purposeful, repetitive movements that are inappropriate to the situation. They may be identified as hysterical type reactions. Lip smacking and knee slapping are examples of this type of repetitive activity. The episode lasts longer than a petit mal seizure and the child will have no recollection of the incident. These seizures are occasionally referred to as temporal lobe seizures.

Focal seizures are those that emanate from a particular portion of the motor strip in the cerebral cortex. If the seizure continues, it spreads to other portions of the body and loss of consciousness occurs. This phenomenon of the seizure activity "marching" up the motor strip is referred to as a Jacksonian episode. It is important for the nurse to document where the first seizure activity originates.

Diagnosis

The diagnostic tool that is most commonly used to confirm a seizure disorder is electroencephalography. However, it is possible that an individual with an abnormal electroencephalogram (EEG) may not have seizures, and that some children with known seizure episodes may exhibit a normal pattern on an EEG.

Other diagnostic tests that may be performed include blood chemistry analysis and electrolytes in order to rule out imbalances of a metabolic nature. A CAT scan may also be performed in order to determine the presence or absence of a specific lesion that could cause the seizures.

Nursing Care

During the period of diagnosis, the parents and child need a great deal of support. They also need factual information regarding the diagnosis of a seizure disorder and its implications. Careful written and verbal instructions for intervention during a seizure should be provided, with ample opportunity given for questioning.

Prior to the EEG, all medication is withheld from the child for a period of twenty-four hours. Immediately before the EEG is to be performed, chloral hydrate is given to the young child for sedation. It is important to organize the child's care and, after the sedative is administered, to control the environment in order to promote maximal effectiveness of the drug. Prior to and after the EEG, the child's hair must be shampooed. This is done before the procedure to avoid any aberrant conduction because of sweat or oils in the hair. Afterward, the shampoo removes the electrode paste which otherwise would become increasingly difficult to remove with the passage of time.

An explanation of the EEG must be provided using language that is appropriate for the child's developmental level. School-aged children who have been exposed to monster movies on television may have a difficult time expressing their fears about the procedure and may be uncooperative during the procedure. Afterward, they may need time to talk out what has happened to them. Drawing is also an acceptable means of sharing their feelings.

Care During a Seizure

If a child knows that a seizure is imminent, either because of a distinct aura or a vague feeling of uneasiness, the child should lie down on a protected surface. A padded tongue depressor should be placed in the mouth after checking for and removing any gum or food. Tight clothing is loosened, particularly around the neck and waist.

During the seizure, restraint of the child should be avoided but the head and limbs should be protected from injury. Bumper pads may be used on the bed of a small child who is prone to seizures. If possible, the head should be turned to one side to prevent aspiration.

After the seizure, the child should be allowed to rest or to sleep as long as necessary. Forcing the individual to awaken is not helpful. Ice may be used to relieve the postseizure headache.

Seizures that occur repeatedly, one after another, for thirty minutes or more without the patient regaining consciousness are referred to as status epilepticus. This type of seizure activity should be documented and the physician notified. An anesthetic or heavy doses of a sedative may have to be given in order to interrupt the seizure pattern.

Anticonvulsant Medication

Phenytoin (Dilantin) is one of the drugs that is commonly used for grand mal seizures. It is usually given after meals to reduce the side effects of nausea, vomiting, and diarrhea. Skin eruptions may occur. When it is given for a long period of time, gingival hypertrophy often occurs. To prevent such problems, the child should be taught proper oral hygiene and should have regular dental care. Phenobarbital may be administered along with the Dilantin. The effectiveness of the drug is measured by blood levels.

Valproic acid (Depakene) is one of the newer drugs used in children to treat seizure disorders. It has been particularly effective with status epilepticus and seizures that are uncontrolled with other drug combinations.

Limitations

Minimal restrictions should be placed on the child's activity level. Physical activity seems to prevent seizures, rather than cause them, and for this reason, activity is encouraged. Some individuals may be restricted from participating in activities in which a head injury is possible, such as diving or contact sports.

A driver's license for the adolescent with a seizure disorder is limited or restricted. Most states require documentation of a two-year period without seizures, issuing a renewable six-month permit in those cases.

Long-term Considerations

Both parents and children should know that the seizure pattern frequently changes with the advent of puberty. This does not necessarily mean that the seizures will not occur, or that they will intensify, it simply means that the pattern will change in some way.

SUMMARY

The majority of the conditions discussed in this chapter on the care of the school-aged child are chronic or long-term disease processes. Diabetes, glomerulonephritis, rheumatoid arthritis, brain tumors, and epilepsy, among others, are all chronic problems that require ongoing evaluations of health care needs and alterations in the treatment program. In working with children with these conditions, it is imperative that the nurse assist the family in establishing long-range goals and working toward their achievement. It is also important for the nurse to provide ongoing support and encouragement during hospitalizations, as well as in outpatient or clinic settings. Education of parents and child is especially important with each of these conditions.

Legg-Calvē-Perthes disease, cryptorchidism, rheumatic fever, and precocious puberty are all acute problems at some point. They may or may not become long-term or chronic problems for the child, depending on when they occur. Nursing care is directed toward identifying the child with acute problems and then preventing long-term or chronic disability.

SUGGESTED ACTIVITIES

- Organize a panel discussion on juvenile diabetes. Include on the panel a child with juvenile diabetes, the parent of a juvenile diabetic patient, and a nurse involved in a clinic or hospital unit giving direct care to juvenile diabetics.

- Request a physical therapist to demonstrate to your class the proper method of carrying out range of motion exercises on a child with rheumatoid arthritis. Include information about the various methods which can be used in the home setting to relieve joint stiffness.

DISCUSSION TOPICS

1. Identify and discuss methods of providing support for the parents and family of a child terminally ill with a brain tumor.

2. Select one of the agencies providing information or assistance to families on one of the diseases discussed in the chapter. Determine what is provided by the agency, as well as what the eligibility requirements include.

REVIEW

A. Matching. Match the symptoms in Column I with the disease in Column II.

Column I	Column II
1. Weight loss, glycosuria, polydipsia, polyphagia	a. Rheumatoid arthritis
2. Unilateral limp with pain referred to hip or knee	b. Rheumatic fever
3. Swollen, painful joints with marked immobility	c. Diabetes mellitus
4. Fever, joint pain and possible carditis following a streptococcal infection	d. Glomerulonephritis
5. Painless hematuria and hypertension	e. Legg-Calvé-Perthes disease

B. Multiple choice. Select the one best answer.

1. Ellen is a nine-year-old girl who is newly diagnosed as having juvenile diabetes. As you are teaching Ellen and her parents prior to discharge, you remind them that one to three months after hospitalization,
   a. insulin requirements may increase.
   b. insulin requirements may remain the same.
   c. insulin requirements may decrease.
   d. none of the above.
2. Ellen is regulated on 20 units of NPH insulin administered at 8:00 AM daily. She should be instructed to carry which of the following items with her once she returns to school?
   a. Her insulin and syringe and a lump of sugar
   b. A diabetic identification card and two cubes of sugar
   c. A candy bar and urine testing kit
   d. A lump of sugar and her syringe
3. Sally is a 12-year-old girl who was readmitted to the hospital with rheumatic fever accompanied by Sydenham's chorea. Symptoms of Sydenham's chorea include
   a. orthopnea, cyanosis, and pain.
   b. emotional instability and purposeless movements.
   c. swollen ankles and an elevated temperature.
   d. joint pain and epistaxis.
4. Another common name for Sydenham's chorea is
   a. Still's dance.
   b. Hansen's disease.
   c. St. Vitus' dance.
   d. Huntington's syndrome.
5. John is a six-year-old boy who is being treated for undescended testicles. One of the conservative methods of treatment for cryptorchidism involves the use of
   a. estrogen and progesterone therapy for one to two weeks.
   b. pituitary hormone therapy for two to three weeks.
   c. antibiotic therapy for four to five weeks.
   d. gonadotropin therapy for six to eight weeks.

6. The conservative method is unsuccessful and John undergoes an orchiopexy. His immediate postoperative care should include
   1. routine postoperative monitoring of vital signs.
   2. application of ice to the area.
   3. prevention of fecal contamination.
   4. avoidance of any disturbance of the rubber band taped to the thigh.

   a. 2, 3 and 4 c. 3 and 4
   b. 1 and 2 d. 1, 2, 3 and 4

7. Sam is an eight-year-old boy of average height and weight. He was admitted to the hospital with a chief complaint of pain in the right knee and limping of several weeks' duration. These symptoms are suggestive of
   a. a slipped femoral capital epiphysis.
   b. Legg-Calvē-Perthes disease.
   c. congenital dislocation of the hip.
   d. osteogenesis imperfecta.

8. Which of the following statements about Legg-Calvē-Perthes disease are true?
   1. The period of pathologic changes and subsequent healing may take two to three years.
   2. The avoidance of weight-bearing is the most important aspect of the treatment.
   3. The inability to abduct the right leg more than ninety degrees is of diagnostic significance.
   4. The disease is caused by a recessive gene and is characterized on x-ray studies by ribbonlike bone shadows and multiple fractures.
   5. Its incidence is greatest in the Black population.

   a. 1 and 2 c. 1, 2, 3, 4 and 5
   b. 3 and 4 d. None are true

C. Short answer. Briefly respond to the following statements.

1. List interventions that can prevent joint destruction in patients with juvenile rheumatoid arthritis.
2. List the nursing observations that should be made in a patient who has had a grand mal seizure.

BIBLIOGRAPHY

Altshuler, Anne, Marie K. Butz, and Jane Meyer. "Even Children Can Learn Clean Self-Catheterization." *American Journal of Nursing*, Vol. 77 (January, 1977), pp. 97–101.

Banlon, C. "The Child With Diabetes." *Issues in Comprehensive Pediatric Nursing*, Vol. 3 (September, 1978), pp. 21–35.

Bruya, Margaret A., and Rose Homan Bolin. "Epilepsy: A Controllable Disease, Part 1. Classification and Diagnosis of Seizures." *American Journal of Nursing*, Vol. 76 (March, 1976), pp. 388–392.

Bruya, Margaret A., and Rose Homan Bolin. "Epilepsy: A Controllable Disease, Part 2. Drug Therapy and Nursing Care." *American Journal of Nursing*, Vol. 76 (March, 1976), pp. 393–397.

Crittenden, Mary R., et al. "Taking It Day By Day: When Children Undergo Hemodialysis and Renal Transplantation." *Children Today*, Vol. 6 (May–June, 1977), pp. 6–9.

Friedland, C.M. "Learning Behaviors of a Preadolescent with Diabetes." *American Journal of Nursing*, Vol. 76 (January, 1976), pp. 59–60.

Guthrie, D. "Exercise, Diets and Insulin for Children with Diabetes." *Nursing 77*, Vol. 7 (February, 1977), pp. 48–54.

Guthrie, D. "Debbie Got Attention – The Hard Way." *Nursing 75*, Vol. 5 (November, 1975), pp. 52–54.

Guthrie, D. "Helping the Diabetic Manage His Self Care." *Nursing 80*, Vol. 10 (February, 1980), pp. 57–64.

Guthrie, D. "The Pangs and the Pains of Adolescence: Diabetes in Adolescence." *American Journal of Nursing*, Vol. 75 (October, 1975), pp. 1740–1744.

Guthrie, D., et al. "Juvenile Diabetes Mellitus." *Nursing Clinics of North America*, Vol. 8 (December, 1973), pp. 587–603.

Guthrie, R., and D. Guthrie. *Nursing Management of Diabetes Mellitus.* New York: C. V. Mosby Company, 1977.

Hite, A.F., et al. "How to Spot the Vicious Cycle of Insulin Rebound." *RN*, Vol. 42 (July, 1979), pp. 44–47.

Kiser, D. "The Somogyi Effect." *American Journal of Nursing,* Vol. 80 (February, 1980), pp. 236–238.

Lee, J. "Care and Management of the Adolescent Juvenile Diabetic." *Pediatric Nursing,* Vol. 4 (May–June, 1978), pp. 42–45.

Lorick, M., et al. "A Diabetic Child is Still a Child – With Diabetes." *RN,* Vol. 38 (October, 1975), pp. 39–43.

Melber, Sheryl, Martha Leonard, and William Primack. "Hemodialysis at Camp." *American Journal of Nursing,* Vol. 76 (June, 1976), pp. 938–940.

Millspaugh, Delight, et al. "Providing Services for Adolescents Who Live With Seizures." *Children Today,* Vol. 76 (September–October, 1976), pp. 7–9+.

Rodman, Morton. "Drugs for Treating Epilepsy." *RN,* Vol. 35 (September, 1972), pp. 63–65.

Ruskin, T.W. "Juvenile Diabetes Mellitus: A Reassessment of Etiology, Clinical Assessment and Therapy." *Journal of Nursing Care,* Vol. 11 (March, 1978), pp. 8–11.

Smith, M. "Meeting the Needs of Diabetic Youths and Their Families." *Children Today,* Vol. 3 (January–February, 1974), pp. 28–29.

Spring, E. "Diabetes Mellitus in Children." *Nursing Care,* Vol. 8 (March, 1975), pp. 9–11.

Swift, Nancy. "Helping Patients Live With Seizures." *Nursing 78,* Vol. 8 (June, 1978), pp. 24–31.

Witty, K. "Young Diabetics in Your Practice – Juvenile Diabetes." *Patient Care,* Vol. 9 (May 1, 1975), pp. 32–41.

Chapter 24

Health Care Problems Requiring Infection Control

OBJECTIVES

Upon completion of this chapter, the student will be able to

- describe the type of health care problems that require infection control techniques.
- identify appropriate nursing interventions that can be used in care of children with communicable health problems.
- compare the various types of isolation techniques used, as well as the nursing responsibilities involved in the care of children with the common diseases of childhood.

COMMUNICABLE DISEASES

Communicable diseases are those that are transmitted from one person to the other, either directly or indirectly. To care for the patient effectively, the nurse must know

- what type of organism is present.
- how the organism resides in the patient.
- what portal of entry and exit the organism uses.
- whether the organism can survive outside the host.
- what precautions must be taken to care for the patient.

This information will dictate the nurses' responsibilities in relation to the patient and to the prevention of the spread of this disease.

ISOLATION TECHNIQUES FOR COMMUNICABLE DISEASES

In the past, isolation techniques were enforced rigidly, almost in a ritualistic manner. Little thought was given to the criteria just mentioned. The technique was the same for all patients, regardless of the knowledge of the organism or its transmissibility.

The basis for present techniques is the prevention of spread of the disease by interrupting the chain of events that lead to communicability. The technique varies somewhat from agency to agency, depending on whether the equipment is disposable or reusable.

Requirements for Isolation

Specific requirements may be identified for each type of isolation technique. Isolation requirements involve the wearing of specific clothing, such as masks, caps, gowns, and gloves; the creation of a noncontaminated area around the patient, as would be achieved by placing the patient in an isolation room; and the proper disposal of wastes that harbor the organism.

A mainstay of every isolation technique is careful hand washing. This is done before and after every contact with the patient. Either soap and water or a bactericidal preparation may be used. Regardless of the preparation used, the mechanical cleansing of the hands is

(A)

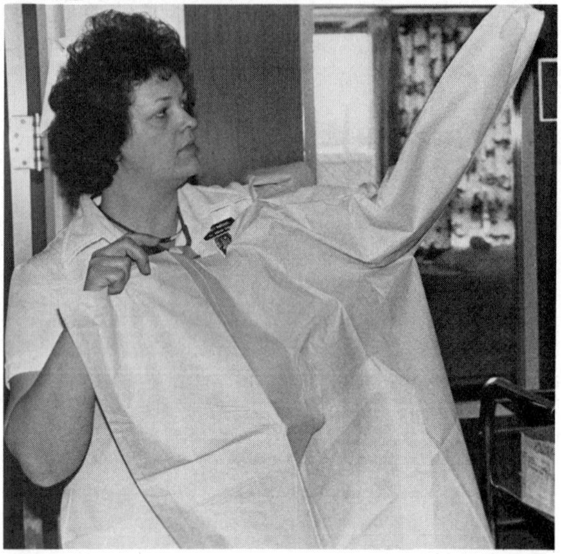

(B)

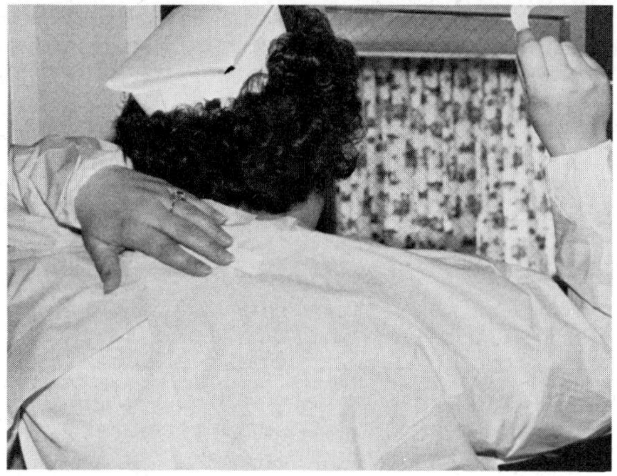

(C)

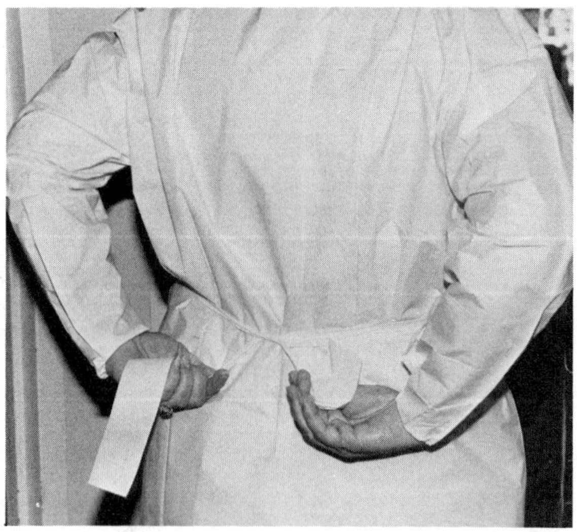

FIG. 24-1 A disposable gown is donned outside the door of the isolation unit *(A)*, the tape tab at the upper back is fastened securely *(B)*, and the back of the gown is overlapped before tying securely *(C)*. This ensures complete coverage.

the greatest deterrent to the spread of communicable disease.

Masks are used in those diseases that are spread through droplet infection via the respiratory tract. These diseases include mumps, pertussis, and rubella. After wearing the mask, it is important for the nurse to handle it only by the ties. The mask must be changed when it becomes moist. To be effective, the mask should be changed every twenty to thirty minutes. Some disposable masks must be changed as often as every five minutes to preserve their effectiveness. The mask should be applied so that it covers the nose and mouth completely, or it is of no protective value. Masks are not reusable and should be discarded immediately upon leaving the patient's room.

Gowns are used to protect the nurse's clothing from contact with any type of contaminated excreta. It is important to protect any clothing that might carry pathogens. Disposable gowns are worn once and then discarded. They are removed and changed any time they become wet. They are never worn outside the immediate isolation environment, Figure 24-1.

Gloves are an additional precautionary measure used in those diseases that may be easily transmitted by hand contact. The use of gloves does not, however, obviate the need for careful and thorough hand washing when caring for patients in isolation. Clean, disposable gloves are generally used, Figure 24-2. If a procedure such as a dressing change must be performed, sterile gloves are used.

Disposal of contaminated equipment and supplies such as linen and trash, from an isolation unit requires a double-bagging technique and the involvement of two people. Wearing the appropriate garb, the person inside the isolation unit ties or secures the contaminated bag of equipment or linen. It is then taken to the open door of the unit or the adjacent utility area. Another individual outside the isolation unit holds open the second clean bag, keeping a wide cuff of the bag over the hands to protect them from contamination, Figure 24-3. The

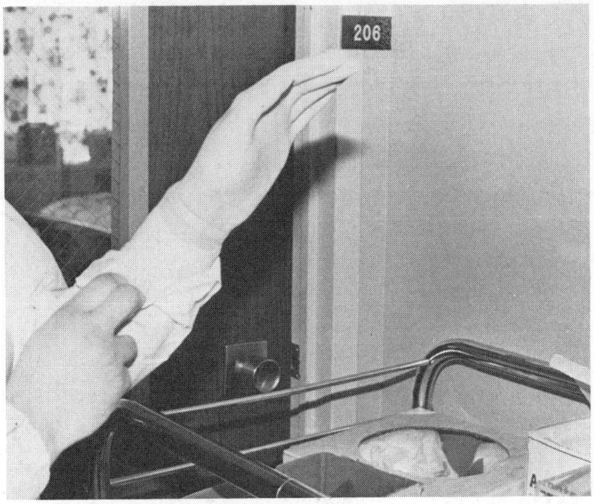

FIG. 24-2 Disposable gloves should be worn with the cuff overlapping the wrist portion of the gown by approximately 1 inch.

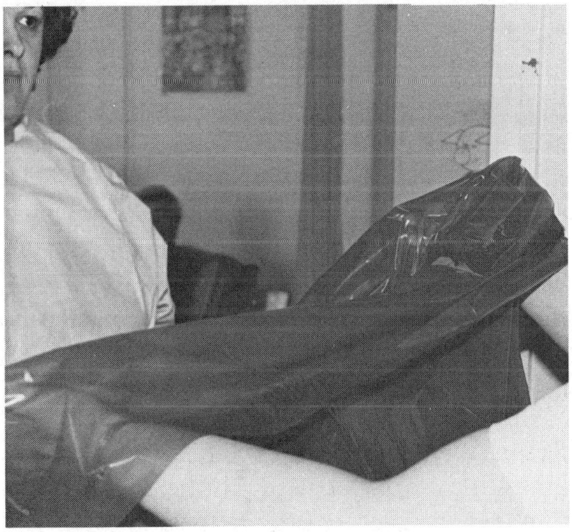

FIG. 24-3 Nurses outside the isolation unit can collect contaminated supplies by placing their hands well beneath the folded cuff of the disposable bag.

individual inside the isolation unit then places the contaminated bag upside down, into the clean bag. The person outside the unit then closes the bag, secures it, and labels it so that it is properly handled. The bags should be intact and should be made of a material that is impervious to moisture, such as plastic.

Types of Isolation

The classification system that is most commonly used to identify the various types of isolation was devised by the United States Public Health Service. The types of isolation are categorized as strict, respiratory, enteric, wound and skin, discharge precautions, and protective isolation. These classifications were developed by the Center for Disease Control. They emphasize control of the disease, not the patient.

Strict Isolation. Strict isolation, or complete precaution, is used for diseases such as smallpox, vaccinia, and rabies. The patient is kept in a private room with the door closed at all times. Anyone entering the isolation area must wear a gown and mask. In addition, gloves are worn by all those who have direct contact with the patient or with any items in the room that might carry the organisms. Special precautions are necessary for the handling of dishes, linens, and secretions.

Respiratory Isolation. Respiratory isolation requires the use of a mask by all who enter the patient's room. A private room, the door of which is kept closed, is also necessary for this patient. Secretion precautions are also taken. It is important to teach the patient the proper method of tissue use so that large numbers of organisms are not coughed or sneezed into the environment. Diseases such as mumps, rubella, and pertussis require this type of isolation.

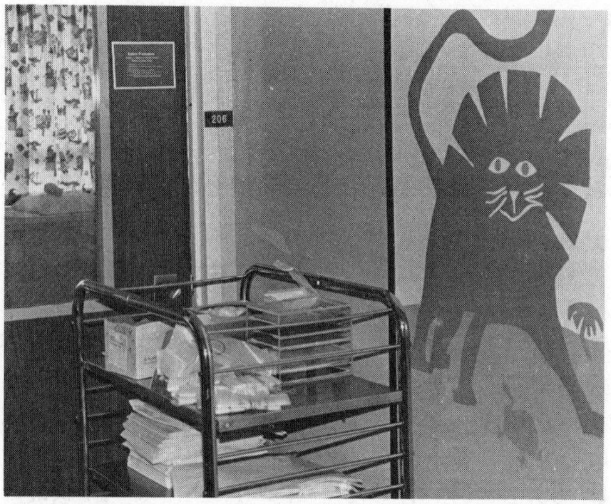

FIG. 24-4 An enteric isolation unit setup. Note the sign on the door and the placement of all necessary equipment on a cart immediately outside the isolation unit.

Enteric Isolation. Enteric precautions require the use of gowns and gloves by those in direct contact with either soiled linen or feces, Figure 24-4. This type of isolation is used for all diseases that are spread by the fecal-oral route, including bacterial gastroenteritis and salmonellosis. Hand washing is extremely important in order to break the contamination cycle. Patients must be taught to wash their hands carefully before eating, as well as before and after elimination.

Wound and Skin Precautions. Wound and skin precautions involve the use of gowns for any direct contact with the patient. In addition, any contact with infected body areas or dressing changes requires the use of gloves. Masks are also required for dressing changes, and special precautions must also be taken with any instruments used for the dressing change. Impetigo and infected burns are among the conditions that require this type of precautionary isolation.

Discharge Precautions. Discharge precautions reflect a knowledge of the secretions that contain the infective organisms. If skin lesions contain these organisms, the nurse must dispose of the dressings by the double-bagging technique. If oral secretions carry the organisms, as in patients with scarlet fever, the nurse must teach the patient to dispose of tissues in a waxed or plastic bag that is sealed prior to disposal. Excretion precautions require careful hand washing after any contact with the patient or with the secretions.

Protective Isolation. Protective isolation, or reverse isolation as it is often called, is used for those patients who must be protected from the organisms of others. Typically, it is used for children with leukemia who have severe bone marrow depression or those who are receiving immunosuppressives. A sterile gown, gloves, mask and cap must be worn during any contact with the patient. In some hospitals, the patient in protective isolation is kept in a room with laminar airflow. Life islands may also be used to protect these patients. Life islands consist of germ-free plastic tents that surround the patient. Contact with the patient is established through the use of the attached gloves, similar in concept to the port holes in incubators.

DIPHTHERIA

Diphtheria is one of the communicable diseases that is seldom seen because of massive immunization efforts. It is a highly contagious disease that is spread through the respiratory tract. Its peak incidence is in the fall and winter months.

Classification and Symptoms

The disease can occur in a variety of distinct forms, each affecting a specific area. The various types include nasal, pharyngeal and tonsillar, laryngeal, and nonrespiratory diphtheria. The latter type affects the eyes, ears, and skin and is very rare and difficult to diagnose.

The nasal form of the disease is relatively mild. Initially, the symptoms are those of the common cold. The distinguishing feature is the increased viscosity of the nasal secretions and the formation of the characteristic whitish-gray membrane over the nasal surfaces.

The pharyngeal and tonsillar varieties may occur together or separately. This form begins, as do many other diseases, with a low-grade fever, malaise, and anorexia. A membrane forms within the first few days and is considered to be diagnostic. Along with the appearance of the membrane, there is cervical lymphadenopathy and a disproportionate or very elevated pulse rate. The membrane persists for about four days and then begins to slough. Respiratory obstruction can occur if pieces of the membrane are aspirated into the respiratory tract.

The laryngeal form is far more serious than the other types and is associated with severe symptoms from the onset. The child appears to have some form of croup as aphonia, retractions, and a barky cough are noted. The presence of the characteristic membrane identifies the disease. The possibility of respiratory obstruction is great in this child because of the position of the membrane in the respiratory tract.

Treatment, Prevention, and Nursing Care

Treatment for all forms of the disease includes the use of diphtheria antitoxin, antibiotics, and supportive treatment. The antitoxin carries additional risks because it is made of horse serum. Skin testing with a test dose is mandatory to determine the likelihood of a sensitivity reaction. This testing should be done only when equipment is available for intervention should anaphylactic shock occur. All such equipment and medications should be readily accessible prior to the administration of the test dose.

Use of the biologic preparation to immunize against the disease is preferable. It is available in a combined vaccine, diphtheria-pertussis-tetanus, and is given at two-month intervals during infancy, followed by booster doses later. The adult form of the preparation is a diphtheria-tetanus combination and is administered as a booster every ten years after the age of six years. More adult cases than pediatric cases occur because adults do not generally maintain their immunization status.

Nursing care of this child includes isolation, antibiotics, and supportive care based on the specific problems of the child. The antibiotics used are broad-spectrum ones, such as the penicillins and tetracyclines. Hypersensitivity to medications should be identified in the initial assessment. Throughout the treatment the child is observed for any specific side effects of the drug used.

Supportive care includes an assessment of the child's respiratory status and hydration. The involvement of all or limited areas of the respiratory tract indicates the need for careful ongoing assessment for changes as well as extension of the disease. Increased amounts of easily tolerated fluids at frequent intervals aids in maintaining hydration. Careful cleansing of the nares from the viscid secretions is especially important in the younger child. The nurse must also be alert to the potential of respiratory obstruction as the membrane begins to slough near the end of the first week.

MUMPS

Mumps is one of the communicable diseases that is spread through the respiratory tract. In some individuals, the disease is so mild that it goes unnoticed. Even in these individuals, the disease can be spread to others, and active immunity will develop.

Symptoms

The swelling of the parotid gland is the major symptom of the disease. The swelling occurs both behind and in front of the ear so that the lobe is displaced outwardly. It may also affect the submaxillary and sublingual areas. Fever is usually present the day prior to the swelling and continues for five or six days. The virus is shed during the time that the temperature is elevated and for several days afterward.

Treatment, Prevention, and Nursing Care

Immunization is available for this disease in either a single vaccine or a combined one. The combined vaccine is administered along with the measles and rubella vaccines. It is usually deferred until the child is one year of age in order to avoid neutralization by maternal antibodies. The vaccine is not recommended for any child who is allergic to eggs or neomycin, or for those children receiving immunosuppressive therapy.

Nursing care is related to the disease symptoms. Rest and control of the child's fever are important. Fluids should be encouraged to aid in decreasing the temperature. Food or fluids that are highly spiced or seasoned, or those that are very sour should be avoided.

Complications

Complications that can occur include oophoritis or orchitis, and occasionally, encephalitis. The complications occur more commonly in adults than in children.

PERTUSSIS

Pertussis, or whooping cough, is also spread through the respiratory tract. Although it is thought of as a respiratory disease, it does not occur at the time of the peak incidence of most respiratory infections. The disease occurs in the spring and summer, and affects girls more often than boys.

Symptoms

The disease occurs in three relatively long stages. The first is the catarrhal stage, which lasts one or two weeks. During this time, the child has coryza, a dry cough, fever, and anorexia. The child may also sneeze frequently and exhibit excess tearing, or lacrimation.

The second stage is called the paroxysmal stage. It lasts from one to two months and is identified by its associated attacks of violent coughing. During these attacks, the child usually vomits and becomes cyanotic. These attacks may occur as often as forty to fifty times a day, and may lead to exhaustion.

The third stage, or the convalescent stage, lasts up to two years after the initial onset of the disease. The coughing spells occur less frequently, but they may recur at any time in the presence of a respiratory infection. Convulsions may also accompany this stage.

Treatment, Prevention, and Nursing Care

Prevention is accomplished through the use of the combined diphtheria-pertussis-tetanus vaccine early in infancy at the prescribed intervals.

The treatment includes the use of pertussis immune globulin to shorten the period of communicability. Antibiotic therapy is also used to eradicate the organism. Humidified oxygen and gentle suctioning are used in the initial stages because of the thick, viscid secretions. Adequate fluid and nutritional intake are of importance because of the frequent vomiting with coughing episodes. Any stimuli that provokes coughing is avoided if at all possible.

The nursing care of affected children includes respiratory isolation, measures to prevent aspiration during an attack, and observation and care during seizures. All other care is symptomatic and dependent on the stage of the child's disease.

Complications

Complications for individuals who have had the disease include both respiratory and neurologic problems. In those children who have had a seizure, brain damage may be present.

RUBELLA

Rubella is a communicable disease that is viral in origin. The disease develops fourteen to twenty-one days after the child has been exposed to the virus. It is commonly referred to as German measles.

Symptoms

Characteristic symptoms of the disease include headache, a low-grade fever, coryza, anorexia, pharyngitis, and conjunctivitis. These symptoms are generally mild and precede the development of a rash. Lymphadenopathy, or enlarged lymph nodes, occurs in the cervical, suboccipital and postauricular areas. Shortly after this lymph node enlargement, the rash will be evident. The rash begins in the area of the face and spreads to the feet. It lasts about three days, after which it begins to fade in the same sequence as it occurred. Occasionally, it lasts as long as five days. In some children, the rash may be seen on the soft palate. These spots are referred to as Forschheimer's spots.

This virus can be transmitted to others from seven days prior to the appearance of the rash to five days afterward. The period of greatest communicability is the three-day period preceding the appearance of the rash.

Prevention

Prevention of the disease is always preferable to curing the illness. If the mother of a child has not been immunized or has not had the disease, the child should be given the vaccine prior to one year of age. This child is not protected even passively. If the mother has active immunity, however, the vaccine should not be given until after the first year of the child's life. This is to prevent passive maternal antibodies that may be circulating in the child's bloodstream from inactivating the vaccine.

Treatment and Nursing Care

The child with this disease is usually not hospitalized unless the child has another health problem. However, if this child manifests the disease during the course of hospitalization, the child must be isolated in respiratory isolation. This type of isolation is used because the virus is spread via secretions in the nose and throat.

Treatment of the disease is symptomatic. Nursing care involves maintaining the isolation technique, maintaining bedrest for the child, and providing comfort. Darkening of the room may be necessary if the child has photosensitivity. Soft foods and increased fluids are helpful in maintaining intake when the child complains of a sore throat. Frequent use of mouthwash and gargles promotes comfort. Diversional activities also should be provided for this child.

Complications

The disease presents few problems in children. However, in the adult, it may cause encephalitis, arthritis, and purpura. It can have a direct effect on the fetus of a mother who is unprotected and who contracts the disease. The greatest risk is during the first and second month of the pregnancy. The damage to the fetus may include brain and liver disorders, bone lesions, and sight and hearing defects. Any infant born after contracting the disease will continue to shed the virus in all secretions, including urine, stools, and blood, for months. Vaccination is required in order to prevent these birth defects from occurring.

RUBEOLA

Rubeola is frequently called seven-day measles or hard measles in order to differentiate it from rubella. It is viral in origin and generally occurs during the latter part of winter and the early part of spring. It is highly contagious and has an incubation period of ten days.

Symptoms

The symptoms of fever, coryza, cough and conjunctivitis, as well as lethargy, occur prior to the development of the rash. The symptoms become gradually more severe. At this point, Koplik's spots appear on the mucous membranes of the mouth. These are reddened areas with greyish blue centers that are first seen in the area of the molars. They gradually spread throughout the mouth, including the area of the palate. Koplik's spots are unique to rubeola and are considered a diagnostic sign. One to two days later, the skin rash will appear around the hairline and spreads down to the feet. The rash will begin to fade after five days.

Prevention and Nursing Care

Immunizations are available for this disease. They may be given as a combined vaccine with rubella (measles-rubella) or with both rubella and mumps (measles-mumps-rubella). Again, vaccination is deferred until twelve months of age in order to prevent neutralization by the circulating maternal antibodies. Any tuberculin tests that are done on the child must be performed prior to the immunization, as the rubeola vaccine will cause a false-positive reaction for up to two months after its administration.

As with rubella, the nursing care is symptomatic. Respiratory isolation is maintained.

Complications

Complications that may occur include middle ear infection, pneumonia, and encephalitis. The encephalitis may result in mental retardation.

VARICELLA

Varicella, or chickenpox, is another of the childhood communicable diseases that is caused by a virus. The virus is from the varicella-zoster group. The incubation period is fourteen to twenty-one days after exposure.

Symptoms

The initial symptoms of varicella prior to the development of the rash include malaise and fever. The lesions begin as macules and progress to papules and vesicles, eventually becoming crusted. The lesions erupt in clusters, initially on the head and on the mucous membranes. All lesions proceed through the same sequence. However, the rash does not break out at the same time in all body regions. Because of this, it is possible to see lesions in various stages at any one time. The greatest concentration of lesions occurs on the trunk with less on the extremities.

The rash is pruritic. The child should be kept from scratching the lesions so as to prevent bacterial infection and subsequent scarring. The disease is communicable until the last lesion has dried and formed a crust. This may be as long as three weeks in some children.

Treatment and Nursing Care

Immunizations are not currently available for this disease, but research is being conducted on an active vaccine. Immune serum globulin (Varicella-Zoster immune globulin) that provides passive immunity for those at risk is available.

Respiratory isolation is maintained for these patients. Antipruritic ointments may be ordered for the lesions. The child must be prevented from scratching or rubbing the lesions if at all possible.

Complications

Complications include a hemorrhagic form of varicella that can occur in individuals receiving steroids. This form may be fatal in both children and adults. Encephalitis is another fatal complication. Symptoms of central nervous system involvement may occur three days to one week after the onset of the rash.

TETANUS

Tetanus can occur in all age groups. The organisms enter through breaks in the skin caused by wounds. It can be a particular problem in patients with burns, in those who have undergone orthopedic surgery, and in infants whose umbilical stump has not been cared for appropriately.

Symptoms

The first sign of the disease is a tightening of the muscles of the jaw. The muscular tightening progresses to severe muscle spasms. The patient's face assumes a characteristic appearance called risus sardonicus, or sardonic grin. At this point, the jaws are immovable, hence the common name of lockjaw.

Treatment and Nursing Care

The inability to move the jaws, as well as to control secretions, necessitates a tracheostomy and intravenous therapy. The patient with tetanus should be placed in a quiet, darkened environment as any stimuli may precipitate spasms or possibly, seizures.

The treatment involves the use of tetanus immune globulin obtained from humans or the tetanus antitoxin made from horse serum. The toxins produced by the organism must be neutralized. Some form of penicillin is used to kill the organism itself.

Immunization is available in combined diphtheria-pertussis-tetanus vaccine, as well as in the adult form of tetanus-diphtheria vaccine. When emergency treatment is required, the patient or family member may be asked about immunization. Whether the patient receives another dose of the tetanus toxoid will depend on the number of immunizing doses received, the type of wound, and the number of years since the last dose. Because the organisms can live in the intestinal tract, as well as in the soil, contaminated wounds are a major problem.

TUBERCULOSIS

Mycobacterium tuberculosis is the causative organism of tuberculosis. The organism is usually 1 to 5 microns in size. Because of its minute size, it is not filtered out in the respiratory tract, but enters the alveoli directly.

Transmission of the Disease

Transmission of the disease is by inhalation of the droplet nuclei or minute aerosol droplets that are produced when the individual with tuberculosis coughs, sneezes, or speaks. In the past, it was thought to be transmitted by any contact with an infected person or with any contaminated inanimate objects, or fomites, that the individual touched. Dishes, letters, and books were commonly destroyed after the patient handled them. It was also thought to be inherited at one time.

A primary infection occurs when the organism enters the body. Individuals with decreased resistance, poor nutrition, and other chronic diseases are particularly susceptible. Very young children may contract the disease from contact with infected individuals in the home. Older children or young adults may contract the disease outside the home.

A secondary infection may occur later in the child's life. It may be a response to exposure to large numbers of tubercle bacilli or it may result from the child's decreased resistance at the time. Whatever the reason, the organisms multiply rapidly and the child's defense mechanisms are overwhelmed.

Symptoms

The child may be asymptomatic, but usually has mild constitutional symptoms that are characteristic of a respiratory infection. Other children may have nonspecific symptoms, such as weight loss, fatigue, anorexia, and elevated temperatures during the afternoons. Some of the children may also have a productive cough and may show signs of hemoptysis. Night sweats, or diaphoresis, may or may not be seen in the child. When infants contract the disease, their growth may be stunted over a period of time, unless the disease is treated.

Diagnosis

Diagnostic testing is completed in three stages: tuberculin skin tests, chest radiography, and gastric washings for culture. The tuberculin skin tests involve the use of either the Mantoux test (intradermal) or the Tine test (multiple puncture). The Mantoux test uses a testing substance called purified protein derivative (PPD), which is a form of tuberculin protein. A test dose of 0.1 cubic cemtimeter is injected intradermally after the forearm has been cleansed, Figure 24-5. A small bleb is produced

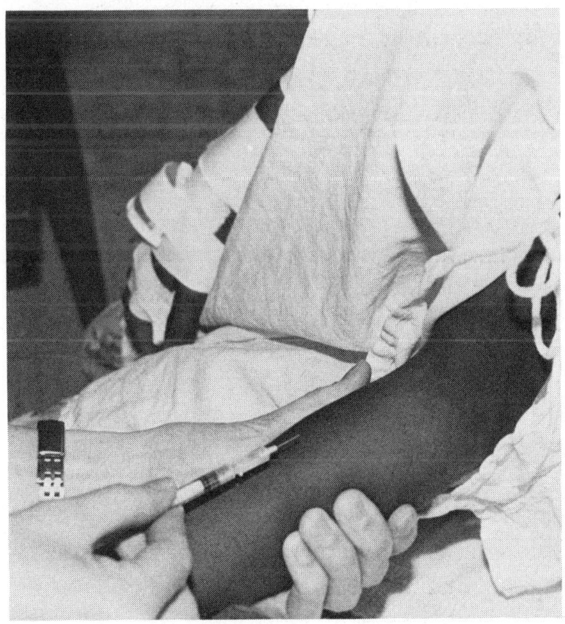

FIG. 24-5 An intermediate dose of PPD is injected into the volar surface of the forearm.

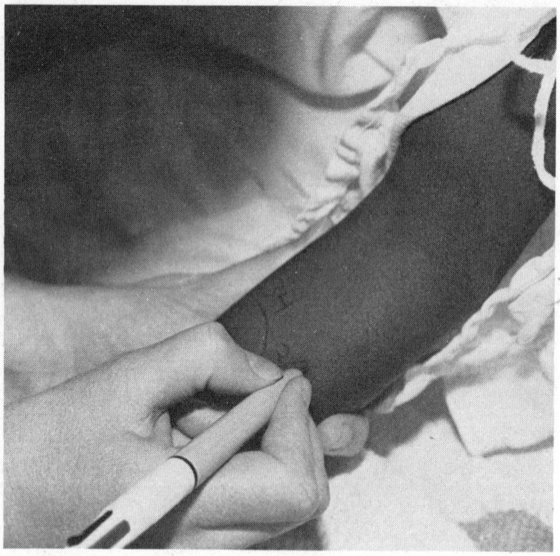

FIG. 24-6 The site is marked with a circle. The date, time, and initials of the person doing the test are noted.

and the site is marked as to date and time, Figure 24-6. This site is inspected forty-eight hours after injection and the amount of induration and erythema is measured exactly. An area of tissue response or hypersensitivity to the tuberculin protein measuring 10 millimeters or more is considered to be diagnostic. A response of 5 millimeters or more is highly questionable.

The Tine test involves the use of a disc with four prongs that are coated with concentrated tuberculin substance. The volar surface of the arm is cleansed and the disc is applied. The site is circled and dated. The reaction is observed in forty-eight hours. An area of response around any of the puncture sites that is greater than 2 millimeters is considered to be a positive reaction. A positive reaction to any of these tests simply means the individual has been exposed to the tuberculosis organism and has developed a hypersensitivity to it.

A chest radiograph is usually done as a follow-up to a positive skin test. The chest x-ray study may be negative, or it may show the presence of pulmonary lesions. In young children, the disease may be very widespread and the entire lung may be involved. This is referred to as miliary tuberculosis. It is often fatal because of the acute and overwhelming nature of the infection.

Gastric washings are used to obtain organisms for culture. Children rarely cough up sputum that contains viable organisms. Instead, the child swallows the secretions. For this reason, gastric lavage is carried out in the early morning prior to breakfast. The culture may take three to eight weeks before the results are known.

Treatment

Once the diagnosis has been established, the treatment regimen is begun. The child is considered to be infectious only during the diagnosis and first few weeks of the chemotherapeutic program. During this time, respiratory isolation is maintained. Methods to control the transmission of organisms include the use of tissues to control the spread of droplet nuclei during coughing or sneezing, proper and adequate ventilation to decrease the number of organisms present, the use of ultraviolet light to kill the bacilli in the droplet nuclei, and the establishment of an effective regimen of chemotherapy.

Chemotherapy. Most health departments recommend the use of chemotherapy for any individual who has reacted negatively to one of the intradermal tests and on a subsequent test reacts positively. This is particularly important for all children, especially teenagers, who are at high risk.

Drugs that are utilized to treat tuberculosis include isoniazid (INH), para-aminosalicylic acid (PAS), ethambutol (EMB), and streptomycin. These drugs are considered for initial or primary treatment. They are always used in combination to prevent the development of resistant strains of the organism. Other drugs that may be used for retreatment or to treat resistant strains include pyrazinamide, ethionamide, cycloserine, viomycin, and rifampin.

Isoniazid is one of the most commonly used drugs. A side effect of the drug is neurotoxicity. For this reason, pyridoxine or vitamin B6 may be administered with isoniazid.

Many of the antituberculosis drugs may be given as one large dose of medication in the morning rather than in partial doses throughout the day. For older children who attend school, this increases the compliance with the drug regimen.

The effects of chemotherapy are rapid. A decrease in the amount of coughing, as well as in the amount of sputum present, will be evident. There will also be a corresponding decrease in the number of organisms present in the sputum.

Nursing Care

Hospitalization of the child permits the establishment of a definitive diagnosis. Also, during this period adequate treatment measures and guidelines for follow-up evaluations are instituted. During the hospitalization, the child, if old enough, and the parents should be taught as much as possible about the transmission of the disease, the rationale for the medications and other treatment measures, and the importance of uninterrupted drug administration. Also during this time, family members and others in the home should be tested to determine the original source of infection.

During the period of treatment, the child should be protected from other infections, particularly respiratory infections, that could create an additional stress for the child. The child's diet should supply extra protein, as well as vitamins, to aid in the healing process.

Nurses caring for children with tuberculosis should carefully assess their developmental level and should assist their parents in maintaining the child's level of functioning. This may be particularly difficult for school-aged or adolescent children who are separated from their peers during the process of hospitalization and who may not be able to return to school immediately. For younger children, particularly infants, the nurse should determine the child's level of achievement and encourage the parents to pursue those activities that enhance the growth and development of the child.

GASTROENTERITIS

Gastroenteritis is an inflammation of the stomach and the small and large intestine. It is most easily recognized by the two major symptoms of vomiting and diarrhea. It can occur in any age-group but infants are most severely affected and have greater problems with the resulting dehydration.

Both bacteria and viruses can be the causative agents for the disease. Some of the bacteria include E. Coli, Salmonella, and Shigella. The viruses which are responsible for the rapid-onset types of gastroenteritis include the enteroviruses, such as the ECHO viruses. Parasites and funguses are also causes, although less common.

Symptoms

The typical symptoms include anorexia, nausea, vomiting, and diarrhea. The severity of the symptoms ranges from mild to severe. The child with moderate to severe symptoms also develops dehydration as a result of excess fluid loss combined with the inadequate fluid intake. An elevated temperature and tachypnea significantly increase the insensible losses and add to the problem of dehydration.

The stools excreted by the child are loose or liquid in consistency and often green in color, denoting the rapid transit time through the gastrointestinal tract. Mucus or blood may also be present in the stools. The stools may be expelled forcefully after abdominal cramping or pain. This can occur as frequently as fifteen to twenty times per day in severe cases.

Assessment

The initial history provides assessment data related to the actual losses, the current intake of the child, and specific signs related to dehydration. The actual losses include the number and frequency of the stools as well as their appearance and consistency. The frequency and the amount of vomitus is also a part of the actual loss. The presence or absence of a temperature elevation and its duration would also be considered.

The assessment of the child's intake is important in two areas: the type and amount of liquids consumed and the ingestion of inappropriate substances that may have caused the onset of gastroenteritis. Because of illness the child may have been given inappropriate items to cure the problem. Formulas, such as boiled skim milk, were used in the past with diarrheas and actually increase the child's dehydration because of the concentration of sodium and the renal solute load. Milk or milk products contaminated with substances such as salmonella may cause gastroenteritis in several family members.

The actual assessment of the child for dehydration comes about through the history as well as through the phyisical examination. Through the history the parent may be able to identify weight loss. The parent would need to have an accurate measurement of previous weights to compare with the current one. A loss of ten percent indicates dehydration. A history of reduced urinary output is also significant. Other physical signs indicating fluid loss greater than five percent include loss of skin turgor, sunken fontanelles, dry mucous membranes, absence of tears, and decreased urinary output. A greater than ten percent fluid loss is indicated by a rapid pulse, decreased blood pressure, sunken eyeballs, and cool, dry extremities. Losses of more than fifteen percent are indicated by distinct changes in the level of consciousness. This child is usually quite lethargic, and may show beginning signs of shock and circulatory failure. When these children have dehydration greater than five percent, continuing vomiting, and loose stools, the children are usually admitted to the hospital for treatment beginning with fluid replacement.

Treatment

Initially, the treatment in the hospital includes placing the child in a room by himself or herself and instituting enteric precautions to eliminate the spread of the organism. If the child has been vomiting, he or she is usually placed on nothing by mouth for at least twelve hours. If the child shows signs of dehydration, intravenous therapy is instituted for fluid replacement.

The diagnostic work includes an anal swab and stool culture to identify the causative organism; an assessment of the electrolyte status and kidney functioning with the sodium, chlorides, potassium and blood urea nitrogen; and an identification of metaboli changes with the CO_2 combining power and the pH level. The hematocrit would indicate hemoconcentration. The urine specific gravity is also monitored closely.

Once the child is able to tolerate oral fluids, he or she is kept on clear liquids and the intravenous fluids are gradually decreased as the oral intake increases. The diet then progresses to an easily tolerated restricted diet such as the BRAT (bananas, rice, applesauce, tea) diet. Because of the high incidence of lactose intolerance following gastroenteritis, the formula is often withheld until ten days after recovery.

Nursing Care

The nursing care begins with a careful assessment of the child's status on admission to the unit. Some agencies use the assessed items on a checklist along with weight, intake and output, and specific gravity. In this way all items can be reassessed at periodic intervals for better accuracy.

Monitoring of intravenous or oral fluid intake is a major responsibility. It is the responsibility of the physician to calculate and order the fluids, however the nurse should be aware of the methods used for calculation to help reduce the possibility of error. Intravenous infusions should all be run with small amounts of fluid being run into a Buretrol or volume control device and monitored with an infusion pump. This permits better control over the volume administered to the child. Documentation of intake and output is a must with all of these children.

Administration of oral fluids is limited in this situation to clear liquids in small amounts. Initially, oral electrolyte solutions such as Pedialyte and Lytren may be used. Other clear liquids that may be used include ginger ale which has had the carbonation removed, Jello water (made with double the recommended amount of water), and Gatorade. The fluids are administered in small amounts (5 to 15 cubic centimeters every half-hour) and gradually increased as the child tolerates the fluids. If the child is receiving both intravenous and oral fluids, maximum limits should be established to prevent fluid overload from occurring. Some physicians establish a total fluid limit and the nurse then decreases the intravenous intake as the child's oral intake begins to increase, still maintaining the accepted limits. This method allows more flexibility in the child's care and allows the child to return to a more normal method of feeding.

Infection control is very much a part of this child's care. Maintenance of the enteric precautions is a must. This is usually continued until forty-eight hours after the child has had the last diarrhea stool. During this period, careful handwashing is necessary to prevent the transmission of the disease to others. Assessment of the intravenous site every shift is also a part of infection control.

Protection of the child's perineal area from the frequent loose stools is a necessity. This area is cleansed carefully after each stool. Expose the area to the air for fifteen to twenty minutes afterward. In some agencies there are routine orders for a topical antibacterial or antifungal ointment to be applied if the area shows obvious signs of skin breakdown.

Parent education is an important aspect of this child's care. The parents or caregivers are taught what to do at the first sign of illness of this type. Emphasis is placed on maintaining the child on clear liquids and what would be acceptable types of liquids. Breast milk is the only exception to this regimen. Identification of a fever and accurate temperature measurement is stressed. The signs of dehydration are also identified so that the parent will recognize when to seek help. Avoidance of any medication to stop the diarrhea is emphasized as this masks signs of dehydration such as weight loss. Signs of lethargy, blood in the stool and diarrhea persisting more than twenty-four hours in an infant are all indications for calling the physician.

BACTERIAL MENINGITIS

Bacterial meningitis is an inflammation of the coverings of the brain and spinal cord caused by a specific organism. The affected child may have had an infection such as tonsillitis, otitis media, or sinusitis, involving the nasopharynx. Other predisposing factors include congenital defects of the central nervous system.

Signs and Symptoms

Initial symptoms include irritability, lethargy, an elevated body temperature, chills, vomiting, and a stiff neck. In some children, meningococcemia or a petechial and purpuric rash may be associated with this disease. A bulging anterior fontanelle is present in about half of the infants with the disease.

Diagnosis

The diagnosis is made on the basis of the child's history, physical examination, and a lumbar puncture. The spinal fluid is analyzed for a cell count and sugar and protein levels. A culture and sensitivity is done to identify the causative organism. The white blood cell count in affected children is greater than 1000, the sugar is less than forty percent of the blood sugar, and the protein level is elevated.

Treatment

Immediately after the lumbar puncture, the child should be given intravenous medications to combat the disease. Ampicillin and chloramphenicol are commonly used for this purpose. Weekly blood studies are mandatory when chloramphenicol is used because of its depressant action on the bone marrow. Once the specific organism has been identified, one of the drugs may be discontinued, depending on the results of the sensitivity study.

Nursing Responsibilities

Nursing care for this child includes the use of careful isolation techniques, with respiratory precautions, as this disease is transmitted via the nasopharynx. The child should be observed carefully for any signs of seizure activity. Seizure precautions, such as taping a padded tongue blade to the top of the bed and ensuring that an airway is readily available, should be taken. Suction and oxygen should also be available and ready for immediate use. The sides of the child's crib or bed should be padded with blankets or bumper pads to prevent injury during a seizure.

If a seizure occurs, the child should be protected from injury, but should not be restrained forcibly. If possible, the padded tongue blade should be inserted at the onset of the seizure activity. If the child's jaws are already clenched, do not attempt to insert the tongue blade as such forcible insertion may cause damage. Any saliva or vomitus should be suctioned in order to maintain a patent airway. Any tight clothing should also be loosened at the onset of the child's seizure activity. Oxygen may be used if cyanosis occurs. The child should be allowed to rest following the seizure.

Observations that should be documented following the seizure include any known precipitating factors, the type of seizure (tonic or clonic movements) and its location on onset, and any loss of consciousness. Notations should also be made regarding the respiratory pattern and any periods of apnea and cyanosis. The length of the seizure activity, the responses of the child and any motor impairment afterward should also be documented. Antipyretic and anticonvulsant medications may be ordered for the child and should be administered appropriately to prevent further seizure activity.

Care of the child with bacterial meningitis also includes the use of cooling sponges or hypothermia blankets, frequent monitoring of vital signs, and careful monitoring of the intravenous therapy and intake and output. Isolation is required until the child's temperature remains normal for forty-eight hours.

Complications may arise from this disease. They include the formation of a brain abscess; death from increased intracranial pressure; visual, hearing, or speech disturbances; and hydrocephalus. As the child recuperates, he or she should be observed carefully for any residual problems of this nature.

INFECTIOUS MONONUCLEOSIS

Infectious mononucleosis is an acute viral infection caused by the Epstein-Barr virus and affects the lymphatic system of an individual. The adolescent has a higher incidence of the disease, although it can occur in the younger school-aged child and is often seen in the young adult population.

Signs and Symptoms

The major symptoms include fever, sore throat, enlarged lymph glands, and fatigue. Other signs of the disease include hepatosplenomegaly, a rash similar to that seen with German measles, and right upper quadrant pain. It occurs more commonly in the fall and winter months.

The virus is present in the oral secretions of the individual. It is spread by direct contact with the saliva, hence its common name of the "kissing disease." It is not highly contagious.

Diagnosis

Diagnosis is confirmed by several laboratory tests. A blood smear for white blood cells usually identifies twenty percent of the lymphocytes as being enlarged. A heterophil antibody agglutination test (Monotest) may confirm the diagnosis but usually not early in the disease. There are also specific antibody tests for the Epstein-Barr virus.

Treatment

The treatment is symptomatic. Steroids may be used in severe cases. Adequate rest, a nutritious diet, and sufficient fluid intake are all helpful. Aspirin is often used to relieve the discomfort. Mouthwash and gargles are used for the sore throat. Strenuous exercises and heavy lifting are to be avoided for four to six weeks after the onset because of the possibility of rupturing the spleen.

Nursing Responsibilities

Nursing care in the hospital setting would involve secretion control, implementation of rest, and relief of discomfort from the pharyngitis.

A school-aged patient can usually follow directions regarding proper disposal and handling of tissues. Covering the mouth when coughing or sneezing is also identified for the patient. Handwashing is emphasized after handling contaminated tissues.

Activities are limited to provide for maximum rest. As the adolescent improves, the importance of the additional rest must be stressed. Overwork, lack of sleep, and stress can often be identified by the individual as precipitating the episode.

Inspection of the mouth gives a clue to the severity of the pharyngitis. Petechiae present on the midpalate are often evident as well. Mouthwashes and gargles often provide some relief from the discomfort. Frequent offering of nutritious snacks may be better tolerated than large meals.

The patient should be taught that the fatigue will persist for some time and that adjustments in activities must be made. The physician should be notified immediately if the patient experiences upper quadrant pain that radiates to the shoulder as this may indicate rupture of the spleen.

INFESTATION DISEASES

Infestations of both parasites and insects may produce relatively few symptoms in children. These infestations can occur in children of any age. Young children who are less apt to adhere to basic hygiene practices may be prone to pinworm infestations. In school-aged children, infestations of lice or scabies may be common.

ROUNDWORM INFESTATIONS (ASCARIASIS)

One of the most common helminthic infections in children is ascariasis. Mild roundworm infections are often asymptomatic. Severe infection with roundworms, however, can cause anorexia, weight loss, irritability, nausea and vomiting, and intestinal colic. As the larvae of the *Ascaris lumbricoides* migrate in the body of the infected individual, symptoms of asthma, intestinal obstruction, and intussusception may occur. The child also may have eosinophilia, urticaria, and other allergy-type symptoms.

This parasite is found in warm climates. The larvae are present in soil contaminated by another infected person. To become infected, the child must ingest the infective egg. The egg may be consumed as the child places contaminated fingers, food, toys, or dirt in the mouth. The frequency with which children defecate where they are playing adds to the prevalence and spread of roundworm infestations.

Diagnosis

The diagnosis is confirmed on the basis of stool specimens obtained from the infected child on several consecutive days. These worms may also be recovered from vomitus if the larvae have migrated to the lungs.

Treatment

Treatment involves the administration of an anthelmintic preparation. Piperazine citrate (Antepar and others) is given in a dosage ranging from 1.0 gram to 3.5 grams, depending on the child's size. This dose is repeated on two consecutive days. Pyrantel pamoate (Antiminth) is another preparation that may be used. It is given in a single dose of 10 milligrams per kilogram of body weight. The maximal dose for this drug is 1 gram. Mebendazole (Vermox) is also effective, but one tablet must be taken twice a day for three consecutive days.

Nursing Considerations

Concerns for the nurse include the possibility of other family members being infested. Both children and adults should be aware of the importance of using appropriate toilet facilities to avoid spreading this hazard. Known sites of contaminated soil should be turned under. Careful hand washing before eating or handling food and after toileting is also preventive.

PINWORM INFESTATIONS (ENTEROBIASIS)

Enterobius vermicularis, commonly known as the pinworm, is ingested as an egg from a contaminated individual. These pinworms hatch in the duodenum and migrate to the area of the appendix. The female travels outside the anus to lay thousands of eggs in the perianal area during the night. The presence of these eggs causes intense pruritus. After scratching, the child's hands become contaminated with the eggs. If left unwashed, the eggs are then reingested, and the cycle of reinfestation continues.

Symptoms

Symptoms in the child may be vague. Pruritus in the anal region is the most common sign of the infestation. It may be so severe that secondary bacterial infections develop. In the girls, eggs may also be deposited in the vagina, causing intense perivaginal itching and vaginitis.

Diagnosis

The diagnosis is confirmed by the presence of ova or worms. A transparent tape test is the best method for diagnosing pinworms. A tongue blade is wrapped with tape, sticky side out. It is then applied to the perianal area in the early morning hours. The presence of the eggs on the tape can then be documented microscopically.

Other family members may also be checked for pinworms. Usually, the entire family is treated because of the ease of transmission of pinworms.

Treatment

The drug of choice is pyrvinium pamoate (Povan), administered in a single dose of 5 milligrams per kilogram of body weight. The drug causes stools, urine, and vomitus to turn bright red. It will stain the clothing and, to the untrained observer, may appear to be blood. Other medications, such as Antepar, Antiminth, and Vermox, may also be used.

Nursing Care

In the hospital setting, the nurse assists in identifying children with pinworms. These children are kept in a room by themselves and special handling of all bed linens and clothing is required. It is important for the nurse to avoid shaking clothing and linens as the eggs may become airborne and can be ingested by anyone in the immediate environment. The nurse should avoid removing the child's night clothes over his head.

The nurse should teach the parents and child how to avoid reinfection after treatment. The child's fingernails should be kept short. All family members should wash their hands carefully upon arising, before meals, and after toileting. Children should not be permitted to scratch the anal area. To enforce this, mittens may be used to cover the hands, and the diaper should be applied snugly. All underwear, bed linens, and pajamas should be washed in very hot water in order to kill the eggs. The child's underwear should be changed daily. The heat from a clothes dryer is also effective in killing the eggs.

In discussing the medication regimen, the nurse should emphasize the importance of adhering to the correct dose. The parents should be told not to increase the dose that is ordered. The parents should also be told of the possibility of retreatment in two weeks to one month. This eliminates any eggs that may have hatched since the original treatment.

LICE (PEDICULOSIS)

Pediculi, or lice, can affect any part of the body. The term *pediculosis capitis* refers to those that are present on the head. Pediculosis corporis designates an infestation of the trunk of the body. Pediculosis pubis refers to an infestation of the pubic area, the least common form of lice in children.

Signs and Symptoms

Lice are identified by the presence of transparent, oval, whitish egg cases, or nits, that are firmly attached to the hair shaft. These may be seen on any hair-bearing area of the body. The head is the most common site in children. Lice are spread by the sharing of combs, hats, and other items.

The intense itching produced by the lice may cause the child to scratch the area, often breaking the skin, which leads to irritation and crusting. Bacterial infection then results in the formation of pustules.

Treatment

Treatment involves the use of gamma benzene hexachloride (Kwell) shampoo. One ounce of the preparation is used to make a thick lather which is kept on the hair for four to five minutes. It is then rinsed off and the wet hair is combed with a fine-tooth comb. Particular attention is given to the base of the hair, close to the scalp. Treatment may be repeated once after a week has elapsed. It is important to emphasize that the parents follow the treatment directions carefully, as excessive use of the preparation may result in its absorption through the skin and subsequent neurotoxicity. The liquid pediculicide Rid can also be used according to package directions.

All clothing is laundered in hot water or dry-cleaned to eliminate the lice. Entire families are often treated for this condition, rather than just isolated members, because of the close contact with the infected person within the home. Items, such as sleeping bags, may be sprayed with a preparation called R & C spray. Families should be reminded that this spray is for inanimate objects only and should not be used on humans or pets.

SCABIES

The cause of another infestation present in some children is the itch mite (*Sarcoptes scabiei*). The female mite burrows under the skin to lay her eggs, choosing areas where the skin is moist, as well as thin, like the abdomen and between the fingers and toes.

Symptoms and Diagnosis

The tracks left in the skin are visible, as are the lesions that result from bacterial infection caused by intensive scratching. The diagnosis of scabies is made by skin scrapings and microscopic visualization of the mite.

Treatment

Treatment includes a hot bath and the application of gamma benzene hexachloride (Kwell) lotion which should remain on the skin for twenty-four hours before being rinsed off. The lotion is applied in a thin layer to all body surfaces from the neck down. Clean clothing is then donned. The child is usually retreated after ten days. All clothing is either laundered in very hot water or is dry-cleaned. All infected members of the family are treated at the same time to prevent reinfestation. Crotomiton (Eurax) cream or lotion may also be used in two separate applications twenty-four hours apart.

SUMMARY

When caring for a child with a communicable disease, precautions and isolation procedures are only as effective as the staff members who use them. Each nurse must be familiar with the mode of transmission for each condition and must then use the appropriate isolation or protective techniques correctly. Periodic review of the procedures for each of the conditions is important.

SUGGESTED ACTIVITIES

- Demonstrate the proper garb for each of the various types of isolation. Include in your presentation a demonstration or discussion of the proper method of removing waste items from the unit.
- Research activities and responsibilities of the Center for Disease Control in Atlanta, Georgia. Compare those activities with those of your local health department.
- Visit your local health department. Report to your class regarding those activities involved in prevention of disease. Investigate the procedure carried out when the food or water supply is suspect in the spread of disease.

DISCUSSION TOPICS

1. Discuss strategies that may be used to relieve the social isolation of a child who must be maintained in strict isolation. Identify appropriate activities for each age-group.
2. Identify and discuss a teaching plan for the parents and family of a child with severe gastroenteritis.

REVIEW

A. Matching. Match the disease in Column I with the appropriate type of isolation in Column II. (Items in Column II can be used more than once.)

Column I	Column II
1. Gastroenteritis	a. Strict
2. Impetigo	b. Enteric
3. Mumps	c. Respiratory
4. Scarlet fever	d. Wound and skin
5. Rabies	e. Discharge precautions
6. Diphtheria	f. Protective
7. Uninfected burns	
8. Salmonella	
9. Pertussis	

B. Multiple choice. Select the one best answer.

1. Jason is a five year old suspected of having pinworms. You know that the adult female pinworm migrates out of the anus and deposits the ova on the perianal area. The ideal time to do a cellophane tape test for collection of the ova is
   a. at bedtime after he has had a bath.
   b. in the early morning before he gets up.
   c. after he has had a bowel movement.
   d. only after he complains of pruritus.
2. Pyrvinium pamoate (Povan) is the drug used for Jason's treatment. A side effect of which parents and child should be aware is the
   a. bright red color of stools and vomitus.
   b. feeling of nausea after administration.
   c. black tarry color of the stools.
   d. constipation that occurs with use.
3. The most common type of tuberculosis found in children is
   a. tuberculosis of the bone.
   b. miliary tuberculosis.
   c. primary tuberculosis of the lung.
   d. tuberculosis of the spine.
4. Skin tests which would indicate a sensitivity to the tuberculin protein are
   a. PPD and Tine test.
   b. cultures and sensitivity tests.
   c. gastric washings and cultures.
   d. BCG tests.

C. Short answer. Briefly respond to the following statements.

1. List the nursing observations to be made for a child admitted to your unit with gastroenteritis with dehydration.
2. List the interventions for an adolescent with infectious mononucleosis.

BIBLIOGRAPHY

Alexander, Steven R., et al. "Childhood Vomiting and Diarrhea: Fending Off Severe Dehydration." *Patient Care,* Vol. 12 (May 15, 1978), pp. 198–224.

Bielan, Barbara. "What That Rash Really Means." *RN,* Vol. 42 (February, 1979), pp. 58–63.

Brown, Marie. "What You Should Know About Communicable Diseases and Their Immunizations, Part 1. Rubella, Roseola, and Rubeola." *Nursing 75,* Vol. 5 (September, 1975), pp. 70–72.

Brown, Marie. "What You Should Know About Communicable Diseases and Their Immunizations, Part 2. Polio, Diphtheria, Pertussis, and Tetanus." *Nursing 75,* Vol. 5 (November, 1975), pp. 55–60.

Castle, Mary. "Isolation: Precise Procedures for Better Protection." *Nursing 75,* Vol. 5 (May, 1975), pp. 50–57.

Green, David, et al. "Infectious Mononucleosis or a Mimic?" *Patient Care,* Vol. 11 (January 15, 1977), pp. 54–74.

O'Grady, Roberta, and Thomas Dolan. "Whooping Cough in Infancy." *American Journal of Nursing,* Vol. 76 (January, 1976), pp. 114–117.

Peterson, Lois D., and Juanita H. Green. "Nurse-Managed Tuberculosis Clinic." *American Journal of Nursing,* Vol. 77 (March, 1977), pp. 433–435.

Robinson, Alice M. "Pulmonary TB: Not Quite a Disease of the Past." *RN,* Vol. 38 (February, 1975), pp. 77–82.

Vaughan, Victor C., et al. *Nelson's Textbook of Pediatrics.* Philadelphia: W. B. Saunders Company, 1979.

Chapter 25

Fractures and Their Treatment

OBJECTIVES

Upon completion of this chapter, the student will be able to

- describe the nursing care of a child who has had a cast applied.
- differentiate between the various types of traction used with children.
- identify the various parts of the traction apparatus that must be checked frequently as a part of the child's care.

Fractures can occur in any child. However, the school-age and adolescent child are at greater risk because of their level of independence. These children spend a great deal of time away from the home, often in unsupervised play. Peer approval is actively sought, and often leads to dares to prove strength or agility.

FRACTURES

The fractures that occur in children are as varied as those that occur in adults. The various types include simple, compound, comminuted, impacted, and greenstick fractures, as well as epiphyseal separations, Figure 25-1. A *simple fracture* involves a clean break of the bone, without splintering or fragmentation and with no external wound. A *compound fracture* is one in which an external skin wound leads directly to the site of bone fracture. A *comminuted fracture* is one in which the bone is shattered or splintered in many pieces. These fractures may be difficult to heal. An *impacted fracture* is one in which a broken bone or bone fragment is firmly wedged into another bone. The term *greenstick fracture* is used to describe a bone that is

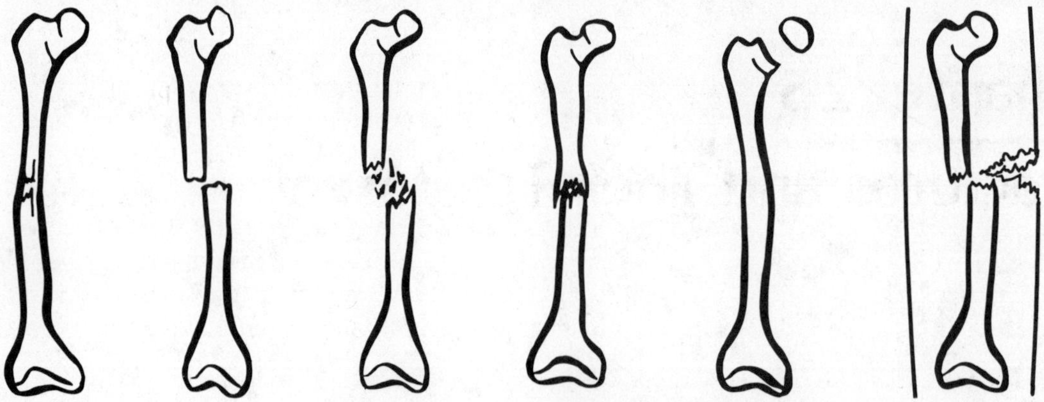

FIG. 25-1 Types of fractures

partially bent or twisted on one side and incompletely broken on the other. These fractures are commonly seen in children. Their appearance resembles the splintered and twisted appearance of a young tree branch that has been broken. *Epiphyseal separations* occur when the shaft of the bone and the growth point separate as a result of trauma. This occurs exclusively in children. It is of particular concern because damage to the epiphyseal plate may alter the growth rate, causing asymmetry.

Symptoms

The symptoms associated with a fracture include loss of movement, pain over the site of the fracture, swelling, discoloration or bruising and unusual or inappropriate movement. Crepitus, which is air in the subcutaneous tissues, may be felt at the fracture site in some children. The involved body part should not be manipulated to document impaired or abnormal movement because of the potential for additional damage to the bones or soft tissues surrounding the fracture site.

Casting

Usually, after reduction of the fracture, a cast is applied to maintain proper alignment and to immobilize the part until healing has occurred. The nurse may be involved in the application of the cast.

Application of the Cast. First, the involved body part is gently cleansed and dried. A circular piece of stockinette is then cut to fit over the body part. A layer of soft cotton, such as sheet wadding, is applied over the stockinette to ensure that it is smooth. The plaster rolls are immersed in warm water until the bubbling stops, then squeezed to remove excess moisture. They are then applied over the area and smoothed to shape the cast. The cast is applied in such a way as to immobilize the moveable joint immediately above and below the fracture site.

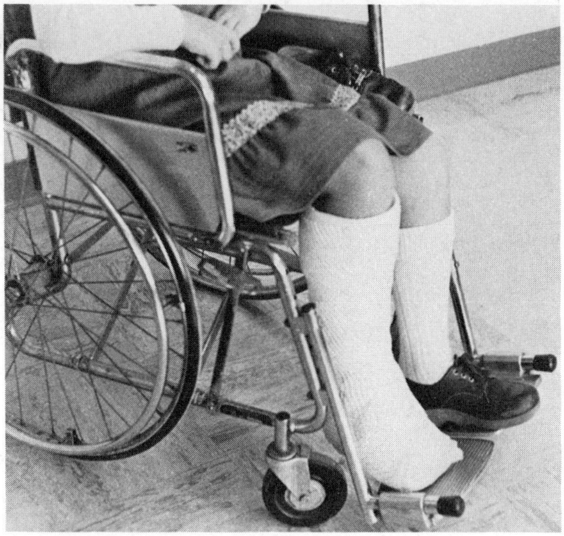

FIG. 25-2 Hexcelite short leg cast. Note the porous appearance of this plastic casting material.

In the case of the newer plastic casts, the material placed against the skin is foam, and a nylon stockinette is used, Figure 25-2. Both the cast and the protective material facilitate drying after swimming and showering. One type of plastic casting material is heated in a special water bath of 140° F and then blotted gently before application. Another type requires the use of an ultraviolet light to cure the material following application.

Plaster casts are dried by exposure to air. They take about twenty-four to forty-eight hours to dry completely, whereas plastic casts take only a few hours to dry. Drying can be hastened by the use of a hair dryer on a low setting or the use of a heat cradle for the child with a body cast.

Handling the Cast. During the drying period, care must be taken to handle the cast gently, using the palms of the hands, not the fingertips, to position the patient. The cast should be exposed to the air as much as possible to facilitate the drying process. The child's position should be changed every two hours, especially in the case of a body cast, to allow the posterior portion to dry at the same rate as the anterior portion, Figure 25-3. The equal exposure of both sides to air prevents the cracks that can develop when one side of the cast dries more rapidly than the other side.

FIG. 25-3 A hip spica cast is supported with pillows to facilitate the drying of the posterior portion.

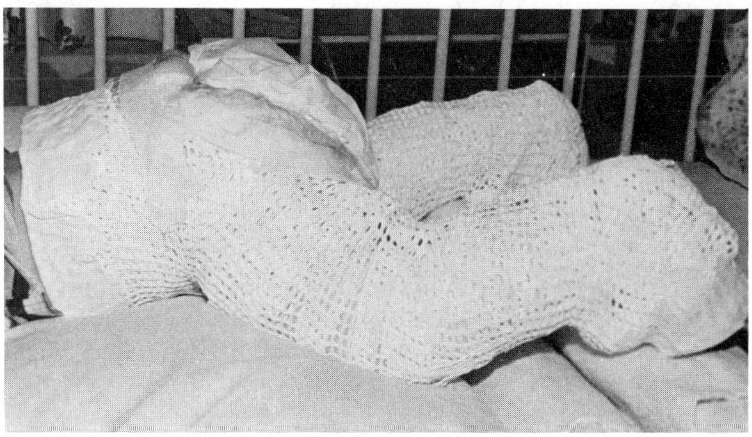

Nursing Care. *Neurovascular status.* The nursing care of children with casts should include a careful assessment of their neurovascular status. The nurse should periodically check the skin at the distal portion of the cast. Is it warm to the touch? Is it a normal color? Do the nails blanch and then return to normal rapidly when they are compressed briefly? Is there any evidence of edema or swelling? The extremities should be compared for equality in size. If there is any question, a tape measure may be used to measure the diameter of the part. The exact site of the measurement should be marked. This measurement is then used as a baseline for future assessments. The nurse should also determine whether the child can flex, extend, and separate the digits. Inability to do so may indicate edema or neuromuscular damage. Does the child complain of numbness or tingling in the body part? Often, such children describe a sensation of "pins and needles" pinching them. Does the child verbalize pain or does the behavior indicate the presence of pain?

Skin care. The child may complain of itching rather than actual pain. Some consideration must be given to the condition of the child's skin. Any excess plaster on the skin must be removed before it causes irritation or actual breakdown. Any sharp edges on the cast should be trimmed and then petaled with narrow strips of adhesive tape or moleskin tape, Figure 25-4. Are there any dented portions of the cast that could cause skin irritation in areas that are not visible? These dents may occur if care is not taken when lifting and turning the patient with an incompletely dried cast.

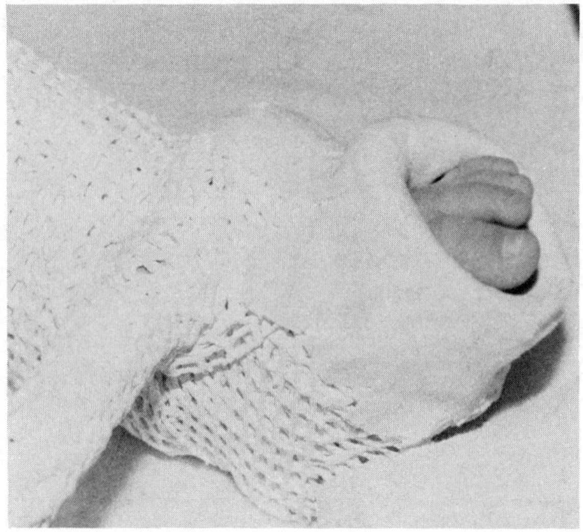

FIG. 25-4 The area around the toes has been petaled with strips of moleskin.

Body Alignment and Mobility. Proper body alignment should be maintained in patients with casts. When the patient has been turned, are all the body parts supported in a neutral position? Is the cast supported adequately with pillows or pads to prevent undue stress in certain areas? If the child with a long leg cast or body cast is lying prone, have provisions been made to avoid undue pressure on the toes? Allowing the child's toes to extend over the foot of the mattress or over the edge of the Bradford frame may be helpful. If a short arm or long arm cast is involved, is the part supported adequately when the patient is ambulating? The application of a sling maintains body alignment and prevents the part from becoming increasingly edematous, Figure 25-5. If the child's movement is grossly impaired because of a cast on the arm or leg, additional supervision and assistance may be needed to compensate for the instability caused by the additional weight of the cast.

Nutrition, Elimination, and Sensory Input. For children whose casts drastically

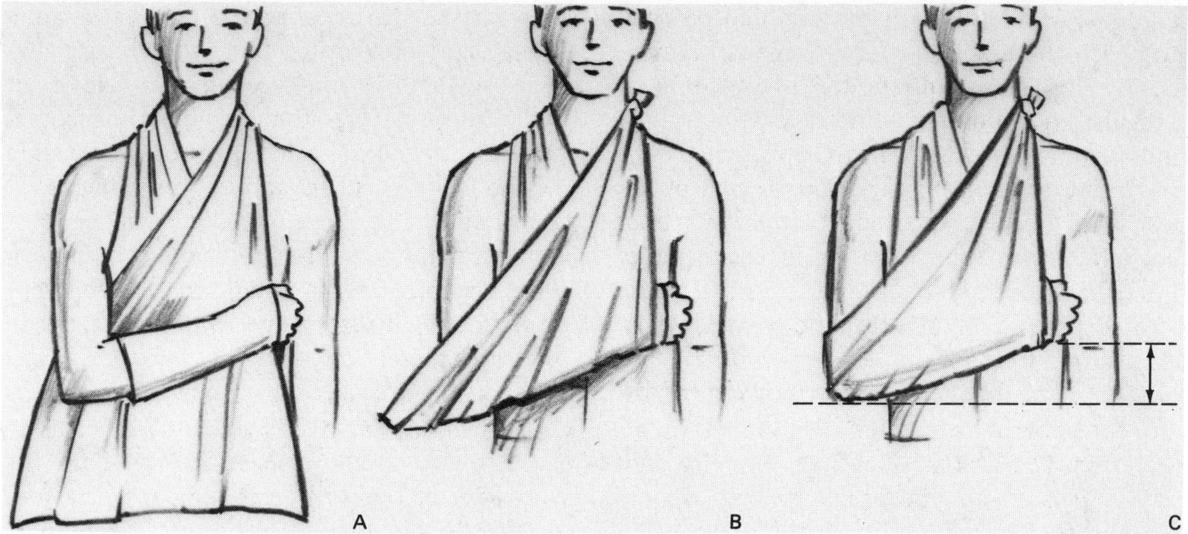

FIG. 25-5 Application of a sling. Note the positioning of the hand above the elbow level in order to prevent edema.

inhibit mobility, special consideration must be given to an adequate intake and output. The child's nutritional intake should include not only the basic four food groups, but also increased amounts of protein and vitamin C in order to enhance the healing process. Fluid intake should be maintained according to the child's normal weight. Roughage, in the form of raw fruits and vegetables, should be included in the diet to aid in the elimination process, as well as to meet minimum daily requirements. The nurse should monitor the child's urinary and fecal output. Urinary tract infections may develop as a result of inadequate output, or urinary retention. Irritability and abdominal discomfort or loss of appetite may signal constipation in the child.

Sensory deprivation may occur in any child, but it may not be recognized as a potential problem in the child who is immobilized in a cast. Especially for a previously active child, a body cast and its resultant limitations may be overwhelming. In the hospital situation, as well as in the home, the child's surroundings should be varied periodically. This may be accomplished by using a cart or a spica bug, or even a large wagon, to transport the child to another room — the playroom or sunroom, for example — outside the usual limited environment. This also provides the child with an opportunity to socialize with other children. School-aged children in casts who are exposed to the handicaps and limitations of other children in the playroom environment may then be more tolerant of their own limitations.

Postoperative Care. In those children who have undergone some type of surgical correction prior to cast application, it is imperative that the nurse initially inspect the cast on an hourly basis. Any signs of bleeding or drainage should be noted. When a child returns to the unit from surgery, any areas of bleeding should be circled and the time and date noted. In this way, additional drainage or bleeding can be easily identified and assessed.

Parent Teaching. The parents should be told to check the cast daily for any type of musty odor. This may indicate the presence of a pressure area underneath the cast. It may also indicate the presence of food items deteriorating inside the cast. Food is a particular problem with children, as they often stuff food particles inside the cast without realizing the potential danger.

For those children in a body or leg cast who are not toilet trained or who have regressed in their toilet training, it is important to protect the perineal area with some type of waterproof material that can be changed easily. Plastic may be used, as long as one edge is tucked securely under the cast with the help of a tongue blade, if necessary, and the other end is fastened to the outside of the cast, Figure 25-6. The child's parents should be shown how to change this protective material, thus avoiding any odor caused by urine or stool being impregnated in the cast.

Areas of skin irritation may develop even when the cast edges have been petaled. Parents should routinely inspect the skin around the cast for redness or irritation using a flashlight. Use of powders and lotions should be avoided. Powders act as irritants and may cause additional skin breakdown beneath the cast. Lotions soften and lubricate the skin. However, under the cast edges, the skin not only becomes softer, it also breaks down from the moisture of the lotion, causing additional problems for the child.

Initially, therefore, after the cast application, the skin edges should be wiped every four hours with isopropyl alcohol to toughen the skin, thereby reducing irritation. This can be continued twice daily in the home situation as a routine part of the child's care.

Parents should inspect the cast daily for any signs of breaks or softening in the cast, as well as to document correct cast size. Some casts may become threadbare from the child's activity. In other cases, particularly in very young children, the cast may have to be changed every ten days to two weeks to accommodate the child's growth rate. Parents are taught to measure the cast for adequate room by inserting one finger between the cast and the skin in various areas. One finger's breadth is an acceptable amount of room between the cast and the child's skin, Figure 25-7. The parent can then decide, on the

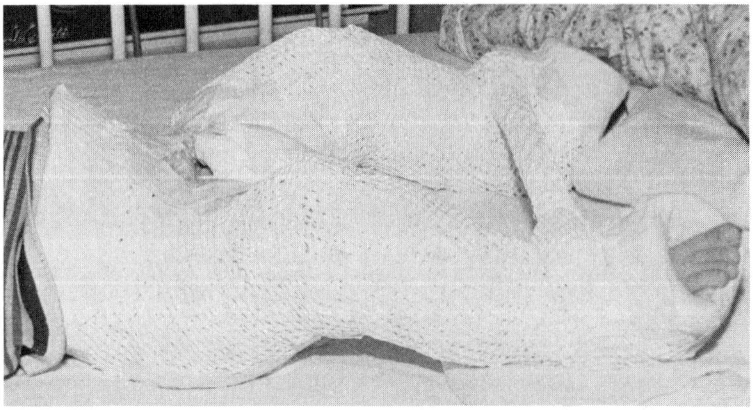

FIG. 25-6 The perineal area of the cast has been petaled and covered. The diaper is inserted into the cast opening.

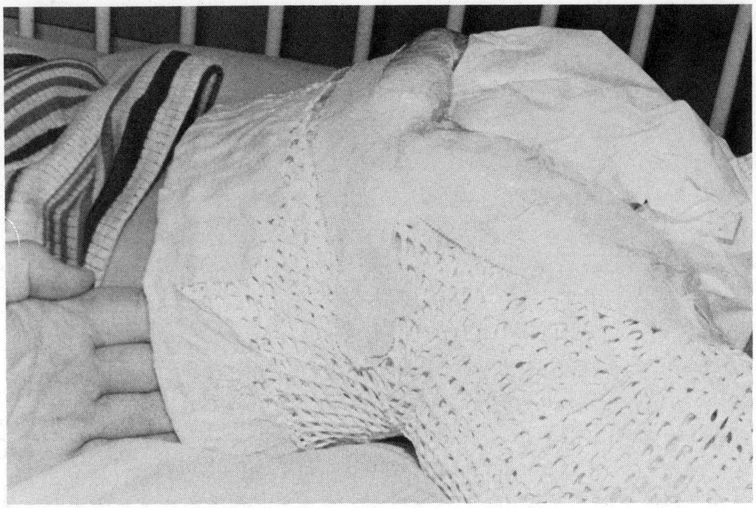

FIG. 25-7 The parent should be taught how to inspect the cast for tightness.

basis of this measurement, whether the physician should be notified. It may be necessary to reapply or adjust the cast in order to avoid compromising the child's neurovascular status.

Traction

In many children, traction is used as an intermediate step after the injury and before the application of a cast. Traction may be used to promote or maintain body alignment, to reduce muscle spasm, to reduce the fracture or dislocation, or to immobilize the part until casting takes place.

Traction is of two types: skin and skeletal. With skin traction, force is applied directly to the skin surface. This may be accomplished through the use of adhesive strips in the case of an extremity; or with a canvas or cotton halter in the case of cervical or pelvic traction. Skeletal traction involves the use of force applied directly to the bone through the use of Kirschner wires, Steinmann's pins, or Crutchfield tongs. For every pound of traction exerted, an equal amount of countertraction, or opposing force, must exist. This may be achieved in a variety of ways. For instance, by placing the foot of the patient's bed on blocks, the patient's body acts as the countertraction in Buck's extension traction. The term *balanced,* when referring to traction, implies the use of both vertical and horizontal traction to achieve the desired result. Usually, the vertical traction line is one-half the horizontal plane. Both forces combine to produce the desired result.

General Considerations. Nurses are not usually responsible for setting up the traction apparatus but they are responsible for checking it on each shift, or more often, in order to maintain the patient's prescribed therapeutic regimen.

The weights of the traction should hang free and away from bedclothes, chairs, or tables. The amount of weight providing the traction should be specified in the physician's orders and should be checked during the routine assessment, particularly when caring for children. The weights should be safely located or protected so that they are not hazardous to the patient. They should not be removed or altered unless there is a specific order to do so.

Traction ropes should be aligned and in good condition. This means that the ropes should be unfrayed and free of unnecessary knots or kinks. The knots that secure the weights should be reinforced with adhesive tape to prevent any slipping.

The pulleys should also be checked. The rope should be located in the groove of the pulley. The pulley itself should be freely moveable and supporting the rope properly, without undue noise. A drop of mineral oil may be used to lubricate the pulley if necessary.

The body alignment of the patient should be maintained. The line of the traction should follow the long axis of the bone, Figure 25-8. The bed should also be checked for the proper position. Can it be raised or lowered? Should the foot or head of the bed be raised at a specific angle? What limitations does the child have with regard to positioning and mobility while in traction? The physician may allow the head of the bed to be raised for meals only, or not at all. This should be clarified. In pediatrics, maintaining the proper position for traction may necessitate the use of a jacket restraint for a brief period of time.

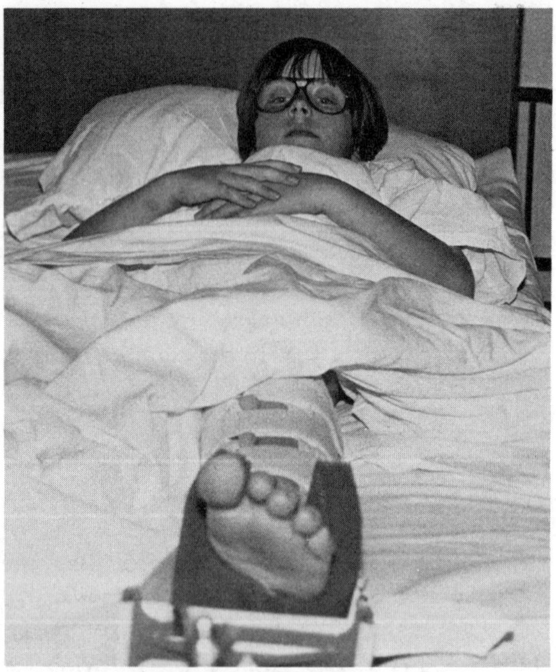

FIG. 25-8 Body alignment may be checked by standing at the foot of the child's bed.

Bryant's Traction. Bryant's traction is one form of skin traction that is utilized for young children with fractures of the femur, Figure 25-9. It is a vertical suspension traction whereby both of the child's legs are attached to an overhead traction frame so that the child's legs form a ninety-degree angle with the body. It is used only for children younger than two years of age who weigh less than 40 pounds. The weights that are used are generally rather light (four to five pounds for each extremity). In the case of a small infant, weights may not be used at all. Instead, the infant's legs are anchored securely to an overhead frame. Position and alignment are maintained with a jacket restraint or a special harness. Countertraction is provided by the child's body weight. Special concerns with this type of traction include skin irritations, maintenance of the position, and possible circulatory problems.

Skin irritation may develop rapidly in the area where the traction tape is applied to the skin. This area should be checked whenever the traction is assessed, usually every four hours along with vital signs. The bandage anchoring the traction tape, as well as the neurovascular status of the feet, should also be checked. The slightest redness or blistering

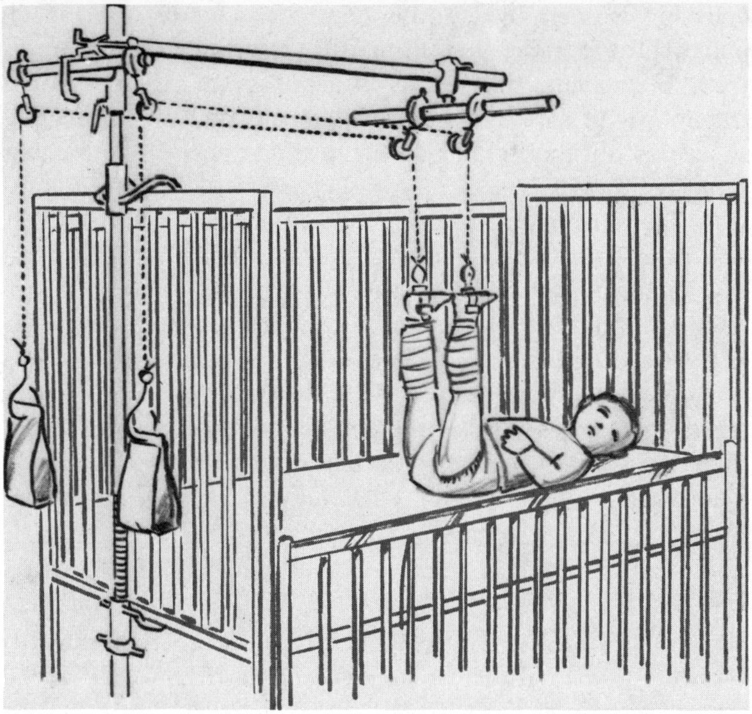

FIG. 25-9 Bryant's traction

should be reported immediately before further skin breakdown occurs.

Maintenance of this position is sometimes very difficult for the child. Some children may have just begun to achieve a high level of mobility and will be frustrated by the restraints imposed by the traction. The buttocks of the child should be raised slightly off the mattress. A flattened hand should be able to pass between the buttocks and the mattress. In some health care agencies, the child is not permitted to wear a diaper while in this type of traction. The movement necessary to secure the diaper is thought to be detrimental to the healing process. A soft blanket or draw sheet pulled across the child's waist may be sufficient restraint for some children. Others require a jacket restraint in order to maintain the position.

The associated circulatory problems relate to the suspension of the feet and the legs. The bandages and traction tape may slip or shift position, causing undue pressure on the dorsum of the foot or on the heel. The feet should be checked frequently for blanching, areas of discoloration or pallor, and also for the presence or absence of sensation. Undue pressure on the peroneal surface can cause footdrop. In heavier children, blood pressure should be monitored on a regular basis, as this position may precipitate hypertension.

Diversional therapy is important for any child, but it is crucial for young children in Bryant's traction. These children are somewhat isolated because of their position, as their view of the world is primarily lateral. Music boxes, mobiles, and soft stuffed toys appropriate for the age level are helpful. If diversion is not provided, they may pick and pull at the bandages securing the traction tape. Ultimately, this results in a release of traction, with pain or discomfort to the child, as well as possible trauma to the healing fracture site.

The nurse must feed this child carefully. The head should be raised slightly or turned to one side. The danger of aspiration is very real. The child should be encouraged to eat and take fluids, but should not be force-fed because of the possibility of vomiting. Constipation may also be a problem for this patient because of the position that must be maintained.

Russell's Traction. This type of traction is used in children with knee problems and hip fractures, Figure 25-10. It involves traction to the lower leg and the use of a sling for the knee. The sling should be high enough so that a twenty-degree angle is formed between the child's hip and the bed. The use of pillows under the thigh is acceptable as long as they do not cause external or internal rotation of the leg. The heel should not be resting on either the pillows or the bed. A foot support should be used to prevent footdrop.

Specific areas of concern with this type of traction include breakdown of the skin over the heel and damage to the peroneal nerve with resultant footdrop. The area around the

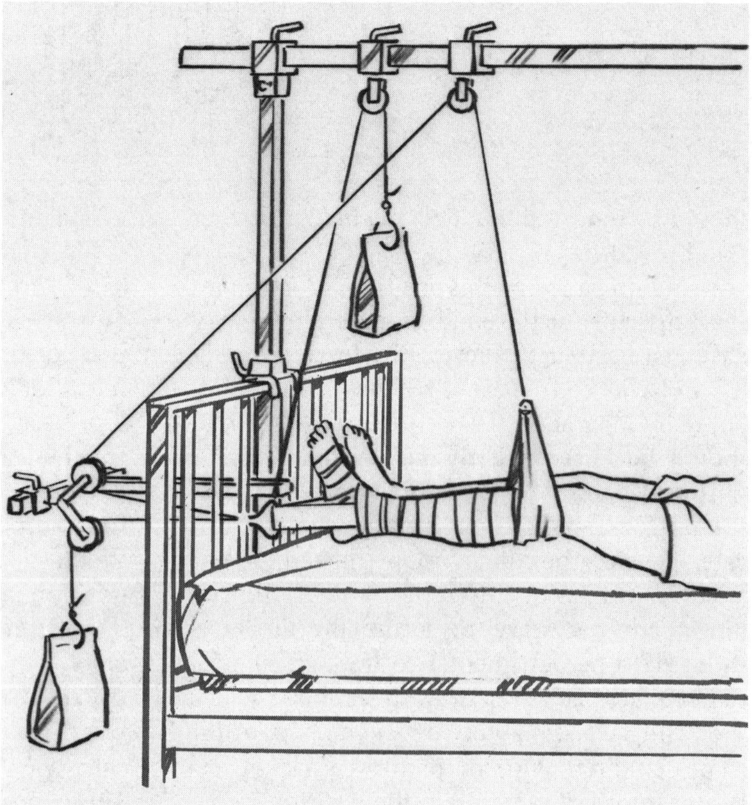

FIG. 25-10 Russell's traction

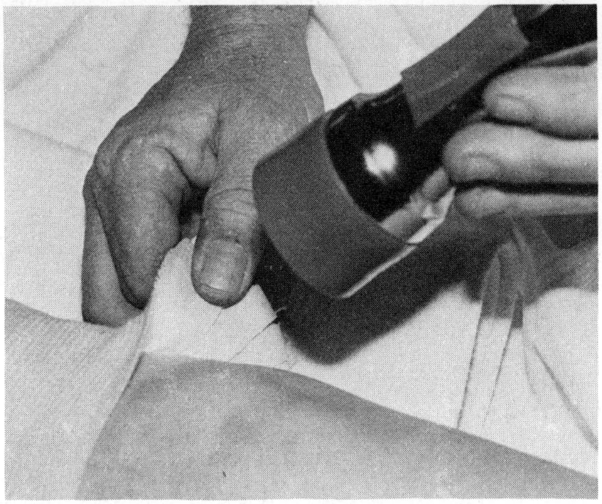

FIG. 25-11 With the aid of a flashlight, the skin under the traction strips is checked for irritation and breakdown.

heel and the popliteal space should be checked at every shift. A flashlight may be used to inspect the skin just under the bandages that hold the traction tape, Figure 25-11. Redness or blister formation may be the first indication of breakdown. Older children may complain of itching in the site and should be cautioned not to scratch or otherwise irritate the area. Foot supports should be applied to both feet. Dorsiflexion and plantar flexion of the affected foot should be done periodically to maintain muscle strength and to prevent other complications.

Balanced Suspension Traction. Balanced suspension traction involves the use of a half-ring Thomas splint and a Pearson attachment, Figure 25-12. It is commonly used for the

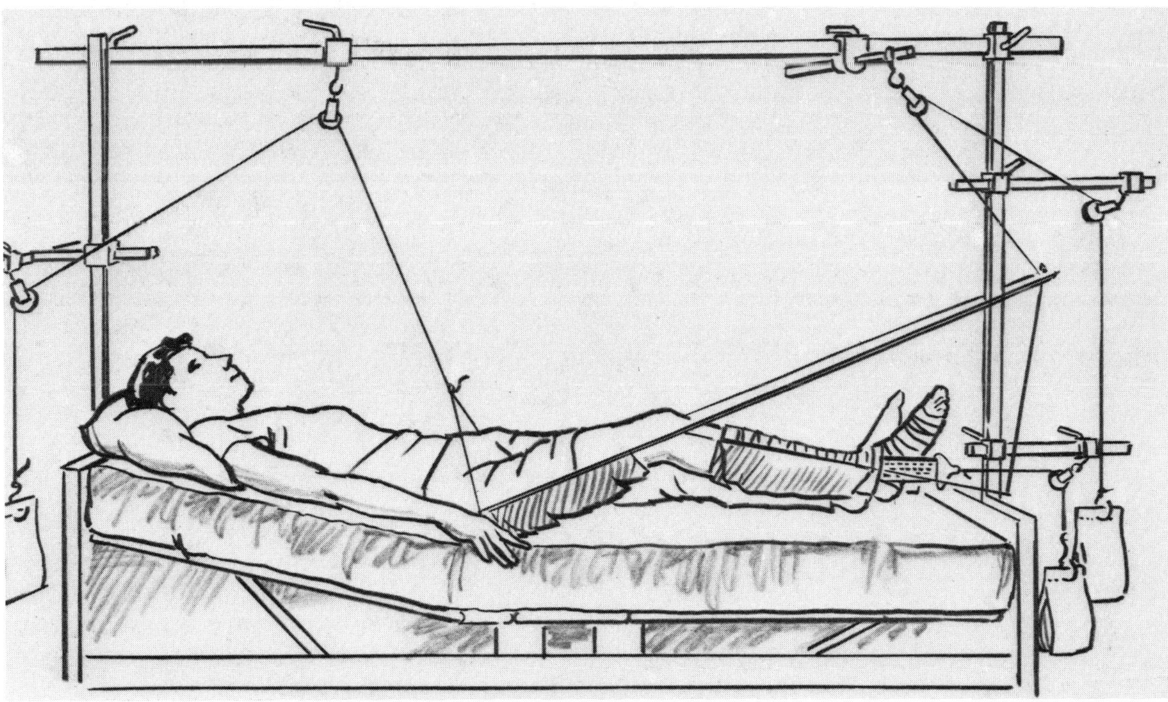

FIG. 25-12 Balanced suspension traction

reduction of femoral fractures in older children. The Thomas splint supports the thigh and the knee. The Pearson attachment supports the leg below the knee in a canvas sling. The knee is flexed at a forty-five-degree angle and the lower leg is kept parallel to the bed. In this type of traction, there are multiple ropes, pulleys, and weights. The nurse should know the correct position for each, as well as the proper weights to be applied.

If the patient is permitted to assist with movement in bed, a trapeze should be provided. Footdrop, skin irritation, and loss of muscular strength are problems that may also arise in this patient. The nurse should check the area around the upper portion of the Thomas splint for skin breakdown.

Dunlap's Traction. Sidearm traction, or Dunlap's traction, is used for reduction of fractures of the upper arm and the elbow, Figure 25-13. Traction is applied to the patient at two sites, the elbow and the hand. The hand is held in a vertical position. The major difficulty with this type of traction is circulatory impairment. The fingers should be checked frequently for pallor, cyanosis, coldness, swelling, pain, or loss of sensation. These signs may be caused by overly tight bandages or too much weight, particularly in the elbow area.

Buck's Extension Traction. Buck's (simple) extension traction involves skin traction to one or both of the lower extremities, Figure 25-14. It may be used to treat muscle spasms

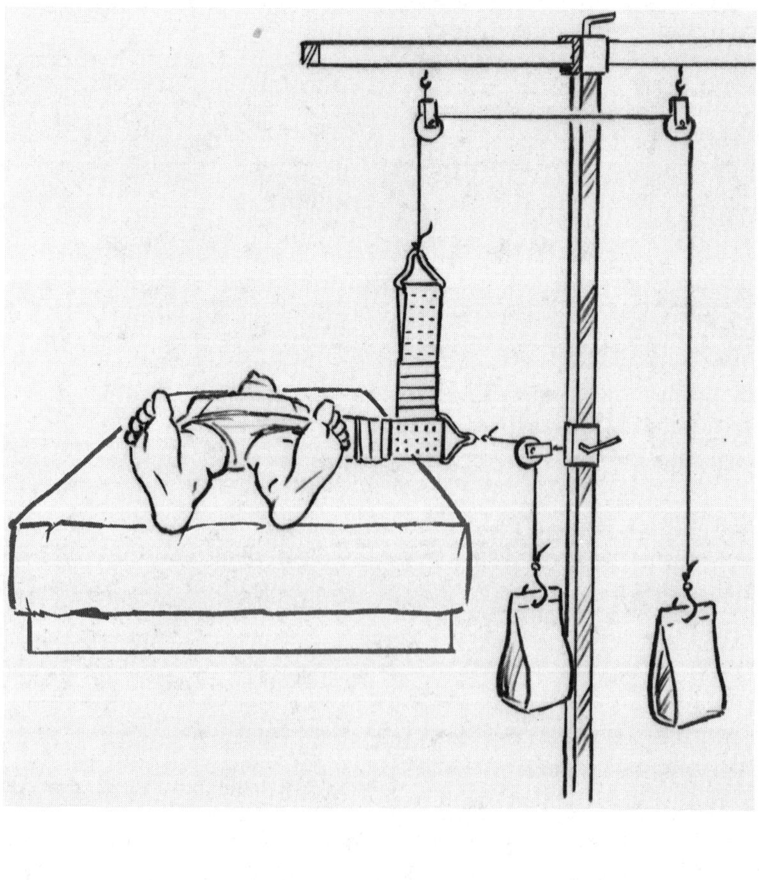

FIG. 25-13 Dunlap's (sidearm) traction

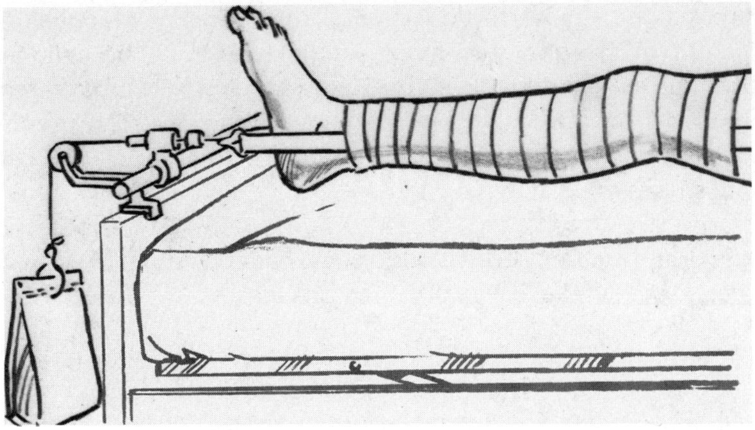

FIG. 25-14 Buck's extension

as well as fractures. Traction tape and bandages, or a fitted foam boot adjusted to the patient with Velcro straps, are applied. A folded towel or bath blanket may be placed under the child's calf and away from the heel to prevent irritation of the heel, Figure 25-15. The foam boot may not conform well to the younger child's foot, and should be checked frequently for evidence of sliding or shifting. This boot can be readjusted by the nurse as necessary, Figure 25-16.

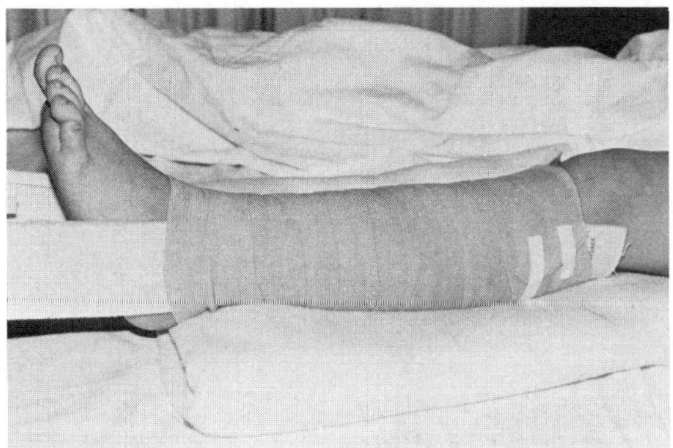

FIG. 25-15 Bath blankets support the leg in Buck's extension traction. Note that pressure on the heel has been avoided.

Skeletal Traction. Traction that is used to apply direct pressure to any part of the skeleton through the use of wires or pins is referred to as skeletal traction. It provides greater traction force than skin traction to treat fractures.

In addition to the usual assessment for problems with the traction itself, special attention must be given to the insertion sites for the traction. A small incision is made in the skin and the wire or pin is applied directly to the bone. The insertion sites are usually dressed with an antibacterial preparation and small sponges. They are inspected on a daily basis for any signs of infection. In the case of cervical traction, the hair on the head should be shaved

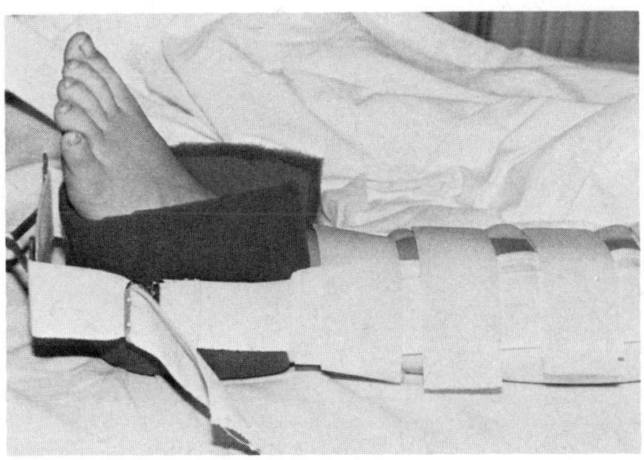

FIG. 25-16 Buck's extension with a foam boot

around the site of the insertion. During the period of traction, the nurse should ensure that the patient's hair does not directly contact the insertion sites, thereby increasing the potential for infection. Careful cleansing of the pin sites is done daily.

Cervical Traction. Crutchfield tongs, halo devices, and Vinke tongs are used in skeletal traction for cervical fractures, such as might occur in automobile or diving accidents. It is advantageous for this patient either to be on a Stryker frame or in a Circolectric bed, Figure 25-17. The patient can then be turned in one single movement every two hours without any possibility of disturbing the traction.

Proper body alignment is essential in the care of these patients. Special care must be

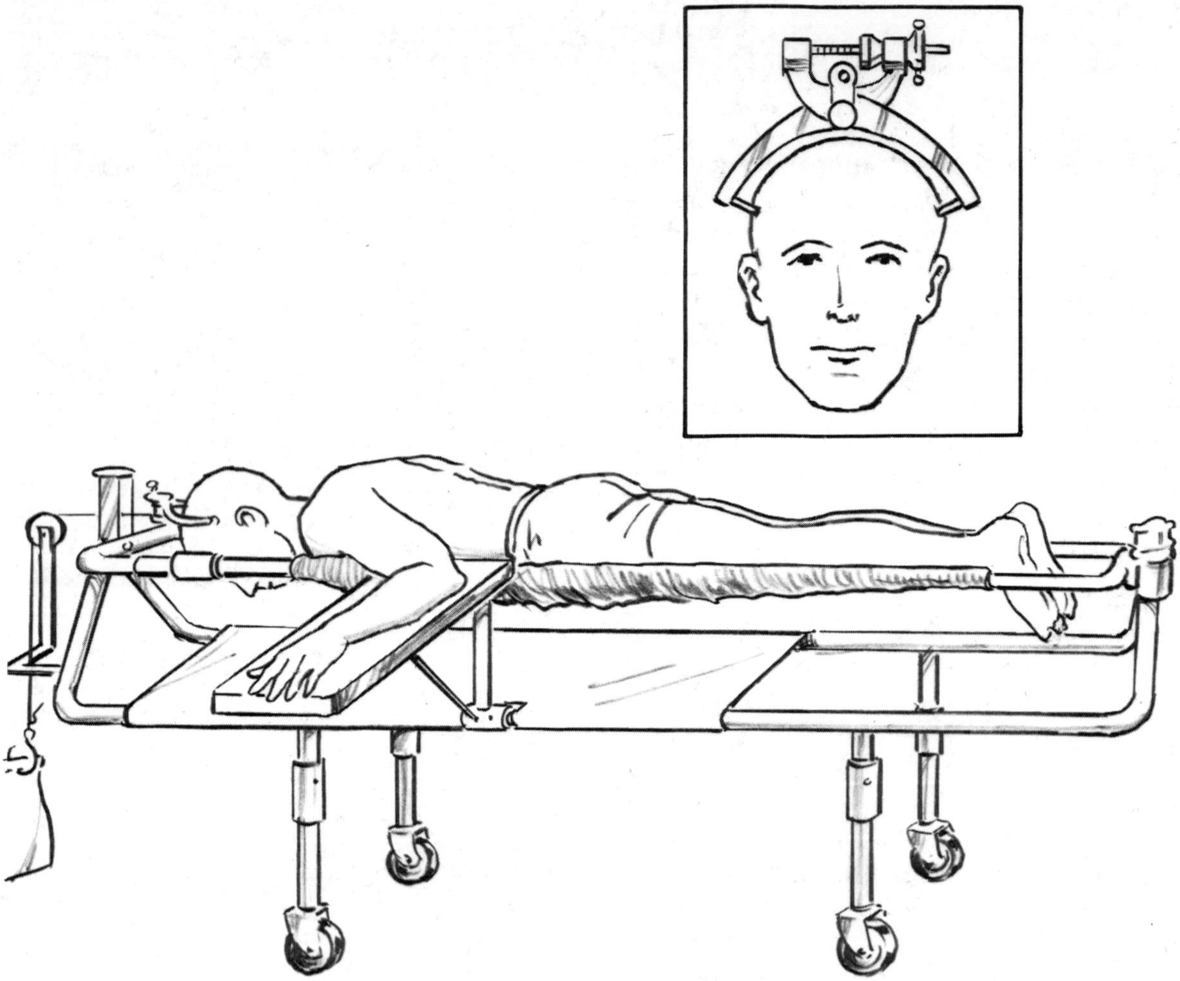

FIG. 25-17 Cervical traction with Crutchfield tongs. The patient is on a Stryker frame. The inset shows how the tongs are applied through burr holes.

taken to prevent pressure areas from developing on the patient's forehead or face as a result of improperly applied turning frames. Pillows may be used to support the arms in proper alignment, as well as to anchor very small patients between the turning frames in order to reposition them.

Braces

Braces are used to correct a deformity, to maintain a corrected position, or to prevent a deformity. They include short leg and long leg braces, bilateral long leg braces with pelvic bands, and the Milwaukee brace. The care for a child in a brace is essentially the same regardless of the type of brace used. The child is expected to wear the brace continuously, allowing one hour per day for skin care. The skin area under the brace should be bathed and dried carefully. Alcohol should be applied to those areas that are prone to irritation. Creams, lotions, and powders should not be used on the skin as they soften it, contributing to breakdown. The patient, if old enough, and the parents should be taught how to care for the skin.

The brace itself should receive routine maintenance on a weekly basis. This includes checking straps, laces, and elastic for signs of fraying or wear. Screws should also be tightened and lint removed. Leather parts should be cleaned with saddle soap and hinges should be oiled, if necessary. With the brace on the child, its length is assessed. Any alterations or adjustments are usually done by the physician or orthotist. The brace should also be inspected at the level of the joints. Does the knee level of the brace fit at the child's knee level? Are the shoes worn unevenly, indicating that the brace has an unequal pull on one side? Are the cuffs overly tight? This may be the first sign of the child outgrowing the brace.

The Jewett brace and the Milwaukee brace both have plastic girdle molds which should be wiped daily with soap and water. These braces are always applied over a cotton tee shirt or a body stocking to protect the underlying skin areas. The upright bars of the Milwaukee brace may be wrapped with strapping tape to prevent undue or excessive wear of the child's clothing.

SUMMARY

A child is usually placed in traction or in a cast because of a traumatic injury. It is important for the nurse to make a complete and accurate assessment of the child's status frequently. The assessment must include an evaluation of the neurovascular status, condition of the skin, and body alignment, as well as an examination for any other problems that relate to immobility. The importance of adequate sensory stimulation of these children should be stressed during parent teaching.

Care of a child in a cast or traction is a unique challenge for the nurse in pediatrics. It requires the reinforcement and encouragement of the child in completing normal developmental tasks as well as in adjusting to a temporary handicap. Care of these children requires a knowledge of the various types of casts, traction, and braces, as well as an awareness of the immediate care needs of the child following injury and the teaching needs of both the parents and the child.

SUGGESTED ACTIVITIES

- Develop a checklist for use by the nursing staff in the care of a child in a cast or in traction. Include the various components of neurovascular assessment, equipment evaluation, planning of daily activities, teaching needs, and diversional therapy.
- Care for a child in traction. Share with your group the type of traction used, the care problems encountered, and the intervention used to resolve the problems.
- Petal a body cast. What type of tape is used and how is it applied? How is the perineal area protected? Involve the parents in caring for the child and evaluate their abilities and their understanding of the rationale for specific care measures.

DISCUSSION TOPICS

1. Share ideas for diversional activities that would be appropriate for a three-year-old and a nine-year-old child in a hip spica cast. Include activities that would help these children adjust to the cast as well.
2. Investigate the requirements for obtaining a tutor for a school-aged child in traction. Is there a fee for the services? How often does the tutor visit the child? What provisions should the nursing staff make for the visits of the tutor to the child?

REVIEW

A. Matching. Match the specific name of the traction in Column I with the general type of traction in Column II.

Column I	Column II
1. Crutchfield tongs	a. Skin
2. Buck's extension	b. Skeletal
3. Bryant's	
4. Russell's with Kirschner wire	
5. Dunlap's	

B. Multiple choice. Select the one best answer.

Situation: Carla, a six-year-old girl, fell off the porch and injured her forearm. Because Carla complained of severe pain in her arm, her mother brought her to the emergency room of the hospital. She had a fracture of the radius very close to the epiphyseal plate. A short arm cast was applied.

1. With pediatric patients such as Carla, there is a great deal of concern for any traumatic injury that involves the epiphyseal plate of the bone. This is because
   a. children's bones are mostly cartilage and take a long time to heal.
   b. children's bones may develop cysts and be easily fractured again.
   c. such injuries may slow or suppress bone maturation and cause asymmetric growth.
   d. such injuries may actually be greenstick fractures resulting in splintering of the bone.

2. As Carla's cast is drying, her nurse remains alert to signs and symptoms of pressure on the nerves and blood vessels. These signs and symptoms include
   1. warmth of the fingers.
   2. coldness of the fingers.
   3. pallor and/or cyanosis of the fingers.
   4. complaints of numbness and/or tingling sensations in the fingers.

   a. 1 and 2 c. 3 only
   b. 2, 3, and 4 d. 1, 2, 3 and 4

3. Certain nursing measures may help to reduce edema in Carla's arm. They include
   1. elevating the arm on a pillow as the cast dries.
   2. splitting or "bivalving" the cast to reduce pressure.
   3. excercising the fingers for a few minutes every hour.
   4. cutting a window in the cast over the pressure area.

   a. 1 and 3 c. 1 only
   b. 2 and 4 d. 1, 2, 3 and 4

4. Carla is to be discharged from the hospital tomorrow. The nurse should instruct Carla's mother to
   1. call the doctor if Carla complains of severe pain.
   2. massage the skin under the cast vigorously with a knitting needle if Carla complains of itching.
   3. make sure Carla does not put anything, such as small toys or candy, inside the cast.
   4. support Carla's arm in a sling to prevent swelling and fatigue.

   a. 1 only
   b. 1 and 2
   c. 2, 3, and 4
   d. 1, 3, and 4

C. Short answer. Briefly respond to the following statements.

1. List the parts of the traction apparatus that should be checked during every shift.
2. Describe the differences between plaster and plastic casts.
3. Describe the daily assessment of a child's cast by a parent.

BIBLIOGRAPHY

Brunner, Lillian S., and Doris S. Suddarth. *Textbook of Medical-Surgical Nursing.* Philadelphia: J. B. Lippincott Company, 1980.

Cohen, Stephen, and Gigi Viellion. "Programmed Instruction: Nursing Care of a Patient in Traction." *American Journal of Nursing,* Vol. 79 (October, 1979), pp. 1771–1798.

Farrell, Jane. "Casts, Your Patients and You – Review of Arm and Leg Cast Procedures." *Nursing 78,* Vol. 8 (November, 1978), pp. 57–61.

Farrell, Jane. "Casts, Your Patients and You – Review of Basic Procedures." *Nursing 78,* Vol. 8 (October, 1978), pp. 65–69.

Hilt, Nancy E., and E. William Schmitt. *Pediatric Orthopedic Nursing.* St. Louis: C. V. Mosby Company, 1975.

Lane, Phyllis. "Home Care of a Toddler in a Spica Cast." *American Journal of Nursing,* Vol. 71 (November, 1971), pp. 2141–2143.

Marlow, Dorothy R. *Textbook of Pediatric Nursing.* Philadelphia: W. B. Saunders Company, 1977.

Meredith, Susie. "Preparing Your Patient to Live With His Cast." *RN,* Vol. 42 (July, 1979), pp. 34–43.

Scipien, Gladys, et al. *Comprehensive Pediatric Nursing.* St. Louis: McGraw-Hill Book Company, 1975.

Section VIII

The Adolescent

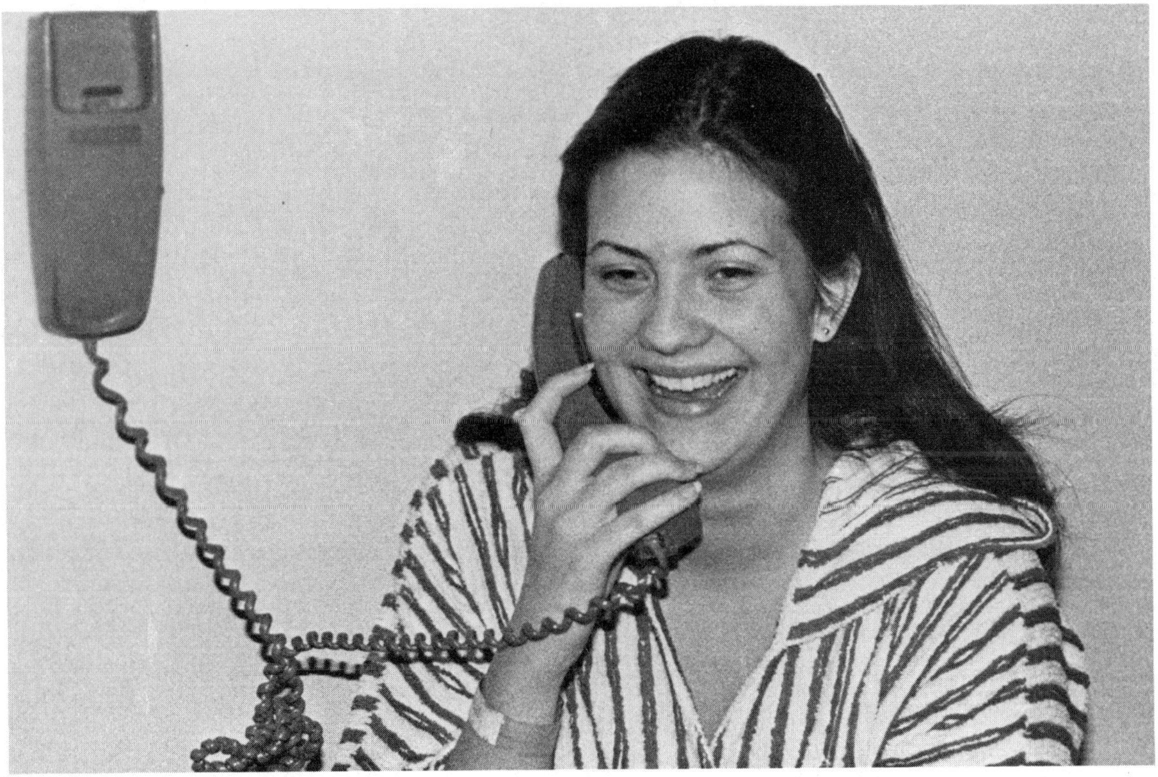

Chapter 26

Growth and Development

OBJECTIVES

Upon completion of this chapter, the student will be able to

- describe the characteristics of physical development in both preadolescents and adolescents.
- identify the emotional and social growth that takes place during the adolescent period.
- list some of the behavioral patterns or problems that produce conflicts during adolescence and suggest possible solutions.

The period of preadolescence and adolescence encompasses the chronological ages of eleven to eighteen years. The eleventh and twelfth years are considered to be part of the preadolescent period, whereas the young person who is thirteen years of age or older is considered to be an adolescent. The period of adolescence is a time of accelerated physical, biochemical, social, and emotional growth.

Assigning a specific chronologic age to a period of development is somewhat misleading, as these changes are dependent on an individual's genetic and nutritional backgrounds, socioeconomic status, and individualized rate of growth. To say that all young men commence puberty at age eleven or twelve years is as erroneous as saying that all young men eat good breakfasts or have blue eyes and blond hair. Rather, the age identified for the onset of certain changes is a mean or an average age at which these changes occur, not an absolute criterion for normal development.

DEVELOPMENTAL TASKS OF THE PREADOLESCENT

The preadolescent or prepubescent period is marked by rapid physical growth. The line of distinction between the preadolescent and the adolescent is puberty, or the ability to reproduce. In the female, this coincides with menarche, or the onset of menstruation. In the male, it is marked by sperm production. The transition from child to man or woman is not instantaneous, but occurs over a period of time and is accompanied by growth and change in many areas.

During preadolescence, a number of developmental tasks are accomplished. Erikson does not divide preadolescence and adolescence, but describes the major task of both periods as learning a sense of identity versus a sense of role diffusion. In this, the young person seeks to know "Who am I?" In the early preadolescent period, youths must adjust to rapid physical changes and personality growth, Figure 26-1. Their relationships with age-mates of both sexes are changing gradually as they move toward heterosexuality. Also in this period, they learn to recognize the expectations of society in regard to their behavior.

This process of "finding oneself" has become more complex in our society as movement has been from a rural to an urban community. In the early 1900s it was not uncommon for marriages at fifteen and participation in full-time jobs rather than school attendance. Adult roles were learned earlier, often by participating in the work role with the parent of the same sex. Now, the single generation households, as well as the distinct separation of the work environment, decreases this participation of the adolescent. Extensive educational requirements for some roles may also increase the period of economic dependency on the parent and slow the process of identity.

According to Piaget, intellectually, preadolescents learn to deal with abstractions.

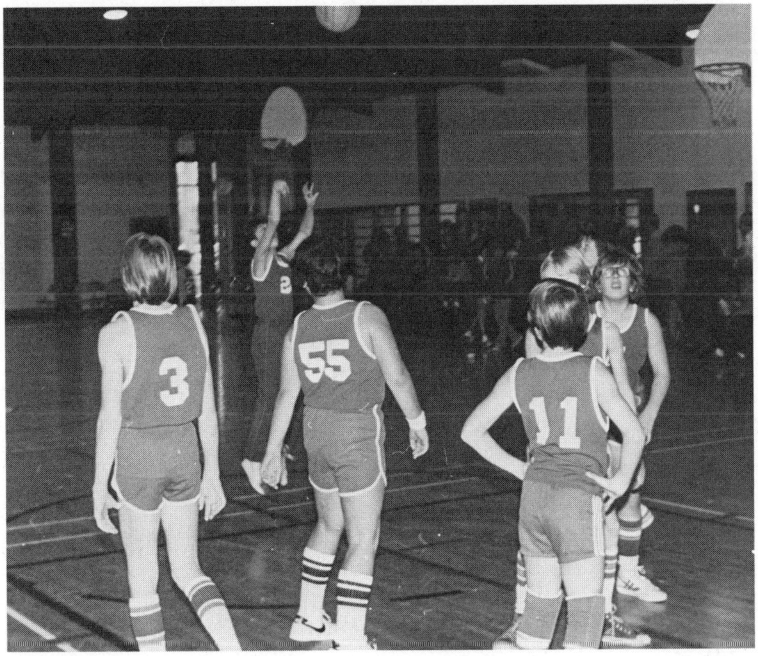

FIG. 26-1 Sports such as basketball provide positive reinforcement of activities with age-mates. Note the differences in muscle mass and size in these preadolescents.

This capability extends through adolescence. It allows the young person to assimilate knowledge and to pose hypothetical problems and their possible solutions. Piaget considers it the last stage of cognitive development, or formal operational thought. It ultimately allows individuals to govern their own lives on the basis of theoretical principles rather than only on their experiences in the environment or learning situation. This stage of cognitive development is marked by the use of inductive and deductive reasoning. It is through this mechanism that the adolescent can realistically look at his parents' behavior and recognize why they made certain choices in life-styles.

DEVELOPMENTAL TASKS OF THE ADOLESCENT

The tasks of the adolescent period may be categorized as early or late, as all are not accomplished at the same time or rate. During the early period of adolescence, young persons usually demonstrate a tendency toward heterosexuality as they begin to assume a masculine or feminine social role. These roles are less clearly demarcated in present culture than in previous ones.

A beginning separation from the family is another task to be achieved as the adolescent grows. Ultimately, this results in the achievement of emotional independence from the parents. The struggle to attain this emotional independence is often marked by confrontation in families as the young person sways between needing and wanting support and staunchly defending his or her independence. Frequently, adolescents will turn to an adult outside the family for support and encouragement, particularly if their family continues to impose restrictions and to thwart their attempts at independence.

Selecting and preparing for a vocation also begins during this period. This process has two basic facets. One involves an occupation or a life work which may require educational preparation. The other is the individual's concept of a state in life, such as single or married. This particular task may extend throughout the period of adolescence and, in some situations, well beyond that period. The young person contemplating a particularly demanding educational program so as to achieve a professional career may deliberately choose a single state until that task is accomplished. He or she may then turn to preparing for marriage and a family. For those who choose marriage, it is necessary for them to establish a mature relationship with a member of the opposite sex.

By the end of this period, adolescents have generally learned to demonstrate socially responsible behavior, Figure 26-2. They are developing the intellectual skills and concepts required for civic competency. They must also acquire a set of values and an ethical system to use as a guide for their own behavior. These

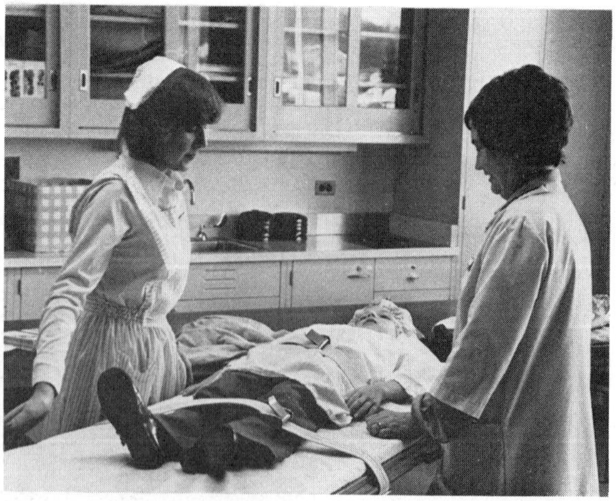

FIG. 26-2 Serving as a hospital volunteer reflects socially responsible behavior as well as a sense of civic duty.

are the ultimate outcomes of Piaget's formal operational thought.

The ability to be economically independent generally occurs in late adolescence or early adulthood. The time at which it occurs depends on occupational goals, education, and motivation. Some studies have indicated that achievement of this task and the ability to hold a full-time job are the only clear markers defining the transition from adolescence to young adulthood. This particular task may not coincide with the chronologic age delineated for this period.

PHYSICAL DEVELOPMENT

The physical growth in the adolescent is highlighted by the changes in height, weight, and body configuration. The slightly overweight, rounded appearance of the preadolescent gives way rather dramatically to the taller, adultlike configuration. During the period of adolescence the male gains between fifteen and sixty-five pounds and increases his height between four and twelve inches, mostly in one rapid spurt. The female increases her weight by fifteen to fifty-five pounds and increases her height between two and eight inches.

The muscles and bones are growing at a rapid pace. The heart and lungs, however, increase more slowly. This slower rate is thought to cause a slight decrease in the oxygen supply and account for the typical fatigue seen in many adolescents. Dietary intake and metabolism are also involved.

The physiologic impetus for pubertal changes is not clearly understood, but appears to arise from the hypothalamus of the pituitary gland. The gonadotropic hormones stimulate the testes to secrete testosterone, and also stimulate the ovaries to secrete estradiol. The secondary sex characteristics are produced by the action of the adrenal cortex and its secretion of androgens. The characteristics are dependent on which hormone is secreted in the largest amount since both are present in differing amounts in each individual.

The estradiol and the testosterone provide a feedback mechanism to the pituitary which results in repression of the growth hormone and resultant closure of the epiphyseal lines and a slowing of physical growth. The epiphyseal closure occurs slowly over a period of time. In the female, skeletal growth is generally completed between sixteen and seventeen years of age. In the average male, skeletal growth may not be completed until seventeen to twenty-one years of age.

In young girls, the physical changes that occur during puberty include: an increase in the transverse diameter of the pelvis; development of the breasts, Figure 26-3; a change in

BREAST DEVELOPMENT IN THE FEMALE

Stage 1
- Prepubescent appearance
- Elevated nipple

Stage 2
- Appearance of breast buds (may be unequal)
- Increased diameter of areola

Stage 3
- Continued enlargement of breast buds and areola
- No separation of contours between breast and nipple

Stage 4
- Secondary mound formed by areola and nipple
- Increased breast size

Stage 5
- Mature appearance
- Recession of areola; projection of the nipple only from the contour

FIG. 26-3 Breast development is one aspect by which sexual maturity is measured in adolescent girls.

PUBIC HAIR DEVELOPMENT IN THE FEMALE

Stage 1
No evidence of pubic hair

Stage 2
Presence of small amount of pubic hair, which is usually straight, sparsely pigmented, and downy
Predominant on labia majora

Stage 3
Darker in color, more coarsely textured, and curlier
More obvious on mons veneris

Stage 4
Thicker, curlier, and coarsely textured
Covers entire mons veneris

Stage 5
Abundant; adult in quantity and type
Present on medial aspect of thighs

FIG. 26-4 The type and distribution of pubic hair is another aspect by which sexual maturity may be rated in girls.

GENITAL DEVELOPMENT IN THE MALE

Stage 1
Prepubescent testes, scrotum, and penis
Similar size and proportion to that present in early childhood

Stage 2
Enlargement of the scrotum and testes
Reddened scrotal skin with rougher texture
Unchanged penile size or only slightly enlarged

Stage 3
Increase in penile length
Increased maturation of testes and scrotum

Stage 4
Increase in penile size and thickness, glans penis more developed
Enlarged, darker scrotum

Stage 5
Adult development in both size and shape

FIG. 26-5 Development of the genitalia is one aspect that determines sexual maturity in adolescent boys.

the vaginal secretions; the onset of menstruation or menarche; and the growth of pubic and axillary hair, Figure 26-4. Both breast development and the distribution of pubic hair have been clearly delineated into distinct stages that represent the normal sequential changes. These stages defined by Tanner, can also be correlated with the average ages at which they occur. Development in the female is considered to be delayed when there is no sign of breast development or breast buds by the age of thirteen years. Menstruation normally occurs within four years of the onset of the pubertal changes.

The physical changes that occur in young boys include: an increase in the size of the penis and scrotum, Figure 26-5; swelling of the breasts, or gynecomastia; growth of hair in the pubic, axillary, and facial areas, Figure 26-6; voice changes; and production of sperm-

PUBIC HAIR DEVELOPMENT IN THE MALE

Stage 1
No evidence of pubic hair

Stage 2
Presence of small amount of pubic hair, which is usually long and straight, and downy in texture
Predominant at the base of the penis

Stage 3
Darker in color, curlier, and more coarsely textured
Sparsely spread over mons veneris

Stage 4
Thicker, curlier, and coarsely textured
More evident over mons veneris

Stage 5
Abundant in amount
Adult in type, texture, and appearance

FIG. 26-6 The type and distribution of pubic hair is another aspect by which sexual maturity may be rated in male adolescents.

atozoa. Tanner also identified the sequential stages of development of the genitalia and pubic hair in the male. Development is considered to be delayed in boys when testicular enlargement is not evident by the age of thirteen and a half years. Any young male who does not show progression in development within four years of the onset of puberty should be evaluated.

Growth patterns are individualized and, as mentioned before, are dependent on the youth's genetic background, nutritional status, and socioeconomic status. Interestingly, those young people who live in inner-city areas mature approximately one and one-half to two years earlier than those living in distinctively rural or middle class communities. Poor nutritional status by itself can retard growth and thwart the stimulation of the normal hormonal function that is necessary for pubertal changes to occur.

A number of physical changes occur in both male and female adolescents. Their rapid changes in height, weight, and body configuration may initially cause some problems with coordination. The rate of growth of the skeletal system may initially exceed that of the muscular system, increasing difficulties with posture, as well as coordination. Hands and feet may appear to be disproportionately large. Diaphoresis, acne, and blushing secondary to vasomotor instability are additional problems that are common to both young men and young women.

EMOTIONAL AND SOCIAL DEVELOPMENT

Influences of the Family

During this period, young adolescents attempt to sort out and develop their own personal value systems. To achieve this end, they test and retest their parents' set of values. They want support and acceptance from the family group, yet often ridicule their beliefs and practices. One of the major sources of conflict may be the activities of daily living, such as bathing. The young person may ignore the parents' suggestion to bathe daily and may refuse to wash his or her hair. If the parents are tolerant of this lapse in hygiene for a period of time, they may soon find the young person bathing daily and even washing the hair twice a day. The personal values ultimately will be based on conscience development, the ability to think abstractly, the ability to make judgments, and recognition of alternatives in a given situation.

The battleground that adolescents use is the home situation. The war that is fought is over their need to be independent and to separate themselves gradually from their families. Adolescents who ridicule their parents' beliefs and activities while in the home situation often highly praise the same beliefs and activities outside the home. Most authorities believe that without these clashes, the young person would never be able to complete the task of separation and achieve independence from the shelter of the family.

This separation is often inappropriately considered to be an event; in actuality, it is a gradual process that may extend over a lifetime. The adolescent, when challenging an attitude or value, is seeking clarification or separation on that issue alone, not on all the values of the parents. During this period, the young person has a continuing need for the parent to set limits; as well as to allow for some emotional independence.

Relationships with Peers

The relationship of adolescents with their peer group is one of reaffirmation of their own goals, attitudes, and beliefs. Peers are chosen for their similarities. The ability of adolescents to function is enhanced by the stability of the peer group. However, their level of achievement may be reduced significantly if, because of delayed development or nonconformity, acceptance by the peer group is lacking.

The peer group provides a stabilizing influence for young adolescents. It reinforces their sense of self-esteem and, to some extent, replaces their families as they test standards and values. The groups reflect their own social and ethical codes. Conformity to the group is mandatory. This may be either a positive or a negative force, depending on the standards set by the group. The peer group involved in delinquent behavior functions in the same manner as that involved in more constructive pursuits, but their standards are different. The time spent in "just talking" allows the group members to cope with changes and reinforces the acceptance of individual members of the group.

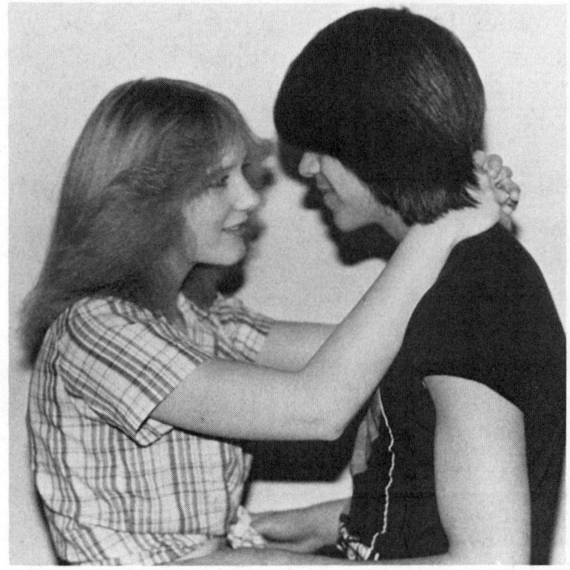

FIG. 26-7 Developing comfortable relationships with the opposite sex precedes selection of a mate.

Development of Sexual Identity

Throughout this period, adolescents are involved in establishing their sexual identities. This process begins with the establishment of satisfactory relationships with the peers of their own sex. Gradually, they learn about those of the opposite sex and move toward establishing a comfortable relationship with them, Figure 26-7.

Prior to actual dating, adolescents begin to show an interest in the opposite sex as evidenced by teasing, less negativism, and more conversational contact. During this period, "crushes" are quite common, and the object of the crush may be totally unaware of the interest. Much of this behavior is fantasized and precedes the establishment of heterosexual activities.

Parents should be aware that they serve as strong role models for the initial patterning of behavior toward the opposite sex. This does not mean that they are the chief source of verbal instruction regarding sexuality, but rather that they are observed in their interactions within the family grouping.

The information presented to young people, as well as their parents, must be factually correct. Parents may convey incorrect or misleading information because of superstition or lack of knowledge. The nurse can help, both in providing information and in correcting misinformation.

Development of Personal Identity

In the process of developing a distinct personality, the behavior of adolescents is marked by great variations and fluctuations. These variations may be evident from day to day, as well as hour to hour. Extremes of behavior are generally a response to a perceived threat or injury.

In one situation, the adolescent may be a "ball of fire" exhibiting tremendous energy and stamina on a project in which he or she is interested. A few hours later, the same individual may be found lying on a bed, staring at the ceiling, and daydreaming for long periods. Many parents perceive the first situation as normal ambition and the second as pure laziness.

Characteristically, the adolescent has periods of irritability. These are in response to increased levels of tension. The adolescent feels real or imagined pressures from many areas, including school, home, and peer group. Many of the pressures also come from within, as in the fear of failing or looking silly in a group situation.

Some of this increase in tension may result from the heightened expectations for the period of adolescence. The intensity built up by the many "firsts" that occur such as the first date, the first kiss, the first dance, and the first driver's license may contribute to unreasonable expectations. These expectations are built in and may be a source of dissatisfaction if the event does not match up to the fantasy.

Occasionally, adolescents carry out aggressive acts against an authority figure as a means of asserting their own individuality. They may break windows or do other damage to property as they act out their anger toward adults. This is more common as a part of peer group activity rather than as an individual action.

All adolescents go through a period of egocentric behavior. During the early years of adolescence, these young persons act as if they were on stage before what is referred to as an "imaginary audience." They believe that everyone is looking at them judging everything they do, wear, and say. It is a period during which adolescents are subjected to many painful moments until they develop a stronger self-identity and some stable personal relationships with others.

The second half of the period of egocentricity is called the "personal fable." They feel that no one has ever experienced anything similar to their own experiences. The problem with this concept is that it prompts some adolescents to take increased risks. For example, an adolescent boy may fantasize or actually consider himself to be immortal and incapable of dying. To prove his point, he may flaunt death by driving at excessive speeds. Likewise, an adolescent girl may convince herself that she cannot get pregnant despite a firmly established sexual relationship. This may be why some adolescent girls deny their pregnancy until labor is imminent.

Concept of Body Image

The adolescent's body image is closely tied to both the personal and the sexual identity. The frequent inspections in the mirror looking for blemishes, trying out a new hairdo, and practicing the application of makeup are part of an adolescent girl's life-style. The young male may be busy evaluating the growth of hair on his upper lip and flexing his muscles in front of the same mirror.

The goal of both of these adolescents is to look like everyone else in the peer group. This includes a desire to mature at the same rate so that all members demonstrate increased height at about the same time, have similar breast development (females), and undergo voice changes in the same manner (males). This need for conformity extends to the appearance which indicates a degree of masculinity or femininity.

The young person deviating from the norm by either early or late maturation may not be accepted. Early maturation is usually better accepted and this individual assumes a leadership role in the group. Teasing or exclusion from the group is particularly painful.

The inordinate amount of time spent in grooming confirms the desired body image. It also permits a certain degree of role-playing behavior as adults are imitated. The body image is also displayed visually to confirm the degree of development.

Participation in Sports

The majority of adolescents participate at some time in an organized sport, either as a recreational pursuit or as a program through high school physical education classes. The emphasis on participation in many areas has overshadowed the fun and exercise portion. Intense competition is often fueled by parents and coaches to the detriment of the adolescent.

This young person is highly motivated and his need for self-esteem drives him to unrealistic limits in achievement of a goal. Losing the competition is not only loss of a game but often a compromising of one's self-esteem and possible rejection by peers, parents, and others.

The ideal program requires health screening prior to participation, all adolescents to play in every game, provisions for conditioning and fitness prior to play, and restrictions of contact-collision sports to those fifteen and older. The coaches should be knowledgeable regarding the playing rules and potential safety problems. They should also avoid verbal abuse and the use of punitive measures for poor performance.

The type of sport selected should be of the adolescent's choice, with parental consent. The adolescent's size, stamina, and interest should all be a part of the decision. Adolescents' awareness of the time commitment and the sacrifices involved is important. Their self-concept should be sufficiently developed so that bench-warming and a string of losing games are not a threat.

PROBLEMATIC ISSUES

Problems of Chronic Illness

Some consideration needs to be made for the adolescent with long-term or chronic health problems. This individual has the same needs as all adolescents but may inadvertently have only negative reinforcement from peers and adults in the environment.

The typical adolescent rebellion in these young people often extends to the diagnosis itself. The adolescent with juvenile diabetes mellitus, for example, may begin to eat and drink as he pleases in open defiance of the prescribed dietary intake and insulin requirements. The adolescent with cystic fibrosis abandons the nebulizer and chest physiotherapy as being "for little kids." The young person with rheumatoid arthritis refuses the use of assistive devices or the anti-inflammatory medication. Certainly these rebellious behaviors have more serious implications for these adolescents because of their illnesses. For each one it is a retesting of the reality of the diagnosis and then a reaffirmation of the prescribed treatment.

The disease process may also interfere with growth, causing a slower sequence of physical development and often a less positive body image. Weakened physical condition and the care needs related to some conditions may force continued dependency on parents. Parents often reinforce this continued attachment process.

Adults can make positive contributions to this young person's life by emphasizing realistic, attainable goals. The focus should be on assets, strengths, and positive interest.

The school setting occasionally becomes the source of negative reinforcement through policies or procedures that apply to all without any adaptation. The young person needing chest physiotherapy during the school day may find the school nurse does not have the authority to do percussion and postural drainage. Family members may then need to come to the school to carry this out. Medications which must be given with the noon meal, such as enzymes, anti-inflammatory agents, or even antibiotics, are often a source of problems. The emphasis on drugs in the schools makes any of these children suspect for carrying the prescribed medications with a lunch. Medications are often required to be turned in to the health clinic in the morning and retrieved at lunch to be taken with the meal. The same process is repeated on a daily basis. Adolescents are also vulnerable to emotional damage from the teacher who does not understand their needs and singles them out because of absence or illness.

Fears of death and disability are very real to these adolescents. At a time when others are worried about careers, these adolescents may be thinking about survival. When another young girl may fantasize about her future family, this young person may fear marriage because of the hereditary implications of a particular disease.

The approach to the special problems of this group of adolescents has to be in acceptance of their particular needs. Adjustments can and must be made to allow them to grow. Health care workers who anticipate these problems in dealing with adolescents can have a positive impact on their lives. Continuity of care should extend into the school as well as into the home and community setting of this individual.

The Hospitalized Adolescent

The nurse working with the adolescent must provide flexible limits in providing health care. Information that is given to the young person should be in realistic and understandable terms. Support and guidance are provided by aiding the individual in making choices as well as sorting out information. Many adolescents need to hear information about health care problems away from the parent to allow them an opportunity to voice their own concerns.

In the hospital setting the adolescent's privacy should be maintained and respected. This includes providing a personal space, time alone, and confidentiality. The personal space may be only a corner of a room but is to be respected. Encouraging the adolescent to hang up cards, posters, and other decorations confirms the personal identification with the owner. Time to be alone is as necessary in the hospital as it is in the home setting. The young person's ability to cope with stress is dependent on the coping mechanisms; privacy promotes coping. Confidentiality permits the adolescent freedom to share information without the threat of repercussions from home and a different value system.

The freedom to make choices should be encouraged as much as possible. Selection of food, daily care routines, and time for treatments allows the adolescent a sense of control over his environment.

Some provisions should be made for the support of the peer group. Adjustments in visiting hours and the encouragement of telephone support systems are helpful. In the long-term facility, peer groups may be newly established as a result of group meetings and social activities promoted for the various age-groups.

Problems of Sexual Involvement

Adolescents in our society are exposed to widely differing views on sexuality. Their increased exposure to a sexual revolution has a bearing on this. A more permissive attitude toward nonconforming life-styles and altered marriage standards prevails. Adolescents frequently engage in sexual activities, not as an expression of a permanent commitment between two mature individuals, but rather to re-emphasize their own self-worth. In this process, they may delude themselves by thinking that they are "in love."

Adolescents also receive mixed messages from their parents regarding sexual behavior. When a parent tells a young girl not to get pregnant, the message that is conveyed is "it's all right to do, but don't get caught." The young person with an insufficiently developed value system may be unable to say "no" to a person of the opposite sex or to stand up against the standard practices of the peer group.

Teenage pregnancy, in or out of a marriage, carries its own set of complex problems. The pregnancy itself causes a degree of social isolation for the young girl even though she may remain in an alternative classroom situation in the schools. Many simply leave school with the intention of completing the work at a later date. The later date seldom arrives as the young mother is caught up in caring for the child, maintaining a home, and securing employment. Regardless of intellectual or socioeconomic status, a distinct termination or limitation of life's choices occurs prior to the pregnancy.

An early marriage generally limits the occupational choices available to individuals, decreases their income level, and increases their potential for unemployment because of a limited education. Young people involved in the marriage are socially isolated from peers and their school friends and must seek out a new social group to provide the support needed.

Problems in Substance Abuse

The term *substance abuse* refers to the inappropriate use of both alcohol and drugs. The media often lends support to the concept that the prolific use of drugs and alcohol is an acceptable adult behavior when, in fact, it is not. The young person may become involved in substance abuse as a part of the rebelliousness of the adolescent period or in an attempt to experience what is perceived as adult behavior, Figure 26-8. Other adolescents may turn to either drugs or alcohol for relief from problems, not recognizing that the problems will continue to exist and that the drugs or alcohol will likely compound them, Figure 26-9.

The nurse should participate in educating adolescents regarding this problem. Initially, the nursing responsibility is the identification of those young persons with a problem of this nature. As a member of the treatment team, which may include therapists, counselors, teachers, and social workers, the nurse assists

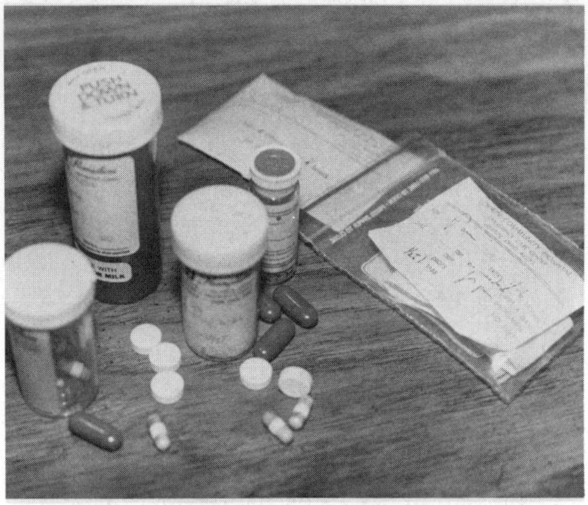

FIG. 26-8 The availability of a wide variety of prescription and nonprescription drugs within the home provides an opportunity for abuse.

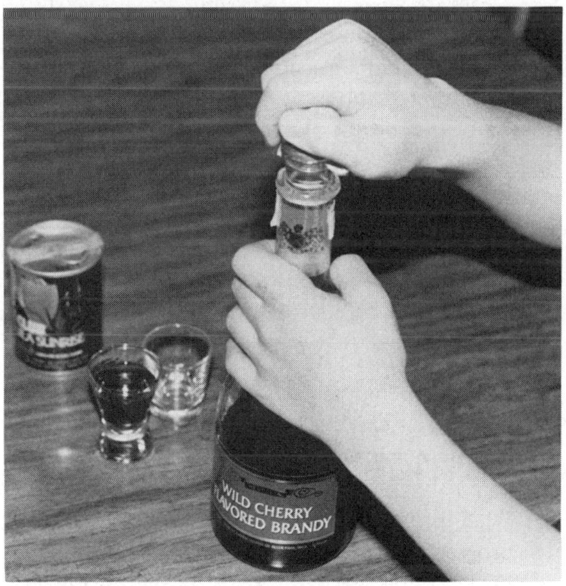

FIG. 26-9 Adult drinking patterns may influence a young person positively or negatively with regard to the use of alcoholic beverages.

in assessing the problem, as well as in meeting the individual's other health needs. The nurse may also serve as the liaison between the family and the adolescent. Ideally, the family is involved in the treatment program as well.

In anticipation of the existence of these problems, all nurses involved in delivering health care to young people should participate in the education of parents regarding drug and alcohol abuse and what can be done about the problem. They are also in a position to provide support to parents with regard to the growth and development of young people, as well as acceptable standards for behavior.

Approaches to the Adolescent

In the health care setting as well as in the home, the adolescent needs both restrictions and privileges. When restrictions are imposed, they should be coupled with an alternate privilege. In the hospital setting, the restriction of bedrest might be coupled with extended television viewing on certain evenings.

Demands for freedom are best coupled with a responsibility. The juvenile diabetic patient who would like to visit a friend on another unit should be responsible for either reporting his or her whereabouts to the staff or using a sign-out and sign-in sheet.

It is important for others to spend time with the adolescent in an honest exchange of ideas and attitudes. This is the ideal opportunity to provide sincere compliments, as well as praise and reassurance. In the hospital setting, reinforcement of positive behavior in an adolescent may be accomplished by arranging regular fifteen-minute periods of interaction with a staff person whom the adolescent respects.

The staff nurse should intervene if the adolescent is being ridiculed, humiliated, nagged, or ignored. Any of these approaches, either on the part of the staff or on the part of the parents, will only further reinforce the predominantly negative self-concept of the adolescent. The nurse can also teach parents how to provide the adolescent with consistent, positive support. In many areas, programs referred to as Parent Effectiveness Training groups, are available. These groups emphasize positive relationships and support for all age-groups, with minimal attention being given to negative behavior that may occur.

During the period of hospitalization, some provision should be made for continued support from the peer group. This may be maintained and facilitated by flexible visiting hours, telephone contacts, letter writing, or taped messages. The method used depends on the length of the hospital stay and the severity of the adolescent's illness.

SUMMARY

The period of adolescence is a time of intense growth in physical, social, and emotional areas. Adults frequently see it as a trying period, emphasizing the negative behavior that is exhibited. An adolescent may be more "tolerated" by parents than understood.

The tasks for this developmental period are involved and complex. Adolescents need the consistent support of an adult to provide encouragement and to act as a sounding board in their development of a value system. The peer group provides an avenue for reinforcing the standards and values identified by the adolescent as important.

Health problems in adolescents may be related to the physical growth that accompanies the pubertal changes. They may also be attributed to the stress and anxiety of this period of growth and development. Many problem areas for the adolescent revolve around those activities that are perceived as adult – sexual activity, alcohol, and drug abuse for instance. Without consistent supportive relationships, these problem areas provide a rich source of negative behavior.

SUGGESTED ACTIVITIES

- Compare two hospitalized adolescents. Chart their height and weight on growth charts. Assess which developmental tasks they have completed and which they are still in the process of achieving. Ask them to share their feelings with you regarding the opposite sex, their peer group, their school, and their relationship with their parents.

- Care for an adolescent in your assigned hospital. Determine what measures are taken to promote and maintain peer support for this young person. What suggestions does the adolescent have for more activities? How did you implement your knowledge of adolescent growth and development in this situation?

DISCUSSION TOPICS

1. Discuss the effects of a hereditary or chronic disease on the developmental tasks of the adolescent. What can the parents do to assist the young person to achieve these tasks?

2. What information is included in the sex education programs offered in the elementary and junior high schools in your area? Is the information presented appropriate for each grade level? Are the parents involved in any way in the development or presentation of the program?

REVIEW

A. Matching. Match the event or activity in Column I with the stage at which it occurs in Column II.

Column I	Column II
1. Growth spurt	a. Preadolescent
2. Menarche	b. Adolescent
3. Production of sperm	
4. Maturing relationship with age-mates	
5. Selecting and preparing for a vocation	
6. Adjusting to rapid physical changes	

B. Multiple choice. Select the one best answer.

1. Julia is a thirteen-year-old girl who is very self-conscious about her appearance. This egocentric behavior that is typical of adolescents is attributable to
   a. the associated growth spurt and voice changes.
   b. the concepts of an imaginary audience and the personal fable.
   c. their negative attitude and behavioral fluctuations.
   d. the development of pubic hair and the breasts.

2. Julia's menarche occured at the age of eleven. The physical changes that should be apparent by now in Julia include
   a. a growth spurt.
   b. an increase in breast size.
   c. the spread of pubic hair.
   d. all of the above.

3. Changes that will occur in both Julia and her fourteen-year-old brother Harry include
   a. changes in body configuration.
   b. acne.
   c. blushing.
   d. all of the above.

4. The peer groups to which Julia and Harry belong provide
   a. an opportunity to test standards and values.
   b. ideas for negative social behavior.
   c. opportunities to conform to a group.
   d. a means of escaping from their parents.

C. Short answer. Briefly respond to the following statements.

1. Name three factors parents should know about an adolescent's establishment of a sexual identity.
2. List four aspects of the nursing approach for the care of an adolescent.

BIBLIOGRAPHY

Anderson, Claudia. "Adolescent Pregnancy." *Issues in Comprehensive Pediatric Nursing,* Vol. 2 (July–August, 1976), pp. 42–49.

Anderson, Frances J. "The Developmental Experience of Adolescence." *Issues in Comprehensive Pediatric Nursing,* Vol. 2 (July–August, 1976), pp. 1–16.

Blades, Sandra. "Clinical Notes on Adolescent Drug Abuse." *Issues in Comprehensive Pediatric Nursing,* Vol. 2 (July–August, 1976), pp. 59–64.

Cannon-Bonaventre, Kristina, and Janet Kahn. "Interviews with Adolescent Parents: Looking at Their Needs." *Children Today,* Vol. 8 (September–October, 1979), pp. 17–19.

Daniel, William, et al. "Adolescent Medicine: Your Patient From Puberty to Maturity." *Patient Care,* Vol. 13 (October 15, 1979), pp. 64–105.

Fox, Greer L. "The Family's Influence on Adolescent Sexual Behavior." *Children Today,* Vol. 8 (May–June, 1979), pp. 21–25.

Graf, Christina M. "Sex and the Adolescent." *Issues in Comprehensive Pediatric Nursing,* Vol. 2 (July–August, 1976), pp. 31–41.

Green, Morris. "Adolescent Health Care." *Children Today,* Vol. 8 (September–October, 1979), pp. 8–11.

Johnson, Thomas R., et al. *Children Are Different: Developmental Physiology.* Columbus: Ross Laboratories, 1978.

Kandell, Netta. "The Unwed Adolescent Pregnancy: An Accident?" *American Journal of Nursing*, Vol. 79 (December, 1979), pp. 2112–2114.

Lipsitz, Joan S. "Adolescent Development: Myths and Realities." *Children Today*, Vol. 8 (September-October, 1979), pp. 2–7.

Marlow, Dorothy R. *Textbook of Pediatric Nursing.* Philadelphia: W. B. Saunders Company, 1977.

Mercer, Ramona T. *Perspectives on Adolescent Health Care.* Philadelphia: J. B. Lippincott Co., 1979.

Moore, Kristin A., et al. "Teenage Motherhood: Its Social and Economic Costs." *Children Today,* Vol. 8 (September–October, 1979), pp. 12–16.

Newman, Barbara M., and Philip R. Newman. *Infancy and Childhood: Development and Its Contexts.* New York: John Wiley and Sons, 1978.

Notaro, Carol. "Adolescents and Alcohol." *Issues in Comprehensive Pediatric Nursing,* Vol. 2 (July–August, 1976), pp. 50–58.

Shearer, Jay D. "The Adolescent Wheelchair Athlete. *Pediatric Nursing,* Vol. 3 (September–October, 1977), pp. 20–22.

Selekman, Janice. "Cystic Fibrosis: What is Involved in the Home Treatment Program for These Children, Adolescents, and Young Adults." *Pediatric Nursing,* Vol. 3 (March–April, 1977), pp. 32–35.

Smith, Nathan J. "Sports Medicine." *Pediatric Nursing,* Vol. 5 (January–February, 1979), pp. 39–46.

Vaughan, Victor C., et al. *Nelson's Textbook of Pediatrics.* Philadelphia: W. B. Saunders Company, 1979.

Chapter 27

Health Care Problems

OBJECTIVES

Upon completion of this chapter, the student will be able to

- describe the nursing care and treatment of an adolescent with one of the sexually transmitted diseases.
- compare the health care teaching that is provided for the adolescent with scoliosis who wears a brace with that provided for the adolescent who is placed in traction prior to surgery.
- identify the types of emotional disturbances that might occur in the adolescent period and describe the nursing approach to such problems.

The health problems that occur in the adolescent are a reflection of the growth and changes that are taking place. The typical orthopedic problem is that of scoliosis. Acne represents a common integumentary disorder. The adolescent population is somewhat responsible for the rising rates of venereal diseases, indicating increasing sexual activity in this age-group. The infections so common in the younger child are not as common in the adolescent. Social and environmental factors may trigger emotional problems and substance abuse.

SCOLIOSIS

Scoliosis refers to a lateral curvature of the spinal column. The definition, by itself, does not clarify whether rotation of the spinal column or deformities of the vertebrae are present.

Classification

Scoliosis may be classified in a number of ways. The most common classification involves a division into postural, acquired, and congenital malformations. Postural scoliosis is the result of habit or improper function and is correctable, if identified early. The acquired type involves a structural deformity that is related to growth, trauma, or paralysis. The congenital category includes those malformations that arise from a faulty germ layer that causes fusion of ribs or vertebrae, resulting in inadequate development. These children require corrective surgery at very early ages, usually during the toddler period.

In the general screening process of school-aged children, some degree of scoliosis is detected in about ten percent of those examined. Of this group, only two percent actually require surgical correction. Slightly more females than males belong to this latter group.

Affected individuals are usually first identifiable by their poor posture, but there are few other symptoms. A history of fatigue-related pain is frequently elicited. Almost all of these individuals derive some pain relief from lying down, which provides mechanical relief.

Diagnostic Screening

Spinal curvature may arise at any point along the vertebral column. It can occur in the cervicothoracic, thoracic, thoracolumbar, or the lumbar area. Examination is undertaken with the patient wearing a minimum of clothing, usually undershorts for the boys and bra and underpants for girls. The gait is observed, as is the position of the head, trunk, and extremities from front, back, and side. On observation of the child from the rear, the head should be over the tailbone, the shoulders equal, the hips level, and the flanks equal. Particular attention should be given to the amount of air space noted between the arms at the sides and the waist, Figure 27-1. Any extra

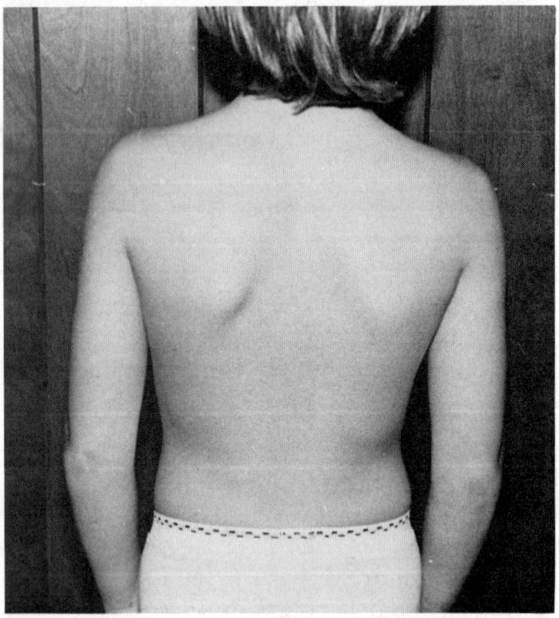

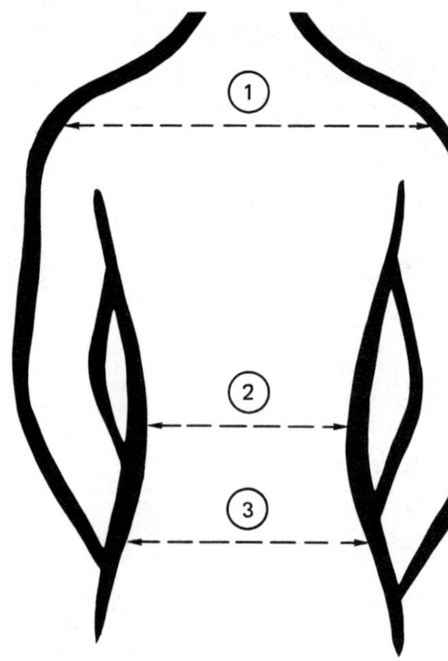

FIG. 27-1 The air space is more visible on the right than on the left. Also note the elevation of the left shoulder and the prominence of the left scapula. Comparison of each of these three areas is made with the patient in an upright position.

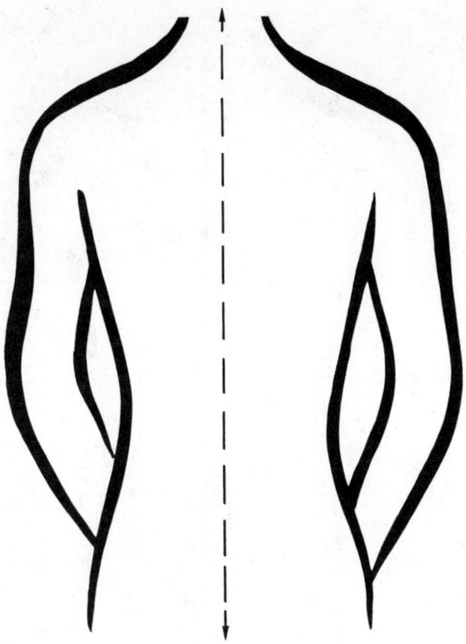

FIG. 27-2 Alignment of the trunk is assessed by using a plumb line that extends from the occiput.

creases in the flank area should also be noted. (These creases are more obvious in slightly overweight individuals.) The child is then asked to bend forward with the hands down and fingertips slightly touching. The back is observed from the side, as well as the rear. In patients with scoliosis, a posterior rib hump is evident. With the child in an erect position, a plumb line extending from the occiput may also be used to check for trunk alignment, Figure 27-2.

Early detection is of major concern. Prompt detection and treatment prevents the development of more severe deformity and complications. It is important to determine whether there is a familial history of scoliosis. This is an indication for the screening of all siblings, especially prior to and during the growth spurt. Young people should be screened prior to the growth spurt and on a continuing basis until the period of spinal maturity is completed. The growth spurt and the period of spinal maturity occurs earlier in Black and Spanish Americans than it does in Caucasians.

If the problem is left untreated, the possible complications range from mild to severe. The cosmetic deformity is often a major concern for adolescents and young adults. The functional disability persists and may become a greater problem in later life. The rotation of the spine, along with the accompanying changes in the ribs, can produce severe problems. Pulmonary complications, as well as cardiac complications, such as right-sided failure and cor pulmonale, may be the end result of severe uncorrected scoliosis.

Treatment

The various modes of treatment that are used for scoliosis include exercises alone, braces or casts used in conjunction with exercises, skin or skeletal traction, and surgical correction. The treatment of choice is dependent on the degree of curvature that exists at the time of the initial diagnosis. If the curvature is twenty degrees or less, an exercise program is initiated and the child is observed closely to determine whether the scoliosis is progressing. For a curvature of greater than twenty degrees but less than forty degrees, the treatment of choice involves the use of braces, and may include traction. Any curvature that is greater than forty degrees indicates the need for surgery. Traction is used prior to surgery and casting is used afterward to maintain the correction. Despite conservative methods such as exercises and bracing, the progression of curvature in some children necessitates surgical intervention.

The particular treatment used also depends on the cause of the scoliosis. The child with a congenital curvature benefits from early surgical intervention even as early as one or two years of age. Growth potential also has a bearing. Rapidly progressing curvature in a child who has not yet reached skeletal maturity will probably dictate surgical correction. Conversely, another young person with minimal, slowly progressive scoliosis or one who has almost reached skeletal maturity, would probably do very well with bracing alone.

Types of Braces

The three types of braces used to treat scoliosis include the Milwaukee brace, the Orthoplast jacket, and the Boston brace. There are specific indications for each. All of the braces are considered to be active devices in that, with exercises and normal activity, pressure is created laterally and traction exerted longitudinally to achieve the correction.

Milwaukee Brace. The Milwaukee brace is comprised of a chin rest and a pelvic girdle which are connected by three vertical bars. A holding pad attached to the brace also provides pressure on the side of the convex curvature. The brace is constructed for and fitted precisely to the individual. The chin rest or neck ring, the pelvic band, and the holding pad are made of leather. The uprights are made of metal, Figure 27-3.

Once the brace has been properly fitted, the child is instructed to wear it for twenty-three hours per day. The remaining hour is specifically used for skin care and exercises performed without the brace. The brace is removed to allow for bathing. The skin must be dried carefully afterward, and alcohol should be applied to any areas where the brace is likely to cause skin irritation. Lotions and ointments are avoided as they cause softening of the skin and further irritation or breakdown. A tee-shirt or body stocking that fits well is applied between the skin and the brace. The uprights of the brace may cause excessive wear on clothing, so they are usually wrapped with a heavy strapping tape. Most young people find it more comfortable to wear clothing one size larger than their usual size.

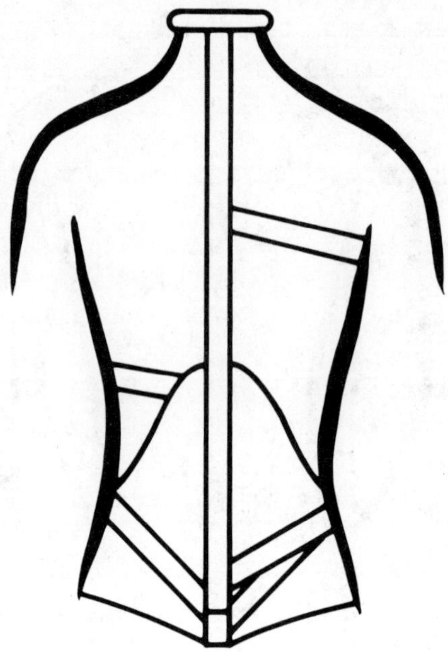

FIG. 27-3 Front view of a Milwaukee brace

The exercise program is carried out both with and without the brace. It involves pelvic tilts, spine extension, push-ups, and sit-ups. Each exercise is usually repeated ten times several times per day according to the instructions of the physical therapist. Minimal restrictions are placed on the activities of these patients. They are encouraged to be as active as possible with the brace. Only two activities must specifically be avoided. These are body contact sports, because of the danger of injuring someone with the metal brace, and the use of a trampoline.

Swimming is encouraged as an active exercise. The child is not permitted to dive from the springboard, but shallow dives from the side of the pool are permitted. Sitting at the side of the pool is to be avoided. Because these patients do not wear a brace while swimming, when they get out of the pool, they are encouraged to lie flat rather than risk increasing vertebral stress as a result of incorrect posture.

Adjustment to the school setting may take a period of time. The neck of the young person wearing the Milwaukee brace is extended and held in a forward position. In the school setting, these students need a desk top that can be elevated and tilted to allow them full usage. When changing classrooms, these children should be given extra time as it takes them longer to traverse a corridor. They must turn their bodies completely in order to see to their left or right. Initially, their balance may also be slightly impaired because of the weight of the brace.

In the home setting, studying may be facilitated by the use of prism glasses. However, some young people are unable to adjust to these glasses because of persistent nausea or perceptual problems. For those who are able to adjust, the glasses may also be used for work in the classroom setting. When studying at home, many of these young people find it easiest to lay prone across their bed with their textbook on the floor or on a low foot stool. This provides a comfortable position and allows them to read easily.

Orthoplast Jacket. The Orthoplast jacket is a molded plastic jacket that provides the same type of corrective force as the Milwaukee brace. The difference is in the cosmetic appearance of the brace, Figure 27-4. The jacket does not extend above the clothing, nor does it have a neck ring or chin rest. It therefore allows mobility of the head and eliminates some of the problems associated with the Milwaukee brace.

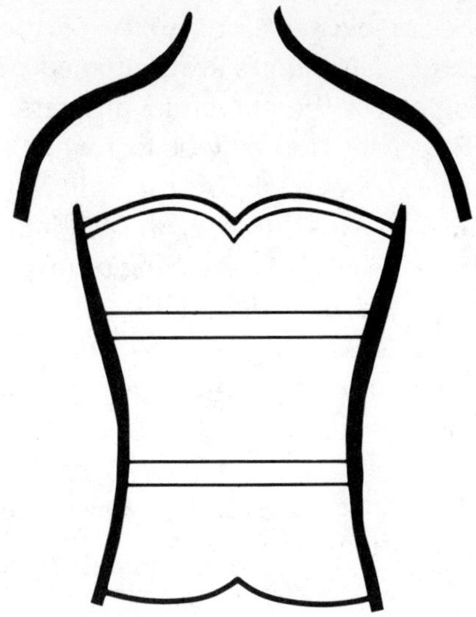

FIG. 27-4 An Orthoplast jacket for correction of scoliosis

Boston Brace. The Boston brace is similar in purpose to the Orthoplast jacket and to the Milwaukee brace. It is used to correct kyphosis and lordosis. It uses a molded pad over the sternum to assist in the correction of the kyphotic hump.

Casting

The Risser turnbuckle cast may also be used to treat scoliosis, but it requires long-term hospitalization. It is a full body cast with wedges cut over the convexity of the spinal curvature. The hinges are tightened periodically to correct the curve in a progressive fashion. The correction may be lost when the cast is removed. With all of the other methods available, this is seldom used. The immobility problems, as well as the long-term problems of care, make this a very difficult type of correction for the young person to accept. Other casts that may be applied include the Risser localizer jacket, the surcingle cast, and the Cotrel E-D-F cast (elongation-derotation-flexion). The latter two correct the rib hump as well as the spinal curvature.

Traction

Traction is often used in these patients prior to surgical correction of the scoliosis. Cotrel's traction or halo-femoral traction is used for this purpose. The patient is maintained in the traction for a period of three to four weeks prior to surgical correction. The major purpose of these methods is to stretch the curvature, muscles, and soft tissues preoperatively. The traction alone is not considered to be corrective.

Cotrel's Traction. Cotrel's traction is a specific type of skin traction consisting of a head harness and a pelvc band or girdle. A specially designed leather head halter is applied. It is constructed so that the pull or pressure is on the occiput rather than on the chin as it would be with cervical traction. A leather harness is applied to the pelvic area to provide the traction at the foot. Foot slings or a foot bar are often added to the traction so that the flexion and extension exercises can be carried out to increase the spinal stretching. The weights are increased gradually, and may be the equivalent of 100 pounds of traction when the child is using the foot bar and pushing to increase the extension.

This type of traction is released for skin care and bathing only. It is imperative that this child remain flat in bed at all other times. Careful skin care is a necessity at the chin area, as well as at the iliac crests. Alcohol is used to toughen these areas. Powders and lotions are avoided, as with all casts and traction. A modified form of Cotrel's traction may be maintained for four to six months at home prior to surgical correction. Parents can be taught to apply it and to assess for skin and pressure problems.

Halo-femoral Traction. Halo-femoral traction is a type of skeletal traction that is also used to treat scoliosis prior to surgical correction. It is used in those patients with curvatures of more than sixty degrees. Insertion of four pins into the skull connected by a metal ring and distally into the femurs or tibias involves a short operative procedure. In addition to the usual care of a child in traction, special care must be given to the insertion sites of each of the pins. This includes cleansing with hydrogen peroxide and application of Betadine. Some also use alcohol-saturated sponges around the pins. These sponges are changed on a daily basis.

One variation of this type of traction includes the insertion of pins into the pelvic bones instead of the femurs. The pins are then attached to a pelvic hoop. Additional metal bars may be used to increase the traction by increasing the distance between the halo and the pelvic traction bands. The use of a mechanical turning frame is necessary for the care of these children.

Neurovascular assessment for the child in halo-femoral traction is extremely important as cranial nerve function may be impaired. Neurovascular assessment is, therefore, done once or twice per shift. An early sign of this functional impairment is loss of lateral gaze. These children are placed on a Stryker frame to facilitate care. A Circolectric bed may also be used. Adaptation to either of these pieces of equipment takes a period of time and patience. Immobility is frightening to children and enhances their fears, even with adequate explanations and preparation.

Surgical Intervention

Surgical intervention is used when adequate correction is not achieved with bracing and exercises, and in those patients with extreme curvature of greater than forty degrees. The goal of surgical treatment is to achieve a structurally balanced spinal column with an alignment that will be maintained permanently.

Surgical correction involves the use of internal and external fixation and instrumentation, as well as spinal fusion or arthrodesis. The specific type of correction used is dependent on the age of the child, the type of curvature, its location, the response to bracing, and other associated complications.

Some of the most common types of fixation involve the insertion of Harrington rods and the use of Dwyer screws and cables. These methods are used in conjunction with spinal fusion. The surgery is often performed in several stages in order to achieve optimal correction. This is always the case in rigid deformities. The first stage involves spinal release and application of skeletal traction. The second stage of the correction involves instrumentation and spinal fusion. Usually, the maximal result achieved is a fifty-percent correction.

Preoperatively, a number of tests are performed. Radiographic assessment includes full-length standing, anteroposterior, and lateral films to determine the degree of curvature and the effect on spinal balance. Bending films are also frequently done for these children. A myelogram is done in any child with congenital scoliosis to rule out other anomalies of the nervous system. An intravenous pyelogram is also done on these children because of the high incidence of associated anomalies of the urinary tract.

Pulmonary function tests are used to identify the degree of impairment or compensation. These are also used to predict the need for ventilatory assistance postoperatively. Hematologic studies and urinalysis are routinely done.

Once the surgical intervention is carried out, the child is cared for on a Stryker frame. The extensive nature of the surgical correction usually necessitates the use of an indwelling Foley catheter, a central venous pressure line, and cardiac monitoring. Some children are also on assisted ventilation with an endotracheal tube for a period of time, depending on pulmonary ventilation.

A Risser localizer cast is applied to this patient one to two weeks after the surgical correction, Figure 27-5. This is worn for three months after the surgery and then changed. At that time, a shorter cast may be applied if the correction is being maintained and good healing has taken place. This second type of cast may be worn for three to six months before removal and regular follow-up is continued for three to five years afterward.

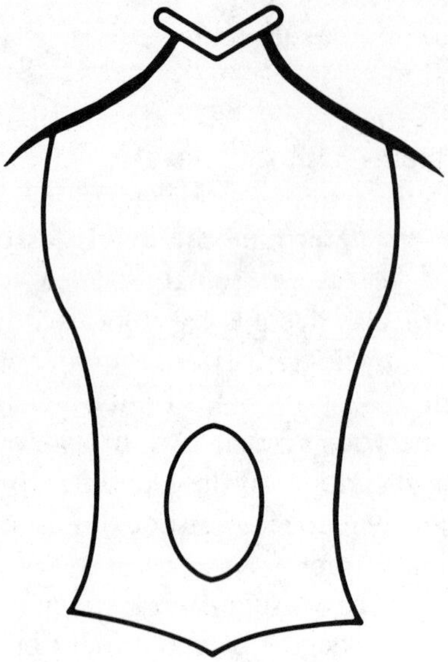

FIG. 27-5 A Risser localizer cast is used postoperatively for the adolescent who has undergone a spinal fusion or insertion of a Harrington rod.

Assisting Children and Parents

Helping the child and the parents adjust to the problem of scoliosis begins with the initial diagnosis and the information provided at that time. Booklets and teaching aids, as well as detailed explanations and the opportunity to ask questions, are extremely important. The information can be presented in several short sessions and repeated as necessary. In the interim, the parents and child have the booklets to use for reference.

It is helpful to use pictures to demonstrate particular types of casts, as well as the preoperative and postoperative appearance of the patient. The use of dolls for the demonstration of cast applications helps the young person look at casting more realistically.

Care of the brace, the exercise program, and the skin and hygienic care are the responsibility of the adolescent. It is also essential that the parents be taught this regimen for reinforcement purposes so that they may assist the young person whenever necessary. For the very young patient with congenital scoliosis, the therapeutic program is the primary responsibility of the parent. Skin and cast care, as well as assessment, are taught to the parents prior to hospital discharge.

For the child who must have surgery, the parents and child are taught logrolling techniques, use of a bedpan, transfer techniques, and hygienic care when necessary. These are all taught in the preoperative period when the child is least uncomfortable. In the early postoperative period, the parent may be reluctant to assist with care because of the fear of causing pain.

Fears must be addressed by the staff, as the parents and child may avoid any mention of them. These children frequently fear needles and injections. They should know that these will be kept to a minimum in the postoperative period. They are used as necessary to keep the child comfortable for the first several days, and then oral pain medications will be used.

Intrusive procedures, such as blood work and enemas, are also upsetting. The child should know what is going to be done and when. Enemas can usually be replaced by the use of suppositories and stool softeners. Diet can also be regulated to aid in elimination. The child should be told how he or she can help to avoid elimination problems.

Diversional activities are essential for these patients. In the hospital setting, the child-life worker can help provide emotional support as well as outlets for emotional expression. Occupational therapy activities are also used in this fashion. Tutoring may begin in the hospital or may commence in the home setting. This too, provides diversion, as well as promoting the child's education. Maintaining peer contact by telephone and visits is also a necessity for the adolescent.

With all of these children, it is imperative that the nurse emphasize the need for ongoing care of a long-term nature. In every part of the child's care, the nurse must encourage open and honest communication with the child and the parents. Other persons involved in this dialogue may include the school nurse, the public health nurse, and the social worker.

Family compliance to the therapeutic regimen is usually enhanced when the various aspects of care and the referrals are handled by a primary care nurse or one individual assigned to the child and family. This individual has an opportunity to understand the child's care fully and can also oversee any referral procedures. This system also provides a single person who can be contacted for clarification of questions and assistance with problems.

Financial assistance may be available to many of these families through the state Crippled Children's Services, the Easter Seal Society, and other federal sources. Private insurance covers some costs, but it frequently does not cover all expenses. The family may then be left with financial difficulties it may not be able to handle. This should be discussed openly with the family in order to eliminate this potential reason for noncompliance with the treatment.

REYE'S SYNDROME

Reye's syndrome is a type of encephalopathy caused by fatty liver degeneration. It was first described in 1963 and its incidence appears to be increasing across the country. The months of January and February have the greatest incidence of the disease.

Symptoms and Stages of the Disease

Characteristically, the onset of the disease occurs two to five days after a viral illness. It most commonly follows episodes of influenza B, Coxsackie, ECHO, and varicella viruses. The child's condition initially appears to be improving, but sudden persistent vomiting develops, accompanied by stupor, delirium or irrational behavior, seizures, and coma. The child's condition deteriorates rapidly, and death from cerebral edema may ensue if the disease is not recognized in time.

Specific stages of the disease have been identified. During stage I, the child is stuporous but is arousable for short periods when stimulated. The level of coma deepens in stage II; the child responds to painful stimuli with decorticate or flexion posturing. In stage III of the disease, the child assumes a position of decerebrate or hyperextension posturing. This may be either continuous or only upon painful stimuli. Spontaneous respirations are still present at this point. During stage IV, the child becomes flaccid with no spontaneous respirations or pupillary reflexes, Table 27-1.

Characteristically, blood studies reveal a high level of blood ammonia and an elevated SGOT level. A lumbar puncture reveals increasing intracranial pressure but normal spinal fluid

TABLE 27-1 Stages and Treatment of Reye's Syndrome

STAGE	SIGNS	TREATMENT
I	Persistent vomiting Confusion Stupor Delirium Arousal by stimuli for short periods Spontaneous respirations Hyperactive reflexes Positive Babinski reflex	Hypertonic intravenous glucose Intravenous fluids provided at maximum 2/3 of maintenance level for 24 hours Transfer to regional center for care
II	Stupor Responds only to painful stimuli Decorticate posturing Spontaneous respirations	Elective intubation done Osmotic diuretics given to reduce cerebral edema
III	Spontaneous respirations Hyperventilation secondary to central nervous system problem Responds only to deep pain stimuli Decerebrate posturing	Subarachnoid screw may be used to monitor intracranial pressure changes 2 volume exchange transfusions may be used every 12 hours
IV	Flaccid Absent pupillary reflex No spontaneous respirations	Mechanical ventilator used May reach this stage rapidly from onset

components. No organism is cultured, such as might be found with bacterial meningitis.

Treatment

These children are cared for in an intensive care area, preferably in regional pediatric centers. The total goal of the treatment is to reduce the cerebral edema. Mannitol or other osmotic diuretics and steroids are used intravenously. Hypertonic glucose is administered to control the edema as well as to supply the glucose that the depleted liver cannot provide.

Exchange transfusions are administered to reduce the elevated blood ammonia levels. These are done at twelve-hour intervals. Approximately one pint of blood is needed for every five pounds of body weight per day. The blood that is transfused must be fresh or no older than forty-eight hours because of the rising ammonia levels in the stored blood.

Mechanical ventilation is used with most of these children. It may be either assisted or total, but it is intended to maintain optimal levels of oxygenation for the child. While the child is on a respirator, paralytic agents are not used as they eliminate the pupillary reflex, which is part of the neurologic assessment.

Other forms of treatment for the child might include the use of a subarachnoid screw to monitor increased intracranial pressure. A craniectomy, or removal of a portion of the skull, may be performed. The bone is then frozen for later use. This allows the brain to expand in response to the edema thereby avoiding the effects of the pressure exerted by the skull.

Nursing Care

Total nursing care is required for this child. Great emphasis is placed on careful assessment of the child's changing condition. Neurologic checks are done every fifteen to thirty minutes. The nursing care also involves monitoring intravenous therapy, tracheostomy care, working with a respirator, and providing a great deal of emotional support for the family.

The suddenness of the disease onset makes it difficult for the family to cope with the worsening situation, particularly since the child was seemingly recuperating. The family should be reassured that, when diagnosis and treatment are instituted early, the chances for recovery are good. A long convalescence is associated with this disease, but the child can then usually achieve complete recovery. During this period of convalescence, physical therapy has an important role in strengthening muscles and maintaining range of motion until the child is able to assist actively and ultimately ambulate independently.

Recent studies indicate two other aspects of care which should be of concern to nurses. The use of salicylates for temperature control in the child with varicella is not recommended because of the increased incidence of Reye's Syndrome. Phenothiazines used in some children may also be implicated. Residual speech and learning disabilities may occur in infants one year of age and younger with the disease. Any child who has been in a coma may suffer brain damage which results in developmental delays, motor impairment, and possible retardation.

SEXUALLY TRANSMITTED DISEASES

In the past, this particular group of diseases was collectively referred to as venereal disease. Current terminology encompasses additional diseases that are also transmitted through sexual contact. The traditional list of such diseases includes gonorrhea, syphilis, chancroid, lymphogranuloma venereum, and granuloma inguinale. The current term of sexually transmitted diseases includes such entities as genital herpes, pediculi, scabies, monilial vaginitis, and trichomonas infections.

Adolescents comprise only twenty percent of the population, but account for over half of the cases of sexually transmitted diseases. Many cases are not treated and others are not reported, although they may be treated. Adolescents often do not seek medical attention. Many deny the existence of the problem or wait until the symptoms are so severe that they cannot be ignored. By this time, the disease may have spread extensively, and new sexual contacts may have acquired the disease. Only three of the major sexually transmitted diseases are discussed in this chapter: gonorrhea, syphilis, and genital herpes.

Gonorrhea

According to statistics from the Center for Disease Control in Atlanta, gonorrhea is the number one reportable disease. It is known in street language as "the clap," "the drip," and "the dose." The disease is transmitted exclusively by sexual contact, with pharyngitis and proctitis reflecting alternate modes of sexual behavior. Gonorrheal conjunctivitis or ophthalmia neonatorum is the only form that is not transmitted in this fashion. Instead, it is transmitted via the vaginal canal during the birthing process.

The organism responsible for the disease is a gram-positive diplococcus, *Neisseria gonorrhea.* It thrives on the moist, warm mucosa of the human body. The incubation period ranges from one day to thirty days, with the average incubation being about a week. The diagnosis is made on the basis of cultures obtained from the infected individual.

Many individuals with the disease are asymptomatic or have minor symptoms which are ignored. This is particularly true in females who may experience dysuria, increased vaginal discharge, and lower abdominal discomfort. None of the complaints may be severe enough to cause the young person to seek out medical assistance. In males, the symptoms are more obvious. They may notice a purulent discharge from the urethra, and pain or discomfort on urination, as well as urinary frequency, are usually present. Vague constitutional symptoms, such as malaise, headache, and low-grade fever, may also be evident. In some females, pelvic inflammatory disease is the first sign of the problem.

Diagnosis and Treatment. Smears and cultures are done to identify the infective organism. In the female, the smears are obtained from the cervix, vagina, and Skene's and Bartholin's glands. In the male, smears are obtained from the urethra and the rectum. Several considerations must be made by the nurse in obtaining the specimen. The speculum used to obtain the smear in females may not be lubricated with anything other than warm water. The sterile-tipped applicator should be held against each of the sites for several seconds to allow absorption of some of the organisms. The swab is then rolled in a large Z pattern on a Thayer-Martin or Transgrow medium, Figure 27-6. Both of these are selective antibiotic media which allows gonococci to grow. Thayer-Martin culture plates should be taken to the laboratory immediately for incubation. The Transgrow bottle contains a special cap which provides an increased carbon dioxide environment.

Treatment of both males and females involves the administration of 4.8 million units of aqueous procaine penicillin G in two injection sites. Bicillin is not recommended for use as it does not achieve a sufficiently high level of tissue saturation to kill the organism. For this

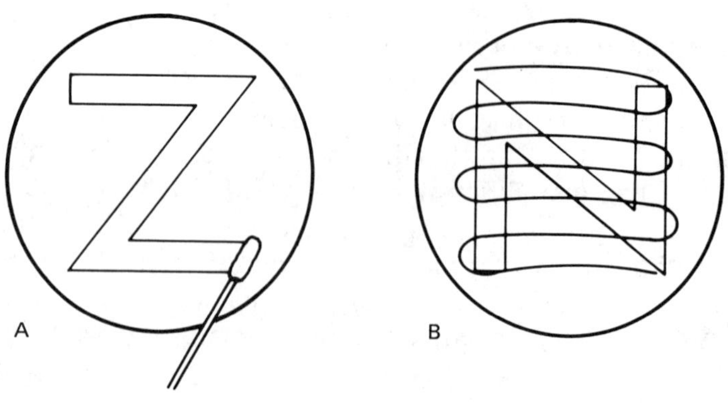

FIG. 27-6 Thayer-Martin culture. ***A)*** **Immediately roll the swab on the Thayer-Martin media in a large Z pattern.** ***B)*** **Cross-streak the plate with a sterile wire loop. (This may be done by laboratory personnel.)**

same reason, patients are given 1 gram of probenecid one-half hour prior to the injection. This drug slows the excretion rate of the penicillin through the kidneys and promotes higher blood levels of the drug. All patients should return to the clinic or doctor's office in one week to have a repeat smear and culture taken to determine the effectiveness of treatment.

In those individuals who are sensitive to penicillin, one of the tetracyclines is usually substituted. The dosage varies according to the specific preparation. Doxycycline, or Vibramycin, is given orally in a dose of 200 milligrams initially and then 100 milligrams at bedtime. An additional 100 milligrams is given twice a day for three days thereafter.

It is important for the nurse to explain the transmission of these diseases to the patient, as well as the method of treatment. Many individuals incorrectly assume that one case of the disease creates an immunity to it. The sexual contacts of the individual should also be treated, or the vicious cycle of treatment and subsequent reinfection will be repeated. Venereal disease clinics have specially trained individuals who interview the patient and who identify the contacts in an attempt to break this cycle.

Syphilis

Syphilis is a sexually transmitted disease that is only slightly less prevalent than gonorrhea. It is fourth on the list of reportable communicable diseases. The disease is caused by a spirochete, *Treponema pallidum.*

Syphilis has a comparatively long incubation period, with the average being twenty-one days. The incubation period for the secondary stage is an average of forty-six days. The disease may be transmitted during both the primary and the secondary stages if treatment is not initiated.

Stages. In the primary stage of syphilis, the site of penetration of the mucosa leaves a painless, indurated ulcer called a chancre. This single lesion can occur anywhere on the mucous membranes of the genitalia, rectum, lips, or mouth. It may not be noticed by the individual when it occurs on the cervix. The serous discharge from this ulcer is highly contagious. If untreated, this lesion disappears spontaneously in three to twelve weeks.

The secondary stage occurs six weeks to six months after the initial contact. This is a highly infectious stage and is characterized by a maculopapular rash, alopecia, fever, headache, and malaise, Table 27-2. Generalized lymphadenopathy can also occur and the disease may initially be mistaken for hepatitis or

TABLE 27-2 Stages of Syphilis

EARLY STAGE (Communicable)
Primary Stage
Chancre at entrance site of organisms
Fever
Slight weight loss
Enlarged regional lymph nodes
Secondary Stage
Maculopapular rash
Pharyngitis or laryngitis
General lymphadenopathy
Enlarged spleen and liver
Alopecia
Condylomata lata (wartlike lesions) on moist surfaces
LATE STAGE (Not communicable)
Occurs four years after the original infection
Tertiary Stage
Skin lesions – gumma, tumors, or ulcers
Bone lesions – destruction and deformity of any bone
Arthritis – monoarticular
Charcot's joint – disintegration of knee
Cardiovascular changes – aortic aneurysm
Neurologic changes – Tabes dorsalis; locomotor ataxia

kidney disease. Wartlike lesions called condylomata lata may appear on moist surfaces of the body. These are not the same as genital herpes and should not be confused with them.

Diagnosis and Treatment. Diagnosis is confirmed only after certain diagnostic tests are completed. The standard screening test is the VDRL (Venereal Disease Research Laboratory) or RPR test. The advantages of this type of test are its ease of performance and low cost. The major disadvantage is the possibility of false-positive reactions. Immunizations and recent febrile illnesses may cause an erroneous positive reaction.

An examination of the serum obtained from the chancre may also be done under a dark-field microscope, if available. The examiner must be skilled at distinguishing the organism, as spirochetes are often present normally, particularly in the mucosa of the mouth.

The FTA-ABS (Fluorescent Treponema Antibody Absorbed) test is a specific test that will yield a positive reaction early in the primary stage of the disease. Its disadvantages are that the test is difficult to perform and that it remains positive after the treatment is completed.

The treatment that is recommended for primary and secondary syphilis by the Center for Disease Control and that is carried out in the venereal disease program of most health departments includes:

- Benzathine penicillin G, 2.4 million units intramuscularly, one-half dose in each buttock, or
- Procaine penicillin G in oil PAM, 2.4 million units in divided doses at first session plus 1.2 million units twice in three-day intervals for a total dose of 4.8 million units, or
- Aqueous procaine penicillin G, 600,000 units intramuscularly daily for eight days, for a total dose of 4.8 million units.

In allergic patients, 500 milligrams of tetracycline is given orally four times a day for fifteen days for a total dose of 30 grams.

Repeat physical examinations are scheduled for these patients at three-month intervals during the first year and six-month intervals thereafter during the second year. By the end of the second year, the results of the VDRL test should be near normal if the patient has not been reinfected in the interim.

If left untreated, the disease progresses to the third stage, with involvement of the cardiovascular and neurologic systems. The disease is not infectious, but the damage is turned inward and any system may be affected.

GENITAL HERPES

Herpes virus Hominus (HVH) Type 2 is the virus associated with the occurrence of genital herpes infections in adolescents. The initial exposure to the organism usually produces systemic symptoms of fever, enlarged lymph nodes in the pelvic area, and dysuria. The cervix is the primary site of the infection in the female along with the vagina and the vulva. In males the lesions are located anywhere on the penis and occasionally on the scrotum.

The acute form of the disease is self-limiting and does not last beyond two weeks. Reinfection occurs, however, because many individuals carry this virus in an occult state. The reoccurrence often has no obvious signs of the infection with the lesions being limited to the cervix.

The diagnosis is made on the appearance of the vesicular lesions. A Papanicolaou smear with a special stain may be used or a tissue culture.

There is no specific treatment at this time. Phototherapy with the use of a proflavine dye is effective for some. Warm baths provide some relief from the discomfort.

Sex education and counseling are particularly important for the sexually active adolescent. Counseling should include support and encouragement for the young person to continue treatment and follow up until the organism is eradicated. The newest antiherpes agent is acyclovir (Zovirax).

Disease Control

The control of these diseases is primarily through education of the public, particularly adolescents and young adults. The changing attitudes in our society toward sexuality have a bearing on this education. In some areas, the flow of information regarding these diseases is hampered in the schools. Parents may protest the dissemination of information of this nature. Unfortunately, the parents do not always freely share this information with the young people who need it.

Some young people who are sexually active are afraid to share their concerns about having these diseases. They may seek medical attention only after the disease has been spread to others. The straightforward presentation of factual information is helpful to them. In some situations, this information may be better received if it is presented by the peer group rather than by adults.

In many states, juveniles may seek treatment at venereal disease clinics without the need for parental consent or notification. This policy encourages the juvenile to seek help early in suspected cases of venereal disease. Unfortunately, this method alienates some parents, particularly those who have a strong need for control within the family system.

ACNE VULGARIS

Acne vulgaris is the most common of all adolescent health problems, occurring in as much as ninety percent of the adolescent population. It occurs at the onset of puberty and may continue into the early adult period. It is caused by the action of hormones that are activated at the onset of puberty. These hormones stimulate the sebaceous glands. Excess sebum that is secreted into the hair follicle opening, bacteria that break up the fatty acids, and the irritating effect of the fatty acids on the skin then combine to produce comedones. The open comedones, or those without an epithelial covering, are commonly called blackheads or "zits" and are highly visible because of their coloring. The closed comedones, which have a thin epithelial covering, are often called whiteheads. If the rupture of the follicle walls is near the dermis, it produces larger lesions, such as pustules. When the rupture is deeper, a cyst or nodule is formed which can ultimately lead to scarring.

Patient Teaching

The emphasis of patient teaching should be on early treatment and care for the adolescent in order to prevent more serious problems. Cleansing of the skin, control of oiliness, and reduction of skin trauma are positive health care activities that can be used by the adolescent. In more severe cases, treatment by a dermatologist may be necessary.

Cleanliness of the skin is ensured by washing the face thoroughly several times a day. Adolescents should be instructed to lather thoroughly but gently for at least one minute.

They should then rinse the face carefully and repeat the procedure. A clean washcloth should be used each time this is done. Cleansing soaps that are recommended for acne may be used with this procedure. Afterwards, a drying agent may be applied to those areas that are unusually oily.

Along with this routine, the adolescent should avoid touching the face with the hands, if at all possible. The hair should be washed frequently and kept away from the face. Adequate rest and avoiding extreme physical stress also help to control acne.

Medical Treatment

Mechanical removal of both blackheads and whiteheads may be accomplished with the use of a comedo extractor. The face should be washed carefully and warm towels applied to facilitate the extraction. Use of the comedo extractor eliminates the temptation of the adolescent to pick or squeeze at the skin, thereby causing further skin trauma to adjacent areas. The face is washed carefully following the extraction procedure. The comedo extractor is then washed and stored in alcohol.

Severe types of inflammatory acne should be treated by a physician. Oral administration of tetracyclines may be the treatment of choice for some. Others may use intralesional injection of corticosteroids. Surgical incision and drainage is necessary for some lesions. An acid form of vitamin A can also be used topically to produce peeling and subsequent normal tissue repair.

After the period of acute acne has subsided and adolescence is completed, scars or pitting may be visible on the skin. This can be improved with the use of planing techniques or some form of dermabrasion. These techniques are limited to the superficial pitted scars.

EMOTIONAL DISORDERS

The period of adolescence can be one of turmoil for any individual. It is a period during which limits are tested and stretched, values are weighed, and physical growth is turbulent. Adolescents are seeking to establish their own separate identities, and in the process, need to evaluate the attitudes and values of their families. Many times this evaluation causes conflict.

Depression

One of the emotional problems seen in the adolescent is depression. The statistics related to accidents and suicides or attempted suicides support this premise. Adults frequently refuse to recognize that a young person may be depressed, sometimes so severely that an attempt is made to take their own life. In retrospect, many adults remember the adolescent years as ones of school activities, sports, dating, and new friends. They may remember only the happy times, forgetting the pain of not being asked to the dance, the silent telephone, and the laughter or ridicule of the peers.

Signs of Depression. The nurse should be able to recognize the signs of depression in children and seek help for them if they cannot or will not seek it for themselves. Children who are sad and look unhappy frequently complain about everything that happens to them. They may verbalize their dissatisfaction, blaming others for their feelings. These children are often unable to complete a project. When they do complete one, they may be unable to accept the fact that they have done it successfully.

Other children may feel rejected and unloved. These feelings might be evident in conversations regarding siblings or their relationship to their parents. Their feelings frequently cannot be shared with others. These young persons may have poor self-concepts, seeing themselves as having no value or little worth. Behavioral patterns, as well as conversations, may reflect this attitude.

Other adolescents may frequently act out their feelings in a negative manner. This may not be identified as depression initially because the adult recognizes only the disruptive behavior, not the underlying mechanism or the cry for help. Adolescents may suddenly become "class clowns." Defense mechanisms allow them to disregard their own feelings. Their very real fear is thus converted to laughter and giggling, which is more socially acceptable.

In some, the depression takes on a provocative or aggressive quality. These individuals are often involved in fighting with others, fighting itself being a self-destructive behavior. Overt delinquent behavior, such as drug abuse, may be seen. Such adolescents may have a criminal record and be well-known to the local police because of this type of behavior. This self-punitive or self-destructive behavior may initially be labeled by others as accident-proneness without the recognition of depression as the underlying cause.

Depression "equivalents" may be more easily recognized in adolescents than other signs of depression. Most are similar to those patterns seen in adults. They include insomnia, eating disturbances, somatization, obsessive-compulsive behavior and problems with bladder and bowel control.

Insomnia. The young person with insomnia sleeps only one to three hours per night. The remainder of the time is spent prowling the house or wandering about. Much of the time is spent in fantasizing. This daydreaming or fantasy life becomes more enjoyable than coping with the realities of depression and real life.

Eating Disturbances. The eating disturbances associated with depression may involve both excesses and insufficiencies. Severely obese adolescents have learned, as infants, that when they are unhappy and cry, the parents provide a bottle or a cookie or other food item. In later life, when they are depressed, they may provide themselves with a piece of pie or ice cream to alleviate their unhappiness.

The other extreme involves adolescents who envision themselves as being unacceptably overweight when, in fact, they are almost emaciated in appearance. This disorder is properly termed anorexia nervosa. Its incidence is increasing in middle and upper class families in this country.

Somatization. Somatization involves the use of recurrent aches and pains as socially acceptable reasons for failing to carry out one's responsibilities. These conditions include headache, dizziness, abdominal pain, and nausea. Because pain is so subjective, one cannot discount another's complaint. Adolescents are sometimes admitted to hospitals to determine the cause of chronic problems of this nature. The basis may be physiologic, but it can also be caused by depression.

Obsessive-Compulsive Behavior. The obsessive-compulsive individual carries out a ritual or routine many times throughout the day. This ritualization is similar in nature to the magic beliefs of the early school-aged child. It is a protective device and must be carried out in precisely the same manner every time. Adolescents who count to ten before speaking, or who wash their hands repeatedly before touching anything, are typically affected by this problem.

Bowel and Bladder Problems. Disturbances with bladder and bowel control are termed enuresis and encopresis, respectively. Enuresis is bedwetting, which is seen in children or adolescents who are well beyond the usual period of toilet training. It may continue despite the lack of any evidence of pathologic problems such as anomalies. Encopresis is similar, but involves fecal soiling. These conditions are both seen in older children, as well as in adolescents. These problems serve to isolate these children further because the conditions are unacceptable to the peer group.

Nursing Intervention

The nursing approach used with these patients involves the establishment of trust before all else. At the beginning of the treatment period, adolescents often test the nursing staff to the limit. They may exhibit anger and resentment in response to the care and concern demonstrated by the staff. The approach of the staff must be consistent, with a limited number of individuals directly involved in care of these adolescents. This enhances the consistency of both the approach and the communications. It also prevents these young patients from being overwhelmed by the number of staff members involved. Sharing confidences is often easier if only a few staff members are privy to them.

It is important for the staff to structure the care of these adolescents. The day should have a sense of routine to it, with limits set on waking and bedtime hours, as well as on tasks that must be accomplished. These tasks may include such activities as dressing, bedmaking, and studying. The structured schedule should include exercise or some other means of releasing energy that is acceptable to that particular adolescent, Figure 27-7.

PATIENT ACTIVITY CONTRACT

The following schedule and activities must be planned with your nurse. Exceptions or changes can be made with the approval of your nurse. Both of you must sign the contract at the bottom.

Get up by ______ AM

Get dressed by ______ AM

Take medication at scheduled times: ______ AM ______ PM

Participate in group meetings.

Participate in occupational therapy.

Exercise on the unit twice a day for 15 minutes.
Exercise chosen: ______________________________

Study or do homework at the following times: ______ AM ______ PM

Be in bed with lights off by ______ PM.

Patient ______________________________

Nurse ______________________________

FIG. 27-7 Contractual agreements with the adolescent patient allow some choice in planning care and activities and provide consistency in the expectations and evaluation of the entire nursing staff.

During the period of hospitalization, it is important for the adolescent to maintain the positive peer relationships that have already been established. If this is an impossibility, the nursing staff may be able to help the adolescent form peer relationships with other patients.

Throughout the delivery of care, the nurse must avoid assuming the role of the parent. Care plans should be developed in cooperation with the hospitalized adolescent rather than imposed upon him or her. Such impositions can destroy trust relationships that may have taken a considerable period of time to build. Throughout this period, the adolescent should know that the nursing staff members are not going to act as surrogate parents. Their relationship will end at the end of the hospitalization, although the patient may come back to visit staff members later.

The emotional upheaval that occurs in some adolescents does not occur in all adolescents. It is not a necessary part of the growth stage for each young person. However, when a young person expresses a desire to do away with themselves, it must be recognized as a cry for help.

Medical Treatment

During hospitalization, treatment for depression may involve psychotherapy as well as medications. The two major types of medications include the monoamine-oxidase inhibitors (MAO inhibitors) and the tricyclic antidepressants. The MAO inhibitor group includes such drugs as phenelzine (Nardil) and isocarboxazid (Marplan). Nursing care for an adolescent taking MAO inhibitors includes monitoring the vital signs, watching particularly for an increase in the blood pressure. The diet is restricted. All foods containing tyramine, one of the essential amino acids, are eliminated, as are foods that are aged or fermented. This group of drugs cannot be immediately followed by substitution with a tricyclic antidepressant. There must be a time lapse of at least three weeks to allow for complete excretion of these drugs.

The tricyclic antidepressants, such as amitryptyline (Elavil) and imipramine (Tofranil), also have specific nursing responsibilities associated with them. The side effects are similar to those of the anticholinergics, including dry mouth and alteration of vital signs. Both constipation and urinary retention may signify a need for reduction of the dosage.

It takes a period of time for any of these drugs to achieve a therapeutic effect. During that initial period, the adolescent must be placed in a protective environment and observed closely to prevent a possible suicide attempt. This surveillance is unusually stressful for these adolescents as it is in direct conflict with their need for privacy.

ANOREXIA NERVOSA

Anorexia nervosa is a disease of psychosocial origin characterized by starvation and excessive weight loss. It is much more common in girls than boys, occurring in a ratio of ten to one.

Some therapists have identified specific criteria for the diagnosis of anorexia. The person is usually under 25 years of age. The weight loss that occurs is 25 percent or more of total body weight. The individual has a distorted attitude toward eating, food, or weight which overrides both hunger and reason. There is an absence of any medical illness or psychiatric illness that would account for the weight loss. The person also has at least two or more of the following symptoms: bulimia, lanugo, amenorrhea, periods of overactivity, and bradycardia. Initially, the young person may undergo a great deal of diagnostic work in order to identify a nonexistent endocrine, metabolic, or gastrointestinal problem that is perceived as the cause of the severe weight loss.

Other factors which contribute to the disease include the young person's inability to live up to family expectations. Low self-esteem combined with an unrealistic idea of perfection cause the youngster to see this excess weight loss as desirable. The value society places on slenderness reinforces the self-starvation and weight loss.

These patients often describe a lack of control over their own lives. Maintaining the diet demonstrates to the world that they have control. This rigid control is maintained in spite of parental urging, threats, and punishment. Each break in the diet or mouthful of food taken beyond what is considered acceptable by the adolescent evokes a renewed vigor in maintaining the diet with even more restrictions.

A rapidly changing body increases the anxiety of this young person. Sexual fears that are not recognized, bodily changes of puberty, and new feelings about physical development also play a part.

One of the behaviors that is identified by the family or which may be observed on the hospital unit is a fanatic determination to avoid weight gain. The parent may give a description of the daily meal plan of the adolescent as no breakfast, plain lettuce for lunch, and a piece of fruit or several tablespoons of vegetables for supper. Forcing the adolescents to eat usually results in trips to the bathroom where hidden food is disposed of or self-induced vomiting occurs. This latter behavior may eventually result in a binge-purge pattern of eating great amounts of food followed by vomiting, laxatives, and enemas to eliminate the food. Extreme exercise programs are often used to avoid weight gain.

Denial is very much a part of this young person's behavor. These individuals refuse to see the seriousness of the weight reduction and its consequences, insisting that there is nothing wrong. This denial extends to the body image, as well; they see themselves as "too fat," when in the mirror they appear cachectic from weight loss.

Treatment involves establishing a therapeutic environment in which patients feel a sense of control over their lives and a new pattern of learned behaviors which aid in interactions with family and peers. Behavioral modification is an important tool for treatment of the malnutrition. Psychotherapy for the family group as well as the young person deals with the emotional problems.

The goals for treatment are the development of good eating habits, an acceptable weight gain, an improved physical appearance, and improvement in emotional status and interpersonal relationships. In the hospital setting, these goals take two to four months to achieve with follow-up care as an outpatient.

Nursing Care

Upon admission to the unit, time is spent in careful assessment of the physical status of the patient. Current weight is documented and weighing is done in only a hospital gown. Vital signs including blood pressure are taken. Bradycardia, a subnormal temperature, and low blood pressure are common findings. The basal metabolic rate is low. The skin is usually dry, with poor turgor and little subcutaneous tissue. Downy hair (lanugo) often covers the normally hairless parts of the body — for example, over the buttocks. A lack of secondary sex characteristics appropriate for the person's age is a common finding. Poor muscle tone and function as well as constipation are also usually present.

The goals and rewards are set by the therapist and explained to the patient at the beginning of the program. Emphasis is on the patient's ability to control what food is eaten, how much weight is gained, and what privileges are received. Reinforcement is on a daily basis in an immediate and consistent but nonpunitive way.

Goals for weight gain are usually established at 1/4 to 1/2 pound per day. Hyperalimentation and nasogastric tube feedings may be done initially for the severely malnourished patient. Acceptable weight gain is rewarded with privileges such as using the phone, sending mail, wearing personal clothing, and removal of time restrictions for completion of meals.

Initially, highly manipulative behavior may be used by the patient to continue losing weight. Hiding or discarding food as well as vomiting may occur. The patient may be consuming excessive amounts of water or hiding weights on the body prior to weighing in the morning. Denial, lying, and cheating are common behaviors that must be handled. One staff member on each shift should have decision-making responsibility for this patient. Any changes in privileges, routines, or care are transmitted in writing. This avoids being entrapped by the patient's manipulation. Frequent team conferences aid in maintaining both consistent and effective care for this patient. Long-term therapy both in and out of the hospital is usually necessary for successful treatment.

A national organization of patients and families which provides for education about this problem is the National Association of Anorexia Nervosa and Associated Disorders, Highland Park, Illinois 60035.

SUMMARY

The health problems of adolescents range from mild cases of acne to severe depression. Each of the health problems considered in this chapter directly affects a specific system. Each in its own way has implications not only for the body image, but also for the individual's self-concept.

Physically, adolescents may be an adult size, but emotionally, they seldom are. For this reason, nursing care for each of the health problems identified must be directed toward relieving much of the emotional distress, as well as caring for the physical or emotional problem presented by the patient.

SUGGESTED ACTIVITIES

- Visit a venereal disease clinic within the local health department in your area. Determine the services that are offered and the requirements for receiving help.
- Care for an adolescent with one of the conditions discussed in this chapter. Describe the care and treatment used and compare it with that presented in the text.
- Tour a hospital where adolescents are treated for scoliosis. Note the clinic facilities for screening, as well as the methods of treatment observed.

DISCUSSION TOPICS

1. Discuss the impact of traction, braces, and costs on an adolescent's concept of body image.
2. Identify ways to improve the self-esteem of adolescents who are hospitalized for any of the health problems discussed in this chapter.

REVIEW

A. Matching. Match the description in Column I with the disease in Column II.

Column I	Column II
1. Lateral curvature of the spinal column with or without rotation	a. Syphilis
2. Encephalopathy characterized by increased intracranial pressure	b. Gonorrhea
3. Venereal disease diagnosed by cultures on a Thayer-Martin media	c. Scoliosis
4. Viral infection which produces vesicles on the cervix	d. Genital herpes
5. Disease caused by the *Treponema pallidum*	e. Reye's syndrome

B. Multiple choice. Select the one best answer.

1. Jim is a fifteen-year-old boy who asks your advice about painful urination and a "whitish discharge" from the penis. You recognize this as the usual signs of
   a. syphilis.
   b. genital herpes.
   c. Reye's syndrome.
   d. gonorrhea.

2. Jim (from question 1) is diagnosed and treated at a local clinic. Follow-up care should include the following instructions:
   a. Return in one week for a repeat culture and smear.
   b. Remain on medication for at least one month.
   c. Tell him he is now immune to future exposures of the disease.
   d. Return for a blood test twice a year.

3. A classmate of Jim's developed Reye's syndrome. Common characteristics of Reye's syndrome include
   1. a predominance in children who are two to sixteen years old.
   2. a preceding viral-type illness that lasts two to five days.
   3. a maximal duration of one to two weeks.
   4. intractable vomiting.
   a. 1 and 3
   b. 1, 3 and 4
   c. 2, 3 and 4
   d. 1, 2 and 4

4. Characteristic laboratory findings in patients with Reye's syndrome include
   a. elevated SGOT, elevated blood ammonia, and increased intracranial pressure.
   b. decreased blood sugar and elevated triglycerides.
   c. elevated cholesterol, elevated blood ammonia, and hyperglycemia.
   d. decreased blood ammonia, hypoglycemia, and elevated cholesterol.

C. Short answer. Briefly respond to the following statements.

1. Describe the cleansing techniques a nurse might teach an adolescent with acne.

2. List what information might be included in the preoperative teaching for an adolescent who will have a Harrington rod inserted for scoliosis.

3. Name five behavioral patterns that may indicate an emotional disturbance in an adolescent.

BIBLIOGRAPHY

Anderson, Beverly. "Carole, A Girl Treated With Bracing." *American Journal of Nursing,* Vol. 79 (September, 1979), pp. 1592–1597.

Anderson, F. J. "The Developmental Experience of Adolescence." *Issues in Comprehensive Pediatric Nursing,* Vol. 1 (July–August, 1976), pp. 2–16.

Brown, M.A. "Syphilis and Gonorrhea." *Nursing 76,* Vol. 6 (January, 1976), pp. 71–74.

Brown, William J. "Acquired Syphilis – Drugs and Blood Tests." *American Journal of Nursing,* Vol. 71 (April, 1971), pp. 713–715.

Cantrell, Dee. "Scoliosis: Screening Potential Victims." *RN,* Vol. 39 (November, 1976), p. 55.

Christopherson, Edward R., and Raoul Berman. "Encopresis Treatment." *Issues in Comprehensive Pediatric Nursing,* Vol. 3 (October, 1978), pp. 51–66.

Claggett, Marilyn Smith. "Anorexia Nervosa: A Behavioral Approach." *American Journal of Nursing,* Vol. 80 (August, 1980), pp. 1471–1472.

Evans, Jane C., and Carolynn E. Singleton. "Acne: The Scourge of Adolescence." *Issues in Comprehensive Pediatric Nursing,* Vol. 1 (July–August, 1976), pp. 60–68.

Graf, Christina M. "Sexually Transmitted Disease: A New Look at an Old Problem." *Issues in Comprehensive Pediatric Nursing,* Vol. 2 (March–April, 1978), pp. 11–20.

Hein, E., and M. Leavitt. "Providing Emotional Support to Patients." *Nursing 77,* Vol. 7 (May, 1977), pp. 38–41.

Hilt, N., and K. E. Schmidt. *Pediatric Orthopedic Nursing.* St. Louis: C. V. Mosby Company, 1975.

Holt de Toledo, Catherine. "The Patient with Scoliosis – The Defect: Classification and Detection." *American Journal of Nursing,* Vol. 79 (September, 1979), pp. 1588–1591.

Holt de Toledo, Catherine. "The Orthoplast Jacket." *American Journal of Nursing,* Vol. 79 (September, 1979), p. 1598.

Kalafatich, Audrey J. *Approaches to the Care of Adolescents.* New York: Appleton-Century-Crofts, 1975.

Lenz, Philomene. "Women, the Unwitting Carriers of Gonorrhea." *American Journal of Nursing,* Vol. 71 (April, 1977), pp. 716–718.

Martelli, Mary Elizabeth. "Teaching Parents About Reye's Syndrome." *American Journal of Nursing,* Vol. 82 (February, 1982), pp. 260–263.

Melton, Janet Howell. "A Boy with Anorexia Nervosa." *American Journal of Nursing,* Vol. 74 (September, 1974), pp. 1649–1651.

Micheli, Lyle J., et al. "The Patient with Scoliosis – Surgical Management and Nursing Care." *American Journal of Nursing,* Vol. 79 (September, 1979), pp. 1599–1607.

Minuchin, Salvador, et al. *Psychosomatic Families: Anorexia Nervosa in Context.* Cambridge, MA: Harvard Universty Press, 1978.

Misik, Irene M. "When the Anorectic Patient Challenges You." *Nursing 81,* Vol. 11 (December, 1981), pp. 46–49.

Nathan, S.W. "Body Image of Scoliotic Female Adolescents Before and After Surgery." *Maternal-Child Nursing Journal,* Vol. 6 (Fall, 1977), pp. 139–149.

Nignona, S. "Scoliosis." *Nursing 77,* Vol. 7 (May, 1977), pp. 50–55.

Page-Goertz, Sallie S., and Lester L. Lansky. "Reye's Syndrome: An Overview of Nursing and Medical Management." *Issues in Comprehensive Pediatric Nursing,* Vol. 1 (May, 1977), pp. 40–56.

Patterson, T. "Scoliosis: Cotrel's Traction and the Risser Cast." *RN,* Vol. 39 (November, 1976), pp. 66–74.

Patterson T. "Scoliosis: The Patient in Braces." *RN,* Vol. 39 (November, 1976), pp. 60–66.

Patterson T. "Scoliosis: The Patient's First Visit." *RN,* Vol. 39 (November, 1976), pp. 58–60.

Richardson, Thomas F. "Anorexia Nervosa: An Overview." *American Journal of Nursing,* Vol. 80 (August, 1980), pp. 1470–1471.

Ross Laboratories. *Common Orthopedic Conditions in Childhood.* Columbus, Ohio: Ross Laboratories, 1973, pp. 38–43.

Schatzinger, Lynn H., et al. "Spinal Fusion: Emotional Stress and Adjustment." *American Journal of Nursing,* Vol. 79 (September, 1979), pp. 1608–1612.

Schmidt, Mary P. W., and Beverly A. B. Duncan. "Modifying Eating Behavior in Anorexia Nervosa." *American Journal of Nursing,* Vol. 74 (September, 1974), pp. 1646–1648.

Strong, Cynthia, and Mary Gavaghan. "Scoliosis and Its Implications." *Issues in Comprehensive Pediatric Nursing,* Vol. 2 (November–December, 1977), pp. 33–45.

Wiley, Loy, et al. "Nursing Care of a Suicidal Adolescent." *Nursing 80,* Vol. 10 (April, 1980), pp. 56–59.

Appendix

APPENDIX A	Normal Vital Signs in Children
APPENDIX B	Nomogram for Computing Total Body Surface Area (BSA)
APPENDIX C	Hematology (Courtesy of Vaughan, V.C.; McKay, R.J.; and Behrman, R.E. *Nelson Textbook of Pediatrics,* 11th ed. Philadelphia: W. B. Saunders Co., 1979.)
APPENDIX D	Urinalysis (Courtesy of Vaughan, V.C.; McKay, R.J.; and Behrman, R.E. *Nelson Textbook of Pediatrics,* 11th ed. Philadelphia: W. B. Saunders Co., 1979.)
APPENDIX E	Lumbar Cerebrospinal Fluid (Courtesy of Vaughan, V.C.; McKay, R.J.; and Behrman, R.E. *Nelson Textbook of Pediatrics,* 11th ed. Philadelphia: W. B. Saunders Co., 1979.)
APPENDIX F	Declaration of the Rights of the Child
APPENDIX G	Voluntary Health Agencies
APPENDIX H	Denver Developmental Screening Test (Courtesy of William K. Frankenbury, M.D., and Josiah B. Dodds, Ph.D., University of Colorado Medical Center)
APPENDIX I	Recommended Daily Dietary Allowances (Courtesy of the National Dairy Council)
APPENDIX J	Growth Charts (Adapted from the National Center for Health Statistics; Courtesy of Ross Laboratories)

APPENDIX A. NORMAL VITAL SIGNS IN CHILDREN

AGE	PULSE Average	PULSE Range	RESPIRATIONS (Average)	BLOOD PRESSURE (Average)
Up to 1 yr	120	80–160	30	90/61
2 yr	110	80–130	25	96/65
4 yr	100	80–120	23	99/65
6 yr	100	75–115	21	100/56
8 yr	90	70–110	20	105/57
10 yr	90	70–110	19	109/58
12 yr	Girls, 90	70–110	19	113/59
	Boys, 85	65–105		
14 yr	Girls, 85	65–105	18	118/61
	Boys, 80	60–100		
16 yr	Girls, 80	60–100	17	122/78
	Boys, 75	55–95		

APPENDIX B. NOMOGRAM FOR COMPUTING TOTAL BODY SURFACE AREA (BSA)

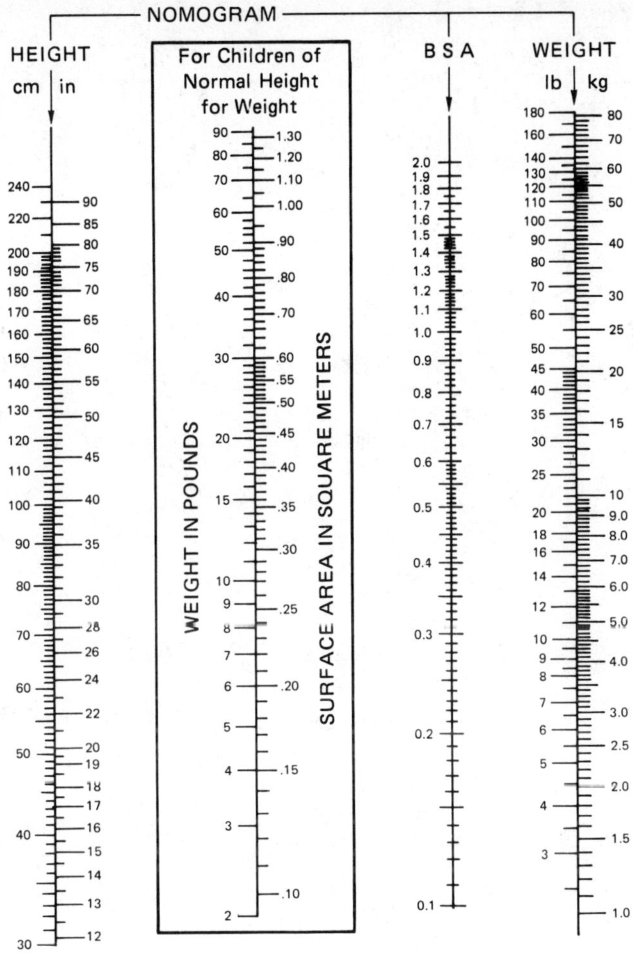

BSA is indicated where straight line that connects height and weight levels intersects BSA column or, if patient is about average size, from weight alone (enclosed area). (Modified from data of E. Boyd by C. D. West. From Shirkey and Barba.)

APPENDIX C. HEMATOLOGY

DETERMINATION	AGE/SEX	NORMAL RANGE
(whole blood unless otherwise indicated)		
Hematocrit (PCV)	Cord	50–60%
	Newborn	53–65
	Neonate	43–54
	Infant	30–40
	Child	31–43
	Thereafter: M	42–52
	F	37–47
Hemoglobin*	Cord	14–20 g/dl
	Newborn	15–22
	Neonate	11–20
	Infant	10–15
	Child	11–16
	Thereafter: M	14–18
	F	12–16
Hemoglobin, fetal (HbF)	Newborn	40–70% of total
	Neonate	20–40
	Infant	2–10
	Thereafter	1–2
Hemoglobin, A_1	Child/adult	5.3–7.2% of total hemoglobin
Hemoglobin, A_{10}	Child/adult	3.5–5.1% of total hemoglobin
Nucleated RBCs	Cord	250–500/mm^3
	Day 1	200–300
	Day 2	20–30
	Thereafter	0
Osmotic fragility (fresh specimen) (50% hemolysis)		0.42–0.46% NaCl
Platelet count	Cord	100–290 000/mm^3
	Premature	100–300 000
	Newborn	140–300 000
	Neonate	150–390 000
	Infant	200–473 000
	Thereafter	150–450 000
Red blood cell count (RBC)	Newborn	4.4–5.8 mil/mm^3
	Neonate	4.1–6.4
	Infant/Child	3.8–5.5
	Thereafter: M	4.7–6.1
	F	4.2–5.4
Blood indices		
MCH	Newborn	32–34 pg ($\mu\mu$g)
	Thereafter: M	27–31
	F	27–31
MCV	Newborn	96–108 fl (μ^3)
	Thereafter: M	80– 94
	F	81– 99
MCHC	Newborn	32–33%
	Thereafter: M	32–36
	F	32–36
Reticulocyte count	Cord	3.0–7.0% total RBC
	Newborn	1.1–4.5
	Neonate	0.1–1.5
	Infant	0.5–3.1
	Thereafter	0.0–2.0
Sedimentation rate (ESR) (uncorrected)	Newborn	0–2 mm/hr
	Neonate/Child	3–13
	Thereafter: M <40 years	1–15
	>40	1–20
	F <40	1–20
	>40	1–30

White blood cell count (WBC)†

	Total mm^3	*$\bar{X}$% neutrophils*	*$\bar{X}$% lymphocytes*
Newborn	9000–30,000	61	31
1 wk	5000–21,000	45	41
4 wk	5000–19,500	35	56
6–12 mo	6000–17,500	32	61
2 yr	6200–17,000	33	59
Child/Adult	4800–10,800	60	30

*During the neonatal period, hemoglobin measurements from capillary blood are 2–3 g/dl greater than those in blood obtained by venipuncture.

†Eosinophilia (up to 20% of white blood cell count) may occur normally in infancy.

Used with permission of Vaughan, V.C.; McKay, R.J.; and Behrman, R.E. *Nelson Textbook of Pediatrics*, 11th ed. Philadelphia: W.B. Saunders Co., 1979.

APPENDIX D. URINALYSIS

DETERMINATION		AGE/SEX	NORMAL RANGE		
Addis count	Leukocytes		<10		
	Erythrocytes		< 5		
	Casts		occasional hyaline		
Colony count, colonies/ml urine (fresh specimen)			*Clean Catch, Midstream**	*Catheter-ization*	*Suprapubic Bladder Puncture*
		Infant/Child	< 1,000	100	0
		Thereafter	<10,000	100	0
Microscopic	Leukocytes		0–4 per high-power field		
	Erythrocytes		rare per high-power field		
	Casts		rare per high-power field		
Osmolarity		Premature/Newborn	50– 600 mOsm/l		
		Thereafter	50–1400		
		Thereafter	>850 (after fluid restriction)		
pH		Newborn/Neonate	5.0–7.0		
		Thereafter	4.8–7.8		
Protein	qualitative		Negative		
	quantitative		10–100 mg/d (higher after strenuous exercise)		
Specific gravity, random		Newborn/Infant	1.001–1.020		
		Thereafter	1.001–1.030		
		Thereafter	>1.025 (after fluid restriction)		
Sugar, qualitative (including glucose)			Negative		
Volume		Newborn/Neonate	50– 300 ml/d		
		Infant	350– 550		
		Child	500–1000		
		Adolescent	700–1400		
		Thereafter: M	800–2000		
		F	800–1600		

*Pure cultures with colony counts >100,000 are considered diagnostic in adults, whereas colony counts of >10,000 are usually considered diagnostic in children. Intermediate counts must be interpreted relative to the clinical situation. For females, the physician must be aware of the cleanliness and care used in collecting the specimen. Urine obtained by means of a plastic collection device or by voiding into a container without prior preparation of the patient is usually contaminated, and has limited usefulness in evaluating the possibility of urinary tract infections.

Used with permission of Vaughan, V.C.; McKay, R.J.; and Behrman, R.E. *Nelson Textbook of Pediatrics,* 11th ed. Philadelphia: W.B. Saunders Co., 1979.

APPENDIX E. LUMBAR CEREBROSPINAL FLUID

DETERMINATION	AGE	NORMAL RANGE		
Albumin/globulin ratio		1.6–2.2		
Albumin, quantitative		10–30 mg/dl		
Calcium		4.2–5.4 mg/dl		
Cell Count		*Polymorpho-nuclear*	$WBCs/mm^3$ *Mono-nuclear*	$RBCs/mm^2$
	Premature	0–100*	0–25*	0–1000*
	Newborn	0– 70*	0–20*	0– 800*
	Neonote, early	0– 25	0– 5	0– 50
	Neonate, late	0– 5	0– 5	0– 10
	Thereafter	0	0– 5	0– 5
Chloride	Newborn Thereafter	108–122 mmol/l 118–132		
Cholinesterase		13–21 mU/ml		
Glucose (40–60% of blood or serum glucose level)	Newborn Infant/child Thereafter	30–80 mg/dl 60–80 40–70		
Immunoglobins		IgG: 0.8–6.4 mg/dl IgA: 0.4–0.6 IgM: Negative		
Lactate		0.1–1.0 mmol/l		
Lactate dehydrogenase (LDH) (1→p; 30°C)	Newborn Child Adult	2.3– 8.4 U/l 0.0–20.0 6.3–30.0		
Magnesium		2.2–3.0 mmol/l		
Pandy test		Negative		
pH (37°C)		7.33–7.42		
Potassium		2.8–4.1 mmol/l		
Protein, total	Premature Newborn Child Adolescent Thereafter	40–300† mg/dl 45–100 10–20 15–30 15–45 (Turbidimetric method) 8–32 (Column method)		
Protein electrophoresis		prealbumin 2.9–5.3% albumin 56.8–68.0 α_1 globulin 4.1–6.4 α_2 globulin 6.2–10.2 β globulin 10.8–14.8 γ globulin 6.1–8.3		
Sodium		138–150 mmol/l		
Specific gravity		1.007–1.009		
Transaminases:				
Aspartate aminotransferase (SGOT, AST; 30°C)		2–10 U/l		
Alanine aminotransferase (SGPT, ALT; 30°C)		None detected		
Xanthochromia		Absent		

*Numbers of cells greater than observed in older infants' CSF occur in many newly born infants who grow and develop normally.

†Values greater than 100 mg/dl are seen in many prematurely born infants (without RBCs in CSF) who grow and develop normally.

Used with permission of Vaughan, V.C.; McKay, R.J.; and Behrman, R.E. *Nelson Textbook of Pediatrics.* 11th ed. Philadelphia: W.B. Saunders Co., 1979.

APPENDIX F. DECLARATION OF THE RIGHTS OF THE CHILD

Preamble

Whereas the people of the United Nations have, in the Charter, reaffirmed their faith in fundamental human rights, and in the dignity and worth of the human person, and have determined to promote social progress and better standards of life in larger freedom.

Whereas the United Nations has, in the Universal Declaration of Human Rights, proclaimed that everyone is entitled to all the rights and freedoms set forth therein, without distinction of any kind, such as race, color, sex, language, religion, political or other opinion, national or social origin, property, birth or other status.

Whereas the child, by reason of his physical and mental immaturity, needs special safeguards, and care, including appropriate legal protection, before as well as after birth.

Whereas the need for such special safeguards has been stated in the Geneva Declaration of the Rights of the Child in 1924, and recognized in the Universal Declaration of Human Rights and in the statutes of specialized agencies and international organizations concerned with the welfare of children.

Whereas mankind owes to the child the best it has to give.

Now therefore,

The General Assembly

Proclaims this Declaration of the Rights of the Child to the end that he may have a happy childhood and enjoy for his own good and for the good of society the rights and freedoms herein set forth, and calls upon parents, upon men and women as individuals and upon voluntary oganizations, local authorities and national governments to recognize these rights and strive for their observance by legislative and other measures progressively taken in accordance with the following principles:

Principle 1

The child shall enjoy all the rights set forth in this Declaration. All children, without any exception whatsoever, shall be entitled to these rights, without distinction or discrimination on account of race, color, sex, language, religion, political or other opinion, national or social origin, property, birth or other status, whether of himself or of his family.

Principle 2

The child shall enjoy special protection, and shall be given opportunities and facilities, by law and by other means, to enable him to develop physically in a healthy and normal manner and in conditions of freedom and dignity. In the enactment of laws for this purpose the best interests of the child shall be the paramount consideration.

Principle 3

The child shall be entitled from his birth to a name and a nationality.

Principle 4

The child shall enjoy the benefits of social security. He shall be entitled to grow and develop in health; to this end special care and protection shall be provided both to him and to his mother, including adequate pre-natal and post-natal care. The child shall have the right to adequate nutrition, housing, recreation and medical services.

Principle 5

The child who is physically, mentally or socially handicapped shall be given the special treatment, education and care required by his particular condition.

Principle 6

The child, for the full and harmonious development of his personality, needs love and understanding. He shall, wherever possible, grow up in the care and under the responsibility of his parents, and in any case in an atmosphere of affection and of moral and material security; a child of tender years shall not, save in exceptional circumstances, be separated from his mother. Society and the public authorities shall have the duty to extend particular care to children without a family and to those without adequate means of support. Payment of state and other assistance toward the maintenance of children of large families is desirable.

Principle 7

The child is entitled to receive education, which shall be free and compulsory, at least in the elementary stages. He shall be given an education which will promote his general culture, and enable him on a basis of equal opportunity to develop his abilities, his individual judgment, and his sense of moral and social responsibility, and to become a useful member of society.

The best interests of the child shall be the guiding principle of those responsible for his education and guidance; that responsibility lies in the first place with his parents.

The child shall have full opportunity for play and recreation, which should be directed to the same purposes as education; society and the public authorities shall endeavor to promote the enjoyment of this right.

Principle 8

The child shall in all circumstances be among the first to receive protection and relief.

Principle 9

The child shall be protected against all forms of neglect, cruelty and exploitation. He shall not be the subject of traffic, in any form.

The child shall not be admitted to employment before an appropriate minimum age; he shall in no case be caused or permitted to engage in any occupation or employment which would prejudice his health or education, or interfere with his physical, mental or moral development.

Principle 10

The child shall be protected from practices which may foster racial, religious and any other form of discrimination. He shall be brought up in a spirit of understanding, tolerance, friendship among peoples, peace and universal brotherhood and in full consciousness that his energy and talents should be devoted to the service of his fellow men.

APPENDIX G. VOLUNTARY HEALTH AGENCIES

Alexander Graham Bell Association for the Deaf
1537 35th St., N.W.
Washington, DC 20007
Education, research, direct services through local groups

Allergy Foundation of America
801 Second Avenue
New York NY 10017
Education, research

American Academy of Pediatrics
P.O. Box 1034
Evanston, IL 60204
Research, education, standards for child care

American Cancer Society, Inc.
219 East 42nd St.
New York, NY 10017
Direct service through local chapters, education, research

American Celiac Society
45 Gifford Ave.
Jersey City, NJ 07304
Education, research, direct services through local groups

American Dental Association
222 East Superior St.
Chicago, IL 60611
Education, research, legislation

American Diabetes Association
1 East 45th St.
New York, NY 10017
Education, research

American Foundation for the Blind, Inc.
15 West 16th St.
New York, NY 10011
Education, research, legislation, local chapters

American Hearing Society, Inc.
919 18th St., N.W.
Washington, DC 20006
Direct services (hearing testing, lip reading, auditory training, speech correction, vocational guidance), education

American Heart Association
7320 Greenville Ave.
Dallas, TX 75231
Direct services through local or regional chapters, education, research, rehabilitation programs for children and adults

American Hospital Association
841 North Lakeshore Drive
Chicago, IL 60611
Education, research, hospital standards, publications

American Lung Association
1740 Broadway
New York, NY 10019
Education, research, direct services through local chapters

American Medical Association
535 N. Dearborn Street
Chicago, IL 60610
Education, research, legislation, publications

American Nurses' Association
10 Columbus Circle
New York, NY 10019
Education, publications, legislation

Arthritis and Rheumatism Foundation
10 Columbus Circle
New York, NY 10019
Education, research

The Candlelighters
123 C Street, S.E.
Washington, DC 20003
Support groups for parents of young cancer patients

Caring P.O. Box 196
Milton, WA 98354
Support group for parents of children with Down's syndrome

Child Welfare League of America
44 East 23rd Street
New York, NY 10010
Publications, standards for care, organization of agencies

Epilepsy Foundation of America
1828 L St., N.W.
Suite 406
Washington, DC 20036
Education, research

Joseph P. Kennedy Foundation
Room 3021
200 Park Avenue
New York, New York 10017
Education, publications, research in retardation

LaLeche League, International
9616 Minneapolis Ave.
Franklin Park, IL 60131
Education, publications, direct services through local groups

Leukemia Society of America, Inc.
211 East 43rd St.
New York, NY 10017
Education, publications, research, direct service through local groups

Medic Alert Foundation
1000 N. Palm
Turlock, CA 95380
Medical identification emblems, information available on a 24-hour basis for emergency treatment

Muscular Dystrophy Association of America, Inc.
810 Seventh Avenue
New York, NY 10019
Education, research, publications, direct aid to victims through local chapters

National Association for Mental Health, Inc.
10 Columbus Circle
New York, NY 10019
Education, research, direct services through clinics

National Association for Retarded Children, Inc.
420 Lexington Avenue
New York, NY 10017
Education, research

National Cancer Institute
Office of Cancer Communications
Bethesda, MD 20014
Education, publications

National Cystic Fibrosis Research Foundation
3379 Peachtree Rd., N.E.
Atlanta, GA 30326
Education, research, direct services through local chapters

The National Foundation – March of Dimes
880 Second Avenue
New York, NY 10017
Education, research, direct services to children under ten years

National Hemophilia Foundation
175 Fifth Avenue
New York, NY 10003
Education, research, direct services through state clinics to victims

National Kidney Foundation
116 East 27th St.
New York, NY 10016
Education, research

National Society for Crippled Children and Adults, Inc.
2023 W. Ogden Ave.
Chicago, IL 60612
Education, research, direct services through state and local chapters

National Society for the Prevention of Blindness, Inc.
79 Madison Ave.
New York, NY 10016
Education, research

National Sudden Infant Death Syndrome Foundation
310 S. Michigan Ave.
Chicago, IL 60604
Education, Research

Parents Anonymous
2810 Artesia Boulevard
Redondo Beach, CA 90278
Services to parents involved with child abuse through local chapters

United Cerebral Palsy Association, Inc.
66 East 34th St.
New York, NY 10016
Education, research, direct services to victims

APPENDIX H. DENVER DEVELOPMENTAL SCREENING TEST

1. Try to get the child to smile by smiling, talking or waving to him. Do not touch him.
2. When child is playing with toy, pull it away from him. Pass if he resists.
3. Child does not have to be able to tie shoes or button in the back.
4. Move yarn slowly in an arc from one side to the other, about 6" above child's face. Pass if eyes follow 90° to midline. (Past midline; 180°)
5. Pass if child grasps rattle when it is touched to the backs or tips of fingers.
6. Pass if child continues to look where yard disappeared or tries to see where it went. Yarn should be dropped quickly from sight from tester's hand without arm movement.
7. Pass if child picks up raisin with any part of thumb and a finger.
8. Pass if child picks up raisin with the ends of thumb and index finger using an overhand approach.

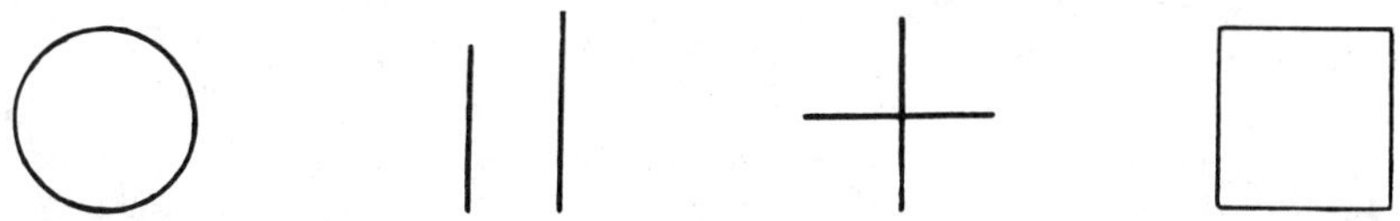

9. Pass any enclosed form. Fail continuous round motions.
10. Which line is longer? (Not bigger.) Turn paper upside down and repeat. (3/3 or 5/6)
11. Pass any crossing lines.
12. Have child copy first. If failed, demonstrate.

When giving items 9, 11 and 12, do not name the forms. Do not demonstrate 9 and 11.

13. When scoring, each pair (2 arms, 2 legs, etc.) counts as one part.
14. Point to picture and have child name it. (No credit is given for sounds only.)

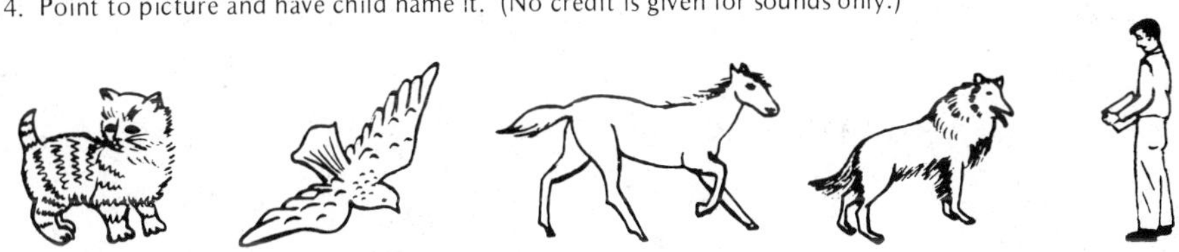

15. Tell child to: Give block to Mommie; put block on table; put block on floor. Pass 2 of 3. (Do not help child by pointing, moving head or eyes.)
16. Ask child: What do you do when you are cold; . . hungry; . . tired; Pass 2 of 3.
17. Tell child to: Put block *on* table; *under* table; *in front* of chair, *behind* chair. Pass 3 of 4. (Do not help child by pointing, moving head or eyes.)
18. Ask child: If fire is hot, ice is ?; Mother is a woman, Dad is a ?; a horse is big, a mouse is ?; Pass 2 of 3.
19. Ask child: What is a ball? . . lake? . . desk? . . house? . . banana? . . curtain? . . ceiling? . . hedge? . . pavement? Pass if defined in terms of use, shape, or what it is made of or general category (such as banana is fruit, not just yellow). Pass 6 of 9.
20. Ask child: What is a spoon made of? . . a shoe made of? . . a door made of? (No other objects may be substituted.) Pass 3 of 3.
21. When placed on stomach, child lifts chest off table with support of forearms and/or hands.
22. When child is on back, grasp his hands and pull him to sitting. Pass if head does not hang back.
23. Child may use wall or rail only, not person. May not crawl.
24. Child must throw ball overhand 3 feet to within arm's reach of tester.
25. Child must perform standing broad jump over width of test sheet. (8-1/2 inches)
26. Tell child to walk forward, heel within 1 inch of toe. Tester may demonstrate. Child must walk 4 consecutive steps, 2 out of 3 trials.
27. Bounce ball to child who should stand 3 feet away from tester. Child must catch ball with hands, not arms, 2 out of 3 trials.
28. Tell child to walk backward, toe within 1 inch of heel. Tester may demonstrate. Child must walk 4 consecutive steps, 2 out of 3 trials.

DATE AND BEHAVIORAL OBSERVATIONS (how child feels at time of test, relation to tester, attention span, verbal behavior, self-confidence, etc.):

DENVER DEVELOPMENTAL SCREENING TEST

Date

Name

Birthdate

Hosp. No.

STO.=STOMACH

SIT=SITTING

PERCENT OF CHILDREN PASSING

25 50 75 90

May pass by report →

Footnote No. → see back of form

Test Item

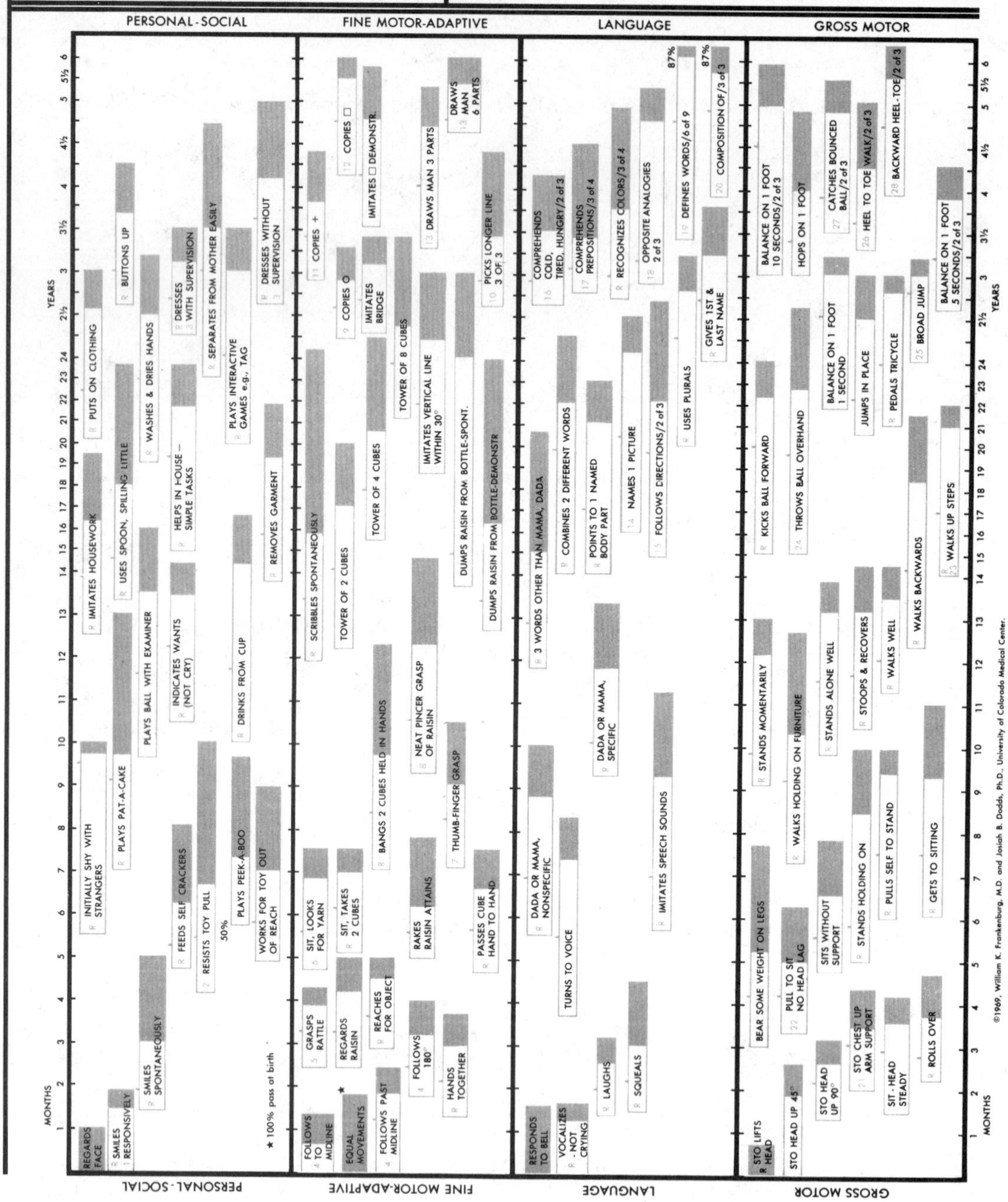

APPENDIX I. RECOMMENDED DAILY DIETARY ALLOWANCES

TABLE I Recommended Daily Dietary Allowances,[a] Revised 1980

Food and Nutrition Board, National Academy of Sciences--National Research Council

Designed for the maintenance of good nutrition of practically all healthy people in the U.S.A.

	Age (years)	Weight (kg)	Weight (lbs)	Height (cm)	Height (in)	Protein (g)	Fat-Soluble Vitamins: Vitamin A (μg R.E.)[b]	Vitamin D (μg)[c]	Vitamin E (mg α T.E.)[d]	Water-Soluble Vitamins: Vitamin C (mg)	Thiamin (mg)	Riboflavin (mg)	Niacin (mg N.E.)[e]	Vitamin B_6 (mg)	Folacin[f] (μg)	Vitamin B_{12} (μg)	Minerals: Calcium (mg)	Phosphorus (mg)	Magnesium (mg)	Iron (mg)	Zinc (mg)	Iodine (μg)
Infants	0.0-0.5	6	13	60	24	kg × 2.2	420	10	3	35	0.3	0.4	6	0.3	30	0.5[g]	360	240	50	10	3	40
	0.5-1.0	9	20	71	28	kg × 2.0	400	10	4	35	0.5	0.6	8	0.6	45	1.5	540	360	70	15	5	50
Children	1-3	13	29	90	35	23	400	10	5	45	0.7	0.8	9	0.9	100	2.0	800	800	150	15	10	70
	4-6	20	44	112	44	30	500	10	6	45	0.9	1.0	11	1.3	200	2.5	800	800	200	10	10	90
	7-10	28	62	132	52	34	700	10	7	45	1.2	1.4	16	1.6	300	3.0	800	800	250	10	10	120
Males	11-14	45	99	157	62	45	1000	10	8	50	1.4	1.6	18	1.8	400	3.0	1200	1200	350	18	15	150
	15-18	66	145	176	69	56	1000	10	10	60	1.4	1.7	18	2.0	400	3.0	1200	1200	400	18	15	150
	19-22	70	154	177	70	56	1000	7.5	10	60	1.5	1.7	19	2.2	400	3.0	800	800	350	10	15	150
	23-50	70	154	178	70	56	1000	5	10	60	1.4	1.6	18	2.2	400	3.0	800	800	350	10	15	150
	51+	70	154	178	70	56	1000	5	10	60	1.2	1.4	16	2.2	400	3.0	800	800	350	10	15	150
Females	11-14	46	101	157	62	46	800	10	8	50	1.1	1.3	15	1.8	400	3.0	1200	1200	300	18	15	150
	15-18	55	120	163	64	46	800	10	8	60	1.1	1.3	14	2.0	400	3.0	1200	1200	300	18	15	150
	19-22	55	120	163	64	44	800	7.5	8	60	1.1	1.3	14	2.0	400	3.0	800	800	300	18	15	150
	23-50	55	120	163	64	44	800	5	8	60	1.0	1.2	13	2.0	400	3.0	800	800	300	18	15	150
	51+	55	120	163	64	44	800	5	8	60	1.0	1.2	13	2.0	400	3.0	800	800	300	10	15	150
Pregnant						+30	+200	+5	+2	+20	+0.4	+0.3	+2	+0.6	+400	+1.0	+400	+400	+150	h	+5	+25
Lactating						+20	+400	+5	+3	+40	+0.5	+0.5	+5	+0.5	+100	+1.0	+400	+400	+150	h	+10	+50

a The allowances are intended to provide for individual variations among most normal persons as they live in the United States under usual environmental stresses. Diets should be based on a variety of common foods in order to provide other nutrients for which human requirements have been less well defined. See p. 23 for heights, weights and recommended intake.

b Retinol equivalents. 1 Retinol equivalent = 1 μg retinol or 6 μg β carotene. See text for calculation of vitamin A activity of diets as retinol equivalents.

c As cholecalciferol. 10 μg cholecalciferol = 400 I.U. vitamin D.

d α-tocopherol equivalents. 1 mg d-α-tocopherol = 1 α T.E. See text for variation in allowances and calculation of vitamin E activity of the diet as α-tocopherol equivalents.

e 1 N.E. (niacin equivalent) is equal to 1 mg of niacin or 60 mg of dietary tryptophan.

f The folacin allowances refer to dietary sources as determined by *Lactobacillus casei* assay after treatment with enzymes ("conjugases") to make polyglutamyl forms of the vitamin available to the test organism.

g The RDA for vitamin B_{12} in infants is based on average concentration of the vitamin in human milk. The allowances after weaning are based on energy intake (as recommended by the American Academy of Pediatrics) and consideration of other factors such as intestinal absorption: see text.

h The increased requirement during pregnancy cannot be met by the iron content of habitual American diets nor by the existing iron stores of many women; therefore the use of 30-60 mg of supplemental iron is recommended. Iron needs during lactation are not substantially different from those of non-pregnant women, but continued supplementation of the mother for 2-3 months after parturition is advisable in order to replenish stores depleted by pregnancy.

TABLE II Recommended Dietary Allowances, Revised 1980

Food and Nutrition Board, National Academy of Sciences—National Research Council, Washington, D.C.

Estimated Safe and Adequate Daily Dietary Intakes of Selected Vitamins and Minerals[a]

	Age (years)	Vitamins: Vitamin K (μg)	Biotin (μg)	Pantothenic Acid (mg)	Trace Elements[b]: Copper (mg)	Manganese (mg)	Fluoride (mg)	Chromium (mg)	Selenium (mg)	Molybdenum (mg)	Electrolytes: Sodium (mg)	Potassium (mg)	Chloride (mg)
Infants	0-0.5	12	35	2	0.5-0.7	0.5-0.7	0.1-0.5	0.01-0.04	0.01-0.04	0.03-0.06	115-350	350-925	275-700
	0.5-1	10-20	50	3	0.7-1.0	0.7-1.0	0.2-1.0	0.02-0.06	0.02-0.06	0.04-0.08	250-750	425-1275	400-1200
Children	1-3	15-30	65	3	1.0-1.5	1.0-1.5	0.5-1.5	0.02-0.08	0.02-0.08	0.05-0.1	325-975	550-1650	500-1500
and	4-6	20-40	85	3-4	1.5-2.0	1.5-2.0	1.0-2.5	0.03-0.12	0.03-0.12	0.06-0.15	450-1350	775-2325	700-2100
Adolescents	7-10	30-60	120	4-5	2.0-2.5	2.0-3.0	1.5-2.5	0.05-0.2	0.05-0.2	0.1-0.3	600-1800	1000-3000	925-2775
	11+	50-100	100-200	4-7	2.0-3.0	2.5-5.0	1.5-2.5	0.05-0.2	0.05-0.2	0.15-0.5	900-2700	1525-4575	1400-4200
Adults		70-140	100-200	4-7	2.0-3.0	2.5-5.0	1.5-4.0	0.05-0.2	0.05-0.2	0.15-0.5	1100-3300	1875-5625	1700-5100

a Because there is less information on which to base allowances, these figures are not given in the main table of the RDA and are provided here in the form of ranges of recommended intakes.

b Since the toxic levels for many trace elements may be only several times usual intakes, the upper levels for the trace elements given in this table should not be habitually exceeded.

GIRLS: BIRTH TO 36 MONTHS
PHYSICAL GROWTH
NCHS PERCENTILES*

NAME ______________________ RECORD # ____________

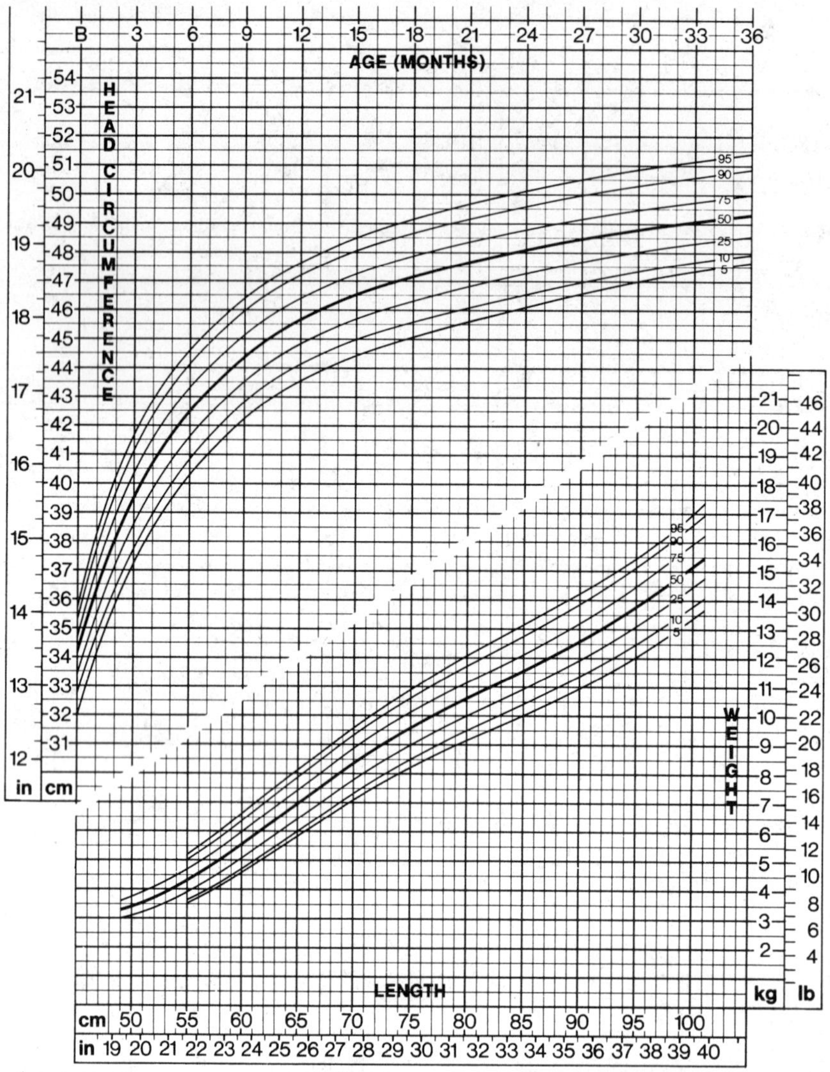

DATE	AGE	LENGTH	WEIGHT	HEAD C.
	BIRTH			

DATE	AGE	LENGTH	WEIGHT	HEAD C.

*Adapted from: National Center for Health Statistics: NCHS Growth Charts, 1976. Monthly Vital Statistics Report. Vol. 25, No. 3, Supp. (HRA) 76-1120. Health Resources Administration, Rockville, Maryland, June, 1976. Data from The Fels Research Institute, Yellow Springs, Ohio.

GIRLS: BIRTH TO 36 MONTHS
PHYSICAL GROWTH
NCHS PERCENTILES*

NAME ______________________ RECORD # ______________

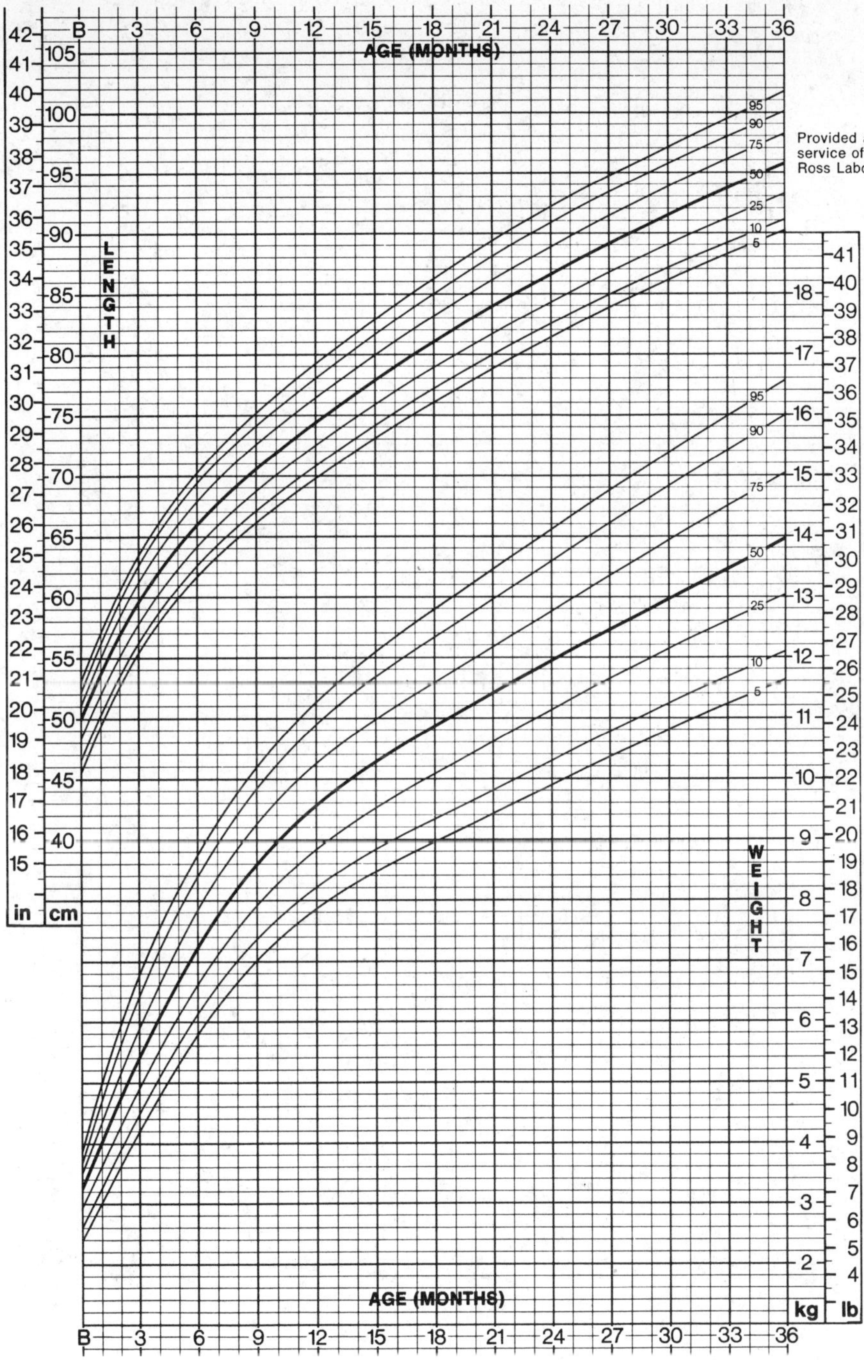

Provided as a service of Ross Laboratories

*Adapted from: National Center for Health Statistics: NCHS Growth Charts, 1976. Monthly Vital Statistics Report. Vol. 25, No. 3, Supp. (HRA) 76-1120. Health Resources Administration, Rockville, Maryland, June, 1976. Data from The Fels Research Institute, Yellow Springs, Ohio.

GIRLS: 2 TO 18 YEARS
PHYSICAL GROWTH
NCHS PERCENTILES*

NAME________________________ RECORD #______________

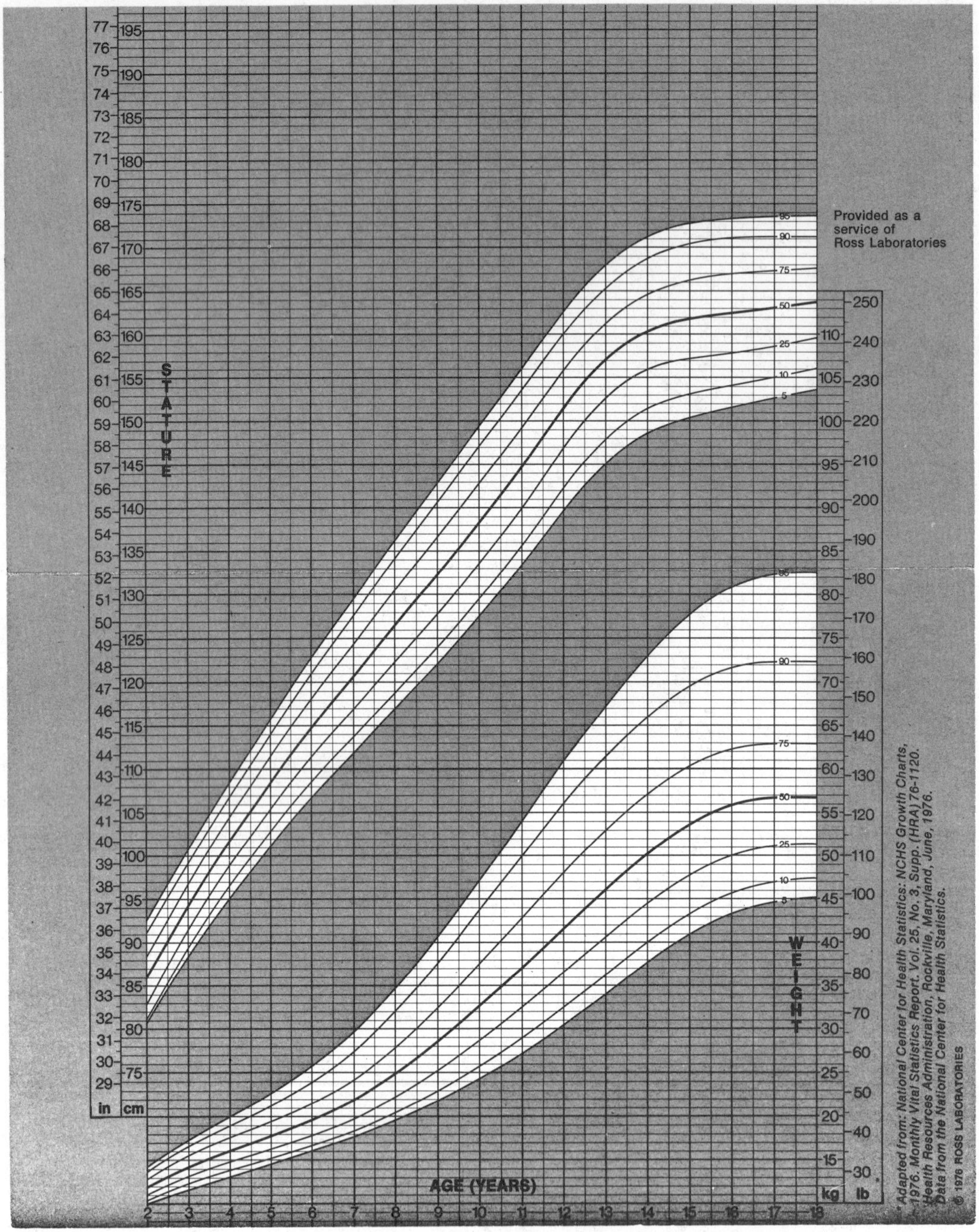

GIRLS: PREPUBESCENT
PHYSICAL GROWTH
NCHS PERCENTILES*

NAME________________________ RECORD #______________

DATE	AGE	STATURE	WEIGHT

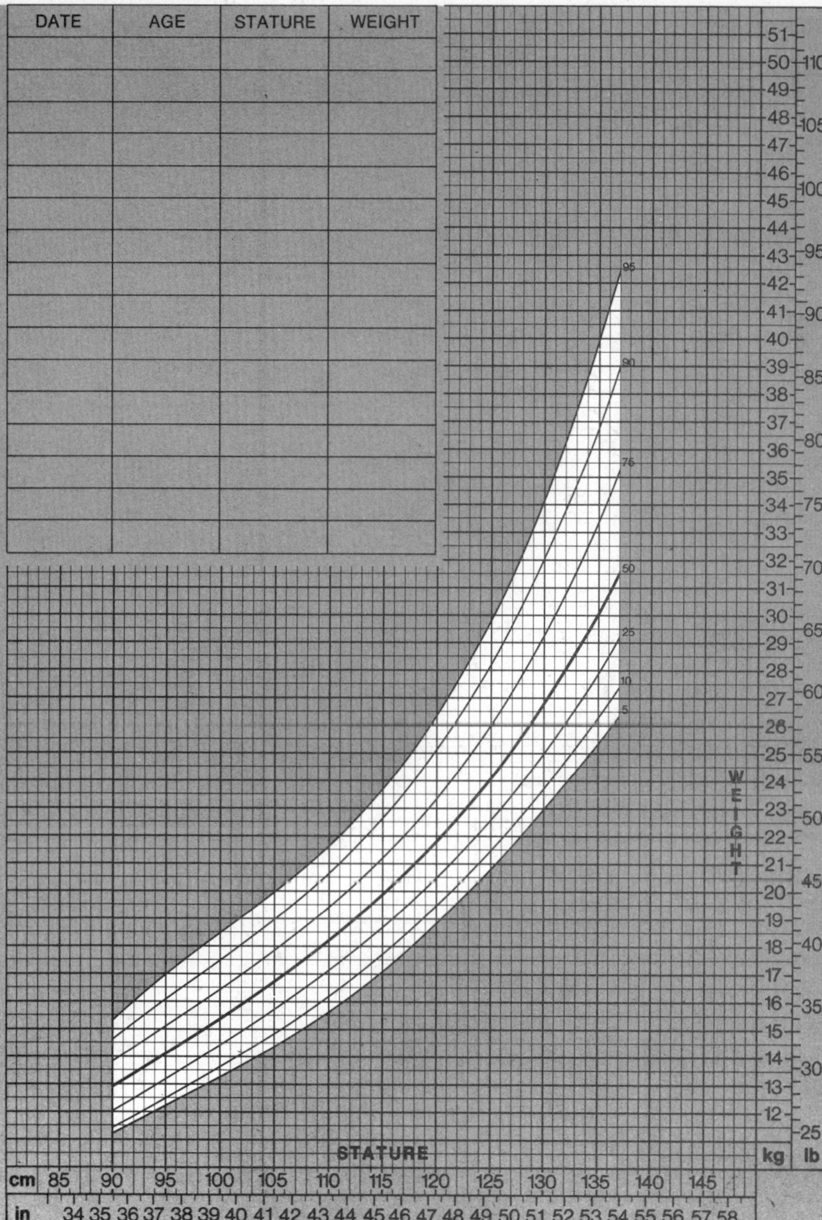

*Adapted from: National Center for Health Statistics: NCHS Growth Charts, 1976. Monthly Vital Statistics Report. Vol. 25, No. 3, Supp. (HRA) 76-1120. Health Resources Administration, Rockville, Maryland, June, 1976. Data from the National Center for Health Statistics.

BOYS: BIRTH TO 36 MONTHS
PHYSICAL GROWTH
NCHS PERCENTILES*

NAME ______________________ RECORD # ____________

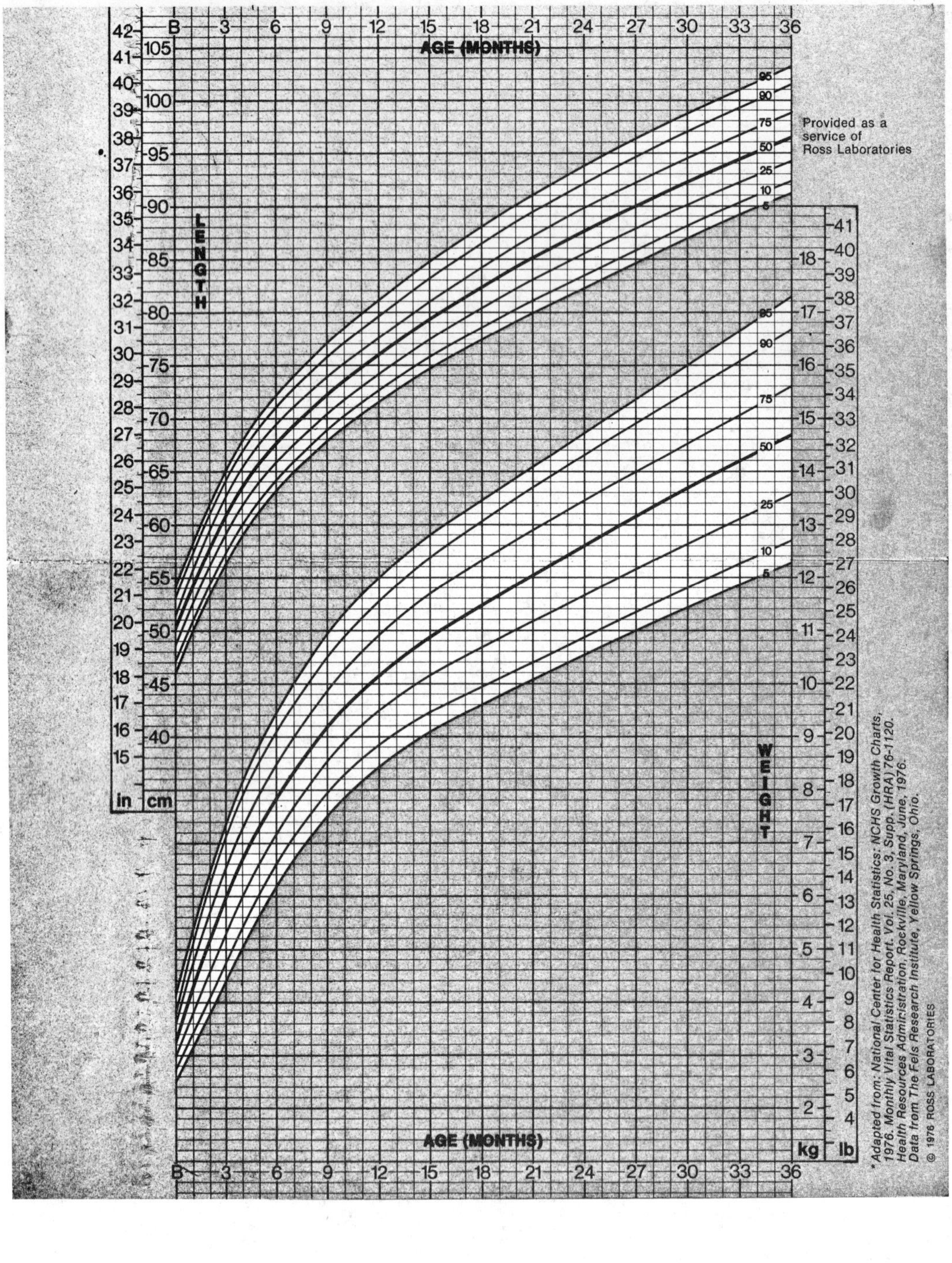

*Adapted from: National Center for Health Statistics: NCHS Growth Charts, 1976. Monthly Vital Statistics Report. Vol. 25, No. 3, Supp. (HRA) 76-1120. Health Resources Administration, Rockville, Maryland, June, 1976. Data from The Fels Research Institute, Yellow Springs, Ohio.

BOYS: BIRTH TO 36 MONTHS
PHYSICAL GROWTH
NCHS PERCENTILES*

NAME ______________________ RECORD # __________

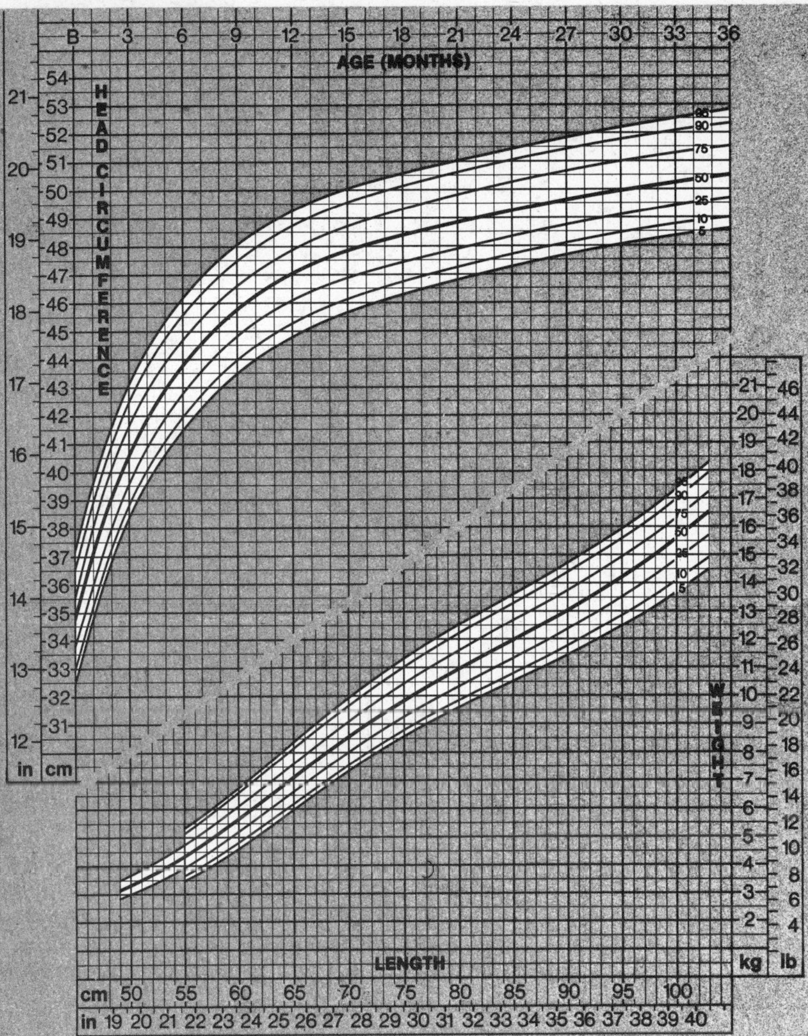

DATE	AGE	LENGTH	WEIGHT	HEAD C.
	BIRTH			

DATE	AGE	LENGTH	WEIGHT	HEAD C.

*Adapted from: National Center for Health Statistics: NCHS Growth Charts, 1976. Monthly Vital Statistics Report. Vol. 25, No. 3, Supp. (HRA) 76-1120. Health Resources Administration, Rockville, Maryland, June, 1976. Data from The Fels Research Institute, Yellow Springs, Ohio.

BOYS: PREPUBESCENT
PHYSICAL GROWTH
NCHS PERCENTILES*

NAME ______________________ RECORD # __________

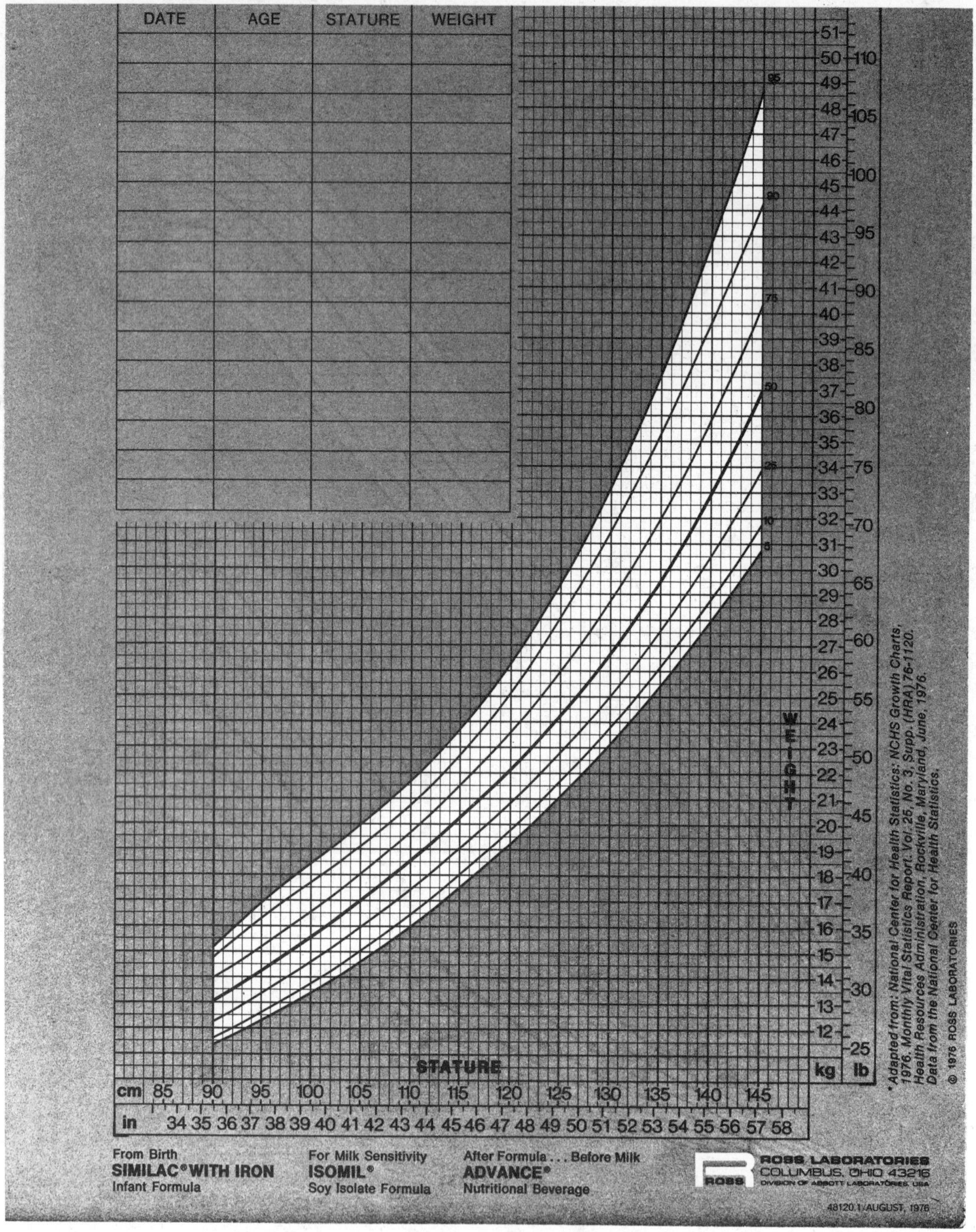

BOYS: 2 TO 18 YEARS
PHYSICAL GROWTH
NCHS PERCENTILES*

NAME________________________ RECORD #____________

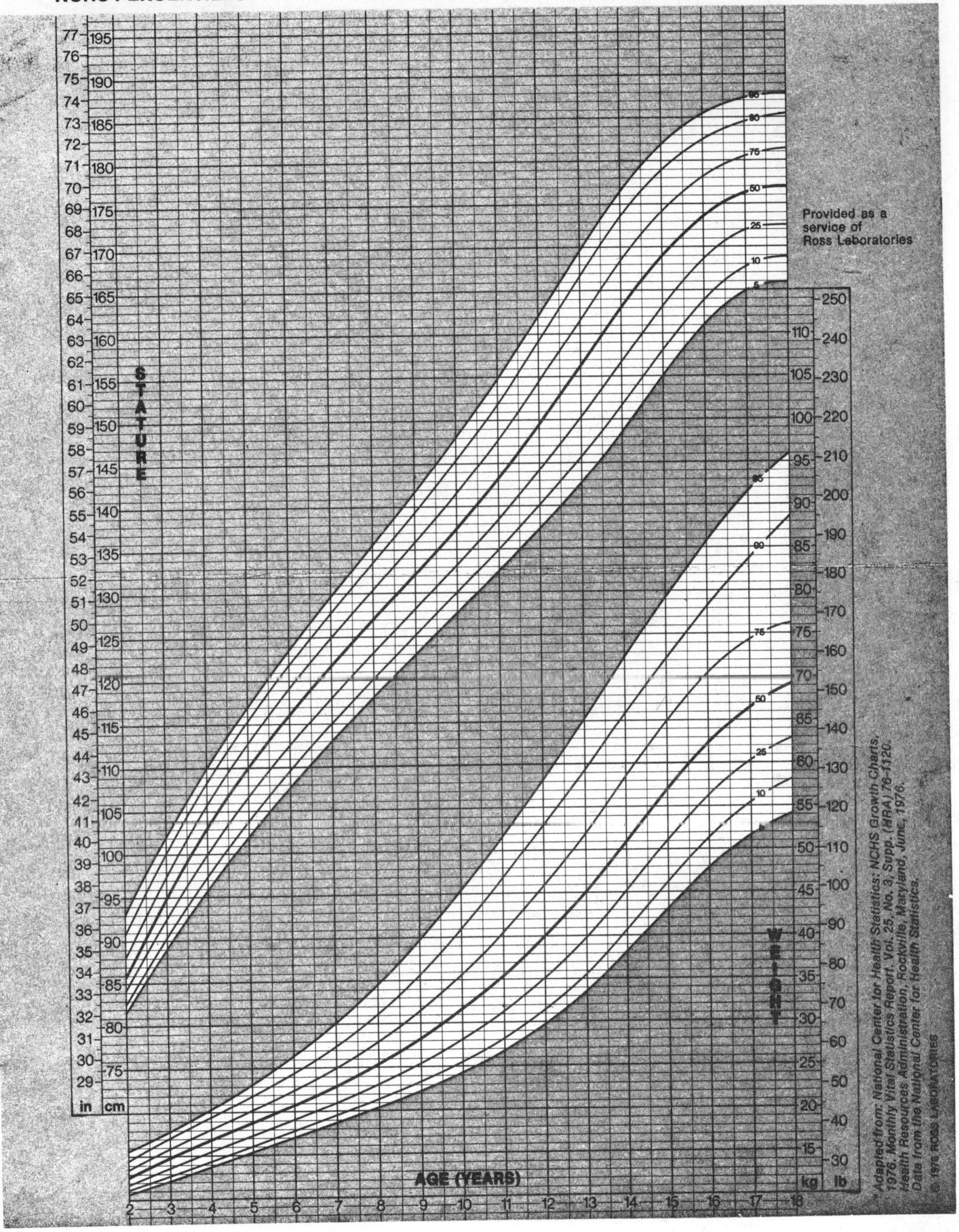

Glossary

Acculturation – The process through which the child acquires the values, attitudes, and beliefs of the family group

Acrocyanosis – Bluish discoloration of the hands and feet seen in normal neonates indicating decreased peripheral oxygenation

Agranulocytosis – A marked decrease in the polymorphonuclear leukocytes present in bone marrow or blood

Allis' sign – Shortening of the affected leg seen in congenital dislocation of the hip

Alopecia – Complete or partial loss of hair observed in children as a response to cancer chemotherapy

Amblyopia – A condition referred to as lazy eye which denotes diminished vision in one eye detected by vision screening

Amnion – The innermost of two fetal membranes which form the amniotic sac

Amniotic fluid – The fluid that surrounds the fetus within the amniotic sac

Anaphylaxis – A severe hypersensitivity reaction to a foreign protein or drug which causes shock and may result in death

Animism – A thought process of young children in which they endow inanimate objects with life and human characteristics

Anomaly – A malformation

Anorexia – Loss of appetite

Anoxia – The absence of oxygen

Anthelmintic – A preparation used to eradicate intestinal parasites

Antibody – A substance produced by the lymphocytes and carried by the immunoglobulins in antagonistic response to a specific antigen

Antigen – A substance, usually protein or polysaccharide, that is capable of producing antibodies. Immunizing agents act as antigens to protect the individual against a disease.

Antineoplastics – Drugs used to treat a malignant growth or tumor

Apgar score – A method of rapid assessment that was devised by Dr. Virginia Apgar and used in the delivery area to evaluate the status of the neonate

Aphonia – Loss of voice

Apnea – Without respirations

Areola – The pigmented area around the nipple

Arnold-Chiari Malformation – A congenital defect of the brain stem and cerebellum in which spinal fluid is obstructed causing hydrocephalus. Most cases of myelomeningocele are associated with this.

Arthralgia – Painful joints

Atelectasis – Incomplete expansion of the lungs

Atresia – Absence of an opening in a hollow body structure, such as esophageal atresia

Auscultation – A method of assessment that involves listening to the sounds within the body

Autism – A condition of early infancy in which the child withdraws from all human contact
Autosomes – A term designating all chromosomes except those carrying the sex characteristics

Barr body – The sex chromatin mass, present only in females, that is derived from one of the X chromosomes
Bilirubin – A substance formed by the breakdown of red cells
Blastocyst – An early stage of embryologic development in which the cell mass has a hollow center with the cells arranged around the outside of the mass
Blood dyscrasia – A condition caused by abnormal substances in the blood
Bonding – Maternal-infant and paternal-infant attachment behaviors that begin at the delivery and have long-range implications for caretaking
Bradycardia – A slow sinus rhythm of the heart, usually 90 beats per minute in the neonate and 70 beats per minute in the child
Brazelton assessment – Refers to the Neonatal Behavioral Assessment Scale, developed by T. B. Brazelton, which provides criteria for assessment of the infant's interaction with the environment
Brown fat – A source of energy for heat production in neonates

Canthus – The angle at either end between the eyelids
Caput succedaneum – Edema of the scalp over the bones of that part of the head that is presented first at delivery
Celiac disease – A disease characterized by an intolerance to gluten that is found in wheat, rye, oats, and barley
Cephalhematoma – A collection of blood between a cranial bone and the periosteum of that bone
Cerebral palsy – A congenital or acquired disorder of the motor pathways of the central nervous system
Cheiloplasty – The surgical reconstruction of the lip, as for cleft lip
Chorion – The outermost layer of the two fused fetal membranes
Clark's Rule – A rule for calculation of pediatric medication dosages based on either body weight or body surface area
Cleft lip – A congenital failure of fusion of the lip
Cleft palate – A congenital failure of the palate to fuse during the embryonic period
Coitus – Sexual intercourse
Colostrum – A yellowish fluid secreted from the breasts prior to the secretion of milk
Cowling's Rule – A rule for calculation of pediatric medication dosages based on the child's age in years
Croup – An inflammation of the larynx
Cushing's triad – The combination of signs which may occur with severe head injury including increased intracranial pressure, arterial hypertension and bradycardia
Cyanosis – A dark blue or purplish discoloration of the skin that denotes an insufficiency of oxygen and increased levels of carbon dioxide

Debridement – Removal of dead tissue from the surface of a burn
Decidua – The term used to designate the endometrium of the uterus during pregnancy
Dermatome – A surgical instrument used to incise a thin layer of skin for use in grafting
Diaphoresis – Profuse sweating
Digitalization – A process in which a Digitalis preparation is used to improve the functioning of the heart
Diplopia – Double vision
Diuresis – Excess secretion of urine usually after medication to achieve this effect
Dominant inheritance – Inheritance of a trait through the gene of one parent only
DPT – Diphtheria-Pertussis-Tetanus vaccine for immunizations
Dubowitz assessment – A set of criteria, developed by L. Dubowitz, M.D., for estimation of gestational age
Ductus arteriosus – The anatomic connection of a small blood vessel between the pulmonary artery and the aorta that is normally present in fetal circulation but which is closed shortly after birth

Ductus venosus – The anatomic connection of a small blood vessel between the umbilical vein and the inferior vena cava that is present in fetal circulation but which closes shortly after birth

Ecchymosis – A large, irregularly shaped hemorrhagic area under the skin which varies in color from deep blue to pale yellow depending on the age of the lesion
Ectoderm – The outer layer of the three germinal layers present in the embryo
Eczema – An inflammatory skin disease associated with allergies
Embryo – The developing conceptus. The term is appropriate for the period from two to eight weeks after fertilization.
Emesis – Vomiting
Entoderm – The inner layer of the three germinal layers present in the embryo
Epispadias – A condition in which the urethral opening is on the dorsal surface of the penis
Epistaxis – Bleeding from the nose
Erythema – Diffuse redness in the skin which may be local or widespread
Eschar – A crust formed by destroyed tissues, such as a burn
Exopthalmos – Abnormal protrusion of the eyeballs

Fertilization – Penetration of the ovum by a single sperm cell
Fetus – The name given to the conceptus the eighth postfertilization week to the time of birth
Fimbria – A fringe-like structure, such as at the distal ends of the Fallopian tubes
Fontanelle, anterior – The diamond-shaped space at the intersection of the sagittal, frontal, and coronal sutures
Fontanelle, posterior – The triangular space at the intersection of the sagittal and lambdoid sutures
Foramen ovale – An opening in the septum between the right and left atria which facilitates fetal circulation, closing shortly after birth
Fried's Rule – A rule for calculation of pediatric medication dosages used for children under one year and based on age in months

Galactosemia – An inborn error of metabolism in which the infant cannot metabolize lactose and galactose because of the absence of a specific enzyme
Genes – Determiners of hereditary traits
Gestational age – The age of the embryo or fetus calculated from the date of the last menstrual period
Glycosuria – The presence of sugar in the urine
Gonad – The sex cell: in females, the ovary; in males, the testis
Grasp Reflex – A reflex present at birth in a normal infant which allows the infant to hold any item placed in his hand and then release it after a brief period
Grunt – The sound caused by partial closure of the glottis. It is used by the infant to prolong the expiratory phase and keep the alveoli from collapsing.

Hemarthrosis – The presence of blood in the joints
Hematemesis – Vomiting of blood
Hematuria – Blood in the urine
Hemochromatosis – A disease characterized by excess iron storage in the liver, pancreas, heart, and gonads causing impaired function
Hemophilia – An inherited disease characterized by abnormal bleeding tendencies
Hepatomegaly – Enlargement of the liver
Heterozygous – Having different alleles for a trait on each gene of a pair
Hirschsprung's disease – Disease caused by congenital absence of the ganglionic cells in the colon. It is also called megacolon.
Histogenesis – The process by which tissues differentiate
Homozygous – Having the same alleles for a trait on each gene of a pair
Hydrocephalus – A condition characterized by rapid head growth secondary to excessive accumulations of cerebrospinal fluid
Hyperalimentation – The infusion of a total nutrient solution to meet nutritional and growth needs
Hyperplasia – An increase in the number of cells
Hypertrophy – An increase in the size of cells
Hypokalemia – Decreased amount of potassium in the blood

Hyponatremia – Decreased amount of sodium in the blood
Hypospadias – A condition in which the urethral opening is on the ventral surface of the penis
Hypovolemia – Decrease in the volume of circulating blood
Hypoxia – Inadequate oxygenation of body tissues

Idiopathic – Refers to a condition or disease without a recognizable cause
Immunoglobulin G (IgG) – The substance that crosses the placenta and provides passive immunity from some diseases
Implantation – Attachment of the fertilized ovum in the uterus
Inborn errors of metabolism – The hereditary lack of a specific enzyme needed for metabolism
Iritis – Inflammation of the iris of the eye characterized by a decrease in vision, excess tearing, and pain

Jaundice – The yellow discoloration of tissues that occurs as a result of deposits of unconjugated bilirubin. It is also known as icterus.

Ketonuria – Presence of ketones (end products of fat metabolism) in urine
Kussmaul's respiration – Deep, rapid respirations characteristically seen in metabolic acidosis

Lactase – The enzyme needed for lactose digestion
Lactose – Human milk sugar
Lanugo – The fine, downy hair that covers the fetus from twenty weeks on
Let-down reflex – A response to oxytocin that allows milk in the alveoli of the breast to flow in the milk ducts
Leukopenia – An abnormal decrease in white blood cells
Log-rolling – A method of turning the patient with trauma or surgery of the vertebral column in which the patient stiffens his back and neck, with arms crossed on the chest, and is rolled to a side-lying position by several individuals
Lunar month – The delineation of a month according to the cycles of the moon, consisting of 28 days

Macewen's sign – A resonant note obvious on percussion of the skull in a child with separation of the cranial sutures from hydrocephalus. It is also called the "cracked pot" sign.
Maslow's Hierarchy of Needs – A system of classification of needs which motivate human behavior that are arranged in an ascending order of complexity. It was developed by Abraham Maslow in 1954.
Meconium – Odorless, tarry stools that are normally passed immediately after birth
Meconium ileus – Paralysis of the gastrointestinal tract secondary to the presence of thick, puttylike meconium. This is seen in infants with cystic fibrosis.
Melena – Tarlike stools due to the presence of blood
Meningocele – Congenital defect in which the meninges protrude through a vertebral defect
Mesoderm – The middle layer of the three germinal layers present in the embryo
M-M-R – Measles-Mumps-Rubella combined vaccine
Molding – The process through which the shape of the fetal head changes to fit the pelvis during labor
Morbidity – A diseased or abnormal condition
Moro reflex – The startle reflex that is normally present in neonates. It involves flexion of the hips and knees and extension and then embracing movements of the arms with the fingers and thumb in a characteristic C shape.
Mortality rate – The number of deaths within a specific population
Morula – A mulberrylike ball of cells present in the early development of the embryo
M-R – Measles-Rubella combined vaccine
Myelinization – The acquiring of a white lipoid sheath over nerve fibers
Myringotomy – An incision into the tympanic membrane for drainage

Necrotizing enterocolitis – A condition of necrosis of the bowel wall caused by lack of oxygenation and infection

Neonate – An infant from birth to twenty-eight days old

Nidation – Implantation of the fertilized ovum

Nystagmus – Constant, involuntary movement of the eyeballs in either a lateral or vertical direction

Oliguria – Diminished urinary secretion

Ophthalmia neonatorum – Infection of the newborn's eyes caused by *Neisseria gonorrhea*

Opisthotonos – The arched, hyperextended position of the body seen in meningitis

Organogenesis – The process by which organs develop in the embryo and fetus

Orthopneic – A respiratory problem in which the individual must sit in an erect position to breathe comfortably

Ortolani's sign – A "click" felt by the examiner's hand over the head of the femur as the leg is flexed and abducted. It is positive in the child with a congenital dislocation of the hip.

Otitis media – Inflammation of the middle ear

Otorrhea – An inflammation of the ear characterized by purulent drainage

Petechiae – Pinpoint hemorrhages that resemble a fine rash. They do not disappear with pressure.

Phenylketonuria (PKU) – An inborn error of metabolism in which the infant cannot metabolize phenylalanine, an essential amino acid present in proteins

Pica – Craving for inedible substances

Plumbism – Also called lead poisoning; involves a toxic response of the body to ingestion or inhalation of lead

Pneumothorax – A collection of air in the pleural cavity which may be large enough to collapse a lung and cause a shift of the mediastinum

Polycythemia – An increased number of erythrocytes

Polydactyly – Extra digits, either fingers or toes

Porphyria – The term for a group of disorders of metabolism involving hemoglobin and characterized by excretion of porphyrins in the urine. It is an autosomal dominant trait and can cause severe illness with ingestion of certain drugs.

Post-coarctation syndrome – The characteristically severe abdominal pains in children who have undergone repair of a coarctation of the aorta. Pain is caused by the increased perfusion of the viscera after correction of the defect.

Projectile vomiting – Explosive or very forceful vomiting

Pruritus – Severe itching

Pseudohypertrophy – An increase in the size of a part with a decrease in function

Pulse pressure – The difference between the systolic and the diastolic blood pressure

Purpura – Purplish blotches in the skin due to hemorrhage seen in some diseases. These do not disappear under pressure.

Pyramidal effect – Side effects such as tremors, rigidity and uncoordinated movements caused by some medications

Respiratory distress syndrome (RDS) – A disease of preterm infants associated with a lack of surfactant in the alveoli; also called hyaline membrane disease

Retrolental fibroplasia – Blindness caused by high concentrations of oxygen administered to an immature infant

Retrusion tongue reflex – The placement of solid food on the infant's tongue stimulates thrusting movements of the tongue which appear as if the infant is trying to spit the food out

Rhinorrhea – A thin watery discharge coming from the nose

Rooting reflex – Stimulation of the infant's cheek will cause him to turn in that direction as if searching for food. It is one of the protective reflexes present in the newborn.

Rule of Nines – A method of rapid determination of percentages of burned surface area applicable to adults (not children)

Scarf sign – An estimation of muscle tone in newborn infants. The arm is pulled across the chest toward the opposite shoulder. In the premature with poor muscle tone the bend of the elbow goes past the chin.

Spina bifida occulta – A congenital malformation in which the posterior portions of the vertebrae fail to fuse
Stepping reflex – Holding the infant upright and allowing the feet to touch the examining table elicits stepping or dancing movements of the feet
Strabismus – Crossed eyes
Stridor – High-pitched, harsh respiratory sounds
Subluxation – An incomplete dislocation of a joint
Sucking reflex – The production of sucking movements in the newborn when anything touches the newborn's lips
Sunset sign – The appearance of the sclera above the iris in infants with hydrocephalus caused by depression of the orbital plate
Surfactant – A substance formed in the alveoli that reduces surface tension and prevents alveoli from collapsing
Syndactyly – Webbing of digits, either fingers or toes

Tachypnea – Rapid respirations; rate depends on age of infant or child
Talipes calcancovalgus A congenital condition in which the foot is flexed and deviates laterally
Talipes equinovarus – A congenital condition in which the foot is extended and deviates medially
T-D – Tetanus-Diphtheria toxoid of the adult immunizing form
Teratogen – Any environmental factor, either chemical or physical, that adversely affects the embryo or fetus
Thrombophlebitis – Inflammation of a vein caused by a blood clot
Tinnitus – Ringing in the ears which may be caused by aspirin overdose
Tonic Neck Reflex – This is a postural reflex in which the infant, while lying on his back, assumes a "fencing position" with arm and leg extended on the same side the head is facing. The other extremities are flexed.
T-O-P-V – Trivalent Oral Polio Vaccine
TORCH organisms – Mnemonic that refers to those organisms that may injure the embryo or fetus in utero
Toxoplasmosis – An infection caused by a protozoa which damages the eyes and nervous system of the fetus causing retardation

Vernix caseosa – A cheeselike substance, composed of secretions of the sebaceous glands and dead epidermal cells, that covers the fetus during the last half of the pregnancy
Vertigo – A sensation of dizziness

Young's Rule – A rule for calculation of pediatric medication dosages based on age in years

Zona pellucida – The protective covering of the ovum
Zygote – The fertilized ovum

Acknowledgments

The author gratefully acknowledges the efforts of the many individuals who contributed to this text. They have each had a significant and unique impact on its development.

Special thanks is extended to the members of the Division of Health Careers, Lorain County Community College, Elyria, Ohio, and in particular, to Robert A. Schloss, M.S., Division Chairman, and Sylvia M. Shepherd, M.S.N., Coordinator of Nursing. The photographic assistance of Gary Romanik of the audiovisual staff is also recognized.

The author appreciates the cooperation of the staff members of the various agencies who offered suggestions and encouragement, and allowed their facilities to be photographed. The assistance of the nursing staffs of the Pediatrics Unit at Lorain Community Hospital and the Newborn Nursery at Allen Memorial Hospital, as well as of the staff from Little People's Palace Day-Care center, is especially appreciated. Additionally, the author's colleagues in the clinical area have offered continued support in the completion of this project.

A word of thanks is also due Judy Clutter and Betty Jo Horn, who typed the original manuscript.

This acknowledgment would not be complete without recognition of all the helpful parents and children. They allowed the use of many photographs and shared a little of their lives with the readers.

The author's students, both past and present, have also shared in the development of the text. Their enthusiasm and inquisitiveness were both a challenge and a delight. Many participated in classroom testing of materials, as well as in the acquisition of photographic material in the clinical setting.

The author wishes to acknowledge the staff at Delmar Publishers Inc., and in particular Susan Wiley, Angela Emmi, and Judy Thorpe. Susan deserves special recognition for her gentle reminders and constant encouragement that kept the project moving and often lifted flagging spirits.

The author wishes to express her gratitude to her husband, children, parents, and other family members for their enthusiasm, suggestions, and direct contributions to this project.

Other contributors included: Department of Health and Human Services (formerly H.E.W.); William K. Frankenberg Director, Child Development Center, University of Colorado Medical Center; Gerber Products Company; McGraw-Hill Company; National Dairy Council; Ross Laboratories; and Wyeth Laboratories.

INDEX